FLOW CYTOMETRY
IN CLINICAL DIAGNOSIS
3rd Edition

Contributors

DAVID F. KEREN, MD
Warde Medical Laboratory
Department of Pathology
Catherine McAuley Health Systems
Clinical Professor of Pathology
University of Michigan
Ann Arbor, Michigan

J. PHILIP MCCOY, JR., PHD
Director of Flow Cytometry
Cooper Hospital
Camden, New Jersey

JOHN L. CAREY, MD
Head, Division of Immunopathology
Henry Ford Hospital
Detroit, Michigan

SAMUEL J. PIRRUCCELLO, MD
Professor of Pathology
Department of Pathology and Microbiology
University of Nebraska Medical Center
Omaha, Nebraska

PATRICIA AOUN, MD, MPH
Assistant Professor of Pathologyr
Department of Pathology and Microbiology
University of Nebraska Medical Center
Omaha, Nebraska

W. ROY OVERTON, PHD
Cytomation, Inc.
Ft. Collins, Colorado

CHARLES WILLIAM CALDWELL, MD, PHD
Professor of Pathology and Anatomical Sciences
Director of Laboratories
Ellis Fischel Cancer Center
Columbia, Missouri

ADAM L. ASARE, PHD
Department of Pathology and Anatomical Sciences
Ellis Fischel Cancer Center
Columbia, Missouri

HARPREET K. MONGA, MD
Department of Pathology and Anatomical Sciences
Ellis Fischel Cancer Center
Columbia, Missouri

DENNIS GRIMAUD
Chief Executive Officer
Scytech, Inc.
Nashville, Tennessee

CHARLES GOOLSBY, PHD
Associate Professor of Pathology
Northwestern University Medical School
Chicago, Illinois

CATHERINE P. LEITH, MB, BCHIR
Department of Pathology and Laboratory Medicine
University of Wisconsin Medical School
Madison, Wisconsin

RICHARD SCHIFF, MD, PHD
Director, Clinical Immunology
Miami Children's Hospital
Miami, Florida

SHERRIE E. SCHIFF, BS
Miami Children's Hospital
Miami, Florida

ROBERT A. BRAY, PHD
Associate Professor
Department of Pathology
Emory University
Atlanta, Georgia

HOWARD M. GEBEL, PHD
Professor
Department of Surgery
LSU Medical Center
Shreveport, Louisiana

THOMAS K. HUARD, PHD
Technical Director of Clinical Immunology
Sparrow Hospital
Lansing, Michigan

JERRY A. KATZMANN, PHD
Department of Laboratory Medicine
Mayo Clinic
Rochester, Minnesota

BRUCE H. DAVIS, PHD
Main Medical Center Research Institute
Scarborough, Maine

JEFFREY S. WARREN, MD
Warthin-Weller Professor
Director, Clinical Pathology
Department of Pathology
University of Michigan Medical School
Ann Arbor, Michigan

IRENE J. CHECK, PHD
Evanston Hospital
Evanston, Illinois

THOMAS E. WITZIG, MD
Department of Internal Medicine
Division of Hematology
Cell Kinetics Laboratory
Mayo Clinic
Rochester, Minnesota

FLOW CYTOMETRY
IN CLINICAL DIAGNOSIS
3rd Edition

Editors

DAVID F. KEREN, MD
Medical Director
Warde Medical Laboratory
Ann Arbor, Michigan

J. PHILIP MCCOY, JR., PHD
Director of Flow Cytometry
Cooper Hospital
Camden, New Jersey

JOHN L. CAREY, MD
Head, Division of Immunopathology
Henry Ford Hospital
Detroit, Michigan

ASCP Press
American Society of Clinical Pathologists
Chicago

Publishing Team
Jeffrey Carlson (design)
Adam Haus (production)
Alyssa Naumann (editorial)
Joshua Weikersheimer (publisher)

Printed in the United States of America

05 04 03 02 01   5   4   3   2   1

Contents

Preface

This third edition of the ASCP Press' text on the use of flow cytometry in clinical diagnosis has been extensively revised and updated. To accommodate the many changes in flow cytometric techniques and in the clinical use of those techniques, we have added the work of 16 new authors and 2 new editors to the present edition. Yet our goal remains constant: to acquaint you with the basic principles of flow cytometry and to provide you with an understanding of how surface marker analysis is used in clinical diagnosis.

To achieve these goals, the first part of the book provides basic technical information about flow cytometry, monoclonal antibodies, DNA ploidy analysis, quality control, database use, and the economics of flow cytometry. The remainder of the book discusses the clinical applications of flow cytometry in a wide variety of settings. Although we discuss some exciting new uses of flow cytometry, such as its molecular applications, our emphasis is the use of these techniques in the diagnostic rather than the research setting. We give the reader perspective on when flow cytometry will provide useful diagnostic information for an individual patient.

Chapters 1-7 provide background information on the technical and organizational aspects of flow cytometry.

Chapter 1 reviews details of immunochemical interactions that serve as the basis for most reagent antisera and cellular reactions in flow cytometry. It also discusses the link between original manual surface marker technologies and the current use of monoclonal antibodies, which accomplishes the same goal in a more precise and quantitative manner.

Chapter 2 describes the principles of flow cytometry, fluidics, optics, computer systems, and distinguishes between clinical and research flow cytometers. It provides background on the basics of gating, the types of fluorochromes available, how fluorochromes work, and the issue of compensation when multiple fluorochromes are used.

Chapter 3 explains how monoclonal antibodies are produced and reviews the results of international workshops that have led to the standardization of cluster designation (CD) nomenclature. It provides a guide to the use of these reagents in studying the maturation and differentiation of lymphocytes, myelocytes, monocytes, natural killer cells, megakaryocytes, and erythrocytes. An appendix serves as a handy reference to the nomenclature and antigen specificity of monoclonal antibodies.

Chapter 4 provides many user-friendly tables detailing operating systems and hardware for processing flow cytometric data, as well as the display capabilities and statistical analyses of available systems.

Chapters 5 and 6 consider quality control and quality assurance and provide many useful examples on the development of a relational flow cytometry database.

Chapter 7 focuses on the economics of flow cytometry, analyzing real numbers to determine when flow cytometry would be a financially viable enterprise—either on-site or through a reference laboratory.

The remainder of the book presents the diverse applications of flow cytometry in the clinical laboratory: from evaluation of patients with lymphoproliferative disorders and immunodeficiency syndromes to uses in allogeneic transplantation, gene therapy and stem cell handling. Other less mainstream applications, such as evaluation of leukocyte function and analysis of DNA content, are considered the last several chapters.

Chapter 8 discusses the merging of flow cytometry and molecular biology. It presents exciting new applications, including flow cytometric analysis of gene rearrangements and expression of the MDR1 gene product that has been associated with multiple drug resistance. The potential use of flow cytometry to sort for pluripotent stem cells may give flow cytometry a new role in gene therapy.

Chapter 9 reviews in detail the use of immunophenotyping in patients with mature lymphoproliferative disorders.

Chapter 10 reviews in detail the use of immunophenotyping in patients with acute leukemia.

Chapter 11 thoroughly reviews the less common, but highly complex flow cytometric evaluation of patients with congenital immunodeficiency syndromes.

Chapter 12 considers the use of flow cytometry and some related techniques to evaluate the immune system in individuals infected with human immunodeficiency virus (HIV).

Chapter **13** discusses the flow cytometry crossmatch and explains how flow cytometry has become the most sensitive method to detect alloantibodies. It also reviews the use of flow cytometry microparticle-panel-reactive antibodies (with an emphasis on the need to use in-house controls) and an intriguing approach to evaluation of cytokine production by flow cytometry to identify patients who may be at risk for acute rejection.

Chapter **14** treats the clinically useful applications of flow cytometry in hematology, such as the detection of fetal erythrocytes and the diagnosis of paroxysmal nocturnal hemoglobulinuria.

Chapter **15** provides a detailed review of the use of flow cytometry to identify and quantify stem cells, contrasting the different monoclonal antibodies used to identify stem cells, and emphasizing the importance of using fluorochromes with high quantum yields to improve detection.

Chapter **16** demonstrates how monoclonal antibodies CD11 and CD18 are used to identify individuals with functional deficiencies in leukocyte adhesion. Through the use of dihydrorhodamine as a sensitive marker of H_2O_2 production, flow cytometry has replaced the relatively subjective nitroblue tetrazolium test for chronic granulomatous disease.

Chapter **17** takes a skeptical look at the use of flow cytometry to explain poorly understood conditions that may have some relationship to immunological phenomena. For instance, some studies suggest the use of flow cytometry as a serologic device to test for the presence of anti-neutrophil cytoplasmic antibody (ANCA). Other studies suggest that immunophenotyping or lymphocyte transformation studies may be useful in such diverse conditions as celiac disease and chronic fatigue syndrome, and even in patients with silicone breast implants. Convincing evidence that these tests are useful in the diagnosis or management of such patients is lacking.

The last 2 chapters discuss another controversial issue, the use of flow cytometry for the analysis of DNA content of neoplasms. When the first and second editions of this book were published, there was considerable enthusiasm for this type of information. Unfortunately, the enthusiasm for this technique has been tempered by the rather poor reproducibility of this technique from one laboratory to the next. Furthermore, the current National Guideline Clearinghouse reports that present data are insufficient to recommend flow cytometry to examine ploidy or S-phase fraction for the management of patients with breast or colorectal cancer. Not surprisingly, many major centers have discontinued performance of this testing except for research. Yet other centers continue to perform these tests, and some clinicians view the information as useful in subcategorizing their patients.

Chapter 18 reviews the current literature on analyses of DNA content, emphasizing the use and problems of the testing for individual patients in the clinical setting.

Chapter 19 provides several helpful comparisons of the studies on several common neoplasms. These tables show the epidemiological evidence of this technique's utility in larger studies and give the reader a framework to help sort out new information on this topic. The development of other marker techniques and more sophisticated cytogenetic and molecular studies will probably decrease the use of flow cytometry for most neoplasms.

Last, we've compiled a handy, extensive appendix of normal ranges for a wide variety of common markers. 95% confidence intervals for most common markers for cord blood, neonatal peripheral blood, pediatric peripheral blood samples, and most common and some uncommon markers for adults are provided. Normal range information is provided for bone marrow samples from adults and children. Furthermore, 95% confidence intervals for surface marker studies on lymph nodes (normal/hyperplastic) are included.

The techniques of flow cytometry continue to expand, and its use in clinical diagnosis has become more clearly defined in the past few years than when the first 2 editions of this book were published. We hope this book serves as a guide to what is currently practical technically and useful for clinical practice.

David F. Keren, MD
J. Philip McCoy, Jr., PhD
John L. Carey, III, MD

1

Background on Surface Marker Assays and Immunologic Reagents

David F. Keren

History and Evolution of Surface Marker Assays

Flow cytometers are remarkable instruments which, together with specific antibody and fluorochrome reagents, allow us to glimpse at the surface, cytoplasm, and DNA content of cells to determine their lineage and to estimate their potential biologic behavior. The first generation of flow cytometers available to clinical laboratories in the early 1980s were clumsy, large, expensive instruments with woefully underpowered computer hardware support and primitive software—basically, they were dinosaurs.

Laboratories brave (foolish?) enough to buy such instruments quickly found that their operational cost was far greater than the usefulness of the data they provided for routine clinical care. However, investigations were launched using these early instruments that resulted in a massive expansion of our knowledge about the biology of hematolymphoid populations and solid neoplasms. Currently, kits are available that permit rapid assays to: enumerate stem cells for allogeneic and autologous hematopoietic progenitor cell transplantation,[1,2] identify fetal cells in maternal circulation,[3] look at cell function,[4,5] estimate autoimmune disease activity,[6,7] follow up transplantation results on patients with paroxysmal nocturnal hemoglobinuria (PNH),[8] and study microorganisms and intracellular events[9,10] in ways that were often laborious or subjective with older technology.

Advances in our understanding of the biology of lymphocytes and neoplasms were sped by the ability to perform more sophisticated appraisal of cell populations by flow cytometry than was possible by the older subjective methodologies. To give the reader perspective on the difficulties of earlier studies of surface markers, this chapter presents some of the older methods by which lymphocytes and monocytes were studied prior to the common use of flow cytometry. The evolution of flow cytometry continues at a rapid pace, with newer, smaller, and more clinically useful instruments replacing older versions.

Flow cytometry has become much more than an extension of examination of the structural features of hematology and tissue pathology. Traditionally, morphological characteristics of peripheral blood cells are used to classify them into groups with functional similarities. For example, the Wright's stain allows us to classify cells into erythrocytes and several types of leukocytes (**Table 1-1**). Unfortunately, morphology alone does not allow us to distinguish between functionally different subsets of lymphocytes. Although many other uses of flow cytometry have been described, by far the most common use of this technology in the clinical laboratory is to enumerate leukocyte subsets and relate the results to leukemias, lymphomas, and immunodeficiency syndromes.[11]

T and B lymphocytes

Lymphocytes are broadly divided into T (thymus-derived) lymphocytes and B (bursal-equivalent) lymphocytes, which are responsible for cell-mediated and humoral immunity, respectively. Prior to the use of flow cytometry in

Table 1-1
Classification of Peripheral Blood Cells by Wright's Stain

Cell Type
Erythrocyte
Lymphocyte
Monocyte
Granulocyte
Neutrophil
Eosinophil
Basophil
Platelet

the clinical laboratory, these cell populations could be distinguished because T lymphocytes have a receptor for sheep erythrocytes, whereas B lymphocytes do not.[12] Today, we know that the sheep erythrocyte receptor is the CD2 molecule (see below) which serves as the natural ligand for the general adhesion molecule CD58 (LFA-3).

B lymphocytes synthesize small quantities of immunoglobulin that become incorporated into the cytoplasmic membrane and serve as a handy differentiator because T lymphocytes do not make immunoglobulin. Prior to the use of flow cytometry, surface immunoglobulin was detected by incubating the cells with a fluorescein-conjugated antibody against human immunoglobulin and examining the cells under a fluorescent microscope. Those cells with fluorescence on their membranes were presumed to be B lymphocytes. Thus, because of their mutually exclusive nature, these 2 surface markers, sheep erythrocyte rosettes (E-rosettes) for T cells (**Figure 1-1**) and surface immunoglobulin (sIg) for B cells (**Figure 1-2**) became the mainstay of the clinical laboratory evaluation of lymphoid populations.

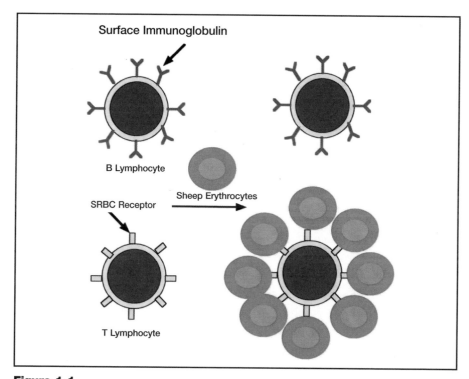

Figure 1-1
B lymphocytes have immunoglobulin molecules on the surface, whereas T lymphocytes have receptors for sheep erythrocytes on their surface. Consequently, when both cells are mixed with sheep erythrocytes, only the T lymphocytes will form rosettes with the red blood cells.

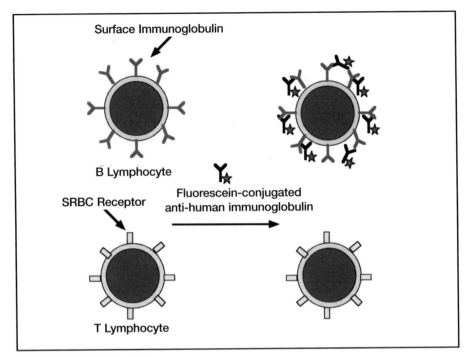

Figure 1-2
When a mixture of B and T lymphocytes is reacted with fluorescein-conjugated antibody against immunoglobulin, only the B lymphocytes will react, if all of the cells are viable.

Although early studies of T and B lymphocytes were less elegant and precise than the characterization of lymphocyte populations by flow cytometry, they did yield several clinically useful pieces of information. For instance, the normal ranges of T and B lymphocytes in the peripheral blood were established. Lymphoid neoplasms were characterized, and the locations of B and T lymphocytes within tissues were determined. By using these techniques on lymphoid tissues from patients with immunodeficiency syndromes, we began to understand the functional significance of the loss of these populations of cells.[13]

Despite these useful bits of information, there were several problems with our early techniques which led to inaccuracies and controversies (**Table 1-2**). For instance, dead T lymphocytes would not form E-rosettes as effectively as live T lymphocytes, resulting in falsely low T cell counts. T lymphocytes at various stages of "activation" had a variety of binding affinities for sheep erythrocytes—thus giving a relatively broad range for "normal" T cells in some samples of cells at various stages of stimulation. Furthermore, dead T cells nonspecifically adhered to fluorescein-conjugated antibodies (regardless of the specificity of the antibody). Therefore, antibodies directed against human immunoglobulin would correctly react with B lymphocytes, but would nonspecifically stick to the dead T lymphocytes, thereby falsely elevating the percentage of B cells in the population (**Figure 1-3**).

Problems with Sheep Erythrocyte Rosette Assays

Because of the many variables involved in the assay, the sheep E-rosette method for quantifying T lymphocytes needed to be very carefully controlled.

Table 1-2
Problems with Early Surface Marker Assays

Too subjective
Viable cells required
False-positive B cells due to Fc binding
False-positive B cells due to lymphocytotoxic antibodies
False-positive B cells due to monocyte phagocytosis
Sheep erythrocytes deteriorated quickly

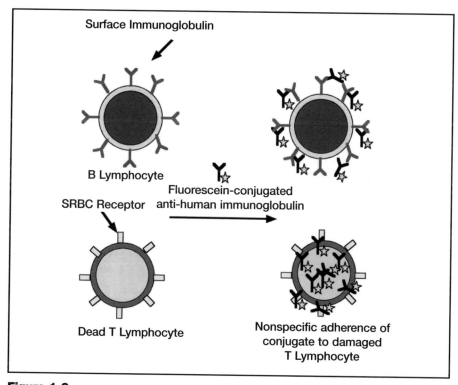

Figure 1-3
Dead cells (whether T or B lymphocytes) will nonspecifically take up fluorescein-conjugated antibodies and will give a false-positive test result for B lymphoyctes.

Fresh sheep erythrocytes were required, because those that had been stored for more than 2 weeks gave poor rosettes. In addition to using fresh sheep erythrocytes, treatment of the red cells with neuraminidase or with the sulfhydryl reagent 2-amino-ethylisothiouranium bromide (AET) was found to enhance their binding to T cells.[14] Under such conditions, most laboratory workers required adherence of at least 3 erythrocytes to the surface of a lymphocyte for it to be counted as a T lymphocyte. However, during counting, different technicians interpreted the number of adherent or closely applied erythrocytes differently. This degree of subjectivity was a problem not easily solved with early methods. Thus there was poor reproducibility from one laboratory to another. Furthermore, at the time these subjective techniques were popular, national quality survey sample programs were not available to provide quality assurance.

Problems with Surface Immunoglobulin Assays

There were also many variables for assays of B lymphocytes. This resulted in gross errors in estimates of the normal numbers of B lymphocytes in different tissues. Some early studies reported that as many as 25% to 30% of peripheral blood lymphocytes were B lymphocytes. Today we know the correct range is much lower. This error resulted from several factors. There was a failure to take into account the fact that T cells, B cells, monocytes, and neutrophils all have surface receptors with various binding affinities for the Fc portion of the immunoglobulin molecule. Because of this Fc receptor, many of these cells bound immunoglobulin from serum (endogenous immunoglobulin), especially when the serum contained circulating immune complexes. Furthermore, because this receptor was not species-specific, it could combine with the Fc portion of the fluorescein-conjugated sheep or rabbit anti-human immunoglobulin used to detect B cells (exogenous immunoglobulin). Another cause for falsely high B cell counts was the presence of lymphocytotoxic antibodies in some patients with autoimmune diseases that reacted with lymphocytes and were detected as surface immunoglobulin. As stated above, immunoglobulin nonspecifically adhered to dead T cells, falsely elevating the apparent B lymphocyte count.

In order to obtain more accurate results, several modifications were made in the techniques to detect B lymphocyte populations (**Table 1-3**). Some of these techniques are still used (though considerably modified) in preparation for flow cytometric analysis. One of the most important modifications was the separation of cell populations that could pose problems if they remained together. For instance, granulocytes, erythrocytes, and dead cells were separated from the mononuclear population of lymphocytes and monocytes by using a density gradient centrifugation on Ficoll-Hypaque.[15]

A second problem was the binding of some reagents to monocytes. Therefore, attempts were made to identify or remove the monocytes in the preparation. There were many methods for performing this task; none was completely successful. Some laboratories incubated the cells to be studied with a suspension of carbonyl iron (which the monocytes would engulf) and used a magnet to remove them. Unfortunately, this would often result in depletion of other populations, especially B lymphocytes. A more popular procedure incubated the samples with latex beads that would be phagocytosed by monocytes. When the cells were examined for fluorescence, a combination of darkfield and phase-contrast microscopy was used to determine if the fluorescing cells contained beads. If they did, they were called monocytes and were not included in the tally of B lymphocytes. Another method to deal with nonspecific absorption of immunoglobulins and immune complexes to Fc receptors employed a wash step with warm buffer[16] prior to staining the sample with fluorescein-conjugated anti-human immunoglobulin.

Lastly, instead of using intact sheep (or rabbit) anti-human immunoglobulin, fluorescein-conjugated F(ab')2 fragments were prepared by digesting the antibody with pepsin. These fluorescein-conjugated F(ab')2 fragments would not bind to the Fc receptors on T lymphocytes, monocytes, or B lymphocytes, but would bind to the B lymphocytes by virtue of the specificity of the Fab portion of the antibody for human immunoglobulin. These more rigorously defined methods allowed a more precise measurement of the percentage of B lymphocytes in the peripheral blood.

Table 1-3
Techniques to Improve T and B Surface Marker Assays

Gradient centrifugation removal of
    Erythrocytes
    Granulocytes
    Dead cells
Separation or identification of monocytes through the use of
    Carbonyl iron
    Latex beads
Removal of nonspecific surface immunoglobulin—warm saline
Use of F(ab')2 reagents to avoid Fc receptor problems
Prevention of endocytosis (capping phenomenon) through the use of
    Metabolic inhibitors
    Ice

However, because the cells were not fixed during those assays, one might obtain false negative results due to the capping phenomenon (endocytosis of the reagent). Once the anti-human immunoglobulin reagents reacted with the antibodies on the surface of the B lymphocytes, the fluorescein-conjugated antibody-surface immunoglobulin complexes formed on the cell membrane would coalesce into small clumps that would migrate to one end of the cell and would eventually be endocytosed. At one stage of this process, the fluorescent molecules would be condensed mainly at one end of the cell and would resemble a cap (**Figure 1-4**). Because this endocytosis and capping was an active physiologic process, it could be interrupted by cold temperatures or enzyme inhibition. Failure to include metabolic inhibitors such as sodium azide or to keep the sample on ice to retard this process often produced false negative results.

Early Markers for Subpopulations of T and B lymphocytes
Through the use of functional studies in research laboratories, it soon became apparent that there were subpopulations of T and B lymphocytes.

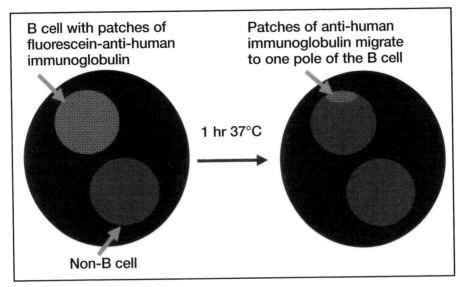

Figure 1-4
In this schematic representation of a darkfield view of a B lymphocyte stained with fluorescein-conjugated antibody and a non-B lymphocyte, the B cell has clusters or patches of bright fluorescence. If the cells are not kept at 4°C, or if metabolic inhibitors (sodium azide) are not added, the patches will migrate to one pole of the cell (right). This process is called capping. If it is allowed to continue, the cap will be endocytosed into the cytoplasm and the fluorescence will be obscured.

Some lymphocytes had cytotoxic capabilities, others could help production of immunoglobulin, while still other populations of cells could inhibit immunoglobulin production. Some lymphocytes were capable of killing tissue culture cell lines, or erythrocytes to which they had never been exposed. These were termed natural killer cells.

Unfortunately, prior to the development of specific CD markers and flow cytometry, accurate enumeration of these populations was very difficult. Because they could only be tested for by the use of laborious and imprecise techniques, they were not measured in most clinical immunology laboratories. Imagine the difficulty we would have in understanding the pathophysiology of acquired immunodeficiency syndrome (AIDS) if we were not able to study lymphocytes by the newer monoclonal surface marker assays such as CD4 and CD8, which we already take for granted.

Although T and B lymphocyte surface marker assays were usually performed on unstained cells in suspension, we had occasion to study populations of cells in intact tissues. The morphology of cells was of particular interest when a mixed population of cells (malignant and reactive lymphocytes) was present. The most straightforward way to study the morphology of these populations was to disaggregate the cells from the tissues, perform rosette assays, centrifuge the cells, and stain them with Wright's stain. The centrifugation step, however, was often disruptive to the rosettes, and cells with less avid binding properties could give false-negative results.

C3 and Fc Rosette Assays

To study the morphology of B lymphocytes, we took advantage of the presence of strong receptors for the third component of complement (C3) and for the C-terminal half of the IgG molecule (Fc). Once sheep erythrocytes were treated with trypsin they no longer bound to T lymphocytes, but were still suitable for use in C3 and Fc rosetting assays. When C3 was attached to these erythrocytes, they formed rosettes with B lymphocytes and monocytes but not with T lymphocytes. These rosette preparations were cytocentrifuged and stained with Wright's stain for study (**Figure 1-5**). B lymphocytes and monocytes could also be stained with erythrocytes coated with IgG (because of the Fc receptor).[17]

Several other techniques were advocated to study subpopulations of B and T lymphocytes. Probably the most useful of these was the test for Fc receptors on T lymphocytes. Although conventional techniques demonstrated Fc receptors for IgG on B lymphocytes and monocytes, no such receptors were initially

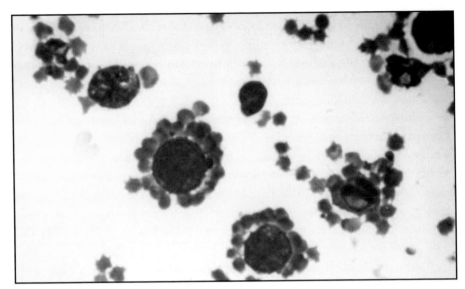

Figure 1-5
Wright-stained sample of B cell lymphoproliferative disorder with C3b receptor rosettes.

found on T lymphocytes. However, by using more sensitive techniques, such as overnight incubation, T lymphocytes were found to have receptors for IgG (Fcγ), IgM (Fcμ), IgA (Fcα), and IgE (Fcε).[18-24] Attempts to categorize diseases other than monoclonal gammopathies in terms of increases or decreases in Fc receptor-bearing cells have provided the medical literature with little useful diagnostic information. While studies that use these receptors still occasionally appear in the scientific literature, these rosetting techniques have been almost completely supplanted by the more specific and reproducible monoclonal antibody markers.

Activated T Cell Rosettes

Another early procedure used to subcategorize T lymphocytes was the "activated" T cell assay. This was a way of distinguishing T cells by the avidity of their receptors for sheep erythrocytes. Active T cells were those T lymphocytes that reacted very quickly (within 5 minutes) with sheep red blood cells. The number of such active rosettes was reported to correlate with the cell-mediated immune function in cancer patients and in patients with immunodeficiency.[24] The usual quoted range was 25% ± 5% (mean ± 1 SD) active rosettes in the peripheral blood. Considering the subjectivity involved in the rosette assays, this was a very ineffective measure of cellular immune status. Even at the height of this assay's popularity, simple skin testing for delayed hypersensitivity was superior.

Enzyme Histochemistry and Tμ Lymphocytes

Enzyme histochemistry continues to provide important clues concerning the types of cells present in a variety of lesions. Myeloperoxidase, Sudan black B, and nonspecific esterase are useful in verifying a myeloid proliferation. While nonspecific esterase stains macrophages diffusely, it was found that a proportion of T lymphocytes had a single dense granule of reactivity with nonspecific esterase in the cytoplasm. This population of T lymphocytes was found to correlate with the subpopulation of helper T cells that had a receptor for the Fc portion of IgM (Tμ cells).[25] This provided a more straightforward method for detecting a population of cells with T-helper function than the clumsy Fc rosette methods.

T and B lymphocytes in Tissue Sections

To study T and B lymphocyte populations in tissue sections in which the architectural relationships of structures were to be preserved, unique modifications of the rosetting techniques were employed that used darkfield microscopy to emphasize the location of the refractile erythrocytes.[26-28] B lymphocytes in tissue sections were detected by virtue of their avid C3b receptors. Although monocytes also had such receptors, they did not react strongly with the C3b-coated erythrocytes used to detect the B lymphocytes (**Figure 1-6**). Monocytes were best detected by staining the tissues with nonspecific esterase,

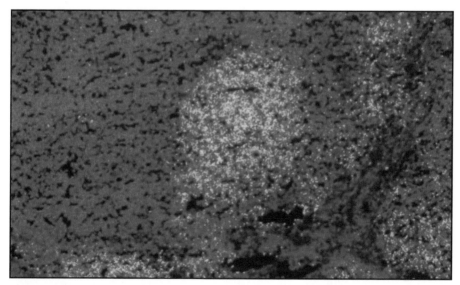

Figure 1-6
Darkfield photomicrograph of a lymph node reacted with C3b-coated erythrocytes that attach to the B lymphocytes in the follicular areas.

but they could also be detected with erythrocytes coated with IgG. This was due to the serendipitously strong interactions of monocyte Fc receptors for IgG with the IgG-coated erythrocytes. The B and T cells with receptors for the Fc portion of IgG were not as avid and would usually give negative results with this test in tissue section.[29]

Detection of T cells in tissue sections was difficult. Although a few laboratories had good success in using sheep erythrocytes on frozen sections of tissue, the techniques were very tricky and many laboratories were not able to get clean backgrounds. The technique for detecting T lymphocytes in tissue sections required that frozen sections be carefully layered with a 1% solution of sheep erythrocytes. Unfortunately, if these sections were allowed to dry for more than 30 seconds, the red blood cells would not adhere properly. On the other hand, if the sections did not dry well enough after sectioning (subjective enough for you?), the tissue would float away during processing (this was before the days of poly-L-lysine, a useful adherent for immunohistochemistry). The author's laboratory always had difficulty with this technique, although we occasionally found weak staining in the T cell areas.

Immunologic Reagents in Flow Cytometry

Fortunately, with the advent of flow cytometry and immunohistochemistry, these subjective, crude assays can now be relegated to the vaults of history and introductory chapters.[30] One key feature of these new techniques is the use of monoclonal antibody technology to ensure epitope specificity. To clarify the use of these new reagents in this text, I review here the nature of antibody-antigen interactions and the preparation of both polyclonal and monoclonal antibodies.

Antibody-Antigen Interactions

Antibody-antigen interactions are highly complex because of the many variables that determine how they occur. This reflects the fact that most antigens have several different structures (called antigenic determinants or epitopes) to which specific antibodies may form. Each antigenic determinant can stimulate several different clones of B lymphocytes that will differentiate into antibody-producing cells. The antibody products of these clones will vary from one another in structure and in their ability to bind to the epitope.

The binding strength of the antibody depends on multiple noncovalent interactions. The following 4 major types of bonds are known to be of importance.

(1) Ionic forces result from the interaction of oppositely charged groups such as R-NH3+ and R-COO-.

(2) Hydrogen bonding is the interaction between a hydrogen atom that is covalently linked to an electronegative atom, such as oxygen, with another nearby electronegative atom.

(3) Hydrophobic bonding is due to the tendency of hydrophobic molecules to exclude ionic groups and water molecules that are between them.

(4) Van der Waals forces concern the interaction of the outer orbital electrons of the reactants. These are normally weak forces, but gain in strength as the reactants come closer.

The basic relationship for antibody (Ab) and antigen (Ag) interaction is expressed as:

$$Ag + Ab \longleftrightarrow AbAg$$

The rate of formation of antibody-antigen complexes (AbAg) is proportional to the concentration of the initial Ab and Ag, according to the law of mass action. Furthermore, the rate of dissociation of the AbAg complex is proportional to the concentration of AbAg. Each particular Ag and Ab has an association constant k1 and each AbAg has a dissociation constant k2. Eventually, the equilibrium point is reached, where no more association or dissociation occurs. At equilibrium, the rates of association and dissociation are represented as:

$$k1[Ab][Ag]=k2[AbAg]$$

The equilibrium constant, or affinity, K, is the ratio of the association constant to the dissociation constant.

$$K=k1/k2$$

By substituting the reactants for k^1 and k^2, the relationship between the affinity and the reactants is more apparent:

$$K=[AbAg]/[Ab][Ag]$$

When half of the available antibody binding sites have combined with antigen, the molar concentration of AbAg must equal the molar concentration of Ab. Thus, these terms cancel out, leaving:

$$K=1/[Ag]$$

Therefore, in the situation described, an antibody's affinity inversely correlates with the concentration of unbound Ag in the solution. High-affinity antibodies possess half of the available binding sites occupied by antigen, leaving very few molecules of free antigen in the solution, whereas low-affinity antibodies require many more free molecules of antigen to be present in solution in order to saturate half of the antibody binding sites.

Serum from an immunized animal has a much more complex relationship with the antigen than the affinity constant described above. It is not just composed of thousands of copies of a single type of antibody molecule directed against one epitope. Most antigens have many epitopes. Consequently, serum from an immunized animal contains many families of antibodies that react with each epitope. Each population of antibodies against each epitope will have a specific affinity constant. Since antigens tend to have many different antigenic determinants (that is, they are multivalent) and antibodies have from 2 to 5 functional combining sites (2 for IgG, 5 for IgM), antibody-antigen interactions are very complex. The strength of a multivalent interaction is greater than the simple monovalent interaction because when one of the antibody combining sites is already attached to a multivalent antigen, it greatly decreases the chances for dissociation and increases the chances for further association of the other antibody combining site that is nearby.

Production of Polyclonal and Monoclonal Antibodies

Polyclonal and monoclonal antibodies are available today from many commercial suppliers. The author will describe the preparation and use of these reagents from both theoretical and practical points of view so the reader will be able to understand why unusual reactions occasionally occur and how to troubleshoot these problems. To produce a polyclonal antibody against an antigen, the antigen should be separated from other potentially immunogenic molecules. When highly purified antigens are used for immunization, it minimizes the number of confusing reactivities that may develop against other antigenic molecules in crude preparations.

Production of Polyclonal Antibodies

Antigen is injected into an animal with an adjuvant, typically complete Freund's adjuvant, to enhance its immunogenicity.[31] The antigen is given at least 2 or 3 times to boost the response of several specific B cell clones. Together with the appropriate regulatory T lymphocytes, these antigen-specific B cells mature into immunoglobulin-secreting plasma cells. Each B cell clone responding to the antigen produces a variable region on the immunoglobulin molecule that can interact with a specific epitope on the antigen. The immunoglobulins from some clones attach with higher affinity to the antigen than do immunoglobulins from other clones. Early on in the immune response, when there are large amounts of antigen present to stimulate the lymphocytes, both low- and high-affinity-producing clones will be stimulated. Later, when only small amounts of antigen are present, B cell clones with high-affinity immunoglobulin receptors are preferentially stimulated because they are more likely to remain bound to the small amount of antigen available. Therefore, serum taken several months after immunizing and boosting a large animal with an antigen generally provides stronger antibodies than serum taken soon after immunization.

Polyclonal reagents are preferred in several laboratory situations. For instance, when examining complex antigens such as human immunoglobulin by immunoprecipitation techniques (eg, immunofixation), a polyclonal antibody is essential. Because there is a huge number of possible combinations of determinants in the immunoglobulins, a monoclonal antibody would be able to react with only one. If that particular determinant is represented in only a minority of the population of immunoglobulins, a highly skewed tally would result. Polyclonal reagents are also preferred here because the products of myeloma may be deficient in one or another region; therefore, a monoclonal antibody directed against such a region would not detect the molecule. Lastly, polyclonal antibodies are the preferred reagents for performing many types of precipitation and agglutination reactions. The multivalency of antigens allows many of the families of polyclonal antibodies to stabilize the precipitation or agglutination. Monoclonal antibodies would only react with one epitope.

A major disadvantage of polyclonal antibodies is their tendency to cross-react. If one is trying to distinguish a subtle difference in a surface antigen on a neoplastic cell versus a normal cell, polyclonal reagents are often very clumsy. The presence of many antibodies against many different epitopes increases the chance of cross-reacting with other cells.

It is also very difficult to have consistent results with polyclonal antibodies because their titers and binding affinities vary from lot to lot. Therefore, polyclonal reagents, though easy to prepare, are problematic, especially when applied to a discrete technique like flow cytometry.

Monoclonal antibodies

Kohler and Milstein created the first monoclonal antibodies when they combined genetic material from B cells with specific immunoreactivity with that of myeloma cells.[32] The resulting clone (hybridoma) was immortal and produced only one antibody product.

Briefly, injecting mice with the antigen of interest stimulates B lymphocytes with the desired specificity. Antigen-specific B lymphocytes from the spleens of these animals are mixed with mouse plasma cell lines that are deficient for the enzyme hypoxanthine/guanine phosphoribosyl transferase (HGPRT) (**Figure 1-7**). The splenic B lymphocytes are fused with the mouse plasma cell tumor line by adding polyethylene glycol (PEG) or another agent to the suspension of tumor cells and spleen cells. Under the culture conditions, only hybrids are able to survive. The resulting clones are grown separately, and the monoclonal immunoglobulins in the supernatant can be tested for the intensity of their reactivity.

Advantages of Monoclonal Reagents

Monoclonal antibodies have several advantages and some disadvantages. A major advantage is reproducibility. The binding strength of monoclonal antibodies should always be the same from one lot to the next, as long as it is from the same clone. Therefore, the only difference from one batch of a monoclonal antibody reagent to the next should be the concentration of the particular antibody produced. Such reliability has resulted in the widespread use of these reagents for both immunohistology and immunochemical detection methods in clinical laboratories. Monoclonal antibodies are also useful because even when they are produced in ascitic fluid, there is relatively little other gamma globulin to cross-react with tissue components. Furthermore, because the vast majority of the product has specificity for the particular epitope of interest, it may be used at large dilutions. This minimizes cross-reactivity (which is virtually always weaker than specific reactivity) and background due to the nonspecific stickiness of proteins present in the fluid.

This ability to stain discrete epitopes with minimal cross-reactivity has made monoclonal antibodies the reagent of choice in flow cytometry, where there are many sites on cell surfaces that may fall prey to the cross-reactivity of polyclonal reagents. These reagents are also a favorite for indirect immunohistology to distinguish one type of tumor cell from another. (Note that rarely they may not react because the epitope in that particular tumor is altered, produced in very small amounts, or not produced at all.)

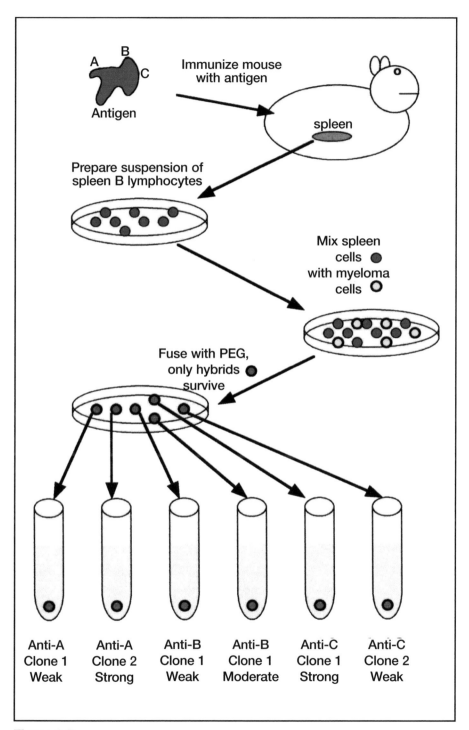

Figure 1-7
Production of monoclonal antibodies (see text for description).

Disadvantages of Monoclonal Antibodies

Monoclonal antibodies do have some disadvantages. It is easy to be fooled into reasoning that because they are monoclonal, they have the "ultimate" specificity. Be assured that monoclonal antibodies from the best manufacturers can give nonspecific results. As stated above, these antibodies bind to a particular epitope, a unique three-dimensional structure. However, like any other antibody, the monoclonal reagent will bind to that epitope even if it is present on the surface of a different antigen. The presence of a similar epitope on other antigens is due to the fact that monoclonal antibodies are specific for a particular epitope, not necessarily for the particular antigen on which the epitope may be found. If that epitope or one that is structurally quite similar is present on other antigens in a tissue, the monoclonal antibody will also react with that antigen. Although monoclonal antibodies are selected for the trait of not binding to other antigens usually present in the same tissues, be aware that such interactions may occur.

Another problem with monoclonal antibodies relates to their exquisite specificity. Each monoclonal antibody can react with only one epitope. So unlike polyclonal reagents where antibodies against many epitopes on an antigen will be present in the reagent, only one site on the antigen will be recognized by the monoclonal antibody. This may be a problem with precipitation and agglutination reactions. Both types of these reactions depend on the formation of multiple antibody-antigen interactions. If there are relatively few epitopes of interest on the surface of a molecule or particle, there is limited availability of sites for interaction to produce the necessary lattice for precipitation or to hold large particles (such as erythrocytes) together in an agglutination reaction. Therefore, monoclonal antibodies alone are generally not good precipitating reagents. Some scientists have suggested the use of a "cocktail" containing several monoclonal antibodies with specificities for several epitopes on an antigen to facilitate these reactions. In effect, one would have a tailor-made polyclonal reagent.

The precise reactivity of monoclonal antibodies can also be a problem in some neoplasms. As discussed above, some immunoglobulin products from patients with multiple myeloma have portions of their immunoglobulin structure deleted from the final secreted product. If the reagent monoclonal antibody your laboratory is using happens to be directed against the deleted epitope, you may grossly underestimate the amount of monoclonal protein present in a patient. This is why polyclonal reagents are preferred for many types of immunoassays. In the future, it is likely that tailor-made monoclonal antibody cocktails of several clones with defined reactivity will be the standard as their cost for production declines and optimal-reacting clones are characterized.

Monoclonal antibodies were originally given names that were relevant to their activity, such as common acute lymphoblastic leukemia antigen (CALLA). Eventually, companies began to name the monoclonal antibodies they marketed, loosely based on their reactivity, such as T4 (helper T cell activity). Since one company could not use the same name as another company for its product, the literature became cluttered with names such as Leu3, T4, and OKT4 for monoclonal antibodies that all reacted with the same antigen. Thankfully, the World Health Organization has come up with cluster designations (CD) to group antibodies that have reactivity for the same antigen. Therefore, the term CD4 is now used for Leu 3, T4, and OKT4.

Correlations of Pre-flow Cell Surface Assays with Monoclonal Markers

B cell monoclonal markers have some similarities with and many differences from the older surface immunoglobulin, Fc, and C3 receptor assays. Although flow cytometry is used occasionally to look at surface immunoglobulin expression on B lymphocytes, this is not the most common method for evaluating the B cell population.

Some of the reagents used for detecting surface immunoglobulin by flow cytometry are still polyclonal reagents. There is a good reason for this. When one is looking at B lymphocyte populations, one is usually trying to determine clonality. This is done by looking for the proportion of k- versus l-bearing cells (normally about 2:1). Some malignancies do not produce the immunoglobulins correctly (hence the term "paraprotein"). Therefore, if the reagents were specific for only one epitope, and that epitope were altered, one could obtain a false-negative result. Polyclonal reagents (usually F(ab')2 fragments) will react with many epitopes and will not give false-negative results if a few are missing.

However, most B lymphocytes are enumerated using monoclonal antibodies against other surface determinants. The monoclonal antibodies against CD19, 20, and 21 all define B cell populations. These monoclonal markers give more information than the surface immunoglobulin alone because subtle differences can be seen in the cell populations. For instance, the CD19 antigen is a 95 kDa membrane glycoprotein expressed on both mature B lymphocytes and on pre-B cells in acute lymphoblastic leukemia. However, it is not entirely specific for the B cell lineage being expressed on follicular dendritic cells. Furthermore, when the B lymphocytes mature to plasma cells, CD19 can no longer be detected. The CD21 marker reacts with a large 145 kDa glycoprotein on mature B lymphocytes. This is the marker for the C3d receptor on B lymphocytes. Both CD19 and CD21 are absent from T lymphocytes. The CD16 marker is the monoclonal antibody that reacts with the Fc receptor for IgG on neutrophils and natural killer lymphocytes (**Table 1-4**). For T lymphocytes, the CD2 marker reacts with a 50 kDa glycoprotein, which, with older techniques, was detected as the sheep red blood cell rosette receptor. Antibodies that detect CD 16 (for Fcγ), CD23 (for Fcε), CD21 (for C3d), and CD35 (for C3b) have replaced the older Fc receptor assays and C3 receptor assays.

Applications of Flow Cytometry in Diagnostic Laboratories

One major advance that has occurred in the past few years is the standardization of cell surface marker measurements. When manual surface immunoglobulin and sheep E-rosettes were the norm, there was little correlation of results between one laboratory and another. Today, through programs such as those offered by the College of American Pathologists, it has been established that there is little difference from one institution to another in results obtained using the more standard monoclonal antibody-detected cells.

As shown in **Table 1-5**, for instance, there was very little variation in the number of CD3 (total T lymphocytes) or CD4 (helper/inducer T lymphocytes) calculated by many different instruments.[33] This interlaboratory standardization has improved precision in the study of both traditional and new markers. This type of comparison is also useful in evaluating newer methods of sample preparation. For instance, such comparisons demonstrated that the lymphocyte subset numbers are equivalent when cells are processed by a rapid, no-wash, whole-blood lysis system, compared with a more laborious manual lysis system.[34] Because of such findings, simple, automated lysis assays have become the standard in most flow cytometry laboratories.

Flow cytometry techniques have been adopted into routine hematology analyzers to improve the quantification of reticulocytes present in a blood sample.[35-37] The manual reticulocyte assay is subjective and therefore liable to wide observer variation.

Flow cytometry has also found a niche in replacing the older thymidine-labeling studies for lymphocyte function. Under appropriate stimulation by certain mitogens or specific antigens, normal lymphocytes will proliferate in culture. Lymphocytes from patients with certain immunodeficiency diseases or exposure to specific antigens will exhibit characteristic responses which, in the

Table 1-4

Correlation of CD Monoclonal Antibody Markers with Older Surface Marker Assays

Cluster of Differentiation	Classic Marker Correlation
CD2	SRBC rosette receptor
CD11	C3bi receptor on granulocytes, monocytes, and natural killer lymphocytes
CD16	Fcγ receptor on neutrophils, basophils, and natural killer lymphocytes
CD23	Fcε receptor on B lymphocytes
CD21	C3d receptor on mature B lymphocytes
CD35	C3b receptor on B lymphocytes, neutrophils, and monocytes

Table 1-5

Interlaboratory Comparison of Total T CD3 and CD3 and
CD4 Dual-Positive Lymphocytes

Instrument	CD3 Positive (1SD)* CD3,CD4	Dual Positive (1SD) BD
FACScalibur	78.4 (2.1)	51.5 (2.6)
BD FACScan	77.5 (3.0)	50.7 (2.9)
Coulter Profile	77.5 (3.6)	50.5 (3.6)
Coulter XL	75.4 (3.1)	49.0 (3.0)
Ortho Cytron Absolute	78.1 (3.8)	50.9 (3.4)
All Instruments	76.9 (3.2)	50.2 (3.1)

Data from CAP Survey FL-01, 1999. (Used with CAP permission.)
*Numbers represent means of results from laboratories responding to survey

past, were measured by the uptake of ^{3}H-thymidine by those cells in culture. These assays, however, were slow and required the use of radioactive labels.

The flow cytometer has attempted to aid surgical pathology by providing objective information about DNA content (ploidy and S-phase). Formerly, one index of the grade of a neoplasm was the mitotic count. This was a very imprecise measurement in which the pathologist would count the number of mitoses per a given number of high-power fields (the size of which varies from microscope to microscope). By the use of the fluorochrome propidium iodide that binds the DNA stoichiometrically, the flow cytometer offers an excellent estimate of the ploidy of a neoplasm and can render a reasonable account of the S-phase fraction of cells in the tumor.[38,39]

However, some of the enthusiasm for the use of flow cytometry to aid the surgical pathologist by providing information about DNA content has been tempered by the poor reproducibility of this technique from one laboratory to the next. The recommendations of the American Society of Clinical Oncology did not endorse the usefulness of DNA ploidy or S-phase assays to monitor therapy for breast and colorectal cancer.[40] This variability in performance of DNA analysis may explain why the growth of this area has been slow compared with that of immunophenotyping. The recent American Society of Clinical Pathologists survey of flow cytometry facilities documented the slow rate of increase in this area of testing.[11] In the author's own laboratory, the requests for this type of testing have declined dramatically in the past few years.

Therefore, although studies of ploidy and S-phase fraction may be useful experimental tools, they do not seem to be part of the routine practice at many centers. The 1999 ASCP survey of current practices in clinical flow cytometry found that DNA analysis was performed most commonly on breast cancers (82% of 75 laboratories using DNA ploidy performed studies on breast cancer), with far fewer laboratories evaluating other types of tissues for DNA content.[11] Indeed, 2 authors of chapters on the use of DNA analysis from our previous edition noted markedly decreased volumes of these assays in their laboratories.

The information from these studies has occasionally provided information that was useful for the prognosis or therapy of patients with those neoplasms. Unfortunately, because of current variations in techniques, types of tissues used for studies (fresh tissue, frozen tissue, paraffin-embedded tissues), and statistical methods for evaluating the significance of the information obtained, there is considerable disagreement about the use of these techniques in surgical pathology today. Nonetheless, some research studies continue to show that under carefully controlled situations, DNA content studies can offer useful predictive information in evaluating dysplasia and carcinoma.[41]

The Just-Barely or Perhaps-Not-Quite-Yet Ready for Prime Time Applications of Flow Cytometry

In the past few years, flow cytometric methods have been used to quantify and classify a diverse array of substances, from cytokines to microorganisms. The incorporation of these techniques into clinical flow cytometry laboratories depends on the role of the institutions where the laboratories are located. Many laboratories, such as those in transplant centers, have already adopted some of these newer techniques. During the next few years, other clinical flow cytometry laboratories will consider incorporating some of these techniques into their routine diagnostic armamentarium. Each institution must determine the utility of these techniques based on the specific applications of these methods to the care of its patients.

Although flow cytometry excels at defining populations on the basis of the expression of certain antigens on the cell surface, until recently, its use in assessing the level of individual cell activation within the population defined by surface markers has been limited. The 1999 ASCP survey on flow cytometry usage in diagnostic clinical laboratories demonstrated that immunophenotyping for CD4 lymphocytes for patients infected with the human immunodeficiency virus (HIV) and immunophenotyping for patients with leukemias and lymphomas were the most common applications (**Figure 1-8**). According to the survey, functional studies such as mitogen stimulation or oxidative burst were uncommonly

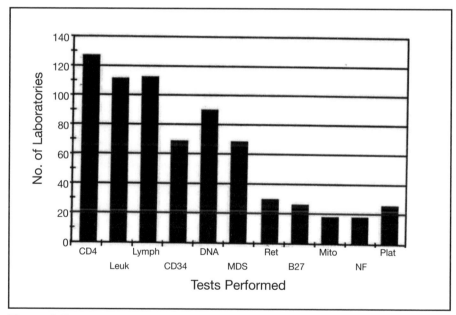

Figure 1-8
The number of laboratories performing various tests by flow cytometry.

Abbreviations: CD4 = CD4+ T-lymphocyte enumeration; Leuk = leukemia immunophenotyping; Lymph = lymphoma immunophenotyping; CD34 – CD34+ stem cell enumeration; DNA = DNA ploidy/cell cycle analysis of various specimens; MDS = immunophenotyping for myelodysplasia; Ret = reticulocyte enumeration; B27 = HLA=B27 determinations; Mito = mitogen stimulation; NF = neutrophil function studies (usually phagocytosis, oxidative burst, or both); Plat = platelet antibody or activation.

performed (**Figure 1-8**).[11] It is likely that this will soon change. New methods allow one to quantify the activation of specific T cell populations by their expression of cytokine receptors and allow the flow cytometric quantification of cytokine secretion.[42] These techniques provide a useful tool for research studies on T cell function. Although reagents for such studies are currently available, the assays themselves require considerable attention to the purification of the cell populations studied and to the methods used to activate the lymphocytes themselves. Considerable variables determine the results of such studies. For instance, the cells may need to be stimulated in vitro. If a single common antigen (eg, tetanus toxoid) is used, it would be able to activate only a relatively small subpopulation of the cells in culture. In contrast, general mitogens such as pokeweed mitogen stimulate a larger population of the cultured cells and thus provide a stronger signal than single-antigen stimulation does.[42] By using specific antibodies against different cytokines and their receptors, one can quantify the response of in vitro populations. These methods have many research applications for studying autoimmune diseases and infections such as HIV. Although it is too soon to recommend the use of these techniques in the clinical flow cytometry laboratory, it is certainly an interesting area to keep track of.

As mentioned above, flow cytometric techniques have found application in many laboratories associated with transplantation programs during the past 10 years.[43] The use of flow cytometry crossmatch to detect donor-specific antibodies prior to or following transplantation can predict the likelihood of an episode of acute rejection.[44,45] This serologic use of flow cytometry as a sensitive serological tool has recently gained momentum.[46] Kashahara et al found that early acute rejection among patients receiving living donor liver transplantation was strongly associated with the presence of antibodies against donor T lymphocytes in ABO-compatible transplants.[46] In this serological use of flow cytometry, the recipient's serum is mixed with peripheral blood mononuclear cells (prepared by density gradient centrifugation). The cells are then reacted with either fluorescein-conjugated anti-human IgM or IgG and evaluated by flow cytometry. In Kasahara's study, all 12 patients who developed detectable antibody experienced acute rejection within one month of the assay. In contrast, only 17.4% of patients who were negative based on this technique had acute rejection within a month. Similarly, Przybylowski et al found flow cytometric detection of IgG and IgM antibodies to be a more sensitive predictor of cardiac allograft outcome than the IgG anti-human globulin crossmatch.[47] For transplantation, flow cytometry may be an effective procedure to assess humoral immunity.

New uses of flow cytometry sometimes follow from new therapeutic interventions for conditions that are difficult to manage. For instance, hydroxyurea and butyrate have been used therapeutically to increase fetal hemoglobin production in the blood in patients with sickle cell anemia.[48] This therapy increases the proportion of cells producing hemoglobin F (F cells), thereby decreasing these patients' need for transfusions. The F cells may be quantified using a fluorescein-conjugated antibody against hemoglobin F gamma chain within fixed, permeabilized peripheral blood erythrocytes. Although earlier techniques were somewhat clumsy, a recent modification by Campbell et al that fixes washed erythrocytes in formaldehyde and glutaraldehyde followed by permeabilization in Triton X-100 allows the process to be performed relatively quickly at room temperature.[49] Their technique has a further advantage in that it may be used to detect other hemoglobin variants. Flow cytometry laboratories may wish to consider using this technique in association with centers with such therapeutic programs.

Flow cytometry has also been used to help define poorly understood conditions such as Tourette's syndrome and obsessive compulsive disorder by taking advantage of the development of mouse monoclonal antibody D8/17 (which was originally prepared to detect an antigen on B lymphocytes of patients with rheumatic fever). Murphy et al found that expression of antigens recognized by D8/17 was significantly more prevalent among individuals with these neurologic conditions than in controls.[50] By applying flow cytometry with D8/17 to peripheral blood lymphocytes from these patients, Chapman et al found a sensitivity of 77% and a specificity of 87% for detecting Tourette's syndrome and obsessive compulsive disorder.[51] The ability to provide this objective confirmatory test may be a boon to research in this problematic area.

The evaluation of microorganisms and their heterogeneity under culture conditions has been improved by the application of flow cytometric methods. Prior to the use of flow cytometry, evaluation of the heterogeneity of bacterial cultures was performed by laborious manual analysis of samples taken at various periods of time. Recently, Zhao et al reported the development of a flow injection system integrated with a flow cytometer.[52] Their system continuously samples bacterial cultures and follows the development of specific events in the populations without operator supervision. Using this technique, they recorded the population distribution of DNA content in a culture of *Saccharomyces cerevisiae*, among other findings. Ultrasensitive flow cytometers have been used to analyze the size of bacterial genome fragments following restriction endonuclease digestion. These methods compare favorably with pulsed-field gel electrophoresis techniques in providing fast, accurate, and linear estimates of the size of DNA fragments for use in identifying the microorganisms.[53] Even the complex process of evaluating viral infection of cells in culture has been facilitated by flow cytometric technique, using a microsphere-based hybridization assay.[54]

Surface marker analysis and cellular function studies have come a long way from the surface immunoglobulin fluorescence and sheep erythrocyte rosettes that enumerated B and T lymphocytes, respectively. Flow cytometry technology has expanded to become a potentially powerful serologic tool as well as one that allows evaluation of microorganisms. Newer, relatively inexpensive instruments, an ever-increasing supply of monoclonal reagents, new fluorochromes available for multicolor analysis, convenient cellular preparation devices, more powerful computers, and improved software available for analyzing data have made flow cytometry an integral technique for the clinical laboratory.

References

1. Olivero S, Alario T, Ladaique P, et al. CD34+ cell enumeration in peripheral blood and apheresis samples, using two laboratory diagnostic kits or an institutional protocol. *Bone Marrow Transplantation.* 1999;23:387-394.

2. Barnett D, Granger V, Storie I, et al. Quality assessment of CD34+ stem cell enumeration: experience of the United Kingdom National external quality assessment scheme (UK NEQAS) using a unique stable whole blood preparation. *Br J Haematol.* 1998;102:553-565.

3. Campagnoli C, Fisk N, Overton T, et al. Circulating hematopoietic progenitor cells in first trimester fetal blood. *Blood.* 2000;95:1967-1972.

4. Collins DP, Luebering BJ, Shaut DM. T-lymphocyte functionality assessed by analysis of cytokine receptor expression, intracellular cytokine expression, and femtomolar detection of cytokine secretion by quantitative flow cytometry. *Cytometry.* 1998;33:249-255.

5. Uchida M, Ichida T, Sato K, et al. Detection of intracelluar interleukin-2 production in peripheral T lymphocytes by flow cytometry in patients with pancreatobiliary malignancies. *J Gastroenterol Hepatol.* 2000;15:1212-1218.

6. Bemer B, Akca D, Junt T, et al. Analysis of Th1 and Th2 cytokines expressing CD4+ and CD8+ T cells in rheumatoid arthritis by flow cytometry. *J Rheumatol.* 2000;27:1128-1135.

7. Kobold ACM, Kallenberg CGM, Tervaert JWC. Leucocyte membrane expression of proteinase 3 correlates with disease activity in patients with Wegener's granulomatosis. *Br J Rheumatol.* 1998;37:901-907.

8. Richards SJ, Rawstron AC, Hillmen P. Application of flow cytometry to the diagnosis of paroxysmal nocturnal hemoglobinuria. *Cytometry.* 2000;42:223-233.

9. Alvarez-Barrientos A, Arroyo J, Canton R, et al. Applications of flow cytometry to clinical microbiology. *Clin Microbiol Rev.* 2000;13:167-195.

10. Musco ML, Cui S, Small D, et al. Comparison of flow cytometry and laser scanning cytometry for the intracellular evaluation of adenoviral infectivity and p53 protein expression in gene therapy. *Cytometry.* 1998;33:290-296.

11. McCoy P, Keren DF. Current practices in clinical flow cytometry. A practice survey by the Amercian Society of Clinical Pathologists. *Am J Clin Pathol.* 1999;111:161-168.

12. Jondal M, Holm G, Wigzell HJ. Surface markers on human T and B-lymphocytes. I. A large population of lymphocytes forming nonimmune rosettes with sheep red blood cells. *J Exp Med.* 1972;136:207-215.

13. Gajl-Peczalska KJ, Park BH, Biggar WD, et al. B and T lymphocytes in primary immunodeficiency disease in man. *J Clin Invest.* 1973;52:919-28.

14. Weiner MS, Bianco C, Nussenzweig V. Enhanced binding of neuraminidase-treated sheep erythrocytes to human T lymphocytes. *Blood.* 1973;42:939-951.

15. Boyumm AA. Isolation of mononuclear cells and granulocytes from human blood. *Scand J Clin Lab Invest.* 1968;21(suppl 94):77-92.

16. Nussenzweig VN. Receptors for immune complexes on lymphocytes. *Adv Immunol.* 1974;19:217-258.

17. Abramson N, Gelfand EW, Jandl JH, et al. The interaction between human monocytes and red cells. Specificity for IgG subclass and IgG fragments. *J Exp Med.* 1970;132:1207-1218.

18. Moretta L, Webb SR, Grossi CE, et al. Functional analysis of two human T cell subpopulations: help and suppression of B-cell responses by T cells bearing receptors for IgM or IgG. *J Exp Med.* 1977;146:184-200.

19. Yodoi J, Ishizaka K. Lymphocytes bearing Fc receptors for IgE. I. Presence of human and rat T lymphocytes with FcE receptors. *J Immunol.* 1980;123:455-462.

20. Lum LG, Muchmore AV, Keren DF, et al. A receptor for IgA on human T lymphocytes. *J Immunol.* 1979;122:65-69.

21. Huddleston JR, Oldstone MBA. T suppressor lymphocytes fluctuate in parallel with changes in the clinical course of patients with multiple sclerosis. *J Immunol.* 1979;123:1615-1618.

22. Moretta L, Mingari C, Webb SR. Imbalances in T cell subpopulations associated with immunodeficiency and autoimmune syndromes. *Eur J Immunol.* 1977;7:696-700.

23. Gupta S, Good RA. Subpopulation of human T lymphocytes. V. T lymphocytes with receptors for immunoglobulin M or G in patients with immunodeficiency disorders. *Clin Immunol Immunopathol.* 1978;11:292-801.

24. Wybran J, Fudenberg HH. Thymus-derived rosette forming cells in various human disease states. Cancer, lymphoma, bacterial and viral infections, and other diseases. *J Clin Invest.* 1973;52:1028-1036.

25. Grossi CE, Webb SR, Zicca A, et al. Morphological and histochemical analyses of two human T-cell subpopulations bearing receptors for IgM or IgG. *J Exp Med.* 1978;147:1405-1417.

26. Whiteside TL. Basic techniques for the detection of human T and B-lymphocytes in tissues. *Clin Immunol News.* 1980;1:1-15.

27. Brubaker DB, Whiteside TL. Localization of human T lymphocytes in tissue sections by a rosetting technique. *Am J Pathol.* 1977;88:323-332.

28. Sakamoto H, Oda T. Studies of human lymphocytes in frozen tissue section; viability and spontaneous rosette formation with sheep erythrocytes. *J Immunol Methods.* 1979;26:325-335.

29. Johnsen JE, Madsen M. Lymphocyte subpopulations in man: ox erythrocytes as indicators in the EA and EAC-rosette tests. Serological and technical aspects. *Scand J Immunol.* 1978;8:247-256.

30. Loken MR, Stall AM. Flow cytometry as an analytical and preparative tool in immunology. *J Immunol Methods.* 1982;50:85-112.

31. Ritchie RF. Preparation of polyclonal antisera. In: Rose NR, Friedman H, Fahey JL, eds. *Manual of Clinical Laboratory Immunology.* 3rd ed. Washington, DC: American Society of Microbiology; 1986:4-8.

32. Kohler G, Milstein C. Continuous cultures of fused cells secreting antibody of predefined specificity. *Nature.* 1975;256:445-497.

33. CAP Survey FL-01, 1999. Cited with permission.

34. Kotylo PK, Sample RB, Redmond NL, et al. Reference ranges for lymphocyte subsets. A comparison of standard vs. rapid whole-blood lysis techniques. *Arch Pathol Lab Med.* 1991;115:181-184.

35. Sandberg S, Rustad P, Johannesen B, et al. Within-subject biological variation of reticulocytes and reticulocyte-derived parameters. *Eur J Haematol.* 1998;61(1):42-8.

36. Charuruks N, Limpanasithikul W, Voravud N, et al. Reference ranges of reticulocytes in adults. *J Med Assoc Thai.* 1998;81(5):357-64.

37. Brugnara C. Use of reticulocyte cellular indices in the diagnosis and treatment of hematological disorders. *Int J Clin Lab Res.* 1998;28(1):1-11.

38. Heiden T, Auer G, Tribukait B. Reliability of DNA cytometric s-phase analysis in surgical biopsies: assessment of systematic and sampling errors and comparison between results obtained by image and flow cytometry. *Cytometry.* 2000;42:196-208.

39. Rijken A, Dekker A, Taylor S, et al. Diagnostic value of DNA analysis in effusions by flow cytometry and image analysis. *Am J Clin Pathol.* 1991;95:6-12.

40. American Society of Clinical Oncology (ASCO) (Tumor Marker Expert Panel). Clinical practice guidelines for the use of tumor markers in breast and colorectal cancer. *J Clin Oncol.* 1996;14:2843-2877.

41. Teodori L, Gohde W, Persiani M, et al. DNA/protein flow cytometry as a predictive marker of malignancy in dysplasia-free Barrett's esophagus: thirteen-year follow-up study on a cohort of patients. *Cytometry.* 1998;34:257-263.

42. Collins DP. Multi-system approach to analysis of T-lymphocyte activation by flow cytometry: utilization of intracellular cytokine expression, cytokine receptor expression, and quantification of cytokine secretion as an indicator of activation. *Clin Immunol Newsletter.* 1999;18:140-145.

43. Bray RA, Lebeck LL, Gebel HM. The flow cytometric crossmatch: dual color analysis of T cell and B cell reactivities. *Transplantation.* 1989;48:834-840.

44. Bray RA. The clinical utility of flow cytometry in the histocompatibility laboratory. *Clin Immunol Newsletter.* 1996;16:10-14.

45. Piazza A, Borrelli L, Buonomo O, et al. Flow cytometry crossmatch and kidney graft outcome. *Transplantation Proc.* 1999;31:1-3.

46. Kasahara M, Kiuchi T, Takakura K, et al. Postoperative flow cytometry crossmatch in living donor liver transplantation. *Transplantation.* 1999;67:568-575.

47. Przybylowski P, Balogna M, Radovancevic B, et al. The role of flow cytometry-detected IgG and IgM anti-donor antibodies in cardiac allograft recipients. *Transplantation.* 1999;67:258-262.

48. Charache S, Terrin ML, Moore RD, et al. Effect of hydroxyurea on the frequency of painful crises in sickle cell anemia. Investigators of the multicenter study of hydroxyurea in sickle cell anemia. *New Engl J Med.* 1995;332:1317-1329.

49. Campbell TA, Ware RE, Mason M. Detection of hemoglobin variants in erythrocytes by flow cytometry. *Cytometry.* 1999;35:242-248.

50. Murphy TK, Goodman WK, Fudge MW, et al. B lymphocyte antigen D3/17: a peripheral marker for childhood-onset obsessive compulsive disorder and Tourette's syndrome? *Am J Psychiatry.* 1997;154:402-409.

51. Chapman F, Visvanathan K, Carreno-Manjarrez R, et al. Flow cytometric assay for D8/17 B cell marker in patients with Tourette's syndrome and obsessive compulsive disorder. *J Immunol Methods.* 1998;219:181-186.

52. Zhao R, Natarajan A, Srienc F. A flow injection flow cytometry system for on-line monitoring of bioreactors. *Biotechnol Bioeng.* 1999;62:609-617.

53. Huang Z, Jett JH, Keller RA. Bacteria fingerprinting by flow cytometry. *Cytometry.* 1999;35:169-175.

54. Defoort JP, Martin M, Casano B, et al. Simultaneous detection of multiplex-amplified human immunodeficiency virus type 1 RNA, hepatitis C virus RNA, and hepatitis B virus DNA using a flow cytometer microsphere-based hybridization assay. *J Clin Microbiol.* 2000;38:1066-1071.

2

Basic Principles in Clinical Flow Cytometry

J. Philip McCoy, Jr.

Introduction

Flow cytometry is the most widely applied member of a family of technologies known variously as automated, analytical, or quantitative cytology. As the term implies, flow cytometry is the measurement (-metry) of cellular (cyto-) properties as they are moving in a fluid stream (flow), past a stationary set of detectors. Technologies similar to, but distinct from, flow cytometry include image cytometry and volumetric cytometry, which will be discussed further below. The melding of such diverse areas of scientific endeavor and technical accomplishments as computer science, laser technology, electronic and microchip development, hydrodynamic focusing and ink-jet technology, optics and light detection, monoclonal antibody production and conjugation, and fluorescent dye development have produced an instrument, the flow cytometer, which is capable of rapid, quantitative, multiparameter analysis of heterogeneous cell populations on a cell-by-cell basis (ie, single-cell analysis).

In this chapter flow cytometry will be presented from the point of view of clinical utility. Technical detail will be included as an aid to understanding the clinical value of the technology. This approach should allow a more informed use of the instrument's capabilities and afford the clinician a base from which to best apply the technology to various clinical problems. It should also provide the technologist with an understanding of the technical aspects of cytometry, which are increasingly obscured by the trend towards automation of these systems. In-depth technical aspects of flow cytometry and flow cytometers will not be discussed; these details have recently been published by others. One excellent reference, written by Dr. H. Shapiro,[1] is entitled *Practical Flow Cytometry*, 3rd ed. Dr. M. A. Van Dilla and colleagues have co-edited a volume in the Academic Press Analytical Cytology Series entitled *Flow Cytometry: Instrumentation and Data Analysis*.[2] This work contains contributions from leaders in the field and represents the state of the art of flow cytometry at a technical level. The reader is also referred to several compendia and reviews if supplemental information is desired.[3-9]

Why Flow Cytometry in the Clinical Laboratory?

Over the past several decades, flow cytometry has evolved from a highly specialized research tool to a commonplace technique for many clinical assays. Clearly the impetus for this change has been the fact that flow cytometry is the only technique which is capable of quantitative measurements of multiple features of individual cells in a rapid, sensitive manner. However, with all it has to offer, flow cytometry should not be envisioned as the quintessential pursuit in diagnostic pathology. Rather, it should be viewed as a powerful and versatile adjunctive tool used by the pathologist to diagnose disease and monitor therapy.

The precise changes that have driven the evolution of flow cytometry from the research lab to the clinical lab are complex, and include dramatic improvements in the cytometers and associated computers, in fluorochromes and monoclonal antibodies, in the development of flow cytometers specifically designed for the clinical lab (discussed later in this chapter), and in our basic understanding of many disease processes. The latter improvements have often resulted from the application of flow cytometry to clinical problems (eg, HIV infection) and at the same time have fueled further applications. It has also become apparent that flow cytometry offers not one but many assays for the clinical laboratory (**Table 2-1**).

Table 2-1

Flow Cytometric Assays Performed in the Clinical Laboratory

Clinical Assays	Examples	References
A. Surface marker analysis	CD4 enumeration	55
(Immunophenotyping)	Leukemia/lymphoma analysis	56
	CD34 enumeration	57
B. Intracellular antigen detection	Tdt	58,59
	Cytoplasmic immunoglobulin	59,60
C. DNA analysis	Ploidy and proliferation	61-67
D. Autoantibodies	Anti-platelet, anti-neutrophil	68-71
E. Neutrophil function	Oxidative burst, phagocytosis	72-76
F. Receptor analysis	Cytokine or estrogen receptors	77-80
G. Gene expression	MDR, oncogene products	81-86

Abbreviations: Tdt=terminal deoxynucleotidyl transferase; IL=interleukin; MDR=multidrug resistance gene

Basic Concepts of Cellular Analysis

Several concepts are central to an appreciation of flow cytometry. The first is that of single cell analysis and the difference between single-cell analysis and population analysis. The quantitation of various noncellular components of body fluids, for example, is typically a population analysis. Serum, urine, and other body fluids, because of the nature of solutes and solvents, are homogeneous; a single analysis of 2 aliquots of the same specimen should give equivalent results. Examples of population analysis are radioimmunoassays (RIAs) or enzyme-linked immunosorbent assays (ELISAs) performed on cells to detect the presence of specific antigens. To perform these studies, large numbers of cells must be assayed (eg, 10^5 or 10^6 per determination) to achieve results within the sensitivity of the method. To determine the amount of antigen per cell, the result of the assay is divided by the number of cells studied, based on the assumption of homogeneous populations. Tissues (or blood or bone marrow), however, are composed of multiple subpopulations of different cell types and/or of similar cell types at different stages of differentiation or functional capability. The goal of flow cytometry is the definition and quantitation of this heterogeneity. In contrast to population analysis, flow cytometry analyzes a population of cells on an individual cell basis, and thus will detect heterogeneity within a population.

Given the concept of single cell analysis in flow cytometry, it is important to realize that cytometers recognize particles, not cells per se. Therefore, 2 cells clumped together, isolated nuclei, or debris will all be recognized by the cytometer. Specific instructions, therefore, must be given to the cytometer to delineate monodisperse cells from other particles so that the data analysis is meaningful. This is often accomplished by "gating," a procedure which will be described later in this chapter.

Finally, the concept of multiparameter analysis must be emphasized. Flow cytometry is not merely an automated method for evaluating staining of a single fluorescent marker, it is a rapid and quantitative way of examining multiple features of individual cells simultaneously. It is not uncommon for a commercially available clinical cytometer to be able to detect 5 or 6 parameters per cell, thus allowing a much more sophisticated correlation to be developed between combinations of parameters and the disease process.

Design and Operation of a Flow Cytometer

In the simplest terms, a flow cytometer operates by causing cells in a fluid stream to pass in single file through a beam of light, usually generated by a laser (**Figure 2-1**). The photons of light that are scattered and emitted by the cells following their interaction with the laser beam are separated into constituent wavelengths by a series of filters and mirrors. This separated light falls upon individual detectors that generate electrical impulses, or analog signals, proportional to the amount of incident light striking the detectors. Each analog signal is converted to a digital signal, a number, which is accumulated in a frequency distribution, or histogram. Therefore, the resultant number is proportional to the amount of light emitted from, or scattered by, the individual cell.

The operating components of a flow cytometer may be divided into the following 3 categories: *fluidics,* including the flow cell and associated fluidics and hydraulics; *optics,* including the light source, optics, and scatter and fluorescence detectors; and the *computer systems and electronics* responsible for signal processing, data collection, and data analysis. Additional systems are included in instruments capable of preparative cell sorting.

Optics of a Clinical Flow Cytometer

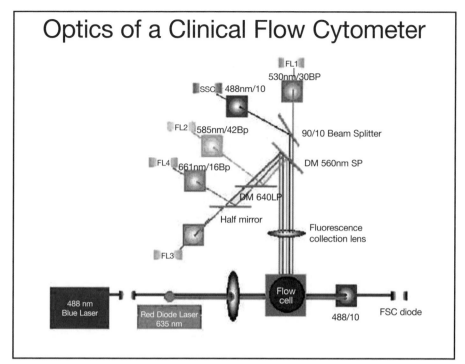

Figure 2-1

A schematic representation of the optical path of a flow cytometer. A single-cell suspension, stained with fluorescent probes, is intersected by a beam of laser light in a flow cell. A series of beam splitters and mirrors separate the light emitted from the flow cells in different wavelengths. An array of detectors collect specific signals that are ultimately digitized to construct histograms. Modified with permission from BD Biosciences, San Jose, CA.
Abbreviations: DM = dichroic mirror; LP = long pass filter; SP = short pass; 488/10 (for example) = 488nm band pass with a band 10nm wide.

Fluidics

A *sine qua non* for flow cytometric analysis is that (with rare exception) the specimen must be presented to the instrument in a monodisperse suspension. In order to analyze the cells, one must establish and maintain a highly controlled fluid stream designed to provide the exact location of the specimen in 3 dimensions. This is achieved in the sample handling compartment by forcing a usually isotonic fluid (called a sheath fluid) under pressure through a conical nozzle assembly geometrically designed to produce a laminar flow (**Figure 2-2**). The nozzle has an orifice 50 to 250 micrometers in diameter through which the fluid exits at a high flow rate, typically 10 meters per second (certain applications require a slower flow rate of 1 meter per second). The sample, in its own isotonic fluid, is introduced into the nozzle through an insertion rod at a higher differen-

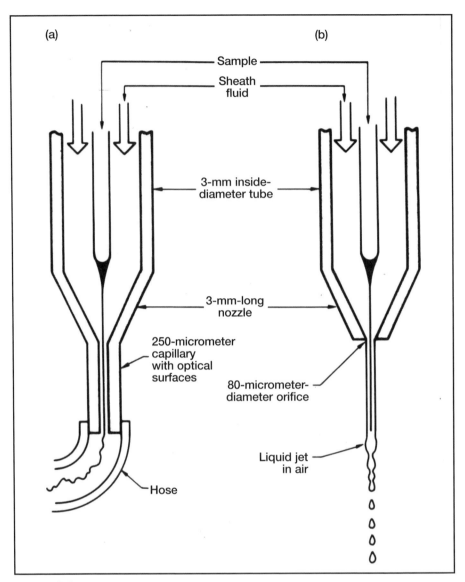

Figure 2-2
Representative cytometer flow chambers. The effect of drag and shearing forces on the sample fluid is minimized by a stable flow of sheath fluid. The coaxial fluid passes through a conical nozzle to the interrogation point. (a) A flow chamber of a cytometer for analysis only, (b) flow chamber for a cell sorter. (From Pinkel and Stovel[87]).

tial pressure than the sheath stream. The laminar flow induced by the nozzle imparts a hydrodynamic focusing effect to locate the sample stream in the center of the sheath stream. Thus, a coaxial stream-within-a-stream is created; the sheath fluid surrounds the sample fluid. Under these conditions, with optimized differential pressure, the sample stream is no wider than the cells it contains.

Optics

All commercial flow cytometers use a light source for the excitation of fluorochromes and the quantitation of intrinsic cellular parameters. This light source is most commonly a laser (or lasers), although arc lamps may also be used for the same purpose. Laser light differs from conventional sources of light, such as incandescent or fluorescent bulbs, in 2 fundamental ways. First, laser light is coherent; all of the waves of light are parallel. Second, laser light is monochromatic (of a single wavelength or frequency representing a single color). Historically, most lasers used in cytometers have been gas ion lasers. Argon, krypton, and helium-neon are examples of the gases used; each gas produces characteristic wavelengths of light. Argon lasers are the most commonly used lasers in clinical cytometers because they produce a strong 488nm line of light that excites many common fluorochromes. More recently, low-power diode lasers have been used in clinical cytometers.

Lasers are inherently inefficient. Hundreds of volts of electricity are required to produce the plasma in the system, while outputs are generally less than a watt. The excess energy is given off as heat. The larger gas ion lasers (in the 1- to 5-watt range) require large volumes of water for cooling (up to 2 gallons per minute). This is an obvious disadvantage because of its cost and the limited availability of large quantities of particle-free water in some locales. Most clinical flow cytometers have more efficient optical systems and can operate with low-power lasers that are air-cooled. These lasers operate in the milliwatt range (around 15mW) and are as useful as the larger lasers for lymphocyte immunophenotyping with many fluorochromes, have a longer life, and require less maintenance. It is now common for cytometers (even small clinical units) to contain multiple low-output lasers, which permit the use of a larger number and variety of fluorochromes.

The point at which the laser beam and the cell stream meet is called the laser interrogation point. The alignment of the light beam with the stream is critical to successful operation of flow cytometers; suboptimal alignment can result in erroneous data collection, presentation, and interpretation. With most large research cytometers, alignment is performed under mechanical control by the operator. Newer clinical instruments reduce or eliminate the need for daily alignment by bonding the flow chamber to the light-sensing optics. Daily quality control checks (described later in this chapter) ensure that the cytometer is functioning properly; any variance requires adjustment by a qualified engineer.

If the flow chamber is constructed in such a manner that the cells enter the laser beam after exiting the constriction nozzle, the sensing is termed jet-in-air, or open; the jet of fluid (stream of cells) is in the air at the interrogation point. On the other hand, if the nozzle terminates with an optical quartz square-tipped cuvette, the sample is interrogated in quartz and is thus a closed system. The closed system is preferable for biologically hazardous specimens and is typically operated at a 1-meter-per-second flow rate. The open (jet-in-air) system allows preparative cell sorting and is generally operated at flow rates of 10 meters per second or higher. The jet-in-air system allows higher analysis rates, whereas the quartz tip system affords more efficient collection of light and is therefore more sensitive (and hence may use a smaller air-cooled laser as the light source for the cytometer). Approaches to maximize light collection include the use of collecting lenses and mirrors bonded to the flow chamber to increase efficiency.[10]

Once a cell has traversed the sample stream to the point that it intersects the light beam, 2 events will occur, assuming that fluorochromes are in or on the cell. First, light from the beam at the incident wavelength will be scattered by the cell in 360°. The dynamics of light scatter are complicated and involve diffraction and reflection of the light by the cell. Briefly, if light scattered along the axis of the laser beam is collected, a parameter known as forward-angle light scatter, the quantity of light is proportional to the size of the particle or cell. This is true if the particle is a homogeneous sphere. Obviously, mammalian cells are neither homogeneous nor spherical, so the relationship tends to break down. In general, however, forward-angle scatter is roughly proportional to cell size. If the scattered light is collected orthogonally at right angles to the laser beam, the parameter is termed 90° light scatter or side scatter. Ninety-degree scatter has been shown to be composed primarily of light that has been reflected from internal structures or membrane undulations. Therefore, this parameter correlates with cell granularity. The properties of forward and 90° light scatter are termed intrinsic properties because they can be measured by cytometric instruments without the aid of exogenous reagents. Those properties requiring additional reagents for analysis are called extrinsic properties.

As an example of intrinsic properties, if one were to analyze a peripheral blood specimen from which the red blood cells have been removed, one would find that lymphocytes, relatively small cells with monotonous cytoplasm and a regular nucleus, exhibit both low forward-angle scatter and low 90° scatter (**Figure 2-3**). On the other hand, granulocytes, larger cells with a multilobed nucleus and many cytoplasmic inclusions, have increased scatter properties. Monocytes show intermediate forward and 90° scatter patterns. The sensitivity of these measurements is such that red blood cells, platelets, lymphocytes, monocytes, and granulocytes may all be resolved.

In the second event that occurs at the laser interrogation point, fluorochromes present on or in the cell absorb the laser light and re-emit the light at a lower energy and longer wavelength. This property is known as fluorescence. It occurs very rapidly, on the order of 10^{-6} seconds. The light produced in the

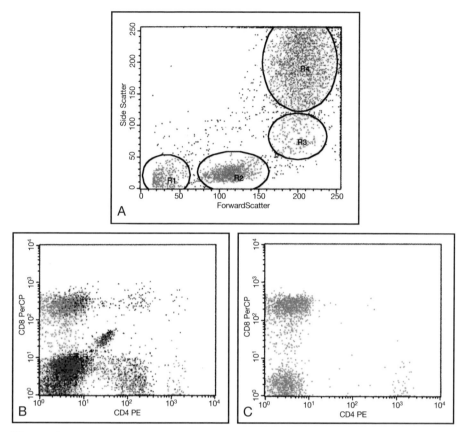

Figure 2-3

(a): A 2-parameter dot-plot histogram illustrating the light-scattering characteristics of whole blood after lysis of the red blood cells. Red (R1) = erythrocytes; green (R2) = lymphocytes; pink (R3) = monocytes; blue (R4) = granulocytes. (b): A 2-parameter dot-plot histogram illustrating the fluorescence of the whole blood preparation (ungated) stained with fluorescein isothiocyanate (FITC)-anti-CD4 and phycoerythrin (PE)-anti-CD8 antibodies. The same colors indicate the same cells as in the dot-plot (a). (c): A 2-parameter dot-plot illustrating the same staining, except here the only cells displayed are those falling inside the lymphocyte (green) gate, as shown in histogram (b).

fluorescence event, like the scattered light, is emitted in 360°. Typically, commercial instruments collect the emitted fluorescent light simultaneously with, and through, the same optical system as the 90° light scatter. Multicolored (multiwavelength) light now enters the detection chamber—the scattered light at the incident wavelength and the fluorescent light at longer wavelengths. The amount of light, or number of photons, is proportional to the amount of fluorochrome present in or on the cell; the more fluorochrome, the more light will be emitted. The multicolored light is separated into its constituent wavelengths (colors), and each wavelength is directed to a different detector. This is accomplished with short- and long-pass filters, which selectively allow only short or long wavelengths of light to pass, or, additionally, with dichroic mirrors (**Figure 2-4**). The short- and long-pass filters are interference or absorption filters, absorbing the light not allowed to pass through. Dichroic mirrors, on the other hand, reflect the light not allowed to pass. In this manner dichroic mirrors may be used to send light of one color to one detector and light of another color to a second detector. For example, a cell preparation may be stained with 2 fluorochromes, one emitting green light and the other emitting red light. A dichroic mirror may be used to direct the incident wavelength light collected as 90 light scatter to a detector that allows the remaining fluorescent light to pass. An interference long-pass filter may then be used to remove any residual laser light from the fluorescent emissions. Now only fluorescent light is in the detector system. A second dichroic mirror may be added further "downstream" in

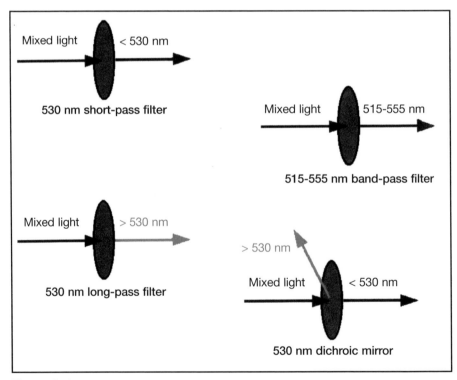

Figure 2-4
How long-pass, short-pass, and band pass filters and dichroic mirrors are used to separate light of differing wavelengths.

the lightpath to separate the longer wavelength red light from the shorter wavelength green light. Thus, the light from each fluorochrome may be physically separated and individually quantitated.

Electronics and Computer Systems

The photons of light impinging upon either the scatter or the fluorescent detectors are converted to electrical impulses proportional in magnitude to the number of photons received. Generally, these impulses are analog signals and vary in magnitude from 0 to 10 volts. Analog signals are then processed in a variety of ways. Either the brightest signal reaching a detector from a given cell is processed, or all the signals from a given cell are accumulated. The former process is known as peak-sense-and-hold signal processing, and the latter is known as integrated signal processing; the total amount of fluorescence emitted by the cell is integrated over the time that the cell is in the laser beam. Consequently, a peak signal represents the single brightest spot on a cell, whereas an integral signal is a measurement of the total cellular fluorescence. In addition to these modes of signal processing, the peak or integral signals may be collected in either linear or log domain. Collection of logarithmic signals affords a broader range of fluorescence detection and more sensitivity in the low fluorescent range, whereas linear signal collection accurately measures the linear differences in fluorochrome binding among cells in a population. Other more esoteric forms of signal processing are available, such as peak width analysis and waveform analysis.

The analog signals produced in the detector systems are converted to digital signals, or numbers, with analog-to-digital converters. The magnitude of the digital signal is proportional to the magnitude of the analog signal and is a function of the instrument resolution. In low-resolution operation, the instruments produce a digital signal with 256-channel resolution; a number from 0 to 255 is the result of the analog-to-digital conversion. Higher resolution data collection may range over 1024 channels.

The electronics associated with the entire signal processing system are designed to ensure correlated cell-by-cell measurement. It is critically important that all the signals associated with a single cell, both scatter and fluorescence, are attributed to only that cell, thus allowing multiparameter cellular analysis. With flow rates of 10 meters per second, it is possible to analyze 10,000 cells per second.

Virtually all data collected from flow cytometers is stored as listmode data. Listmode analysis requires the operator to select the parameters that are to be collected and stored. Then, as each cell is interrogated, the digitized data from each parameter are stored in the computer as a "list," hence listmode. This list is a matrix that contains all the collected data on all the analyzed cells that may subsequently be processed by the computer to form histograms. Listmode analysis is particularly useful in complicated multiparameter analyses with heterogeneous specimens because it is not necessary to make histogram decisions prior to sample analysis, and the data can be reprocessed multiple times.

The dramatic improvements in computers in the past 2 decades have played a major role in flow cytometric assays becoming more commonplace in the clinical environment. Early cytometers had little, if any, computing capabilities, and data were often displayed and stored as 1-parameter histograms generated by strip-chart recorders, or as photographs of the oscilloscope display. Now virtually every cytometer sold is equipped with a dedicated computer that not only collects, stores, and analyzes data, but also assists in controlling the cytometer and monitoring its performance. With the increasing complexity of flow cytometric assays, more extensive data analysis must be performed on larger data files. This extensive data analysis can often limit throughput on the cytometer. In response to this difficulty, considerable effort has recently been devoted to the creation of networks and file transfer systems, as well as stand-alone software, which will permit data to be analyzed on computers other than those dedicated to the cytometer. Similarly, data storage has migrated from small capacity floppy disks to large-capacity media such as CD-ROMs, which permit storage of gigabytes of data. This issue will be further explored in a subsequent chapter of this text.

Clinical versus Research Flow Cytometers

In the late 1980s, manufacturers of cytometers began to market cytometers designed primarily for clinical use. This was accomplished by streamlining research cytometers in several ways-eliminating large, bulky lasers; limiting the capacity of the instruments for assays or procedures seldom conducted in the clinical laboratory (eg, rapid cell sorting); and hardwiring or automating as many of the startup or alignment procedures as possible. The net result of these efforts is easier-to-use instruments that are somewhat more limited in function than large research cytometers. These clinical cytometers are a great advantage in an environment in which a technologist is not dedicated to flow cytometry alone, but must perform numerous laboratory tests on a variety of instrumentation. At the same time, the greatest disadvantage of clinical cytometers is the potential for an improperly trained operator to rely blindly on automated systems without sufficient knowledge of how they operate. Some contemporary clinical cytometers are capable of 4-color analysis in 6 parameters, including forward- and side-light scatter, using 1 or 2 lasers and low-to-moderate-speed cell sorting, if desired. Cell sorting is only rarely used in the clinical laboratory, and optional sorting modules for clinical cytometers are generally not high throughput devices. If high-speed sorting must be performed in the clinical laboratory as a preparative step for other diagnostic or therapeutic purposes, a larger research-style cytometer is probably the instrument of choice.

Other Types of Clinical Cytometry

As mentioned previously, flow cytometry is distinct from a number of other technologies that may be confused with it because of their similar names. These other technologies include image cytometry and volumetric capillary cytometry. Image cytometry captures images of cells or tissues adhered to microscope slides, rather than examining cells flowing past a detector, as flow cytometry does. Volumetric capillary cytometry, a rather new technique,[11,12] detects fluorescent particles present in a capillary tube filled with the specimen to be studied. By scanning a predetermined portion of the capillary for fluorescent particles, one can determine absolute concentrations of fluorescent particles in the specimen.

Mention should also be made of hematology analyzers, which, in many respects, are becoming indistinguishable from what are more classically considered flow cytometers. Many of these analyzers use lasers to measure light scatter of intrinsic cell properties and have the capacity to measure one immunostained parameter. Hematology analyzers also use cells in single-cell suspensions that flow past sets of detectors, thus fulfilling the definition of flow cytometry. However, in practical terms, hematology analyzers are generally used for garnering absolute blood counts and multiple part differentials, but only limited immunostained parameters.

Gating

In addition to the concepts of multiparameter analysis and correlated quantitative single cell analysis, the concept of electronic gating is important to an appreciation of flow cytometry. A gate may be defined as an electronic window encompassing a given region of a distribution set off by upper and lower limits. Gates may be either rectilinear or amorphous and are used to set off a subpopulation from a heterogeneous distribution. To satisfy an inclusive gate, a cell must exhibit the appropriate magnitude of the measured parameter to fall within the window. Gates may be set either as data are collected (ie, as cells are being run through the cytometer)—termed a live gate—or after the collection of data and during subsequent analysis of listmode data. There are advantages to each approach, although the latter permits regating if one desires to reanalyze a sample.

With a peripheral blood sample, it is possible to get a light scatter gate to include only the lymphocyte population by placing upper and lower limits on the forward and 90° scatter distributions (**Figure 2-3**). The instrument can form a histogram of the fluorescence distribution of only the lymphocytes; monocytes and granulocytes will not be included. It is important to emphasize that gates may be set on signals other than forward and orthogonal light scatter. Perhaps the 2 most common examples of use of a fluorescence signal for gating in the clinical laboratory are the use of CD45 (pan-leukocyte marker) antibodies to determine lymphocyte gates[13] and the use of various surface markers to set gates for subsequent analysis of DNA content in various neoplasms.[14]

Particular mention should be made of a gating strategy for bone marrow and peripheral blood using CD45 and side scatter (in log mode, compared with the linear side scatter routinely examined). First described by Stelzer et al,[15] the use of these parameters permits resolution of 8 discreet populations of hematopoietic cells (**Figure 2-5**) rather than the 3 resolved using light scatter alone (**Figure 2-3**).

An additional advantage of gates is that they may be stacked several deep. In other words, one can set several gates for a given analysis. Forward and side light scatter might be used to set a gate around lymphoid cells, then a second gate may be set using 2 fluorescent markers to identify a subset of lymphocytes expressing certain cell surface markers. Subsequent markers may then be examined exclusively on this subset of lymphocytes using the 2 gates simultaneously.

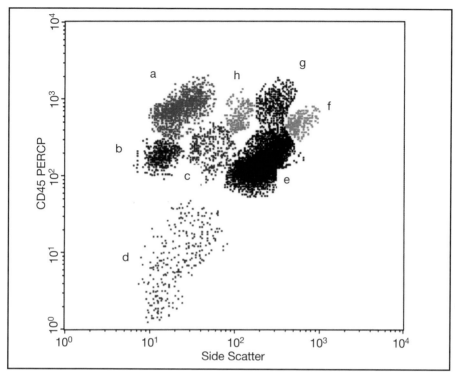

Figure 2-5

An example of CD45/log side scatter gating on human bone marrow. The specimen is resolved into the following populations: (a) lymphocytes; (b) lymphoblasts; (c) myeloblasts; (d) nucleated erythrocytes; (e) myelocytes and metamyelocytes; (f) progranulocytes; (g) mature neutrophils; and (h) monocytes.

Fluorescence and Fluorochromes

Each fluorochrome possesses a distinctive spectral pattern of absorption (excitation) and emission. As noted above, lasers emit monochromatic light (light of a single wavelength). Some lasers are designed to emit a variety of wavelengths, although under normal operating conditions, only one wavelength at a time is emitted. To be of use in flow cytometry, a fluorochrome or chromophore must absorb light at the wavelength or at one of the wavelengths the laser can emit. Not all fluorochromes can be used with all lasers, because each fluorochrome has distinct spectral characteristics and each type of laser produces light of specific wavelengths. Therefore, the choice of fluorochromes to be used in an assay depends on the light source used for excitation (**Table 2-2**).

Typically, with argon-ion lasers a 488nm excitation wavelength is used, which produces a blue to blue-green light. The fluorochrome must emit light at

Table 2-2

Fluorochromes and Dyes Commonly Used in Clinical Flow Cytometry

Excitation Wavelength	Fluorochrome or Dye	Emission Wavelength
488nm (argon laser)	Fluorescein isothiocyanate	530
	Phycoerythrin	580
	Tandem conjugates*	620 or 670
	Propidium iodide	620(broad)
	Peridinin chlorophyll	670
633nm (HeNe laser)	Allophycocyanin	670
	CY-5	670

*Tandem conjugates describe a group of fluorochromes, each of which is comprised of 2 closely bound fluorochromes with distinct excitation and emission spectra. Light excites one fluorochrome, which transfers this light energy to the second fluorochrome, which then emits light at a higher wavelength than possible using the first fluorochrome alone.

a wavelength sufficiently longer than the excitation wavelength so that the 2 colors of light coming from the cell (90° light scatter and the fluorescence signal) may be optically separated with selective filters. The most popular fluorochrome used in immunofluorescence analysis is fluorescein isothiocyanate (FITC), which has an absorption maximum between 450 to 540 nm and an emission maximum of 520 nm. This difference between the absorption and emission wavelengths is known as the Stokes' shift; with all fluorochromes, the wider the Stokes' shift, the more useful it is to the flow cytometrist. If multiple fluorochromes are used, their emission spectra must have minimal overlap so that they can be separately quantitated. Ideally, the fluorochromes would have the same or similar absorption spectra, to allow excitation with a single wavelength of light and a single laser. Typically, in a single argon laser system, phycoerythrin (PE) is used as a second fluorochrome with FITC because it can absorb light from the 488nm line of an argon laser yet has a larger Stokes' shift than FITC (ie, emits most of its light at higher wavelengths than FITC does). Third-color fluorescence is achieved using fluorochromes with a larger Stokes' shift (eg, peridinin chlorophyll protein [PerCP]) or carefully designed tandem fluorochromes (eg, PE-Cy5), which use one fluorochrome to absorb light and a closely coupled second fluorochrome to emit light.

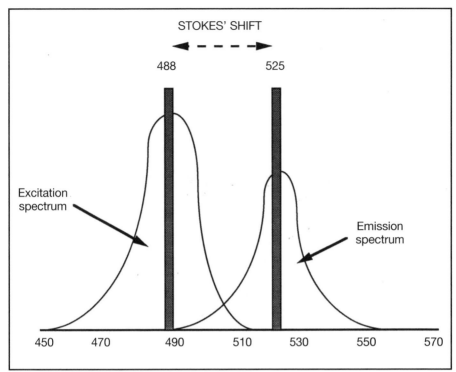

Figure 2-6

Practical examples of how undercompensated (too little of the overlapping signal removed), properly compensated (appropriate amount of overlapping signal removed), and overcompensated (too much signal removed) samples would appear in histogram displays. (From McCoy et al.[34])

Compensation

As multicolor assays become more prevalent in clinical flow cytometry, the need for an understanding of compensation (also called electronic or fluorescence compensation) becomes greater. As discussed above, the basis of 2-color single-laser flow cytometry is the use of 2 fluorochromes that are capable of excitation at the same wavelength, but have different Stokes' shifts, resulting in emissions at different wavelengths. Fluorochromes do not, however, emit at one wavelength, but rather in a spectrum. This quite often results in some overlap (or bleeding) of the emissions of one fluorochrome into the other, which cannot be eliminated by optical filters (**Figure 2-6**). Therefore, the fluorescence from FITC may, and in fact does, give a weak signal in the optical path used to detect PE. This "bleeding-over" is corrected by compensation—an electronic method that subtracts a percentage of the fluorescence signal that is determined to be due to

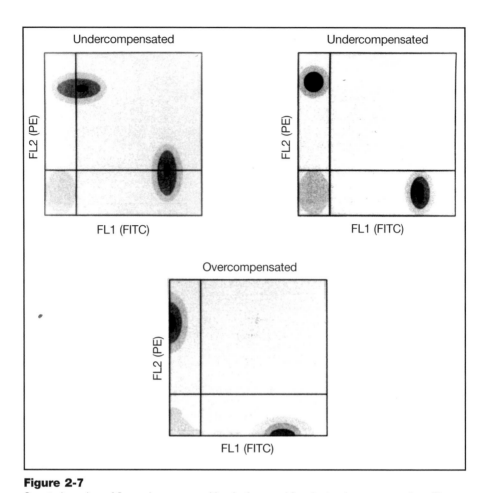

Figure 2-7

Spectral overlap of fluorochromes resulting in the need for electronic compensation. The emission spectra (obtained after excitation with a 488nm laser line) for fluorescein isothiocyanate (FITC) and phycoerythrin (PE) are represented by the left and right curves, respectively. A 530nm band pass filter is used to collect the FITC signal; however, a small portion of the PE signal overlaps into this wavelength. This must be reduced by electronic compensation. Similarly, a 585 band pass filter is used to collect the PE signal, but a portion of the FITC signal "bleeds" into this wavelength and must be reduced by compensation.

spectral overlaps.[16] With many clinical cytometers, automated programs are used to set compensation values; these must be used with caution, however. The amount of compensation required will vary with the brightness of staining and with varying voltages to photomultiplier tubes—in other words, with a number of factors that will affect signal strength. Overcompensation or undercompensation may result from setting compensation values using beads or cells of fluorescence intensity substantially different from the specimens to be analyzed (**Figure 2-7**). This can be checked by analyzing each fluorochrome or marker individually (ie, using one color at a time), but collecting signals from both fluorochromes.

Post-acquisition compensation has been made possible by the introduction of software capable of this task.[17] One advantage of this compensation during analysis is that compensation errors may be avoided, or at least corrected, because only uncompensated data are collected and saved.

Cell Sorting

As mentioned above, many research flow cytometers are capable of preparative cell sorting. This process involves the physical separation of a subpopulation of cells from the main population. This capability evolved from ink-jet printer technology and is elegantly simple in concept. In cell sorters, the flow chamber is seated in a piezoelectric crystal that vibrates in response to a coupled acoustical transducer. The vibration of the crystal is imparted to the flow chamber and causes the stream to form nodes and eventually to break up into droplets. The droplet formation should occur downstream so it does not disturb the laser interrogation point. To engage the sorting mechanism, a logic is established with the computer system that instructs it to look for a cell which satisfies a given sort criteria. These criteria may include gates on any property of any measurable parameter. At the point of laser interrogation, the computer determines whether or not the cell satisfies the sort criteria. If it does, the instrument places an electrical charge of a given polarity on the entire stream. When the droplet containing the cell of interest breaks away from the stream, the entire stream is discharged. The only charged particle in the sample flow is now the droplet containing the specific cell. As the droplet moves downstream at a speed of 10 meters per second, it enters an electrostatic field created by 2 charge plates; one plate carries a negative charge, the other a positive charge. The charged droplet is attracted to the plate of opposite charge and is deflected from the main stream. It is then a simple matter to place a collecting vessel in the path of the sorted droplets. In commercial instruments, 2 different populations may be simultaneously sorted. Cells collected in this manner are viable, may be maintained as sterile, and may be bulk sorted or index sorted and cloned by automatically sorting single cells into the wells of microtiter plates.

To Sort or not to Sort in the Clinical Lab

Some manufacturers have introduced clinical flow cytometers with low-speed sorting capabilities. One example of a low-speed clinical sorter is the FACSort (Becton Dickinson Immunocytometry Systems, San Jose, CA), which uses a mechanical means of sorting cells rather than the traditional jet-in-air approach in which cells are sorted by electrostatic charges. The concept behind low-speed sorters is that they allow the pathologist to correlate morphology with phenotype by sorting small numbers of cells with specified characteristics for later analysis by cytospin preparation. Additionally, sorting may be used as a preparative technique for molecular tests, such as polymerase chain reaction (PCR), where only small numbers of cells are required for study. At this juncture, the long-term reliability of this mechanical design is unproven; however, the ease with which these products can sort would make them highly desirable tools in the clinical laboratory.

High-speed cell sorting can be performed in relatively few, highly specialized clinical flow cytometry laboratories. It is primarily performed in support of stem cell transplantation for stem cell purification or purging of extraneous cells from stem cell preparations. These cytometry sorting protocols vie with other techniques, such as panning and magnetic bead separation, for preparative cell separation in the clinical environment.

Quantitative Flow Cytometry

Flow cytometry by its very design has the ability to quantitate the amount of fluorescence emanating from a cell or other particle. In general, this is an under-utilized aspect of flow cytometry; most users merely determine if a cell (or cells) is positive or negative for expression of a given antigen or receptor. In several clinical situations, such as immunoglobulin light chain expression, the intensity of fluorescence may be useful in distinguishing among different disease processes. Simplistically, this assessment of fluorescence intensity is often subjectively described as "bright" or "dim" staining. The subjectivity of this approach leads to great inter-institutional variability and thus minimizes its use in the clinical environment. It should be emphasized that quantitative flow cytometry does not merely quantitate the number of positive cells for a given marker but also, and most importantly, quantitates the intensity of the fluorescent staining on each cell.

The goal of quantitative flow cytometry is to remove subjectivity from the assessment of fluorescence intensity by using the inherent capabilities of flow cytometers to achieve a more objective assessment. Objective quantitation of the intensity of fluorescent staining is accomplished through the use of a series of standardized beads whose fluorescent properties can be measured in relationship to the specimen in question. These standardized beads may be of different composition, depending on the quantitation desired. For example, standard beads filled with known amounts of soluble fluorescein may be used, with the data reported as the fluorescence proportional to the mean equivalent of soluble fluorescein (MESF).[18-20] Alternatively, standard beads may be coated with an anti-immunoglobulin to capture specific amounts of the fluorochrome-conjugated antibody used for staining the specimen. In this case, intensity of staining is expressed in terms of antibody-bind capacity (ABC). Both approaches require that the technologist make certain assumptions and therefore have a certain amount of controversy associated with them. A thorough discussion of these methods, a definition of terminologies, and proposals for standardization derived from a special conference on this topic, have recently been published.[18-20]

Considerations in Sample Preparation

As stated previously in this chapter, the first requirement of a sample for flow cytometric analysis is that it be in a monodisperse suspension. Failure to meet this requirement results in technical inaccuracies in the data generated and, often, physical blockage of the flow of the sample through the nozzle orifice.

Given a monodisperse sample, the problem becomes defining the conditions that will allow cells to be interrogated for a given property or properties. This involves choosing a dye or fluorochrome conjugate that will mark the desired characteristic of the cell, a light source with a spectrum that will excite the fluorochrome or dye, and filters that will allow the emission wavelengths from the fluorochrome or dye to be detected without interference from extraneous wavelength noise. To simplify this procedure for the clinical laboratory, commercially available reagents are usually supplied with only a limited option for fluorochromes and dyes; similarly, the manufacturers of flow cytometers generally equip their instruments with the filters and lasers required to excite and detect the most commonly used fluorochromes. Commonly used fluorochromes are listed in **Table 2-2.** A recent approach of commercial suppliers of monoclonal antibodies for flow cytometry is the production of kits for multiple marker ("2-, 3-, or 4-color") analysis. These kits are directed toward frequently performed tests, such as determining helper/suppressor ratios of T cells in peripheral blood, and work with commonly used fluorochromes (fluorescein, PE, tandem-conjugates, and allophycocyanin). These kits, while somewhat restrictive in repertoire, offer great advantages; they are prediluted and mixed in predetermined ratios, saving much technical time in the laboratory.

The methods described above rely on probes, such as antibodies, lectins, and various ligands, conjugated to fluorochromes. The probes provide the specificity for interaction with the cell while the fluorochromes provide the fluorescent signal. In other assays, the fluorochrome, or dye, alone provides both the fluorescent signal and the means of specifically recognizing targets or structures of a cell. Common examples of the latter type of staining are some of the methods used for quantitating the DNA content of cells. Propidium iodide, ethidium bromide, acridine orange, 4,6 diamidino-2-phenylindole (DAPI), and Hoechst dyes bind directly to DNA and fluoresce when excited by light of the appropriate wavelength. With certain dyes, notably DAPI and Hoechst dyes, the fluorescence of the dye molecule increases significantly following binding. Other examples of fluorescent dyes include cyanine dyes for the study of changes in membrane potential,[21] fluorescein diacetate for oxidative burst measurements,[22] diacetoxy-2,3-dicyanobenzene for intracellular pH,[23] and a variety of substrates whose enzymes convert from nonfluorogenic to fluorogenic for the measurement of enzymatic activities.[24-29]

In some assays it is of critical importance to identify the staining on only the viable cells in a specimen. In these situations, the cells may be fixed only after the viability staining procedure has been completed (ie, after the dead cells have been identified with stains), because prior fixation will, by definition, kill all cells. Dead cells contaminating the live cell population can be identified using nucleic acid dyes such as propidium iodide or ethidium monoazide.[30,31] This real-time viability assessment offers a great advantage over performing trypan blue staining in parallel with flow cytometric immunophenotyping. Viability assessment as a component of multiparameter analysis will permit exclusion of dead cells from analysis, whereas concomitant trypan blue staining merely excludes specimens with low viability from analysis. In a clinical assay such as CD34 enumeration for stem cell transplantation, knowing the number of viable stem cells is probably more important than determining the total number of CD34+ cells without regard to viability, because only viable cells will engraft.

Other assays, in which the target antigen is sequestered or is found in the cytoplasm or internal organelles, require fixation and/or permeabilization of the cell. As is the case with many other aspects of flow cytometry, the optimal fixative or permeabilizing agent is selected by empirical evaluation. One important aspect of fixation is that many fixatives substantially alter the light scattering characteristics of cells. Therefore, identifying the cells of interest after fixation may be a problem (particularly in mixed populations of cells) when one is accustomed to viewing the light scatter characteristics of unfixed cells. Visual examination of the fixed preparation and the unfixed sample is often useful in determining how the morphology of the cells has been altered during the fixation process.

Absolute Cell Counts by Flow Cytometry

In some clinical assays, such as CD4 enumeration and CD34 evaluation, there is a need to obtain an absolute count of the number of cells of a given immunophenotype, rather than to report the percentage of positive cells only. Historically this was accomplished by obtaining a white blood count and differential on a separate aliquot of the specimen being studied. To perform absolute cell counting in immunophenotyping assays, several manufacturers have developed products that use beads as reference particles. The principle behind this approach is the fact that adding a known number of beads to a predetermined volume of the initial blood (or other fluidic) specimen permits one to calculate absolute cell counts by enumerating the number of beads collected as the cells of interest are analyzed.[32,33] This requires extremely accurate addition of the beads to the specimen, a problem which has been solved in some instances by special, highly precise pipettes, and in other instances by the manufacturers providing test tubes preloaded with precise numbers of beads.

Quality Control

As with other clinical assays, analysis and interpretation of data accumulated by flow cytometry cannot be attempted unless proper attention is directed toward controls and calibration.[34,35] This can be a rather complex undertaking, and, for some assays, completely suitable controls have yet to be devised. The general areas of concern with assays requiring flow cytometric analysis are

(1) proper and reproducible alignment and calibration of the cytometer, (2) the availability of historical databases that demonstrate the distribution of the marker on normal specimens, (3) positive and negative controls performed concomitantly with the clinical test to ensure that the assay is working satisfactorily on a given day, and (4) proper specimen handling and sample preparation. The alignment and calibration of a flow cytometer are usually accomplished with fluorescent beads, nucleated erythrocytes, or both. These procedures are performed not only to ensure that the instrument is properly configured for the desired analysis, but also to minimize the day-to-day variability in analyses. Therefore, particles with constant amounts of fluorescence are run daily, and the laser power and/or high-voltage settings for the photomultiplier tubes (PMTs) are adjusted to bring the fluorescence peak of the particles to a consistent channel; the settings are then recorded in a log book. This reduces the possibility that differences in the staining of cells or markers are due to changes in the ability of the cytometer to detect fluorescence in a consistent manner. Furthermore, records of laser power and voltage settings can delineate long-term trends in the instrument that may be indicative of technical problems, such as a gradual failure of the laser characterized by decreasing light output at a constant voltage.

An historical database is important because it defines the distribution of a marker or markers on normal populations of cells, given a consistent alignment and calibration of the cytometer. Each laboratory should maintain its own database because calibration and staining procedures may vary, which may have an impact upon the apparent distribution of markers. Laboratories should compare their database values to those of other laboratories or those reported in the literature. Significant variation from commonly accepted values necessitates a reexamination of laboratory procedures. Currently, there are programs to establish interlaboratory quality assurance for clinical flow cytometry laboratories through the use of send-out specimens.[36,37]

To ensure that staining and instrumentation are performing properly, blood or other samples (eg, cord blood, bone marrow) from normal individuals are assayed at least daily and must fall within the limits defined as normal by the historical database. Failure of a marker to fall within those limits eliminates the credibility of staining for that marker on that day. Many samples also contain internal controls that can be quickly checked to verify the accuracy of the staining. Does the number of cells staining as T-helper (CD4) plus the number of T-suppressor cells (CD8) roughly equal the number of cells staining with a pan T marker? If multiple markers for T cells, B cells, monocytes, etc, are tested, do they yield similar results? Can all of the cells within a given gate be accounted for by the results of the marker staining?

Mention should be made of the advantages and disadvantages of density gradient and whole blood lysis techniques. Density gradient preparation of lymphocytes may be advantageous (compared with whole blood lysis) when a specimen contains a low percentage of viable lymphocytes, because this procedure yields a semi-purified population of viable mononuclear cells. (However, the real-time viability staining technique described above is generally a better approach for such a specimen.) On the other hand, density gradient preparation is not the method of choice for sample preparation for many leukemic specimens that may contain blast cells with an altered buoyant density. Similarly, density gradients are to be avoided if one wishes to examine the granulocytes as well as the lymphocytes in a specimen. Whole blood lysis techniques are generally considered the preferred preparative technique.[38-40] A potential hazard of lysis techniques is the risk of antigen denaturation by the lysing agent. However, this pitfall can be avoided by testing the effect of lysing reagents on cells known to express the antigen prior to embarking upon routine use of whole blood lysis for preparation of cells for surface marker staining.

The historic use of negative controls consisting of staining cells with nonspecific antibodies of the same isotype as the antibodies directed against the surface marker is coming under question. Traditionally, this procedure had been thought to indicate the amount of nonspecific binding unrelated to the presence of antigen on the cell surface, and was (and is) used by many cytometrists to establish a cutoff point between positive staining and non-specific background staining. Recently, however, the use of such isotype controls has been deemed superfluous, and pathologists are relying instead on the pattern of staining to determine which cells are to be considered positive in multiparameter analyses.[40-43]

A more complicated and as yet incomplete undertaking concerns performing proper controls for markers expressed primarily in malignant cells. The common acute lymphoblastic leukemia antigen (CALLA, J5), for example, is not expressed in normal peripheral blood cells, but it is diagnostic when found in certain types of leukemia. To establish the veracity of staining with reagents to markers like this, laboratories use either cell lines or frozen cells stored from previous samples shown to be positive. Neither approach is without difficulties; cell lines often show high autofluorescence and frozen samples often suffer from low viabilities. An alternative for controls of this nature would be the coating of synthetic beads with the purified antigen to be assayed; however, often the purified antigen is not available.

The analysis of DNA histograms generated by flow cytometry presents requirements different from those of surface marker analysis (**Figure 2-8**). Methods, approaches, and problems encountered in DNA analysis can be found in

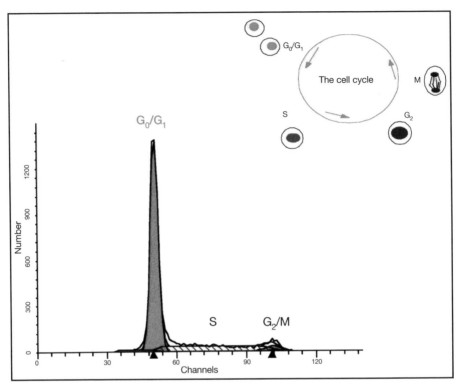

Figure 2-8
A 1-parameter DNA histogram of cell nuclei stained with propidium iodide illustrating the appearance of the G_0/G_1, S, and G_2/M phases of the cell cycle.

subsequent chapters of this book. Generally, DNA is studied for one or both of the following reasons: (1) to determine the presence of aneuploid cells in a population and (2) to determine the percentage of cells in each phase of the cell cycle (ie, the growth rate of the cells). The 2 goals have distinct requirements in terms of data analysis. Ploidy determination relies upon the position of the G_0/G_1 peak of the sample in relationship to the G_0/G_1 peak of control diploid cells derived from the sample species, whereas cell cycling analysis requires the division of the histogram into 3 areas representing the G_0/G_1, S, and G_2/M phases and the integration of the area representing each phase. The determination of ploidy is usually an easier undertaking than accurately assessing cell cycling. The channels representing the maximum G_0/G_1 peak heights of the sample and the control may be delineated either manually or by computer, and aneuploidy is defined as a significant difference between the 2 peaks. Diploid controls usually consist of lymphocytes or thymocytes, and chicken and/or trout erythrocytes are often run in each sample as additional controls to reduce the possibility that apparent shifts in the G_0/G_1 peaks are due to instrument drift or fluctuations in the laser output.[44,45]

Watson[46] has suggested the use of time as a quality control parameter for flow cytometry. In this approach, fluorescence or light scatter data for individual samples may be analyzed chronologically; the time sequence for each bit of information is remembered along with the light scatter or fluorescence data. This allows visualization of instrumental drift within a sample due to a variety of factors, including fluidic and light source faults. Currently, this approach to quality control is not available on flow cytometers designed for the clinical laboratory unless substantial upgrades are made in the computer systems.

High-quality flow cytometry is intrinsically linked to high-quality sample handling and preparation. Collection and transportation of specimens must be conducted in a consistent manner to minimize the introduction of artifacts. Manual differential cell counts should be made of the sample prior to processing and after staining, and these differentials should be compared to those obtained with the cytometer. Additionally, the size, shape, and number of any unusual or blast-like cells should be noted in the manual differential to guide the operator in gating during the flow cytometric analysis.

Safety Considerations

As flow cytometry becomes a clinical discipline, issues of safety and infection control have become increasingly important. The concern over safety revolves primarily around biological hazards; instrument safety regarding stray laser light or high-voltage PMTs is increased in the new generation of clinical instruments, which largely deny the operator access to potentially dangerous conditions.

Biohazards remain an area of great concern in flow cytometry, however. Cytometer operators should take the same precautions that are recommended for individuals in other clinical laboratories: lab coats should be worn at all times, open-toed shoes are to be avoided, the use of needles should be discouraged, safety glasses should be worn, and gloves are recommended if chafing or abrasions are present on the hands. Specimen tubes should be disposed of in biohazard containers, and bleach should be added to the waste fluid containers in the cytometer to act as a disinfectant. Many laboratories prophylactically disinfect cytometers by running bleach or ethanol as sheath fluid for 1 hour a week (not during data acquisition, of course). The best method of avoiding contamination of a cytometer, however, is to not run infectious material through it. To this end, after staining with monoclonal antibodies, fixation of all specimens with 1%-2% paraformaldehyde for a period of at least 2 hours is recommended.

As in virtually all other laboratories, cytometry lab safety issues are subject to regulation by several federal and local agencies. In the US, these include the Occupational Safety and Health Administration (OSHA), and independent organizations such as the College of American Pathologists (which may inspect laboratories in fulfillment of the Clinical Laboratories Improvement Act of 1988 [CLIA 88]).[47,48]

Limitations

Flow cytometry has much to offer the clinical laboratory. It provides a rapid method for detecting and quantitating many features of individual cells. The advantages of this are apparent and need not be reiterated here. However, with all the beneficial aspects of flow cytometry, the technology as currently practiced has shortcomings that limit its application and can actually lead to inappropriate diagnoses.

First, interpretation of flow cytometric data requires morphological and clinical correlation. Certain disease entities (such as pre-B acute lymphocytic leukemia and lymphoid blast crisis of chronic myelogenous leukemia) are virtually impossible to distinguish from one another by immunophenotype alone. High-quality clinical flow cytometric immunophenotyping is performed only in the context of a complete clinical history and an expert morphologic analysis. Flow cytometry performed in a void is of limited use.

Second, there are limitations in the intrinsic cellular properties detected. As described above, the instruments evaluate intrinsic parameters such as forward-angle and 90° light scatter. These light scatter parameters can discriminate among multiple subpopulations within heterogeneous specimens and may be used to set gates for further analysis of each individual population. Although this approach is generally sufficient to elucidate predominant populations of lymphocytes in peripheral blood specimens, its utility with bone marrow specimens or solid tumors rapidly diminishes as the heterogeneity increases. The major components of peripheral blood, with the exception of red blood cells, are usually discretely separable by light scatter analysis, or by light scatter and CD45 fluorescence. However, bone marrow contains a spectrum of cells of varying lineage, maturity, size, and granularity; these components may be more difficult to study as discrete populations. A third intrinsic cellular parameter, axial light loss, has been described, and, if introduced to clinical cytometers, may prove useful in providing better resolution of these populations.[49] Certainly, performing multiparameter analysis using combinations of intrinsic and extrinsic properties (as the CD45/log side scatter gating described earlier does) helps overcome the limitations found in relying on intrinsic cell properties for gating.

Third, flow cytometry is limited by the quality of the specimen examined. One must know what the relationship is between the specimen obtained from the patient and the one analyzed on the flow cytometer. Essentially, this is the "garbage in/garbage out" scenario. A specimen improperly stored or transported may yield inappropriate data not representative of the patient's clinical status.

A fourth limitation is actually pathologists' desire to analyze cells at even faster rates than are currently possible with standard techniques. Most cytometers are relatively high-throughput instruments, but their capabilities are finite. By running cells too rapidly through a cytometer, one risks missing data on relevant cells. While adequate for most clinical situations, the capacity of the average clinical cytometer might be exceeded in attempting to quickly gather large data files for the detection of rare events in minimal residual disease or in sorting large numbers of cells for therapeutic applications. A method of "fluorescence triggering" has proven useful in overcoming these limitations of hardware due to signal processing constraints; it may find wide use in the future.[50]

As stated frequently in this chapter, a necessity for most flow cytometry assays is the availability of single-cell suspensions. Clearly, however, this is not always possible. In solid tissue, disaggregation procedures may lead to perturbations of cell surface structures or cell disruption. In certain cytologic preparations, such as cervical scrapes or stool lavage specimens, debris, mucus, bacteria, and cell clumping combine to present tremendous obstacles to performing satisfactory flow cytometry. An alternative technology in these instances is often image cytometry. Image cytometry, unlike flow cytometry, examines cells on a microscope slide and can cope better with specimens that are not unicellular. Image cytometry application to DNA analysis will be discussed in a later chapter of this text.

Other limitations of clinical flow cytometry concern biology, the chemistry, or the state of medical treatment related to a given application.

The Future

In the decade that has passed since the first edition of this book was published, flow cytometry has continued to evolve as a useful and integral component of diagnostic pathology. Today it is much more practical to perform 6 (or more)-parameter analysis (4 colors plus forward- and side-light scatter) on most specimens than it was 10 years ago. This yields more precise identification of cells than previously possible and thereby increases the utility of flow cytometry in a number of diagnostic applications. The development of more monoclonal antibodies to novel cell markers, convenient low-speed sorting for subsequent microscopic or molecular studies of the cells examined, faster computing systems, and low-cost, high-capacity storage media have all contributed to the growth and refinement of clinical flow cytometry. Almost certainly, developments of this nature will continue over the foreseeable future and will contribute to the evolution of clinical cytometry.

Additional factors may also have an impact on the future of clinical flow cytometry. Principal among these is the increasing realization that standardization of flow cytometric techniques and interpretation of flow cytometric data is crucial in the clinical environment. Several consensus conferences have already been held to discuss these issues,[51,52] and more are being called for.[53] Although some unity has been reached, these consensus conferences also illustrate how little agreement exists in the more subjective areas of clinical flow cytometry such as leukemia/lymphoma immunophenotyping and stem cell enumeration. Clearly, continuing efforts need to be, and will be, made to standardize the practice of flow cytometry in the clinical environment.

One area of future focus will probably be refinement and standardization of quantitative cytometry. There is increasing awareness that, in some instances, the intensity of marker staining may be as important as the enumeration of cells positive for a given marker. Although methods have been described for standard approaches, most clinical laboratories currently use subjective criteria to quantitate staining (eg, "bright," "dim," etc). A more thorough discussion of this need and future possibilities appeared in a recent publication by Purvis and Stelzer.[54]

In many geographic areas, the economics of health care are driving the direction of clinical flow cytometry. A general reduction in the reimbursement for clinical assays has led to a widespread demand for more cost-effective methods of performing clinical flow cytometry. To reduce the cost of the highly skilled personnel required to operate and interpret flow cytometric assays, there has been a trend toward automating as much of these assays as possible. This includes automatic specimen staining devices, automatic specimen loaders, and software-driven data acquisition and analysis. This trend towards automation is likely to continue in the future.

Novel approaches to using flow cytometry in the clinical laboratory may drastically revolutionize the field. A potential example of this is the LabMAP (Multiple Analyte Profile) technology of the Luminex Corporation (Austin, TX). This technology uses 100 spectrally distinct populations of beads, each of which can be resolved on a flow cytometer. Each color of bead may be coated with a different antigen or ligand. Thus, 100 different beads, each with a distinct antigen or ligand, may be assayed. Through the use of a distinct fluorochrome linked to a reporter, these beads can be used to assay a variety of specimens for a variety of analytes (possibly including HIV and hepatitis B seroconversion, multiple cytokines, allergy testing, DNA-based tissue typing, *Herpes simplex* viral load, IgG, IgA, and IgM assays, IgG sub-classification, substance abuse toxicology, hepatitis C viral load, autoantibodies, cardiac enzymes, hCG and AFP, HIV viral load, and the ToRCH panel).

Finally, the trend towards melding flow cytometry with other areas of diagnostic pathology will no doubt progress. Many distinctions between classical flow cytometry and certain aspects of hematology have already disappeared: they will erode further in the future. This will drive changes in instrumentation, and vice versa. As discussed above, a blending of flow cytometry, serology, and virology may well occur in the near future, and, as will be described in a later chapter, many applications of molecular biology may be adapted to flow cytometry-based techniques. Considered together, these endeavors suggest the advent of revolutionary new applications and hardware in the field of clinical flow cytometry over the next decade.

References

1. Shapiro HM. *Practical Flow Cytometry*. 3rd ed. New York, NY: Wiley-Liss, Inc; 1994.

2. Van Dilla MA, Dean PN, Laerum OD, et al. *Flow Cytometry: Instrumentation and Data Analysis*. Orlando, FL: Academic Press, Inc; 1985.

3. Landay AL, Ault KA, Bauer KD, et al, eds: *Clinical Flow Cytometry. Ann NY Acad Sci.* 1993;677.

4. Owens MA, Loken MR. *Flow Cytometry Principles for Clinical Laboratory Practice: Quality Assurance for Quantitative Immunophenotyping*. New York, NY: Wiley-Liss, Inc;1995.

5. Darzynkiewicz Z, Crissman JA. Flow Cytometry: *Methods in Cell Biology.* Vol 33. San Diego, CA: Academic Press, Inc; 1990.

6. Givan AL. *Flow Cytometry: First Principles.* New York, NY: Wiley-Liss, Inc; 1992.

7. Ormerod MG. *Flow Cytometry.* 2nd ed. New York, NY: Springer-Verlag; 1999.

8. Radbruch A. *Flow Cytometry and Cell Sorting.* 2nd ed. New York, NY: Springer-Verlag; 1999.

9. Grogan WM. *Guide to Flow Cytometry Methods.* New York, NY: Marcel Dekker; 1990.

10. Watson JV. A method for improving light collection of 600% from square cross section flow cytometry chambers. *Br J Cancer.* 1985;51:433-435.

11. Dietz LJ, Dubrow RS, Manian BS, et al. Volumetric capillary cytometry: a new method for absolute cell enumeration. *Cytometry.* 1996;23:177-186.

12. Read EJ, Kunitake ST, Carter CS, et al. Enumeration of CD34+ hematopoietic progenitor cells in peripheral blood and leukapheresis products by microvolume fluorimetry: a comparison to flow cytometry. *J Hematother.* 1997;6:291-301.

13. Loken MR, Brosnan JM, Bach BA, et al. Establishing optimal lymphocyte gates for immunophenotyping by flow cytometry. *Cytometry.* 1990;11:453-459.

14. Braylan RC, Benson NA, Nourse VA. Cellular DNA of human neoplastic B-cells measured by flow cytometry. *Cancer Res.* 1984;44:5010-5016.

15. Stelzer GT, Shults KE, Loken MR. CD45 gating for routine flow cytometric analysis of human bone marrow specimens. *Ann NY Acad Sci.* 1993;677:265-280.

16. Loken MR, Parks DR, Herzenberg LA. Two-color immunofluorescence using a fluorescence-activated cell sorter. *J Histochem Cytochem.* 1997;25:899-907.

17. Bagwell CB. Adams EG. Fluorescence spectral overlap compensation for any number of flow cytometry parameters. *Ann NY Acad Sci.* 1993;677:167-84.

18. Henderson LO, Marti GE, Gaigalas A, et al. Terminology and nomenclature for standardization in quantitative fluorescence cytometry. *Cytometry.* 1998;33:97-105.

19. Schwartz A, Marti GE, Poon R, et al. Standardizing flow cytometry: a classification system of fluorescence standards used for flow cytometry. *Cytometry.* 1998;33:106-14.

20. Lenkei R, Marti GE, Vogt R, et al. Meeting Summary: EC, FDA, and Health Canada. *Cytometry.* 1998;33:94-96.

21. Shapiro, HM. Cell membrane potential analysis. *Meth Cell Biol.* 1990;33:25-35.

22. Bass DA, Parce JW, DeChalelet LR, et al. Flow cytometric studies of oxidative product formation by neutrophils: a graded response to membrane stimulation. *J Immunol.* 1983;130:1910-1917.

23. Cook JA, Fox MH. Intracellular pH measurements using flow cytometry with 1,4-diacetoxy-2,3-dicyanobenzene. *Cytometry.* 1988;9:441-447.

24. Watson JV. Enzyme kinetic studies in cell populations using fluorogenic substrates and flow cytometric techniques. *Cytometry.* 1980;1:143-151.

25. Berglund DL, Taffs RE, Robertson NP. A rapid analytical technique for flow cytometric analysis of cell viability using calcofluor white M2R. *Cytometry.* 1987;8:421-426.

26. Kaplow LS, Dauber H, Lerner E. Assessment of monocyte esterase activity by flow cytophotometry. *J Histochem Cytochem.* 1976;24:363-372.

27. Klein D, Indraccolo S, von Rombs K, et al. Rapid identification of viable retrovirus-transduced cells using the green fluorescent protein as a marker. *Gene Therapy.* 1997;4:1256-60.

28. Lorincz M, Roederer M, Diwu Z, et al. Enzyme-generated intracellular fluorescence for single-cell reporter gene analysis utilizing Escherichia coli beta-glucuronidase. *Cytometry.* 1996;24:321-9.

29. Malin-Berdel J, Valet G. Flow cytometric determination of esterase and phosphatase activities and kinetics in hematopoietic cells with fluorogenic substrates. *Cytometry.* 1980;1:222-228.

30. Sasaki DT, Dumas SE, Engleman EG. Discrimination of viable and non-viable cells using propidium iodide in two color immuno-fluorescence. *Cytometry.* 1987;8:413-420.

31. Riedy MC, Muirhead KA, Jensen CP, et al. Use of a photolabelling technique to identify nonviable cells in fixed homologous or heterologous cell populations. *Cytometry.* 1991;12:133-139.

32. Keeney M, Chin-Yee I, Weir K, et al. Single platform flow cytometric absolute CD34+ cell counts based on the ISHAGE guidelines. *Cytometry.* 1998;34:61-70.

33. Bene MC, Kolopp Sarda MN, El Kaissouni J, et al. Automated cell count in flow cytometry: a valuable tool to assess CD4 absolute levels in peripheral blood. *Am J Clin Path.* 1998;110:321-6.

34. McCoy JP, Carey JL, Krause JR. Quality control in flow cytometry for diagnostic pathology. *Am J Clin Path.* 1990;93(suppl):S27-S37.

35. Nicholson JK. American Society for Histocompatibility and Immunogenetics. Quality control in immunophenotyping: U.S. efforts to establish common methodology and their impact. *Eur J Hist.* 1994;38(suppl)7-12.

36. Centers for Disease Control, MPEP Program.

37. College of American Pathologists, Northfield, IL 60093.

38. Babcock GF, Taylor AF, Hynd BA, et al. Flow cytometric analysis of lymphocyte subset phenotypes comparing normal children and adults. *Diagn Clin Immunol.* 1987;5:175-179.

39. Slade HB, Greenwood JH, Beekman RH, et al. Spurious lymphocyte phenotypes by flow cytometry from mononuclear cells prepared by Ficoll-Hypaque. *Ped Res.* 1987;21:318A.

40. Stelzer GT, Marti G, Hurley A, et al. US-Canadian consensus recommendations on the immunophenotypic analysis of hematologic neoplasia by flow cytometry: standardization and validation of laboratory procedures. *Cytometry.* 1997;30:214-230.

41. McCoy JP, Blumstein L, Donaldson MH, et al. Accuracy and cost-effectiveness of a one-tube, three-color method for obtaining absolute CD4 counts and CD4:CD8 ratios. *Am J Clin Path.* 1994;101:279-282.

42. Keeney M, Gratama JW, Chin-Yee IH, et al. Isotype controls in the analysis of lymphocytes and CD34+ stem and progenitor cells by flow cytometry - time to let go. *Cytometry.* 1998;34:280-283.

43. Sreenan JJ, Tbakhi A, Edinger MG, et al. The use of isotypic control antibodies in the analysis of CD3+ and CD3+, CD4+ lymphocyte subsets by flow cytometry. Are they really necessary? *Arch Path Lab Med.* 1997;121:118-21.

44. Vindelov LL, Christensen IJ, Jensen G, et al. Limits of detection of nuclear DNA abnormalities by flow cytometric DNA analysis. Results obtained by a set of methods for sample storage, staining and internal standardization. *Cytometry.* 1983;3:332-9.

45. Jakobsen A. The use of trout erythrocytes and human lymphocytes for standardization in flow cytometry. *Cytometry.* 1983;4:161-5.

46. Watson JV. Time, a quality-control parameter in flow cytometry. *Cytometry.* 1987;8:646-649.

47. Code of Federal Regulations, volume 29, part 1910. Occupational Health and Safety Administration (OSHA), 1998.

48. Code of Federal Regulations, volume 42, part 405. Clinical Laboratory Improvement Amendments (CLIA), 1998.

49. Stewart CC, Stewart SS, Habbersett RC. Resolving leukocytes using axial light loss. *Cytometry.* 1989;10:426-432.

50. McCoy JP, Chambers WH, Lakomy R, et al. Sorting minor subpopulations of cells: use of fluorescence as the triggering signal. *Cytometry.* 1991;12:268-274.

51. Hedley DW, Shankey VT, Wheeless LL. DNA cytometry consensus conference. *Cytometry.* 1993;14(5):471.

52. Braylan RC, Borowitz MJ, Davis BH, et al. US-Canadian consensus recommendations on the immunophenotypic analysis of hematologic neoplasia by flow cytometry. *Cytometry.* 1997;30:213.

53. Johnsen HE. Toward a worldwide standard for CD34+ enumeration? *J Hematother.* 1997;6:83-84.

54. Purvis N, Stelzer G. Multi-platform, multi-site instrumentation and reagent standardization. *Cytometry.* 1998;33:156-165.

3

Hematopoietic Cell Differentiation: Monoclonal Antibodies and Cluster Designation (CD)-Defined Hematopoietic Cell Antigens

Samuel J. Pirruccello
Patricia Aoun

Monoclonal Antibodies

The central and most powerful advancement in the analysis of cell surface marker expression was the development of highly specific monoclonal antibodies (MoAbs) by Kohler and Milstein in 1975.[1] So far-reaching was this technical discovery that Kohler and Milstein received the Nobel Prize in 1984 in physiology and medicine. As with any significant discovery in biology or biotechnology, the production of monoclonal antibody-secreting hybridomas was dependent on a number of earlier technological achievements, including the development of cell fusion techniques,[2,3] the ability to artificially induce plasma cell tumors in the mouse,[4] and the eventual adaptation of plasmacytomas to tissue culture.[5] Monoclonal antibodies are produced from hybridoma cell lines that secrete a single species of antibody to a unique antigen. The advent of laser cytometry and defined monoclonal antibodies has permitted the precise identification and selection of cells by surface marker expression for both research and clinical analysis. Monoclonal antibodies have many advantages as reagents for flow cytometry. They provide (1) an extremely pure immunological reagent that can be produced from a heterogenous antigenic source, (2) homogeneity in antigen-binding affinity and epitope specificity, (3) the ability to select for antibody activity, affinity, and subclass during antibody production, and (4) the ability to produce unlimited quantities of a well-defined and uniform reagent, which allows reagent standardization and quality control.

Cluster Designation (CD) Nomenclature and Hematopoietic Cell Differentiation

International Workshops on Human Leukocyte Differentiation Antigens

Beginning in the early 1980s, a plethora of reports described the production of lineage-specific monoclonal antibodies and characterized the corresponding antigens recognized. Because of the increasing number of laboratories producing monoclonal antibody reagents, it was realized that a universal mechanism for adequately categorizing the antigens being defined by different monoclonal antibody reagents would be a worthwhile goal. In a manner patterned after the human lymphocyte antigen (HLA) workshops, the first International Workshop on Human Leucocyte Differentiation Antigens was held in 1982 in Paris, France.[6] The workshop was designed so that investigators producing monoclonal antibodies could submit their reagents to the workshop committee; the antibodies would then be distributed in a blinded fashion to all laboratories participating in the workshop. The laboratories were required to perform characterization studies of the monoclonal antibodies and to submit their findings to the workshop for correlation and grouping of similar antibodies. As originally defined, a cluster designation (CD) groups antibodies that all recognize the same antigen. The CD assignment, then, in most cases is synonymous with a specific protein-based gene product. Subscripting is used to identify translational modifications of that gene product or unique epitopes. For some CD assignments (eg, CD15), the epitope represents a glycosyl bond and the antigen recognized will include both glycoproteins and glycolipids.

In the first workshop, categorization studies consisted primarily of defining antigen distribution on various cell types by flow cytometry, fluorescence microscopy, or immunohistology. The primary means for definitive assignment of the antibodies was biochemical characterization of the molecular weight of the antigens by radioimmunoprecipitation coupled with statistical cluster analysis. Approximately 150 antibodies were submitted to the first workshop; 15 clusters were defined. By the sixth workshop, held in 1996 in Kobe, Japan, more than 1000 antibodies had been categorized, and 166 CDs were defined in the areas of T cells, B cells, natural killer (NK) cells, myeloid cells, monocytes, platelets, endothelial cells, and activation and adhesion molecules.[6-11] The "flavor" of each of the 6 workshops was defined by the scientific interests of the participants. This further dictated which antigens would ultimately be defined and thus the seemingly random assignments of CDs for any given cell type (see the Appendix at the end of this chapter).

Despite the focus at the first 2 workshops on defining antigens that were restricted by lineage or stage of differentiation, it was quickly realized that these would represent a small handful of antigens for any given cell type. It became apparent at later workshops that some antigens that were previously thought to be lineage-specific may be expressed on minor subpopulations of other cell types. This emerging information has complicated our picture of phenotypic cell identification, but will ultimately lead to a clearer understanding of functional hematopoietic cell biology. Later workshops have focused on the characterization of antigens that are not lineage-specific or are related to cellular activation or adhesion. In addition, studies aimed at identifying the function of antigens defined by a given CD have received major attention. These functional studies have been aided greatly by advances in molecular biological techniques. The use of nonhuman cell lines transfected with human DNA proved to be a particularly powerful approach to confirming antibody cluster assignments at the fourth through sixth workshops.[9-11]

Hematopoietic Cell Differentiation

Hematopoietic cell differentiation is a complex sequence of events in which pluripotential stem cells first commit to either a lymphoid or myeloid lineage, and then develop into mature cells. Mature and immature hematopoietic cells can be distinguished by flow cytometry based on their expression of cell surface antigens and light scatter characteristics. CD45 (the leukocyte common antigen) is expressed by stem cells early in the development of all hematopoietic cells, and the level of expression changes in a characteristic pattern for each lineage during maturation.[12] The pattern of CD45 expression can be used in combination with side scatter characteristics to identify different hematopoietic lineages, a technique generally referred to as CD45 gating.[13] CD45 expression on stem cells is dim, and increases during lymphoid and monocytic maturation, with the greatest intensity seen on mature lymphocytes and monocytes.[12-15] Granulocytic precursors maintain a relatively constant level of dim CD45 expression during maturation, with mature neutrophils expressing slightly higher levels.[13] Precursors that are committed to an erythroid lineage, however, progressively lose CD45 expression during differentiation and terminate in red blood cells that are CD45-negative. Platelets are also negative for CD45, although cultures of megakaryocytes derived from normal human bone marrow specimens have been shown to be CD45-positive, suggesting that CD45 expression is lost during platelet differentiation as in erythroid differentiation.[16]

The use of CD45 gating in combination with additional lineage-specific markers has become a helpful strategy for distinguishing malignant hematopoietic cells from normal populations. This technique is especially useful in the evaluation of minimal residual disease or in specimens that may contain numerous nonhematopoietic elements.[12-15,17-20] Additional differentiation events for T, B, NK, and myeloid cells are summarized below. Changes in normal expression of other lineage-specific markers that have proven useful for immunophenotyping leukemias and lymphomas by flow cytometry are emphasized.[21-23]

T Lymphocytes

T cells originate from committed lymphoid precursors in the bone marrow that are characterized by HLA-DR and CD34 surface expression and terminal nucleotidyl transferase (TdT) nuclear expression.[24-26] These progenitors migrate to the thymus, where they undergo differentiation and maturation (**Figure 3-1**). The exact sequence and details of this T cell migratory process are not entirely clear. Evidence suggests that a small population of T cell precursors seeds the thymus during embryologic development at approximately 7 to 8 weeks of gestation and provide a thymic stem cell from which most succeeding generations of T cells are derived.[26-30] Whether thymic precursors are still pluripotential stem cells, progenitor cells with potential for development into lymphoid cells of multiple lineages (T, B, NK, or dendritic cells), or have already committed to a T lineage is not yet well understood (as is reviewed in reference 30). A portion of the most immature thymocytes (CD3/CD4/CD8 triple-negative) also express CD38, the stem cell factor receptor c-kit (CD117), and low levels of the T-cell-associated co-stimulatory molecule CD28.[31-35] Although the earliest recognizable T cells (prothymocytes) will express the pan-T-cell antigens CD2 and CD7 as well as cytoplasmic CD3, these markers may not be specific for T lineage. Expression of CD2 and CD7 and cytoplasmic CD3 has also been detected in NK cells,[36] and CD7 expression has been identified in human B-lineage fetal bone marrow cells[37] and in normal human myeloid precursors.[38]

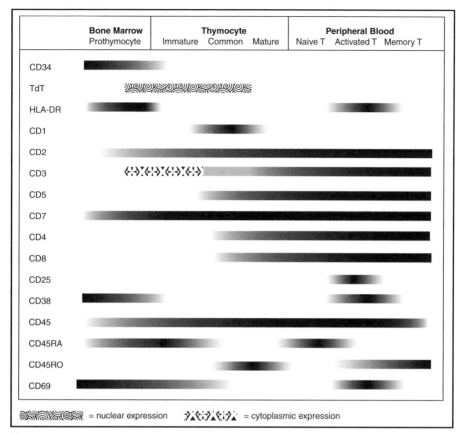

Figure 3-1
T cell differentiation

During thymic maturation the T-cell precursors will undergo genetic rearrangement programs designed to generate functional T-cell receptors which are composed of an alpha- and beta-chain heterodimer in association with the CD3 signaling complex.[28,29] This process is accompanied by the developmental expression of a number of other T cell-associated antigens, including the pan-T cell antigen CD5, the common thymocyte antigen CD1, the helper/inducer cell antigen CD4, the cytotoxic/suppressor cell antigen CD8, and the co-stimulatory antigens CD6, CD27, and CD28.[27,30,35] Expression of CD34 progressively decreases until the earliest stages of low-density T-cell receptor/CD3 expression, when the thymic T cells will co-express CD4 and CD8, and CD34 is absent (ie, the common thymocyte stage).[27,30] Acquisition of common acute lymphoblastic leukemia antigen (CALLA, CD10) expression is another feature of this process. As CD34 expression is down-regulated, CD10 expression transiently increases and then decreases again before surface expression of the T-cell receptor complex begins.[27] The T cells then undergo both negative and positive selection for appropriate context function of the newly expressed T-cell receptors. During this educational process, CD3 surface expression is increased, expression of CD69 and the co-stimulatory markers CD27 and CD28 are progressively enhanced, and either CD4 or CD8 is selected for continued surface expression based on whether the new T-cell receptor is class I or class II major histocompatibility complex antigen (MHC)-restricted.[33] T cells exiting the thymus will therefore be either helper/inducer T cells (CD4+) characterized by MHC class II restriction, or cytotoxic/suppressor T cells (CD8+) characterized by MHC class I restriction. Following CD4 or CD8 selection, CD1 is lost and the CD45 isotype switches from CD45RO to CD45RA.[39] Recent studies also suggest that T cells lose CD69 expression prior to exiting the thymus.[33]

In addition to the predominant population of alpha-beta T-cell receptor-expressing T cells, a minor population of gamma-delta T-cell receptor-expressing T cells are also generated in the thymus. The gamma-delta T cells are the first wave of educated T cells emigrating from the fetal thymus.[40] They represent approximately 3% to 5% of CD3-positive T cells in the peripheral blood and a somewhat higher percentage of resident T cells in the skin, gut, and spleen. In contrast to alpha-beta T cell restriction by classical MHC class I and class II elements, recent attention has focused on the ability of gamma-delta T cells to recognize antigen in the context of the nonclassical MHC class Ib molecules, such as CD1 in humans and Qa and TLa in mice.[41] Furthermore, a high percentage of gamma-delta T cells are capable of recognizing processed heat shock protein antigen,[42] suggesting that these cells may be specialized for recognition of stressed and damaged cells in the skin and gut. The majority of gamma-delta T cells are both CD4- and CD8-negative, while approximately 30% are CD8-positive. Rarely, CD4 is expressed. Specific antibodies are available that can distinguish alpha-beta and gamma-delta T cells based on reactivity with T-cell receptor proteins.

Following thymic selection, less than 1% of the thymus-generated T cells will survive and emigrate into the circulation. These educated T cells may be destined to reside in the epithelium of the gut or skin or comprise the circulatory population, which may later emigrate to lymphoid organs such as the spleen or lymph nodes following antigen stimulation. In the circulation, antigen-naive T cells can be recognized by expression of the CD45RA isoform of CD45.[43] Once T cells undergo antigenic stimulation and activation, differential splicing of the CD45 mRNA results in expression of the CD45RO isoform.[43] These memory T cells represent approximately 30% to 50% of circulating T cells in an adult, with the remainder expressing the naive isoform. Memory T cells gradually increase from 0% at birth to adult levels by the mid- to late teens.[44] Considerable variation in the percentages of these 2 T cell subsets, however, can be demonstrated among individuals. Marked increases in memory T cells have been demonstrated during chronic immune system activation, such as that occurring in patients with autoimmune disorders.[45]

Following antigen stimulation and T cell activation, a number of other antigens may be up-regulated or newly expressed on activated T cells. Some of these antigens represent adhesion molecules that facilitate cell-cell interactions, such as CD44 (HCAM) and CD54 (ICAM-1), or molecules that facilitate cell-substrate interactions, such as the integrins (ie, CD29 or VLA beta-chains and CD49 or VLA alpha-chains). Antigens such as CD27 and CD28 mediate co-stimulatory signals for T-cell activation, proliferation, and cytokine production.[35] Other antigens such as IL-2 receptors (CD25), CD26, CD30, CD40 ligand (CD40L), CD69, and HLA-DR (MHC class II) are also up-regulated during T cell activation. These activation markers may be used clinically to distinguish activation states or detect the presence of transformed T cells, as will be discussed in subsequent chapters.

Natural Killer Lymphocytes

Natural killer (NK) cells represent a phenotypically heterogenous group of non-T, non-B cell lymphocytes characterized by the ability to recognize and kill a wide variety of altered cells, even in the absence of expression of MHC class I or II antigens by the target.[46,47] Recent evidence suggests that NK cells may originate from a common T/NK cell precursor and develop in the bone marrow and/or thymus (as is reviewed in reference 30). The majority of mature and immature NK cells are characterized phenotypically by the expression of the E-rosette receptor CD2 and the pan-T cell antigen CD7. Cytoplasmic expression of CD3 chains in fetal and cord blood NK cells has also been detected.[36,48] Fetal and cord blood NK cells are negative for the NK-associated antigen CD57, but have strong expression of the activation antigen CD69. NK cells, however, do not rearrange T-cell receptor genes, nor do they express the membrane CD3/T cell receptor complex, the pan-T cell antigen CD5, or the helper inducer cell antigen CD4. Mature NK cells are heterogenous for expression of low-density CD8, the Fc gamma receptor CD16 (FcRIII), the neural cell adhesion molecule CD56 (NCAM), and the NK cell-associated antigen CD57. These latter 3 molecules have historically been used to identify NK cells but may also be expressed on subsets of cytotoxic T cells (ie, CD3/T-cell receptor-positive cells). NK cells also typically express CD45, CD45RA, CD38, the lymphocyte function-associated molecules CD11a-c and CD18, and, (upon activation) CD69.[48,49]

Functional features are also important in distinguishing between cytotoxic T cells and NK cells. Most cytotoxic T cells express CD8 and recognize antigens via the MHC class I molecules, resulting in target-specific cell lysis. A minority of cytotoxic T cells expresses CD4 and identifies targets via recognition of MHC class II antigens. In contrast, NK cells can kill target cells in a non-MHC-restricted manner, and activation of the NK cell CD94/NKG and killer inhibitory (CD158 a and b) receptors for MHC class I antigens appears to generally inhibit NK-cell-mediated cell lysis.[50,51]

B Lymphocytes

B cells originate in the bone marrow and therein undergo a primary phase of differentiation. The earliest recognizable B cells express HLA-DR, the pan-B cell antigen CD19, and the stem cell antigen CD34 (**Figure 3-2**).[52-58] A small proportion of marrow CD34-positive B-cell precursors co-express CD19 and the stem cell factor receptor CD117 (c-kit).[59-60] Earlier stages of B cell differentiation that might be characterized by surface HLA-DR and CD34 expression and only cytoplasmic expression of B lineage antigens have been proposed but not conclusively defined. Several other molecules that may be identified as pan-B cell antigens are expressed following B lineage commitment, including CD24, CD72, and CD73. Early B cell precursors will also express cytoplasmic and dim surface CD22, surface CD43, cytoplasmic CD79b, and nuclear TdT. A small proportion of these early precursors may also express dim surface CD20.[58] Acquisition of common acute lymphoblastic leukemia antigen (CALLA, or CD10) expression is another feature of early bone marrow B cell differentiation. This antigen is typically expressed in a window of maturation coinciding with rearrangement and ultimately expression of the immunoglobulin receptor genes. Productive rearrangement of the immunoglobulin heavy chain genes will initially lead to cytoplasmic expression of IgM. The B cells will then rearrange the immunoglobulin light chain genes and, following productive rearrangement, will ultimately express a surface IgM molecule composed of both heavy and light immunoglobulin chains. At this stage, CD34 and Tdt expression is lost. A normal minor subset of immature B cells that express surface IgM and co-express the T cell-associated marker CD5 has also been identified.

Following the acquisition of surface immunoglobulin, bone marrow B cells will lose expression of CD10 and acquire surface expression of CD20, CD22, CD38, CD40, CD74, CDw78, and CD79. This stage of maturation is accompanied by surface expression of IgD and marks the transition from "immature"

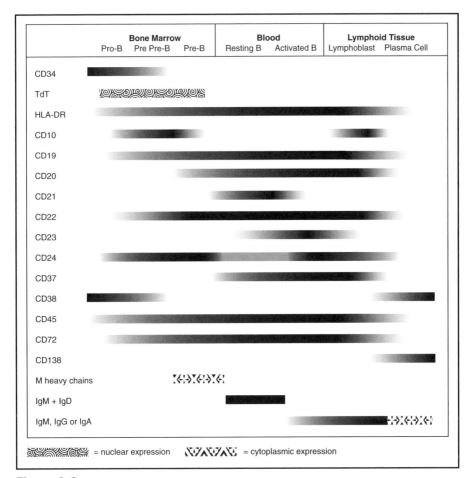

	Bone Marrow			Blood		Lymphoid Tissue	
	Pro-B	Pre Pre-B	Pre-B	Resting B	Activated B	Lymphoblast	Plasma Cell
CD34							
TdT							
HLA-DR							
CD10							
CD19							
CD20							
CD21							
CD22							
CD23							
CD24							
CD37							
CD38							
CD45							
CD72							
CD138							
M heavy chains							
IgM + IgD							
IgM, IgG or IgA							

= nuclear expression   = cytoplasmic expression

Figure 3-2
B cell differentiation

to "mature" B cells. Mature antigen-naive B cells will eventually emigrate to the circulation, at which point they will up-regulate a number of mature B cell antigens, including CD21, CD37, CD39, CD75, CDw76, and low-density CD23. On mature B cells, IgM, IgD, CD79a, and CD79b form the B-cell receptor for antigen binding, whereas CD19, CD21 and CD81 (TAPA-1) form a co-receptor complex that amplifies signals generated by antigen binding to the B-cell receptor.[57,61] Mature B cells also express high levels of bcl-2 protein, which inhibits apoptosis. Resting mature B cells no longer express CD43.

The terminology used for identifying discrete bone marrow stages of B cell differentiation hinges on the immunoglobulin gene rearrangement process and

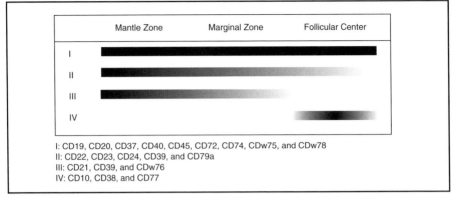

Figure 3-3
Lymph node B cell differentiation

the subsequent cytoplasmic and surface expression of immunoglobulin. In order of maturation, pro-B cells are characterized by germline immunoglobulin genes, pre pre-B cells have rearranged immunoglobulin genes but do not express cytoplasmic IgM, pre-B cells are identified by expression of cytoplasmic IgM in the absence of detectable surface immunoglobulin, and B cells are defined by surface expression of immunoglobulin. This nomenclature has been useful for classifying subtypes of B-lineage acute lymphoblastic leukemia and understanding differentiation of normal B cells. One must keep in mind, however, that hematopoietic differentiation is a dynamic, continuous process, and discrete stages of differentiation are somewhat artificial.

The second stage of B cell differentiation occurs following antigen activation.[61,62] The processes involved include antibody affinity maturation, immunoglobulin class switching, generation of memory B cells, and terminal differentiation of B cells to plasma cells. Once B cells are activated, trafficking to secondary lymphoid tissues occurs, and differentiation ensues in the lymphoid follicles. Characteristic follicular reactivity patterns of the B cell-restricted and associated antibodies have been defined (**Figure 3-3**).[57] The antigens CD19, CD20, CD37, CD40, CD45, CD72, CD74, CDw75, and CDw78 are expressed throughout the lymphoid follicle, including the mantle zone, marginal zone, and follicle center. Antigens CD21, CD39, and CDw76 are expressed on mantle zone and marginal B cells but not on follicular center cells. Antigens CD22, CD23, CD24, and CD79a are expressed strongly on marginal and mantle zone B cells but weakly in follicular center cells. The antigens CD10 and CD77 are restricted to follicular center B cells and are not expressed on mantle or marginal zone B cells. Because of this limited expression pattern,

CD10 (CALLA) has been quite useful in identifying lymphoma cells of follicular origin, as will be discussed in subsequent chapters. The antigen CD38 is weakly expressed in follicle centers.

The events involved in this second differentiation sequence that result in the characteristic reactivity patterns of B-cell antigens are beginning to be clarified.[61-63] Mature, antigen-naive B cells generated in the bone marrow emigrate into the circulation and into lymphoid organs. Upon entering the latter, these naive B cells normally migrate to primary follicles and may return to the peripheral blood if antigen stimulation does not take place. In the peripheral blood, early activation of B cells can be identified by up-regulation of the activation antigens CD23 and CD77. In the paracortical (T-cell) regions of lymphoid organs, activated B cells interact via their surface CD40 receptor with activated helper T cells expressing CD40 ligand (CD40L). Once B cells are activated, they migrate to lymphoid follicles, where further differentiation ensues and the germinal center is formed. In the germinal center, activated B cells acquire expression of CD38 and CD10, and progressively lose surface IgD. These activated and proliferating B cells are morphologically recognizable as centroblasts and occupy the darker region of the germinal center. As centroblasts mature to centrocytes, they lose expression of CD77 and express high levels of the pro-apoptotic receptor protein CD95 (Fas) and low levels of the anti-apoptotic protein bcl-2. Centrocytes do not divide and will undergo apoptosis unless they bind to the B-cell receptor antigen presented by follicular dendritic cells (FDC). Antigen binding results in up-regulation of bcl-2 expression and down-regulation of CD95, with inhibition of apoptosis. Centrocytes selected for survival in this manner move to the light zone of the germinal center, where they become memory B cells. The latter lose CD38 and CD10, and undergo heavy-chain isotype switching from IgM to IgG, IgA, or IgE. Isotype-switching appears to also be mediated by interactions of CD40 on B cells and CD40L on T cells. The remaining resting B cells of the primary follicles form the mantle zone of the secondary follicles and are distinguished by the differential expression of B cell antigens as described above, as well as expression of CD79a, IgM, IgD, and bcl-2.

The terminal differentiation of B cells to plasma cells is the end result of the B cell immunologic response. The molecular events leading to the transformation of B cells to plasma cells are not well understood, but may involve the termination of CD40-CD40L interactions between germinal center B and T cells, in addition to other events.[61,63] The B-cell-to-plasma-cell transformation is accompanied by a loss of the majority of B lineage-restricted and -associated antigens, including HLA-DR, surface immunoglobulin, and CD40. Typically, plasma cells can be demonstrated to express on the cell surface only the activation markers CD38 and CD79a and the high molecular weight isoform of

CD45. Recent studies have also demonstrated that mature plasma cells express syndecan-1 (CD138).[57] The CD138 antigen is a transmembrane proteoglycan which mediates interactions with the extracellular matrix. In human hematopoietic cells, CD138 expression appears to be restricted to normal pre-B cells and mature plasma cells, making it a reliable marker for identification of plasma cells. Terstappen et al[64] demonstrated that a percentage of plasma cells can express CD10 (CALLA) as well as the myeloid lineage antigens CD13 and CD33, explaining earlier reports that described these molecules on multiple myeloma cells. Plasma cells will also express in the cytoplasm complete immunoglobulin molecules of the specific isotype secreted by that cell.

Myeloid Cells

Most myeloid-derived cell types and their precursors express characteristic antigen profiles. The earliest, non-committed hematopoietic stem cell types that have been defined appear to express some combination of CD34, HLA-DR, CD38, and CD117.[31,32,59-60,65-70] Resting (ie, noncycling) stem cells appear to be positive for CD34 but negative for HLA-DR or CD38. Once stem cells are activated to enter the cell cycle, HLA-DR and CD38 expression occurs, regardless of the particular lineage to which the cell commits. As lineage commitment occurs, CD38 expression increases, CD34 expression progressively declines, and lineage-associated antigens appear.[31,70-71] Expression of the stem cell factor receptor CD117 (c-kit) is highest in myeloblasts, erythroblasts, and megakaryocytes, but decreases with differentiation in each of these lineages.[34,59,72-74]

Granulocytes

Myeloblasts are the earliest morphologically recognizable committed stem cells in the neutrophil and monocyte series. Myeloblasts express the stem cell markers CD34 and CD38, HLA-DR, the stem cell factor receptor CD117 (c-kit), and the pan-myeloid antigens CD13 and CD33 (**Figure 3-4**).[31,59-60,67-68,73-78] A recent study has suggested that CD64 (FcRI) is expressed in a subset of CD34- and CD38-positive myeloid precursors in both adult and fetal normal bone marrow, and that it precedes expression of CD15.[69] In the granulocytic line, differentiation to promyelocytes is characterized by loss of CD34 and HLA-DR expression but continued expression of CD13 and CD33 and new expression of CD15. At the early myelocyte stage of differentiation, CD11b surface expression is up-regulated and increases as the cells mature to late myelocytes and metamyelocytes. At the metamyelocyte-to-segmented stage of differentiation, CD16 (FcRIII) expression occurs. Finally, as terminal maturation

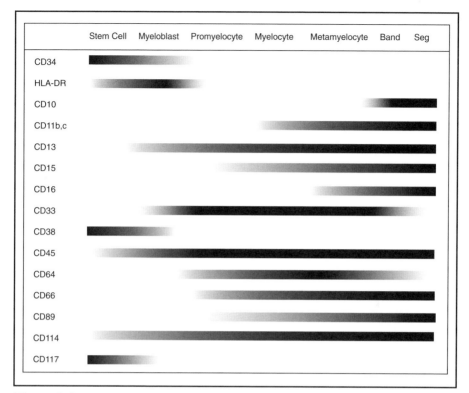

Figure 3-4
Granulocyte differentiation

from bands to mature neutrophils occurs, CD64 is down-regulated and a number of late antigens are expressed, including CD10, CD24, CD32, CD35, and CD65. Mature neutrophils may be weakly positive for CD64 and CD68.

The CD66a,b,c, and d antigens are also expressed at different surface densities early in neutrophil differentiation and are further up-regulated upon neutrophil activation.[78] CD66a is dimly expressed by only promyelocytes and mature neutrophils. CD66b is expressed by promyelocytes and early myelocytes, reaches maximal expression at the late myelocyte and metamyelocyte stages, and then decreases at the band and segmented stages. In contrast, CD66c expression is highest at the promyelocyte stage and progressively declines during maturation as CD11b expression increases. CD66d is expressed only by mature neutrophils. CD66 antigens are up-regulated during activation of mature neutrophils, and may play a signaling role in neutrophil adhesion via interactions with the CD11a/CD18 complex.[78]

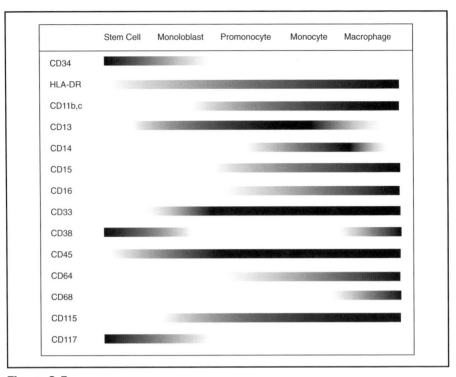

	Stem Cell	Monoloblast	Promonocyte	Monocyte	Macrophage
CD34					
HLA-DR					
CD11b,c					
CD13					
CD14					
CD15					
CD16					
CD33					
CD38					
CD45					
CD64					
CD68					
CD115					
CD117					

Figure 3-5
Monocyte differentiation

Monocytes

Within the monocyte lineage of differentiation, the phenotype of normal monoblasts may be inferred from monoblastic leukemias (**Figure 3-5**).[75,79-81] Recent studies of CD34-positive normal bone marrow cells have been unable to detect CD34-positive precursors that co-express either CD11b or the monocyte-associated antigen CD14, suggesting that the earliest monocyte precursors are most likely morphologically and immunophenotypically indistinguishable from other early myeloid precursors.[31,60,67-70] Monoblastic leukemias are frequently positive for surface expression of tissue factor antigen, which is a very specific marker for monocyte differentiation. As monocytes mature through the promonocyte to mature monocyte stages of differentiation, they lose CD34 and acquire CD11b and CD15. In contrast to the neutrophil differentiation scheme, however, CD11b expression precedes CD15 expression in monocyte maturation, and monocytes retain HLA-DR and CD64 expression. The lipopolysaccharide (endotoxin) receptor CD14 is acquired late in monocytic differentiation and is present on most mature monocytes. Monocytes also express a number of other antigens, including CD4, CD11a,b,c, CD16, CD32 (FcRII), CD35

(CRI), CD64 (FcRI), CD65, CD68, and CD86. Bright CD64 and CD68 are reported to be more monocyte- and macrophage-specific than many of the other monocyte-lineage antigens.[75,78,82] For many of the latter monocyte-associated antigens listed, the timing of antigen acquisition during differentiation has not been well defined. Monocytes will characteristically up-regulate a number of antigens following activation, including CD23, CD25, and CD69.

Megakaryocytes

Megakaryocytes comprise a relatively rare population of normal bone marrow cells. In the megakaryocytic lineage, many of the platelet-associated glycoproteins that were originally defined biochemically were subsequently assigned cluster designations (**Figure 3-6**).[83-85] These include CD9, CD31 (PECAM-1), CD36 (thrombospondin/collagen receptor), CD41a (gpIIb/gpIIIa complex, now generally referred to as CD41/CD61 complex), CD41b (gpIIb only, CD41), CD42a (gpIX), CD42b (gpIb-alpha, which contains a binding site for von Willebrand factor and thrombin), CD42c (gpIb-beta), CD42d (gpV), CD51 (vitronectin receptor alpha-chain), CD61 (gpIIIa), CD62P (GMP-140 P-selectin), CD63 (GP-53), and CD151 (PETA-3). Recent studies have

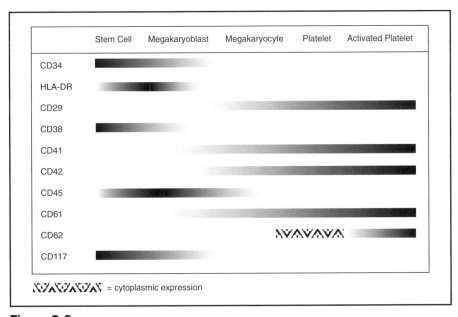

Figure 3-6
Platelet differentiation

reported the presence in normal human bone marrow of minor subsets of CD34-positive cells that also express CD41 or CD61, and possibly represent the earliest megakaryocytic precursors.[67-68,86] Cultures of megakaryocytes derived from normal human bone marrow specimens have been shown to be CD45-positive and CD33- and CD11b-negative.[19] Platelets, however, are negative for CD45. CD117 is expressed by megakaryoblasts and progressively lost during maturation.[34] Other early platelet lineage-associated antigens expressed on megakaryoblasts are CD31 and CD36. As megakaryoblasts mature to early megakaryocytes, the antigens CD42 and CD51 are up-regulated. As the megakaryocytes mature, the VLA antigens characterized by CD29 and CD49b,e,f are expressed. The cytoplasmic expression of CD62P and CD63 also occurs at this stage. These latter 2 antigens, as well as CD117, will ultimately be expressed on the surface of platelets following activation. Expression of CD151 has been demonstrated in both megakaryocytes and platelets.[85] Exact differentiation-related expression sequences for many of the platelet-associated antigens have not been well defined.

Erythrocytes

In the erythrocyte maturation series, several antigens have been used to characterize red cell maturation (**Figure 3-7**).[87] Recent studies of normal human bone marrow indicate that the earliest recognizable erythroid precursors express CD34, CD38, and the transferrin receptor CD71.[31,67-68] CD71 expression precedes glycophorin A expression, shows a sharp increase in antigen den-

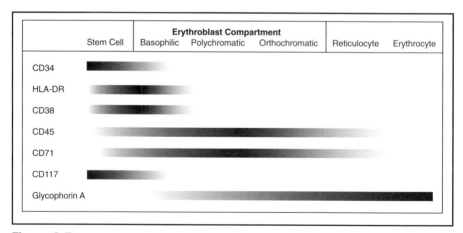

Figure 3-7
Erythrocyte differentiation

sity with erythroid lineage commitment, reaches its highest density levels on early erythroblasts, and then shows an abrupt loss of expression at the late reticulocyte stage of maturation. The stem cell factor receptor CD117 (c-kit) is also expressed on CD34- and CD71-positive erythroblasts.[60,73,74,88] Stimulation of c-kit by stem cell factor in cultures of human bone marrow cells and of an erythropoietin-dependent erythroid progenitor cell line results in growth, suggesting that CD117 plays an important role in erythropoiesis.[70,74,89] In vitro studies have also suggested that this effect may result from the physical association of c-kit with the erythropoietin receptor.[89] As is the case in other myeloid lineages, CD117 levels decrease with erythroid maturation.

Two additional antigens important in characterization of erythropoiesis are the common leukocyte antigen CD45 and the red cell membrane protein glycophorin A. CD45 is expressed maximally on the earliest committed erythroblasts and gradually decreases in density as terminal differentiation to mature erythrocytes occurs. For practical purposes, CD45 density approaches undetectable levels at the reticulocyte stage of differentiation. In the final stages of erythrocyte maturation, glycophorin expression occurs at the erythroblast stage and is maintained through terminal red cell differentiation. Mature, non-nucleated red cells are characteristically glycophorin positive but CD45- and CD71-negative.

Practical Considerations

The major advantage of monoclonal antibodies is reactivity with a single epitope, allowing analysis of the fine antigenic structure of expressed molecules on cells in various stages of differentiation or disease states. The practically unlimited quantities that can be produced permit standardized and quality-controlled reagents for identification of cell markers for investigation or diagnosis. The identification of unique phenotypic markers characteristic of a particular stage of cell differentiation is also useful for structural and functional analysis in more basic investigations.

In using monoclonal antibodies in flow cytometry, several factors should be considered to obtain results that truly reflect fluorescence intensity and the frequency of positive cells. Cell autofluorescence can be estimated by determining the fluorescence of the unstained cells and the background fluorescence of nonspecific binding by including a negative control of a labeled, irrelevant monoclonal antibody. Modulation and internalization of membrane antigens by antibody binding (capping) can be inhibited by staining at low temperatures (eg, 4° C) and including sodium azide 0.05% in the staining buffer.

Immunophenotyping of cells using monoclonal antibodies and flow cytometry is a powerful method for identifying and sorting cells in a mixed population. In order to identify a unique cell population, it may be necessary to use 2 or more different monoclonal antibodies, because some populations of cells can share common epitopes. Thus, one can identify cells by a given repertoire or distribution of expressed epitopes instead of a single and perhaps not exclusive marker.

In flow cytometric applications, one can use either direct or indirect fluorescent techniques.[90] The specific application will determine whether a direct or indirect assay is preferable and what types of secondary fluorescent detector molecules should be used. Indirect staining for antigen detection has the advantage of increased sensitivity because of signal amplification and may be more suitable for detection of antigens expressed at extremely low density. However, because multiple antibody steps are used, background immunofluorescence will also be increased with indirect staining, which may defeat the intended purpose. The authors have found the use of streptavidin-phycoerythrin (PE) or goat anti-mouse-phycoerythrin as secondary conjugates with the appropriate primary antibodies to be the most sensitive technique for the detection of low-density antigens. The use of phycoerythrin has the advantage of both greater quantum efficiency and lower cell autofluorescence than fluorescein isothiocyanate (FITC) at the peak emission wavelengths.[91] For maximum sensitivity it is imperative to have the primary control antibodies matched not only for immunoglobulin class and subclass but also for concentration with the primary test antibody. Concentration-matching of primary control and test antibodies is most critical when one is performing assays for intracellular or nuclear antigens. The use of $F(ab')_2$ secondary conjugates in indirect techniques will also minimize Fc receptor binding and will help maintain low backgrounds for optimal antigen detection.

For most flow cytometric applications of cell surface antigen phenotyping in the clinical laboratory, direct immunofluorescence techniques are desirable. Most commercially available antibodies are offered directly conjugated to fluorescein, phycoerythrin, biotin, or a number of newer dyes and tandem conjugates. The use of directly conjugated antibodies has the advantage of being easily applicable to 2- to 4-parameter analysis as well as whole blood lysis techniques. Multiparameter analysis can increase the amount of information gained from phenotyping by the use of appropriate antibody combinations and will simultaneously decrease labor time by reducing the number of sample tubes required by 50%. Multiparameter analysis, however, requires a greater level of skill in both performance and interpretation of flow results than does single-parameter analysis.

It is imperative that the instrument operators be adept at recognizing discrete populations on 2-parameter histograms, adjusting the sensitivity of fluorescence detectors, and applying color compensation. As in indirect assays, it is important that control antibodies be class-, subclass-, and conjugate-matched to the test antibody combinations when stringent background fluorescence quantitation is required. For multiple antibody combinations in a given phenotyping panel, it may be necessary to run 2 or more negative control tubes to satisfy these requirements. Current use of CD45 gating strategies, however, has obviated the need for multiple background controls in clinical phenotyping.[16-18, 20-22] For surface antigen phenotyping of common antigenic determinants, the authors have not found concentration matching of controls to be as critical as for low-density or intracellular antigens. However, if one is attempting to quantitate extremely low-frequency cells such as CD34$^+$ hematopoietic stem cells in mobilized peripheral blood or bone marrow, concentration matching of negative control and test antibodies is necessary to maximize the signal-to-noise ratio.

For the clinical laboratory interested in phenotypic application of the flow cytometer, a thorough understanding of cell differentiation schemes is crucial. This is especially true when working with acute and chronic leukemias.[92-99] When phenotyping is applied to mature elements in the peripheral blood, a thorough understanding of antigen distribution and potential cell overlap is required to make correct interpretations.[100-102] One must be familiar with the spectrum of possible cell phenotypes in order to be able to identify expansions of major and minor subpopulations of cells. The selection of specific antibodies or antibody combinations by a given laboratory will yield unique profiles based on 2-parameter histograms and the fluorescence intensity of the detected antigens on a given cell type. Familiarity with antibody performance and normal cell patterns and locations on routine histograms is critical to accurate interpretation. One must keep in mind that with hematopoietic malignant cell populations, adherence to accepted phenotypic patterns may be the rule, but malignant cells frequently lose or (less often) gain antigens; one must be prepared to identify these exceptions to the rule.

When designing phenotypic flow cytometry panels to suit a particular purpose, one must choose appropriate monoclonal antibodies that will recognize the antigens of interest. The choice of fluors, whether direct or indirect techniques for antigen detection are applied, and whether lysed or ficolled specimens are used will all influence antibody performance. A great number of manufacturers market monoclonal antibodies, and a considerable price range exists among various manufacturers. Therefore it is important to know your monoclonal antibodies and to develop a clear understanding of the normal phenotypic profiles obtained with antibody combinations chosen for particular clinical applications. Irrespective of price, there may be considerable variability in reactivity for antibodies recognizing the same CD-defined antigenic structure. This is related to variations in affinity, epitope recognition, class of antibody, fluorescent tag, conjugation ratio, and manufacturers' preparation techniques. One should pay attention not only to the percentage of positive cells in the control sample recognized by a given antibody but also to the mean channel of fluorescence for that manufacturer's antibody. The mean channel of fluorescence should be recorded as part of the quality control log for the laboratory. In addition to providing another parameter of day-to-day antibody performance, the mean channel of fluorescence is directly proportional to the antigen density of any given antibody. Most importantly, the ability to identify changes from the expected mean channel of fluorescence for a given antigen may be crucial in correct identification of malignant cell populations.

In conclusion, the development of hybridoma technology and the ability to produce monospecific antibody reagents against defined antigenic structures has had major ramifications in all areas of science and medicine. Furthermore, the standardization of antigen nomenclature by the CD antigen workshops has provided a framework for understanding and applying principles of hematopoietic cell differentiation in clinical practice. The ability of the flow cytometrist to apply these reagents in the clinical setting is dependent on a strong familiarity with normal hematopoietic cell differentiation schemes. In order to consistently identify minor populations of abnormal cells in a mixed cell population, thorough familiarity with the phenotypic profiles expected from normal cells is critical. A clear understanding of what hematopoietic cell differentiation means to flow technology and the potential pitfalls of cytometric analysis will allow the cytometrist to successfully apply flow cytometric analysis to the benefit of clinicians and patients.

References

1. Kohler G, Milstein, C. Continuous cultures of fused cells secreting antibody of predefined specificity. *Nature.* 1975;256:495-497.

2. Okada Y. Analysis of giant polynuclear cell formation caused by HVJ virus from Ehrlich's ascites tumor cells. I. Microscopic observation of giant polynuclear cell formation. *Exp Cell Res.* 1962;26:98-107.

3. Littlefield JW. Selection of hybrids from matings of fibroblasts in vitro and their presumed recombinants. *Science.* 1964;145:709-710.

4. Potter M, Boyce CR. Induction of plasma cell neoplasms in strain BALB/c mice with mineral oil adjuvants. *Nature.* 1962;193:1086-1087.

5. Horibata K, Harris AW. Mouse myelomas and lymphomas in culture. *Exp Cell Res.* 1970;60:61-77.

6. Bernard A, Boumsell L, Dausset J, et al, eds. *Leucocyte Typing.* Berlin: Springer-Verlag; 1984.

7. Renherz EL, Haynes BF, Nadler LM, et al, eds. *Leukocyte Typing II.* New York, NY: Springer-Verlag; 1986.

8. McMichael AJ, ed. *Leukocyte Typing III.* Oxford: Oxford University Press; 1987.

9. Knapp W, Dorken B, Gilks WR, et al, eds. *Leucocyte Typing IV.* Oxford: Oxford University Press; 1990.

10. Schlossman SF, Boumsell L, Gilks W, et al, eds. *Leukocyte Typing V.* New York, NY: Oxford University Press; 1995.

11. Kishimoto T, Kikutani H, von dem Borne A, et al, eds. *Leukocyte Typing VI.* New York, NY: Garland Publishing Inc; 1997.

12. Shah VO, Civin CI, Loken MR. Flow cytometric analysis of human bone marrow. IV. Differential quantitative expression of T-200 common leukocyte antigen during normal hemopoiesis. *J Immunol.* 1998;140:1861-1867.

13. Stelzer GT, Shults KE, Loken MR. CD45 gating for routine flow cytometric analysis of human bone marrow specimens. *Ann NY Acad Sci.* 1993;677:265-280.

14. Borowitz MJ, Guenther KL, Shults KE, et al. Immunophenotyping of acute leukemia by flow cytometric analysis. Use of CD45 and right-angle light scatter to gate on leukemic blasts in three-color analysis. *Am J Clin Pathol.* 1993;100:534-540.

15. Rainer RO, Hodges L, Seltzer GT. CD45 gating correlates with bone marrow differential. *Cytometry.* 1995;22:139-145.

16. Qiao X, Loudovaris M, Unverzagt K, et al. Immunocytochemistry and flow cytometry evaluation of human megakaryocytes in fresh samples and cultures of CD34+ cells. *Cytometry.* 1996;23:250-259.

17. Festin R, Bjorkland A, Totterman TH. Multicolor flow cytometric analysis of the CD45 antigen provides improved lymphoid cell discrimination in bone marrow and tissue biopsies. *J Immunol Methods.* 1994;177:215-224.

18. Sun T, Sangline R, Ryder J, et al. Gating strategy for immunophenotyping of leukemia and lymphoma. *Am J Clin Pathol.* 1997;108:152-157.

19. Lacombe F, Durrieu F, Briais A, et al. Flow cytometry CD45 gating for immunophenotyping of acute myeloid leukemia. *Leukemia.* 1997;11:1878-1886.

20. Wells DA, Sale GE, Shulman HM, et al. Multidimensional flow cytometry of marrow can differentiate leukemic from normal lymphoblasts and myeloblasts after chemotherapy and bone marrow transplantation. *Am J Clin Pathol.* 1998;110:84-94.

21. Bene MC, Castoldi G, Knapp W, et al, for the European Group for the Immunological Characterization of Leukemias (EGIL). Proposals for the immunological classification of acute leukemias. *Leukemia.* 1995;9:1783-1786.

22. Rothe G, Schmitz G, for the Working Group on Flow Cytometry and Image Analysis. Consensus protocol for the flow cytometric immunophenotyping of hematopoietic malignancies. *Leukemia.* 1996;10:877-895.

23. Stewart CC, Behm FG, Carey JL, et al. U.S.-Canadian consensus recommendations on the immunophenotypic analysis of hematologic neoplasia by flow cytometry: Selection of antibody combinations. *Cytometry.* 1997;30:231-235.

24. Kung PC, Goldstein G, Reinherz EL, et al. Monoclonal antibodies defining distinctive human T cell surface antigens. *Science.* 1979;206:347-349.

25. Rieber EP. T-cell section report. In: Knapp W, Dorken B, Gilks WR, et al, eds. *Leucocyte Typing IV.* Oxford: Oxford University Press; 1990:229-383.

26. Terstappen LWMM, Huang S, Picker LJ. Flow cytometric assessment of human T-cell differentiation in thymus and bone marrow. *Blood.* 1992;79:666-677.

27. Van Dongen JJM, Comans-Bitter WM, Wolvers-Tettero WM, et al. Development of human T lymphocytes and their thymus-dependency. *Thymus.* 1990;16:207-234.

28. Campana D. The developmental stages of the human T cell receptors: A review. *Thymus.* 1989;13:3-18.

29. Strominger JL. Developmental biology of T cell receptors. *Science.* 1989;244:943-950.

30. Spits H, Lanier LL, Phillips JH. Development of human T and Natural Killer cells. *Blood.* 1995;85:2654-2670.

31. Terstappen LWMM, Huang S, Safford M, et al. Sequential generations of hematopoietic colonies derived from single nonlineage-committed CD34+ CD38- progenitor cells. *Blood.* 1991;77:1218-1227.

32. deCastro CM, Denning SM, Langdon S, et al. The c-kit proto-oncogene receptor is expressed on a subset of human CD3- CD4- CD8- (triple-negative) thymocytes. *Exp Hematol.* 1994;22:1025-1033.

33. Vanhecke D, Leclerq G, Plum J, et al. Characterization of distinct stages during the differentiation of human CD69+CD3+ thymocytes and identification of thymic emigrants. *J Immunol.* 1995;155:1862-1872.

34. Broudy VC. Stem cell factor and hematopoiesis. *Blood.* 1997;90:1345-1364.

35. Okumura K, ed. T-cell antigens section report. In: Kishimoto T, Kikutani H, von dem Borne A, et al, eds. *Leukocyte Typing VI.* New York, NY: Garland Publishing Inc; 1997:21-123.

36. Lanier LL, Chang C, Spits H, et al. Expression of cytoplasmic CD3z proteins in activated human adult natural killer (NK) cells and CD3z complexes in fetal NK cells. Implications for the relationship of NK and T lymphocytes. *J Immunol.* 1992;149:1876-1880.

37. Grumayer ER, Griesinger F, Hummell DS, et al. Identification of novel B-lineage cells in human fetal bone marrow that coexpress CD7. *Blood.* 1991;77:64-68.

38. Chabannon C, Wood P, Torok-Storb B. Expression of CD7 on normal human myeloid progenitors. *J Immunol.* 1992;149:2110-2113.

39. Fujii Y, Okumura M, Inada K, et al. CD45 isoform expression during T cell development in the thymus. *Eur J Immunol.* 1992;22:1843-1850.

40. Van Dongen JJM, Comans-Bitter WM, Wolvers-Tettero ILM, et al. Development of human T lymphocytes and their thymus-dependency. *Thymus.* 1990;16:207-234.

41. Strominger JL. The gdT cell receptor and class Ib MHC-related proteins: Enigmatic molecules of immune recognition. *Cell.* 1989;57:895-898.

42. Born W, Happ MP, Dallas A, et al. Recognition of heat shock proteins and gdT cell function. *Immunol Today.* 1990;11:40-43.

43. Sanders ME, Makgoba MW, Shaw S. Human naive and memory T cells. *Immunol Today.* 1988;9:195-200.

44. Pirruccello SJ, Collins M, Wilson JE, et al. Age-related changes in naive and memory CD4+ T cells in healthy human children. *Clin Immunol Immunopath.* 1989;52:341-345.

45. Morimoto C, Hafler DA, Weiner HL, et al. Selective loss of the suppressor-inducer T-cell subset in progressive multiple sclerosis. *N Engl J Med.* 1987;316:67-72.

46. Migliorati G, Cannarile L, Herberman RB, et al. Role of interleukin 2 (IL 2) and hemopoietin-1 (H-1) in the generation of mouse natural killer (NK) cells from primitive bone marrow precursors. *J Immunol.* 1987;138:3618-3625.

47. Lanier LL, Phillips JH, Hackett J Jr, et al. Natural killer cells: Definition of a cell type rather than a function. *J Immunol.* 1986;137:2735-2739.

48. Phillips JH, Hori T, Nagler A, et al. Ontogeny of human natural killer (NK) cells: Fetal NK cells mediate cytolytic function and express cytoplasmic CD3ed proteins. *J Exp Med.* 1992;175:1055-1066.

49. Craston R, Koh M, McDermott A, et al. Temporal dynamics of CD69 expression on lymphoid cells. *J Immunol Methods.* 1997;209:37-45.

50. Lanier LL. NK cell receptors. *Ann Rev Immunol.* 1998;16:359-393.

51. Moretta L, ed. Natural killer cell antigens section report. In: Kishimoto T, Kikutani H, von dem Borne A, et al, eds. *Leukocyte Typing VI.* New York, NY: Garland Publishing Inc; 1997:263-329.

52. Loken MR, Shah VO, Dattilio KL, et al. Flow cytometric analysis of human bone marrow. II. Normal B lymphocyte development. *Blood.* 1987;70:1316-1324.

53. Anderson KC, Bates MP, Slaughenhoupt BL, et al. Expression of human B cell-associated antigens on leukemias and lymphomas: A model of human B cell differentiation. *Blood.* 1984;63:1424-1433.

54. Dorken B, Moller P, Pezzutto A, et al. B-cell antigens: Section report. In: Knapp W, Dorken B, Gilks WR, et al, eds. *Leucocyte Typing IV.* Oxford: Oxford University Press; 1990:15-224.

55. Hokland P, Ritz J, Schlossman SF. Orderly expression of B cell antigens during the in vitro differentiation of nonmalignant human pre-B cells. *J Immunol.* 1985;135:1746-1751.

56. Nadler LM, Korsmeyer SJ, Anderson KC. B cell origin of non-T cell acute lymphoblastic leukemia. A model of discrete stages of neoplastic and normal pre-B cell differentiation. *J Clin Invest.* 1984;74:332-340.

57. Mason D, Jones M, eds. B-cell antigens section report. In: Kishimoto T, Kikutani H, von dem Borne A, et al, eds. *Leukocyte Typing VI.* New York, NY: Garland Publishing Inc; 1997:125-262.

58. Ciudad J, Orfao A, Vidriales B, et al. Immunophenotypic analysis of CD19+ precursors in normal human adult bone marrow: implications for minimal residual disease detection. *Haematologica.* 1998;83:1069-1075.

59. Buhring H-J, Ullrich A, Schaudt K, et al. The product of the proto-oncogene c-kit (P145c-kit) is a human bone marrow surface antigen of hemopoietic precursor cells which is expressed on a subset of acute non-lymphoblastic leukemic cells. *Leukemia.* 1991;5:854-860.

60. Strobl H, Takimoto M, Majdic O, et al. Antigenic analysis of human haemopoietic progenitor cells expressing the growth factor receptor c-kit. *Br J Haematol.* 1992;82:287-294.

61. Duchosal MA. B-cell development and differentiation. *Sem Hematol.* 1997;34(suppl 1):2-12.

62. Rudin CM, Thompson CB. B-cell development and maturation. *Sem Oncol.* 1998;25:435-446.

63. Zubler RH. Key differentiation steps in normal B cells and in myeloma cells. *Sem Hematol.* 1997;34(suppl 1):13-22.

64. Terstappen LW, Johnsen S, Segers-Nolten IM, et al. Identification and characterization of plasma cells in normal human bone marrow by high resolution flow cytometry. *Blood.* 1990;76:1739-1747.

65. Civin CI, Banquerigo ML, Strauss LC, et al. Antigenic analysis of hematopoiesis. VI. Flow cytometric characterization of My-10-positive progenitor cells in normal human bone marrow. *Exp Hematol.* 1987;15:10-17.

66. Tassone P, Turco MC, Tuccillo F, et al. CD69 expression on primitive progenitor cells and hematopoietic malignancies. *Tissue Antigens.* 1996;48:65-68.

67. Macedo A, Orfao A, Ciudad J, et al. Phenotypic analysis of CD34 subpopulations in normal human bone marrow and its application for the detection of minimal residual disease. *Leukemia.* 1995;9:1896-1901.

68. Macedo A, Orfao A, Martinez A, et al. Immunophenotype of c-kit cells in normal human bone marrow: implications for the detection of minimal residual disease in AML. *Br J Haematol.* 1995;89:338-341.

69. Olweus J, Lund-Johansen F, Terstappen LWMM. CD64/RcgRI is a granulomonocytic lineage marker on CD34+ hematopoietic progenitor cells. *Blood.* 1995;85:2402-2413.

70. Olweus J, Terstappen LWMM, Thompson PA, et al. Expression and function of receptors for stem cell factor and erythropoietin during lineage commitment of human hematopoietic progenitor cells. *Blood* 1996;88:1594-1607.

71. Terstappen LWMM, Safford M, Unterhalt M, et al. Flow cytometric characterization of acute myelogenous leukemia. IV. Comparison to the differentiation pathway of normal hematopoietic progenitor cells. *Leukemia.* 1992;6:993-1000.

72. Ashman LK, Cambareri AC, To LB, et al. Expression of the YB5.B8 antigen (c-kit proto-oncogene product) in normal human bone marrow. *Blood.* 1991;78:30-37.

73. Broudy VC, Smith FO, Lin N, et al. Blasts from patients with acute myelogenous leukemia express functional receptors for stem cell factor. *Blood.* 1992;80:60-67.

74. Broudy VC, Lin N, Zsebo KM, et al. Isolation and characterization of a monoclonal antibody that recognizes the human c-kit receptor. *Blood.* 1992;79:338-346.

75. Knapp W. Myeloid section report. In: Knapp W, Dorken B, Gilks WR, et al, eds. *Leucocyte Typing IV.* Oxford: Oxford University Press; 1990:747-947.

76. Terstappen LWMM, Safford M, Loken MR. Flow cytometric analysis of human bone marrow. III. Neutrophil maturation. *Leukemia.* 1990;4:657-663.

77. Escribano L, Ocqueteau M, Almeida J, et al. Expression of the c-kit (CD117) molecule in normal and malignant hematopoiesis. *Leukemia and Lymphoma.* 1998;30:459-466.

78. Goyert S, ed. Myeloid antigens section report. In: Kishimoto T, Kikutani H, von dem Borne A, et al, eds. *Leukocyte Typing VI.* New York, NY: Garland Publishing; 1997:927-1108.

79. Griffin JD, Davis R, Nelsen DA, et al. Use of surface marker analysis to predict outcome of adult acute myeloblastic leukemia. *Blood.* 1986;68:1232-1241.

80. Griffin JD. The use of monoclonal antibodies in the characterization of myeloid leukemias. *Hematol Pathol.* 1987;1:81-91.

81. Goyert SM, Ferrero E, Rettig WJ, et al. The CD14 monocyte differentiation antigen maps to a region encoding growth factors and receptors. *Science.* 1988;239:497-500.

82. Krasinskas AM, Wasik MA, Kamoun M, et al. The usefulness of CD64, other monocyte-associated antigens, and CD45 gating in the subclassfication of acute myeloid leukemias with monocytic differentiation. *Am J Clin Pathol.* 1998;110:797-805.

83. Berridge MV, Ralph SJ, Tan, AS. Cell-lineage antigens of the stem cell megakaryocyte-platelet lineage are associated with the platelet glycoprotein complex. *Blood.* 1985;66:76-85.

84. von dem Borne AEGKr, Modderman PW, Admiraal LG, et al. Joint report of the platelet section. In: Knapp W, Dorken B, Gilks WR, et al, eds. *Leukocyte Typing IV.* Oxford: Oxford University Press; 1990:951-1046.

85. de Haas M, von dem Borne A, eds. Platelet antigens section report. In: Kishimoto T, Kikutani H, von dem Borne A, et al, eds. *Leukocyte Typing VI.* New York, NY: Garland Publishing Inc; 1997:623-690.

86. Debili N, Issaad C, Masse J-M, et al. Expression of CD34 and platelet glycoproteins during human megakaryocytic differentiation. *Blood.* 1992;80:3022-3035.

87. Loken MR, Shah VO, Dattilio KL, et al. Flow cytometric analysis of human bone marrow. I. Normal erythroid development. *Blood.* 1987;69:255-263.

88. Papayannopoulou T, Brice M, Broudy VC, et al. Isolation of c-kit receptor-expressing cells from bone marrow, peripheral blood and fetal liver: Functional properties and composite antigenic profile. *Blood.* 1991;78:1403-1412.

89. Wu H, Klingmuller U, Besmer P, et al. Interaction of the erythropoietin and stem-cell-factor receptors. *Nature.* 1995;377:242-246.

90. Jackson AL, Warner NL. Preparation, staining, and analysis by flow cytometry of peripheral blood leukocytes. In: Rose NR, Friedman H, Fahey JL, eds. *Manual of Clinical Laboratory Immunology*. 3rd ed. Washington, DC: American Society for Microbiology; 1986:226-235.

91. Shapiro HM. Parameters and probes. In: Shapiro HM, ed. *Practical Flow Cytometry*. 2nd ed. New York, NY: Alan R. Liss, Inc; 1988:115-198.

92. Griffin JD, Mayer RJ, Weinstein HJ, et al. Surface marker analysis of acute myeloblastic leukemia: Identification of differentiation associated phenotypes. *Blood*. 1983;62:557-563.

93. Knowles DM. Lymphoid cell markers. Their distribution and usefulness in the immunophenotypic analysis of lymphoid neoplasms. *Am J Surg Pathol*. 1985;9(suppl):85-108.

94. Foon KA, Tod RF. Immunologic classification of leukemia and lymphoma. *Blood*. 1986;68:1-31.

95. Knowles DM. The human T cell leukemias: clinical, cytomorphologic, immunophenotypic and genotypic characteristics. *Hum Pathol*. 1986;17:14-33.

96. Coon JS, Landay AL, Weinstein RS. Advances in flow cytometry for diagnostic pathology. *Lab Invest*. 1987;57:453-479.

97. Freedman AS, Nadler LM. Cell surface markers in hematologic malignancies. *Semin Oncol*. 1987;14:193-212.

98. Foucar K, Chen I-M, Crago S. Organization and operation of a flow cytometric immunophenotyping laboratory. In: Santa Cruz DJ, ed. *Seminars in Diagnostic Pathology*. Philadelphia, PA: W.B. Saunders; 1989;6:13-36.

99. Knowles DM. Immunophenotypic and antigen receptor gene rearrangement analysis in T cell neoplasia. *Am J Pathol*. 1989;134:761-785.

100. Babcock GF, Taylor AF, Hynd BA, et al. Flow cytometric analysis of lymphocyte subset phenotypes comparing normal children and adults. *Diag Clin Immunol*. 1987;5:175-179.

101. Remy N, Oberreit M, Thoenes G, et al. Lymphocyte subsets in whole blood and isolated mononuclear leukocytes of healthy infants and children. *Eur J Ped*. 1991;150:230-233.

102. Kotylo PK, Sample RB, Redmond NL, et al. Reference ranges for lymphocyte subsets. *Arch Pathol Lab Med*. 1991;115:181-184.

Appendix to Chapter 3

Cluster Designations for Leukocyte Antigens

Cluster	Specificity	Function	Cell Distribution
CD1a-e*	43-49kDa, HLA class I-like	Antigen-presenting molecule	Thymocyte
CD2	50kDa, LFA-2	T cell activation, CD58 ligand	Thymocyte, T cell, NK cell
CD3	T-cell receptor complex	Antigen recognition	Thymocyte, T cell
CD4	55kDa glycoprotein	HLA class II co-receptor	Stem cell, thymocyte, T cell, monocyte
CD5	67 kDa glycoprotein	CD72 ligand, T cell activation response	Thymocyte, T cell, B cell subset
CD6	105-130 kDa glycoprotein	T cell co-stimulatory molecule	Thymocyte, T cell
CD7	40 kDa glycoprotein	T cell co-stimulatory molecule	Stem cell, thymocyte, T and NK cell
CD8	30/34kDa heterodimer	HLA class I co-receptor	Thymocyte, T cell
CD9	24kDa glycoprotein	Tetraspan-associated molecule	Platelets, pre-B cell, activated T cell
CD10	100kDa, neutral endopeptidase	B cell growth regulation	Pre-B cell, granulocyte
CD11a	180kDa, LFA1, integrin alpha	Intercellular adhesion, co-stimulation	Leukocytes
CD11b	170kDa, mac-1	Adhesion, C3bi receptor	Granulocyte, monocyte, NK cell
CD11c	150kDa, p150	Adhesion, co-stimulation	Monocyte, granulocyte, NK cell
CDw12	120kDa phosphoprotein	Unknown	Monocyte, granulocyte, NK cell
CD13	150kDa, aminopeptidase N	Unknown	Granulocyte and monocyte lineage
CD14	55kDa glycoprotein	Endotoxin ligand, monocyte activation	Monocyte
CD15	Carbohydrate, sialyl Lewis-X	Ligand for E, P, and L selectins	Monocyte, granulocyte
CD16	50-65kDa glycoprotein	Low affinity IgG Fc receptor	NK cell, granulocyte, macrophage

Cluster	Specificity	Function	Cell Distribution
CDw17	120kDa, lactocylceramide	Unknown	Monocyte, granulocyte, platelet
CD18	95kDa, integrin beta-chain	Associated with CD11a,b,c	See CD11a,b,c
CD19	95kDa glycoprotein	B cell maturation and activation	B cell lineage
CD20	33-37kDa phosphoprotein	B cell activation and proliferation	B cell lineage
CD21	110kDa glycoprotein	C3d and EBV receptor	B cell lineage, activated T cells
CD22	130kDa glycoprotein	B cell adhesion and co-stimulation	Mature, resting B cell
CD23	45kDa glycoprotein	IgE Fc receptor	B cell lineage
CD24	35-45kDa glycoprotein	B cell co-stimulation	B cell, monocyte, dendritic cell
CD25	55kDa glycoprotein	IL-2 receptor alpha-chain, T cell activation	B cell lineage, granulocyte
CD26	110kDa gp, dipeptidyl peptidase	T cell co-stimulation	Activated T cell
CD27	55kDa gp, CD70 ligand	Co-stimulatory for T and B activation	Thymocyte, activated T cell, NK cell
CD28	44kDa gp, CD80/86 ligand	T cell co-stimulation	CD45RA+ T cell, B cell subset, NK cell
CD29	130kDa gp, integrin beta-chain	Cell adhesion, VCAM-1 ligand	CD3+ thymocyte, T cell
CD30	105kDa gp, Ki-1/Ber-H2	Negative T cell selection	Leukocytes
CD31	130kDa gp, PECAM-1	Cell adhesion	Activated T, B, and NK cell, monocyte
CD32	42kDa gp, Fc gamma RII	IgG Fc receptor	Platelet, leukocytes
CD33	67kDa gp, sialoadhesin	Unknown	Platelet, leukocytes
CD34	116kDa gp, sialomucin	Cell-cell adhesion	Myeloid and monocyte lineage
CD35	160-285kDa gp, CR1	C3b/C4b receptor	Hematopoietic stem cell
CD36	85kDa gp, GPIIb	Cell adhesion	Red cell, granulocyte, monocyte, B cell
CD37	40-52kDa gp, tetraspan family	B cell signal transduction	Platelet, monocyte, macrophage
CD38	45kDa gp, ADP-ribosyl cyclase	Cell activation and proliferation	Mature B cell
CD39	80kDa gp, ecto-apyrase	Unknown, ATP protection?	Progenitor and activated leukocytes
CD40	48kDa glycoprotein	B cell maturation and isotype switching	Mantle-zone B cell, activated T and NK
			B cell lineage, macrophage, dendritic cell

Cluster	Specificity	Function	Cell Distribution
CD41	120kDa gp, GPIIb	alpha chain of CD41/61, cell adhesion	Platelet and megakaryocyte
CD42a,b,c,d	17–145 kDa multimeric complex	von Willebrand receptor, cell adhesion	Platelet and megakaryocyte
CD43	95–135kDa gp, leukosialin	Anti-adhesion?	Leukocytes
CD44, S, R	85–200kDa glycoprotein	Cell attachment and rolling	Leukocytes
CD45, RA, S, RO	180–220kDa tyrosine phosphatase, LCA	T and B antigen receptor co-stimulatory molecule	Hematopoietic cells, differential isoform expression on T and B cell subsets
CD46	64–68kDa glycoprotein	Inhibits complement activation	Lymphocytes
CD47	50–55kDa glycoprotein	Thrombospondin receptor, adhesion	Hematopoietic cells
CD48	45kDa glycoprotein	Cell adhesion, CD2 ligand	Lymphocyte, monocyte
CD49a–f	125–200kDa gp, VLA 1 alpha-chain	Cell-cell and cell-substrate adhesion	Leukocytes
CD50	115–140kDa gp, ICAM-3	Adhesion, CD11a/CD18 ligand	Leukocytes
CD51	125kDa gp, integrin alpha	Adhesion, vitronectin receptor	Platelet, activated T cell, macrophage
CD52	25–29kDa gp, CAMPATH-1	Unknown	Thymocyte, lymphocyte, monocyte
CD53	32–42kDa gp, tetraspan family	Signal transduction	Leukocytes
CD54	95kda gp, ICAM-1	Adhesion, CD11a,b/CD18 ligand	Activated T, B, and monocyte
CD55	80kDa gp, DAF	Inhibition of complement activation	Leukocytes
CD56	170–225kDa gp, NCAM	Cell-cell adhesion	NK cell, T-cell subset
CD57	110kDa gp, HNK1	Unknown	NK cell, T-cell subset
CD58	40–70kDa gp, LFA-3	Cell adhesion, CD2 ligand	Leukocytes
CD59	19–25kDa gp, MACIF	Inhibits polymerization of C9	Leukocytes, erythrocyte
CDw60	120kDa gp, 9-O-acetyl GD3	T cell co-stimulation	Platelet, T-cell subset
CD61	110kDa gp, GPIIIa	Cell-matrix adhesion	Platelet and megakaryocyte
CD62E, L, P	95–140kDa gp, selectins	Cell homing (L) and rolling (E, P)	Leukocytes, endothelium
CD63	40–55kDa glycoprotein	Unknown	Activated platelet

Cluster	Specificity	Function	Cell Distribution
CD64	72kDa gp, FcgammaRI	High-affinity IgG Fc receptor	Monocyte, macrophage, granulocyte
CD65, s	Poly-N-acetyllactosamine	Unknown	Granulocyte, monocyte
CD66a-f	35-200kDa glycoproteins	Cell adhesion, selectin ligand	Granulocyte lineage
CD68	110kDa gp, sialomucin	Unknown	Leukocytes
CD69	27/33kDa glycoprotein, AIM	Signal transduction, co-stimulation	Activated leukocytes
CD70	29kDa gp, CD27 ligand	T and B cell co-stimulation	Activated T and B cells
CD71	95kDa gp, transferrin receptor	Iron uptake	Proliferating cells
CD72	43kDa gp, CD5 ligand	B cell proliferation and co-stimulation	B cell lineage
CD73	70kDa gp, ecto-5'-nucleotidase	Adenosine availability, co-stimulation	B cell, T-cell subset
CD74	33-41kDa, invariant chain Ii	Intracellular HLA class II sorting	B cell, activated T cell, macrophage
CDw75	Sialoglycan	CD22 ligand, cell-cell adhesion	Mature B cell
CDw76	Sialoglycan	Unknown	Mature B cell
CD77	Gb3, globotriasylceramide	Unknown, CD19 ligand?	Germinal center B cell
CDw78	Unknown	Unknown	Macrophage, B cell
CD79a,b	40/85kDa heterodimer	Antigen receptor signal transduction	B cell lineage
CD80	60kDa gp, B7/BB1	CD28 ligand, T cell co-stimulation	Activated T and B cell
CD81	26kDa gp, TAPA-1 (tetraspan)	B cell signaling complex (CD19/21/81)	Lymphocyte, monocyte
CD82	45-90kDa gp, tetraspan family	Monocyte activation, T cell spreading	Activated leukocytes
CD83	43kDa glycoprotein	Unknown	Dendritic cell
CD84	72-86kDa glycoprotein	Unknown	B cell, platelet, monocyte
CD85	110kDa glycoprotein	T cell activation?	B cell lineage, plasma cell
CD86	80kDa glycoprotein	T cell co-stimulation, CD28 ligand	Dendritic cell, memory B cell
CD87	39-66kDa gp, uPAR	Plasminogen activator receptor	T, NK, monocyte, granulocyte
CD88	43kDa gp, C5a receptor	Granulocyte and monocyte activation	Monocyte, granulocyte

Cluster	Specificity	Function	Cell Distribution
CD89	45-100kDa gp, IgA Fc receptor	Granulocyte and monocyte activation	Granulocyte, monocyte
CD90	25-35kDa gp, Thy-1	Lymphocyte co-stimulation	Stem cell, thymocyte
CD91	600kDa gp, alpha2 mac receptor	Endocytosis of alpha2 macroglobulin	Monocyte, erythrocyte
CDw92	70kDa glycoprotein	Unknown	Monocyte, granulocyte
CD93	120kDa glycoprotein	Unknown	Monocyte, granulocyte
CD94	30-43kDa glycoprotein	NK cell inhibition	NK cell, CD8+ T-cell subset
CD95	45kDa gp, APO-1, Fas	Apoptosis induction	Activated T and B cell
CD96	160kDa glycoprotein	T and NK cell adhesion	Activated T and NK cell
CD97	75-85kDa glycoprotein	Unknown, CD55-associated	Activated T/B, monocyte, granulocyte
CD98	45/80kDa heterodimer	Cell activation, amino acid transporter	Activated leukocytes
CD99, R	32kDa glycoprotein	T cell adhesion	Hematopoietic cells
CD100	150kDa glycoprotein	Lymphocyte co-stimulation	Hematopoietic cells
CD101	120kDa glycoprotein	T cell co-stimulation	Monocyte, granulocyte, activated T cell
CD102	55kDa gp, ICAM-2	Co-stimulatory signal	Resting lymphocyte, monocyte, platelet
CD103	25/150kDa gp, integrin alphaE chain	T cell adhesion in intestinal epithelium	Intestinal lymphocytes
CD104	220kDa gp, integrin beta4 chain	Cell adhesion and migration	Monocyte, pre-T cell
CD105	90kDa gp, TGF-beta R associated	Modulation of TGF-beta R signaling	Endothelial cell, macrophage
CD106	110kDa gp, VCAM-1	Cell adhesion, integrin ligand	Activated endothelial cell
CD107a,b	100-120kDa glycoprotein	Unknown	Activated T and platelet
CDw108	80kDa glycoprotein	Adhesion?	Erythrocyte, lymphocyte
CD109	170kDa glycoprotein	Unknown	Activated T cell, platelet
CD114	130kDa gp, G-CSF receptor	Myeloid cell growth and maturation	Granulocyte lineage, monocyte, platelet
CD115	150kDa gp, CSF-1 receptor	Receptor for M-CSF	Monocyte lineage
CD116	80kDa gp, GM-CSFR alpha-chain	Binding subunit for GM-CSF	Monocyte and granulocyte lineage

Cluster	Specificity	Function	Cell Distribution
CD117	145kDa gp, SCF receptor, C-kit	Stem cell factor binding and signaling	CD34+ stem cells
CDw119	90kDa gp, INF-gamma R alpha-chain	Interferon gamma binding and signaling	Hematopoietic cells
CD120a,b	55/70kDa gp, TNF-R type I/II	Apoptosis, anti-viral responses	Hematopoietic cells
CD121a	75-85kDa gp, IL-1R type I	Interleukin 1 binding and signaling	Hematopoietic cells
CD121b	60-68kDa gp, IL-1R type II	Decoy receptor for interleukin 1	Myeloid cells, B cell, T cell
CD122	70-75kDa gp, IL-2R beta-chain	Component of IL-2R and IL-15R	T cell, B cell, NK cell
CDw123	70kDa gp, IL-3R alpha-chain	Binding subunit for IL-3	Myeloid cells
CD124	140kDa gp, IL-4R	Receptor subunit for IL-4 and IL-13	Hematopoietic cells, T and B cell
CDw125	60kDa gp, IL-5R alpha-chain	Low-affinity receptor for IL-5	Eosinophil, basophil, B cell
CD126	80kDa gp, IL-6R	Binding subunit for IL-6	T cell, monocyte, activated B cell
CD127	65-90kDa gp, IL-7R alpha-chain	Binding subunit for IL-7	Pre-B cell, T cell
CDw128	67-70kDa gp, IL-8R type I	Chemokine receptor for IL-8	Neutrophil, monocyte, NK cell
CD130	130-140kDa gp, cytokine R	Co-receptor for IL-6, IL-11, LIF, CNF	Hematopoietic cells
CDw131	120-140kDa gp, cytokine R	Co-receptor for IL-3, IL-5,GM-CSF	Myeloid lineage, pre-B cell
CD132	65-70kDa gp, cytokine R gamma chain	Signaling of IL-2/7/9/15	Lymphocyte, monocyte, granulocyte
CD134	48-50kDa gp, OX40	T cell co-stimulatory signal	Activated CD4+ T cells
CD135	155kDa gp, FLT3	Growth factor receptor	Pluripotent stem cell, fetal B cell
CDw136	40/150 gp, MSP-R	Growth factor receptor	Macrophage
CDw137	39kDa glycoprotein	Co-stimulator of T cell proliferation	Activated T cell
CD138	65-70kDa gp, syndecan-1	Extracellular matrix adhesion	Pre-B cell, plasma cell
CD139	228kDa glycoprotein	Unknown	B cell, monocyte, granulocyte
CD140a,b	160/180kDa gp, PDGF-R alpha, beta	PDGF binding and signaling	Platelet, monocyte, granulocyte
CD141	105kDa gp, thrombomodulin	Protein C activation	Platelet lineage, monocyte, granulocyte
CD142	45-47kDa gp, tissue factor	Initiation of clotting cascade	Activated monocyte, endothelial cell

Cluster	Specificity	Function	Cell Distribution
CD143	170kDa gp, ACE	Angiotensin and bradykinin cleavage	Endothelial cell
CD144	130kDa gp, cadherin-5	Cell-cell adhesion, contact inhibition	Endothelial cell
CDw145	25/90/110 glycoprotein complex	Unknown	Endothelial cell
CD146	130kDa gp, MCAM	Cell adhesion?	Endothelial cell
CD147	55-65kDa gp, EMMPRIN	Cell adhesion?	Leukocytes, erythrocytes, endothelium
CD148	240-260kDa glycoprotein	Unknown	Granulocyte, monocyte, platelet
CDw149	120kDa glycoprotein	Unknown	Lymphocyte, monocyte
CDw150	75-95kDa gp, SLAM	B cell and dendritic cell co-stimulation	Thymocyte, B cell, dendritic cell
CD151	32kDa glycoprotein	Platelet activation and aggregation	Platelet lineage, endothelium
CD152	33kDa gp, CTLA-4	Negative regulator of T cell activation	Activated T and B cell
CD153	38-40kDa gp, CD30 ligand	CD30 binding and co-stimulation	Activated T cell, macrophage, B cell
CD154	28/30/33kDa gp, CD40 ligand	B cell proliferation and class switching	Activated CD4+ T cell
CD155	80-90kDa gp, PVR	Unknown	Monocyte
CD156	69kDa glycoprotein	Leukocyte extravasation?	Monocyte, granulocyte
CD157	42-50kDa glycoprotein	Pre-B and thymocyte growth signal	Pre-B, pre-T, monocyte, granulocyte
CD158a,b	36,42kDa gp, MHC I receptor	Regulation of NK lysis via MHC I	NK cell, T-cell subset
CD161	40kDa gp, NKR-P1A	Unknown	NK cell, T-cell subset
CD162	120kDa glycoprotein	P-selectin binding/cell rolling	T cell, monocyte, granulocyte
CD163	130kDa glycoprotein	Macrophage differentiation/activation	Macrophage
CD164	80kDa glycoprotein	Precursor cell-stromal cell adhesion	Monocyte, stromal cell
CD165	42kDa glycoprotein	Thymocyte-epithelial cell adhesion	Thymic epithelium, thymocyte, T cell
CD166	100kDa gp, CD6 ligand	Cell adhesion and signaling?	Activated T cell, activated monocyte

4

Software Programs for Flow Cytometry

W. Roy Overton

Perspective

The evolution of computer software programs over the last few decades has been a fascinating process. Early word processing, database, and spreadsheet programs each had a distinctive user interface, which gave each program a unique look and feel. This made each program a challenge to learn, and, once learned, users of a program became very loyal to it because considerable effort and training was required to use a different program. Flow cytometry software was no exception. Early flow cytometry software programs were dramatically different from one another, and switching from one program to another required substantial training.

Today, most software programs have a similar look and feel. Word processing programs from different vendors have become almost identical, as have spreadsheet programs and many other widely used applications. Following the general trend in the software industry, newer cytometry programs are quite similar to one another and use the standard Windows and Macintosh menus and commands, which make them easier to learn and much more user-friendly.

Flow cytometry software programs have 2 main purposes: (1) to acquire data from the cytometer and (2) to analyze these data in a manner useful to most users. Some flow cytometry software is capable of both acquisition and analysis. Increasingly, further handling of flow cytometry data, such as incorporating information into a spreadsheet or a written clinical report, is performed by exporting these data into spreadsheet or word processing programs.

Flow cytometry software will continue to evolve. Programs change not just from year to year, but from month to month. Therefore, the following description of cytometry software is simply a snapshot of how it appears at the moment these words are being written.

Data-Acquisition Software

The design of data-acquisition software is generally dependent on the manufacturer of the cytometer, because most of these programs are also used to operate the cytometer. Therefore, a user of a Becton-Dickinson (B-D) cytometer has little choice but to use CELLQuest software on a Macintosh for data acquisition. Similarly, a user of a Beckman Coulter (BC) cytometer would use Expo software on an IBM-compatible PC, and a user of a Cytomation cytometer would use Summit software on a PC. There are a few exceptions to this general rule, however. The WinFCM program from Applied Cytometry Systems (APS), which runs on a PC with Windows 3.x, 95, or 98, can be used for data acquisition and instrument control on B-D cytometers. Similarly, the Summit program from Cytomation, which runs on a PC with Windows NT, can acquire data from older cytometers made by B-D, BC, Ortho, and Partec. Both Win-FCM and Summit require a hardware interface to acquire data.

All programs with data-acquisition capability, including CELLQuest, Expo, WinFCM, and Summit, can also be used for data analysis on-line or off-line, and hence will be described in greater detail below.

Off-line Analysis Software

Software programs that can be used for routine off-line analysis of flow cytometry data on Macintosh computers include CELLQuest (B-D), FCAP (SoftFlow), FCSPress (Hicks), FlowJo (TreeStar), MacLAS (MSA), and

Table 4-1
Computers and Operating Systems Required for Running Flow Cytometry Software

	MAC OS9	MAC OS8	MAC OS7	PC Win NT	PC Win 98	PC Win 95	PC Win 3.x
CellQuest	✔	✔	✔				
FCAP			✔				
FCSPress	✔	✔	✔				
FlowJo	✔	✔	✔				
MacLAS		✔	✔				
WinList	✔	✔	✔	✔	✔	✔	✔
Summit				✔			
DataMATE				✔	✔	✔	✔
Expo					✔	✔	✔
FCS Express				✔	✔	✔	✔
Flow Explorer				✔	✔	✔	
WinLAS				✔	✔	✔	
WinFCM				✔	✔	✔	✔
WinMDI				✔	✔	✔	✔

WinList (Verity). Software programs for routine off-line analysis on a PC include Summit (Cytomation), DataMATE (ACS), Expo (BC), FCS Express (De Novo), Flow Explorer (Hoebe), WinLAS (MSA), WinList (Verity), WinFCM (ACS), and WinMDI (Trotter). The operating systems that can run these programs are shown in **Table 4-1**. All of these programs can read a Flow Cytometry Standard (FCS) 1.0 or 2.0 data file.[1,2] (Note: A new file standard, FCS 3.0, has recently been proposed.[3]) However, this does not mean that all the programs can read all data files created by the other programs, even though each program is basically using FCS format. This incompatibility is caused by slight deviations from the FCS format during the writing of the data file. It is best to check with the supplier of an analysis program to confirm that it will read data files from other acquisition software.

Displaying Flow Cytometry Data

An essential feature of flow cytometry software is its ability to graphically display cytometry data. Numerous ways of displaying flow cytometry data have

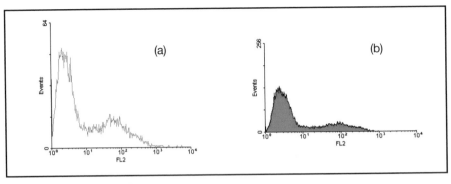

Figures 4-1a and 4-1b
(a) An unshaded, single parameter histogram and (b) a shaded, single parameter histogram from the program WinMDI.

been developed, but not all have become accepted by the cytometry community. The following paragraphs describe the methods that have become most widely used.

A single light scatter or fluorescence parameter is generally displayed as a histogram, as shown in **Figures 4-1a and 4-1b**. These single-parameter histograms, sometimes called univariate histograms, can be unshaded, as in **Figure 4-1a**, or shaded, as in **Figure 4-1b**. In these histograms, the x-axis generally represents the relative intensity of the detected light (in arbitrary units called channel numbers), and the y-axis shows the number of particles, such as cells, associated with each intensity of light. If calibration standards are used, it is possible to convert these arbitrary channel numbers to standardized units. In certain instances it is useful to compare histograms from different data files. An easy way to do that is by overlaying the histograms, as shown in **Figure 4-2**.

Correlated data from 2 parameters, also called bivariate data, can be displayed in several ways. The simplest display of bivariate data is a dot-plot, as shown in **Figure 4-3**. A dot-plot displays the relative light intensity of one parameter on the x-axis and the relative light intensity of the other parameter on the y-axis. The dot-plot does not show the number of particles in each channel, but by examining the distribution of the dots one can identify clusters, which suggest a greater number of particles in those channels. Some programs can overlay 2 dot-plots for comparison, as seen in **Figure 4-4**. When time is collected as a parameter, it is possible to perform kinetics studies, and many programs can produce a dot-plot-type display of kinetics data.

Other methods of displaying bivariate data, such as density plots, contour plots, isometric displays, and isocontours, give a better indication of the number of particles in each channel. A density plot displays 2-parameter data in a way

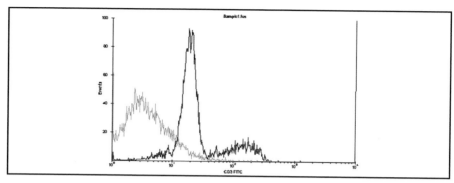

Figure 4-2
Two histograms overlaid using FCS Express.

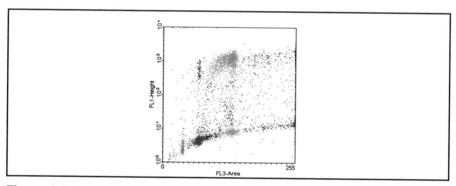

Figure 4-3
A dot-plot display from FCS Explorer.

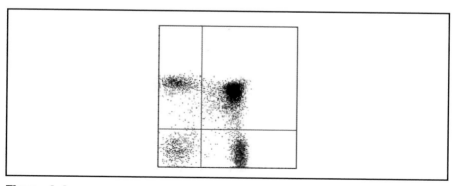

Figure 4-4
Two dot-plots overlaid using FCS Press.

similar to that of a dot-plot, except that colors or shades of gray are used to indicate the number of particles in each location on the density plot, as shown in **Figure 4-5**. Similarly, a contour plot uses concentric polygons to indicate the number of particles in each area of the plot, as shown in **Figure 4-6**. A variation of the contour plot adds dots to the contour to show the distribution of data in areas where the number of cells is below the contour threshold, as seen in **Figure 4-7**. An isometric plot displays 2-parameter data in a pseudo-3-dimensional plot, with the number of cells as the third dimension, as shown in **Figure 4-8**. **Figure 4-9** illustrates a method of data display that combines the contour plot and the isometric display into an isocontour display, which makes the data appear more 3-dimensional than an isometric display or a contour plot. Displaying 3 correlated parameters of flow cytometry data is more challenging, but some programs offer cloud displays like that shown in **Figure 4-10**. **Table 4-2** summarizes which programs offer which types of displays.

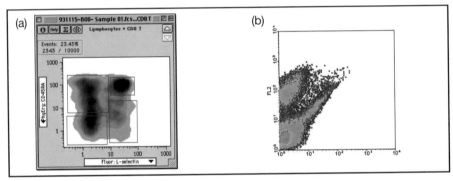

Figure 4-5
(a) A gray density plot from FlowJo and (b) a color density plot from WinMDI

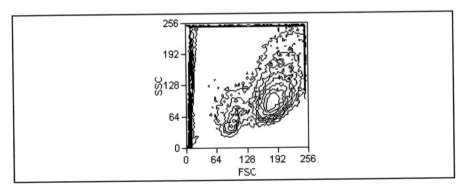

Figure 4-6
A contour plot from Summit.

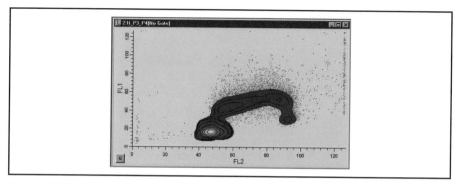

Figure 4-7
Combined contour and dot-plot display from WinList.

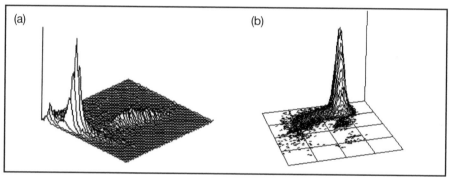

Figure 4-8
Isometric displays from (a) CellQuest and (b) WinMDI.

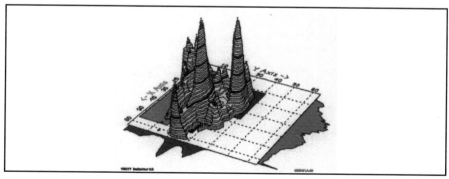

Figure 4-9
An isocontour display from WinList.

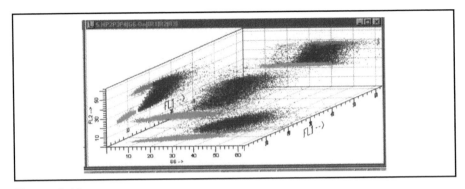

Figure 4-10
A 3-parameter cloud display from WinList.

Analysis of Cytometry Data

A second essential feature of cytometry software is the ability to statistically analyze the distribution of the data. The most basic statistical capability is the ability to compute the percentage of particles and the mean channel of those particles within a given region of the data distribution. All the programs described above can perform these basic computations. For most clinical applications of flow cytometry, those numbers are all that are needed. However, many programs perform other statistical calculations that may be useful for more specialized applications. For example, all of these flow cytometry programs can also compute the coefficient of variation (cv) within a region, which is very important for DNA content analysis. **Table 4-3** summarizes the more extensive statistical tests that can be performed by the various programs.

Software functions have been developed beyond these standard statistical tests to address issues specific to cytometry data. **Table 4-4** summarizes the special methods that are available in software for the analysis of data from flow cytometers.

One cytometry-specific issue is the problem of spectral overlap of fluorochromes. Technicians often deal with this problem by hardware correction, which is called hardware compensation. The main problem with hardware compensation is that the data is then stored compensated, and the compensation can not be altered during later analysis. It is better to store the data uncompensated and use software compensation so that the compensation can be adjusted during analysis. As shown in **Table 4-4**, the programs that can perform software compensation include WinList, FlowJo, and Summit.

Table 4-2
Display Capabilities Available in Cytometry Programs

	Histogram	Dot-plot	Density	Contour	Isometric	Isocontour	Cloud	Kinetics	Overlay
CellQuest	✔	✔	✔	✔	✔			✔	Histogram
FCAP	✔	✔	✔	✔	✔	✔	✔	✔	Histogram Dot-plot
FCSPress	✔	✔	✔					✔	Dot-plot
FlowJo	✔	✔	✔	✔				✔	Histogram
MacLAS	✔	✔		✔		✔			
WinList	✔	✔	✔	✔	✔	✔	✔	✔	Histogram
Summit	✔	✔	✔	✔				✔	Histogram
DataMATE	✔	✔	✔	✔	✔	✔		✔	Histogram
Expo	✔	✔		✔	✔	✔		✔	Histogram
FCS Express	✔	✔	✔	✔					Histogram Dot-plot
Flow Explorer	✔	✔	✔	✔					
WinLAS	✔	✔	✔	✔		✔			
WinFCM	✔	✔	✔	✔	✔	✔		✔	Histogram
WinMDI	✔	✔	✔	✔	✔		✔	✔	Histogram

Table 4-3
Statistical Analysis Available in Cytometry Programs in Addition to Percentile and Mean

	Median	Mode	Full-peak CV	Half-peak CV	SD	Correlation coefficient
CellQuest	✔	✔	✔		✔	
FCAP	✔	✔	✔	✔	✔	✔
FCSPress	✔	✔	✔		✔	
FlowJo	✔	✔	✔	✔		
MacLAS			✔			
WinList	✔	✔	✔		✔	✔
Summit	✔	✔	✔	✔	✔	✔
DataMATE	✔	✔	✔	✔		
Expo	✔	✔	✔	✔	✔	✔
FCS Express	✔	✔	✔			
Flow Explorer			✔			
WinLAS			✔			
WinFCM	✔	✔	✔	✔		
WinMDI			✔			

Table 4-4
Special Features Available in Cytometry Programs

	Software compensation	Ratio	K-S test	Histogram subtract	Overton subtract	Absolute count	Cell cycle	Quant. fluor.	Report
CELLQuest			✔	✔					
FCAP						✔			✔
FCSPress		✔							
FlowJo	✔	✔					✔	✔	✔
MacLAS						✔	✔		✔
WinList	✔	✔	✔	✔	✔		✔	✔	✔
Summit	✔	✔		✔	✔				
DataMATE		✔						✔	✔
Expo		✔						✔	✔
FCS Express		✔		✔	✔	✔		✔	✔
Flow Explorer									
WinLAS						✔	✔		✔
WinFCM								✔	✔
WinMDI									
ModFit							✔		
MultiCycle									
WinReport								✔	✔
QuantiCALC								✔	

A second issue specific to the analysis of flow cytometry data is the examination of 2 fluorescence signals from the same cell in relation to each other. An example of this is the detection of calcium fluxes within a cell. Detection of calcium levels is difficult using only one fluorochrome. This problem has been addressed by using 2 fluorochromes that have inverse responses to intracellular calcium concentration.[4] The ratio of these 2 fluorochromes gives a clearer indication of the calcium level within each cell. Programs that can calculate this ratio are shown in **Table 4-4**.

Yet another key issue in the analysis of some clinical flow cytometry data concerns the distribution of immunoglobulin light chains. The presence of subtle, abnormal distributions of surface immunoglobulin light chains on human B cells has been used for early detection of leukemic B cells. This method, usually called clonal excess,[5,6] uses the Kolmogorov-Smirnov (K-S)[7] test to detect clones of leukemic B cells that perturb the usual distribution of surface Ig. CELLQuest and WinList can perform the K-S test.

Some flow cytometry assays are performed to obtain one value and one value only: the percentage of cells positive for the expression of a given marker. This is true in the clinical laboratory and in the research laboratory. However, this percentage is generally obtained by subjective placement of analysis regions, possibly resulting in erroneous data, especially when the positive population is not well resolved from the negatives (ie, when the positive population displays only "dim" fluorescence). To make this analysis more objective and less prone to error, a method of subtracting a negative control histogram from the test histogram was developed called histogram subtraction.[8,9] This method produces a more objective percentage-positive analysis, but may still overestimate the percentage due to small, random variances in the channel-to-channel distribution of the data. A still more accurate percentage can be obtained by a modification of this method called cumulative or Overton subtraction.[10,11] Overton subtraction performs histogram subtraction, but then eliminates false positives by subtracting negative differences that are brighter than positive differences. Histogram subtraction is found in CELLQuest, and both histogram subtraction and Overton subtraction are found in FCS Express, WinList, and Summit.

In the clinical laboratory, determining the percentage of positive cells may not always be the only desired result from a particular assay. With some assays, such as CD4 enumeration, the absolute count of positive cells per volume of blood is required, usually together with the percentage of positive cells. Several programs listed in **Table 4-4** provide for the calculation of absolute cell counts.

Staining intensity may vary from marker to marker or cell to cell, resulting in more difficult data analysis. As mentioned above, one method of handling this problem is histogram subtraction. Another method is reporting relative fluorescence intensity based on channel numbers of the fluorescence signal. A better approach to analyzing and reporting staining intensity is to quantitate the fluorescence staining through the use of calibrated bead standards.[12] Several programs listed in **Table 4-4** have the ability to convert data to calibrated fluorescence units. QuantiCALC (Verity) is a more automated program written specifically for this kind of quantitative cytometry, and is available in both Macintosh and PC formats.

One of the most useful of these specialized flow cytometry analysis methods is DNA content analysis. As discussed elsewhere in this book, cellular DNA can be stained with any one of a number of nucleic acid-specific fluorescent dyes. The resulting fluorescence is directly proportional to the amount of DNA contained in the cell. Various algorithms may be used to model the possible distributions of DNA content within a population of cells. This enables a pathologist to estimate the percentage of cells that are in the G_0/G_1 phase, S phase, or G_2/M phase of the cell cycle and to determine the percentage of any aneuploid cells while also estimating their cell cycle distribution. Estimation of cell cycle distribution may be performed using either parametric or nonparametric approaches. Cell cycle analysis capability can be found in the WinList and FlowJo programs. There are also 2 programs that were created exclusively for this purpose: ModFit (Verity) and MultiCycle (Phoenix). Both Modfit and MultiCycle are available for the PC and for Mac, although the Macintosh version of MultiCycle is called MacCycle.

In the clinical laboratory, the final product of an assay is generally a report to the ordering physician in either written or electronic form. **Table 4-4** illustrates which programs can generate reports. Some of these have a fairly rigid format for report forms, while others have more flexibility, with options such as the inclusion of histograms. WinReport (Phoenix) is a program that generates a report from cell cycle analysis results produced by MultiCycle. Quite often, data are exported into other programs from which reports can be generated, as will be discussed later.

Automation

One of the greatest costs in the clinical laboratory is that of the highly trained personnel necessary for high-complexity testing. To keep costs as low as possible, and to keep highly trained personnel optimally productive, many of the more repetitive, mundane tasks related to flow cytometry can be automated. One such task is the actual loading of test tubes into the sample intake mechanism of the flow cytometer, followed by collection of the raw data. Because automation of these tasks requires both dedicated hardware custom-designed for a particular model of cytometer and specific software which can interface with both the cytometer and the automatic loading device, this component of automation is, in most cases, utterly dependent on the manufacturer of the cytometer.

Creating the layout of histograms, dot-plots, and text every time a program is run can be quite time-consuming. To address this issue, most programs have been designed to save these layouts, or protocols, as files for repeated use. In some instances, where the software is used to acquire data, these stored protocols may include instrument settings. The capability to store protocols or layouts is found in numerous software programs, including CELLQuest, Data-MATE, Expo, FCAP, FCS Express, FlowJo, MacLAS, Summit, WinFCM, WinLAS, and WinList.

Another time-saving feature available in flow cytometry software is automatic data analysis and printing. Once a layout is created, this feature will sequence through a group of data files, displaying the data, producing the statistical analysis, and printing or exporting the results as appropriate. The programs that have this feature include CELLQuest, DataMATE, Expo, FCAP, FCS Express, FlowJo, MacLAS, WinFCM, WinLAS, and WinList. Taking automation a step further, DataMATE, FCAP, FCS Express, FlowJo, MacLAS, WinFCM, WinLAS, and WinList also have the ability to batch-process data through macros or a programmable batching system. The batch-processing feature gives the user more flexibility in automating the analysis of the data by permitting the user to define the sequence of analytical steps that the software follows.

The creation and adjustment of gating and analysis regions for each specimen can also dramatically slow down the analysis of cytometry data, particularly when there are many data files to be analyzed. Automated gate adjustment addresses this problem and is a feature found in FlowJo, FCAP, and Attractors (B-D), which is a program written for Macintosh for batch analysis of multiple samples. A more powerful solution to this problem is the use of cluster analysis to identify populations of particles or cells that have similar light scatter and fluorescence characteristics.[13] Cluster analysis is a feature of WinLAS and MacLAS.

Exporting Results

All the programs described here can copy graphics into the computer's memory, commonly called the *clipboard*. The images can then be pasted into other applications, such as word processing programs, spreadsheets, and databases. Most flow cytometry programs can also export statistical results for use by other programs such as spreadsheets and databases. Data are often exported to programs such as Microsoft Excel that can be used to generate both clinical reports and ongoing logs of patient results.

Software Suppliers

Applied Cytometry Systems (DataMate, WinFCM)
Phone: +44 (0)1909 566982
Web site (as of August 2001): http://www.appliedcytometry.com

Beckman Coulter, Inc. (Expo)
4300 N. Harbor Boulevard, P.O. Box 3100
Fullerton, CA 92834-3100
Phone: (800) 233-4685 or (714) 871-4848
Fax: (714) 773-8283
Web site (as of August 2001):
    http://www.beckman.com/coulter/Cytometry/expo/default.asp

BioSciences (CellQuest, Attractors)
2350 Qume Drive
San Jose, CA 95131-1807
Phone: (800) 223-8226
Fax: (408) 954-2347
Web site (as of August 2001): http://www.bdfacs.com

Cytomation, Inc. (Summit)
4850 Innovation Drive
Fort Collins, CO 80525
Phone: (800) 822-9902 or (970) 226-2200
Fax: (970) 226-0107
Web site (not verified): http://www.cytomation.com
e-mail: info@cytomation.com

DeNovo Software (FCS Express)
(available from Phoenix Flow Systems)
Web site (not verified): http://www.denovosoftware.com

Ray Hicks (FCSPress)
134 High St.
Harston, Cambridge CB25QD, UK
Phone: +44-0797-4538647
Fax: +44-0870-8595
Web site (as of August 2001): http://www.FCSPress.com
e-mail: Sales@FCSPress.com

R. Hoebe (Flow Explorer)
e-mail: R.Hoebe@amc.uva.nl

Medical Science Associates (WinLAS,MacLAS)
6565 Penn Avenue
Pittsburgh, PA 15206
Phone: (412) 362-9840
Fax: (412) 362-0536
Web site (as of August 2001): http://www.msa.com
e-mail: info@msa.com

Phoenix Flow Systems (MultiCycle, MacCycle, FCS Express)
11575 Sorrento Valley Rd. #208
San Diego, CA 92121
Phone: (800) 886-FLOW or (619) 453-5095
Fax: (619) 259-5268
Web site (as of August 2001): http://www.phnxflow.com
e-mail: info@phnxflow.com

Soft Flow, Inc. (FCAP)
12616 James Road
Minnetonka, MN 55343
Phone: (800) 532-2231
Fax: (612) 945-9913
Web site (as of August 2001): http://www.visi.com/~soft-flow/
e-mail: softflow@wavefront.com

   or

Soft Flow Hungary, Ltd.
Debrecen, Wesseljnyi, 17, Hungary, H4024
Phone: (36) 52-346599 Fax: (36) 52-346599
e-mail: SoftFlow@mail.matav.hu

Tree Star, Inc. (FlowJo)
Phone: (800) 366-6045
Web site (as of August 2001): http://www.treestar.com/flowjo
e-mail: flowjo@treestar.com

Joseph Trotter (WinMDI)
The Scripps Research Institute
10550 North Torrey Pines Road
La Jolla, CA 92037
Web site (as of August 2001): http://facs.scripps.edu/software.html
e-mail: trotter@scripps.edu

Verity Software House, Inc. (WinList, ModFit, QuantiCALC)
45A Augusta Road, P.O. Box 247
Topsham, ME 04086
Phone: (207) 729-6767
Fax: (207) 729-5443
Web site (as of August 2001): http://www.vsh.com
e-mail: verity@vsh.com

References

1. Dean PN, Bagwell CB, Lindmo T, et al. Introduction to flow cytometry data file standard. *Cytometry*. 1990;11:321-2.

2. Anonymous, Data File Standards Committee of the Society for Analytical Cytology. Data file standard for flow cytometry. *Cytometry*. 1990;11:323-32.

3. Seamer LC, Bagwell CB, Barden L, et al. Proposed new data file standard for flow cytometry, version FCS 3.0. *Cytometry*. 1997;28:118-22.

4. Novak EJ, Rabinovitch PS. Improved sensitivity in flow cytometric intracellular ionized calcium measurement using fluo-3/Fura Red fluorescence ratios. *Cytometry*. 1994;17:135-41.

5. Ligler FS, Smith RG, Kettman JR, et al. Detection of tumor cells in the peripheral blood of nonleukemic patients with B-cell lymphoma: analysis of "clonal excess". *Blood*. 1980;55:792-801.

6. Nakano M, Kuge S, Kuwabara S, et al. The basic study on 6-8 imaging by *-curve for the detection of a monoclonal B-cell population in the peripheral blood. *Blood*. 1988;2:1461-1466.

7. Young IT. Proof without prejudice: use of the Kolmogorov-Smirnov test for the analysis of histograms from flow systems and other sources. *J Histochem Cytochem*. 1977;25:935-941.

8. Scher I, Berning AK, Kessler S, et al. Development of B lymphocytes in the mouse; studies of frequency and distribution of surface IgM and IgD in normal and immune-defective CBA/N F1 mice. *J Immunol*. 1980;125:1686-1693.

9. Schipper J, Tilders FJH, Wassink RG, et al. Microfluorometric scanning of sympathetic nerve fibers; quantification of neuronal and extraneuronal fluorescence with the aid of histogram analysis. *J Histochem Cytochem*. 1980;28:124-132.

10. Overton WR. Modified histogram subtraction technique for analysis of flow cytometry data. *Cytometry*. 1988;9:619-626.

11. Overton WR. Reply to Dr. Habermehl. *Cytometry*. 1989;10:494.

12. Stelzer GT, Marti G, Hurley A, et al. Consensus Conference on the Flow Cytometric Analysis of Leukemia and Lymphoma: Report of the Committee on the Standardization and Validation of Laboratory Procedures. *Cytometry*. 1997;30:214-230.

13. Murphy RF. Automated identification of subpopulations in flow cytometric list mode data using cluster analysis. *Cytometry*. 1985;6:302-309.

5

Quality Control and Quality Assurance in Immunophenotyping

Charles William Caldwell

Introduction

The development and natural evolution of new technologies usually begins in research laboratories, but as translational research and medical usefulness are documented, there is a general movement to clinical diagnostic laboratories and ultimately commercialization. As laboratory scientists, we all strive to maintain the highest moral and ethical standards in applying any new technology to diagnosis and patient management. It is in this spirit that laboratorians carefully approach issues of appropriate quality control (QC) and quality assurance (QA) of laboratory procedures such as flow cytometry.

Immunophenotyping (IP) by flow cytometry arose in research laboratories but has found a permanent place in clinical diagnostic laboratories. In general, IP employs the flow cytometer and monoclonal antibodies (MoAbs) to determine biological attributes of cells that help describe states of health and disease. The typical specimen for IP by flow cytometry comprises viable cells capable of being placed into a single cell suspension. Thus, certain limitations on sample handling make flow cytometry somewhat unique as a clinical laboratory procedure; for example, the analytes are usually cells that must be analyzed in a viable state and there are no cellular standards, which differs from clinical chemistry and standard analytes. Nevertheless, many tools of QC, such as longitudinal data representation and cumulative statistics, are still useful. Some of the elements that need to be controlled include instrumentation, specimens, reagents, and preparation/analysis protocols.

The processes of QC and QA present evolving opportunities to improve and standardize patient care. QC is a set of procedures within the laboratory that ensure a valid and reproducible result, whereas QA is the sum of all laboratory functions and procedures that lead to a final correct result. They are dynamic and ongoing processes. Policies and procedures for acceptance of results and remedying problems need to be in place, and there should be a formal review schedule with resultant feedback on all action items. Several national organizations have endeavored to provide guidance in these areas. Although there are divergent opinions on some points, the common goal is improvement in quality. In general, laboratories should apply good laboratory practices, applicable current guidelines, and other standards as available. As specified in the Clinical Laboratory Improvement Amendments of 1988 (CLIA),[1] the laboratory must establish and follow written quality control procedures for monitoring and evaluating the quality of the analytical testing process of each method to ensure the accuracy and reliability of patient test results and reports. Each laboratory must also establish and follow written policies and procedures for a comprehensive QA program designed to monitor and evaluate the ongoing and overall quality of the total testing process. The program should be structured to facilitate recognition of both immediate and potential problems. For any measured or monitored parameter, the laboratory should set and document acceptable ranges of values and appropriate corrective actions to be taken when values exceed these ranges.

Instrument Performance Controls

Issues related to QC/QA of instrument performance differ considerably, dependent in part on whether a laboratory is using a cell sorter or an analytical flow cytometer. Some instruments lend themselves to manual control over a variety of settings and parameters, while others are more self-contained and may not allow certain functions to be adjusted by the operator without assistance from a technical service representative. This chapter will not address specific types of instruments, but rather will focus on the generic issues of measuring

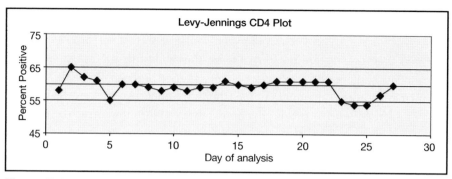

Figure 5-1

An example of a Levy-Jennings plot of CD4 values from normal peripheral blood controls. The line at 60% represents the historical mean, the lines at 55 and 65 represent +/-1 standard deviation, and the actual data points are the daily mean values.

and documenting processes and procedures that should be implemented, as appropriate, in any clinical flow cytometry laboratory.

Reproducible flow cytometric data is dependent on consistent electronic, optical, and fluidic system functions from the instrument. Without such stability, measurements between runs and between days may not be comparable, and some results may not be interpretable. In order to use certain attributes such as fluorescence intensities or approximate light scatter patterns, the linearity and stability of the response over a dynamic range of values is important. Daily monitoring and documentation of selected parameters using standard (or stable) calibrators and controls is necessary to ensure consistency.

Longitudinal monitoring of trends in various parameters, both instrument and noninstrument, are best detected using graphic displays such as Levy-Jennings graphs, whereby the historic mean and standard deviation (SD) are plotted on a daily basis.[2] This method is very useful for detecting drifts in the measured parameter, as well as acute changes. The use of an SD index (SDI) may improve daily analyses of these parameters.[3] The SDI is computed from the difference in the historic mean and the daily value, divided by 1 SD (**Figure 5-1**).

The fluidic component of an instrument is responsible for delivering the cell suspension to the excitation and detection area of the flow cell. When partial or complete obstructions occur in the system, they have the effect of slowing, or even halting, acquisition of events. Therefore, a routine maintenance program aimed at regular cleaning of the fluidic system will help ensure trouble-free operation. Documentation of such maintenance schedules is an important part of a high-quality laboratory operation.

Optical alignment of the light source, sample stream, and detector system is important for reliable collection of event signals. Some of the recent clinically oriented flow cytometers no longer leave this ability to the operator. These instruments contain systems that are factory aligned and usually stable, whereas others may require realignment in the laboratory on a regular basis. Stable fluorescent microspheres or beads are commonly used for monitoring or adjusting the optical alignment of light scatter and fluorescence signals.

Daily monitoring of the mean channel number, coefficient of variation (CV), and instrument settings (gains, photomultiplier tube [PMT] settings, etc) for each measured parameter (fluorescence intensity [FI] or light scatter) under standard instrument settings will allow meaningful graphical representation on Levy-Jennings plots. Acceptable ranges for each parameter should be established and documented, as should any corrective action necessary when these limits are exceeded.

Fluorescence

Fluorescence sensitivity and standardization are necessary to ensure resolution of dimly fluorescent cells and to ensure reproducibility. Sensitivity is typically examined as the signal-noise ratio, or the minimum number of fluorochrome molecules detectable under laboratory conditions. While in the past this determination was very cumbersome and varied with experimental conditions, there are now suppliers of sets of fluorescent microspheres with predetermined numbers of molecules of equivalent soluble fluorochromes, or MESF.[4] The use of these microspheres now allows laboratories to investigate both the linearity and the minimum MESF detectable on a given instrument.

Standardization involves the use of microspheres with stable fluorescence to monitor system performance each day. These reference particles can be placed into a specific region of the fluorescence histogram by adjustments to the PMT high-voltage settings, or gains, if necessary. The mean FI, PMT settings, and CVs may then be recorded on Levy-Jennings plots for further analysis. The goals are to establish reproducible conditions under which the signal-noise ratio is maximized for optimal sensitivity.

In order to employ any quantitative method of measuring FI, it is also useful to ascertain that the response of the detection system is linear over the range of FI measurements expected from clinical specimens. This may be accomplished through a simple method using a set of 4 or 5 fluorescent microspheres of differing FI. These particles should be examined at one PMT voltage setting

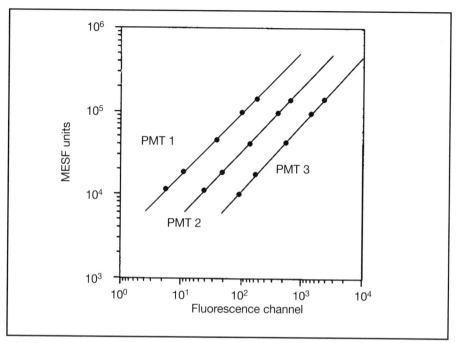

Figure 5-2

Fluorescence measurements from 1 set of 5 fluorescent beads. The measurements were made at 3 different photomultiplier settings.

and the mean position of each peak recorded. The same particles should then be reexamined at additional PMT voltage settings and their positions recorded. Lastly, using log-log graphing paper, plot the fluorescence channel position on the x-axis and the number of MESF units on the y-axis for each set of particles. If the slopes of the lines for each set of particles are roughly parallel, then the response is near linear, and acceptable (**Figure 5-2**). A more detailed method is also explained in the papers of Stelzer et al[4] and others.[5,6]

Fluorescence compensation involves correcting a detection system for spectral overlap that occurs when using certain combinations of fluorochromes that have overlapping fluorescence emission spectra, such as fluorescein isothiocyanate (FITC) and phycoerythrin (PE). The goal is to reliably separate single-stained cells from dual-stained cells. This is necessary to avoid artifactual signals that might erroneously be interpreted as positive or negative signals. Typically, the instrument method is one of electronic subtraction of overlapping signals, or compensation, and is detailed by each manufacturer. The amount of compensation may vary with changes in the electronic gains, PMT settings, or optical filters used. If FI is standardized each day by setting fluorescent particles or stained cells to particular positions on the fluorescence histogram, then fluorescence compensation may not need to be changed unless optical filters are changed.

Color compensation of 2-, 3-, or 4-color systems is automatically set on some instruments and manually set on others. The manual methods involve the use of fluorescent microspheres and/or immunostained cells. Even if microspheres are used for the initial compensation settings, these should be checked with the type of cells under analysis in the laboratory over the expected dynamic range of FI.

Monitoring color compensation may be as simple as daily documentation of the mean FI for each fluorescent particle (or cell) on Levy-Jennings graphs. A range of acceptable values for each type of material should be documented, along with corrective actions to be taken when values exceed the limits (ie, change scratched filter, reset compensation after installation of new laser or power supply). Fluorescence compensation may also be indirectly monitored by simply observing any unexpected changes in the fluorescence patterns of cells under analysis (pattern recognition).

Light Scatter

Fluorescent microspheres provide a means to evaluate instrument parameters independent of biological issues relevant to specimens. Standardization of light scatter signals may be performed as follows.

First, forward-angle light scatter (FALS), side scatter (SS), and the histogram channel position of the microspheres may be determined at constant electronic gain and PMT high-voltage settings and plotted on Levy-Jennings graphs. This procedure detects drifts or failures of the light scatter signal over time. With optimal alignment and standardization, beads from the same lot number should fall in essentially the same channel each day. Variations signal problems in the instrument.

Commercial preparations of fluorescent microspheres are available that provide quantitative levels of FI, thus allowing standardization of FI measurements independent of instrument or laboratory site. Certainly, beads have different light scatter properties and fluorescence than cells, but they still are very useful for standardization. Representative commercial suppliers of fluorescence standards are listed in **Table 5-1**.

Table 5-1
Commercial Suppliers of Fluorescence-Standard Microparticles

Product	Supplier	Location
Flow Set	Beckman Coulter	Miami, Florida
QuantiBrite	BD Immunocytometry	San Jose, California
Quantum Beads	Flow Cytometry Standards Corp.	San Juan, Puerto Rico
Rainbow Beads	Spherotech, Inc.	Libertyville, Illinois

Monitors of Specimen Integrity

One aspect of assuring high-quality results is starting with a high-quality specimen and then appropriately handling the specimen. Although laboratories have little direct control over the biological condition of tissues removed from patients, they are able to influence specimen quality through aggressive education of referring clinicians. Not all types of specimens are appropriate for flow cytometry. In addition to blood, specimens that are typically deemed appropriate for IP evaluation of malignancy include bone marrow, lymphoid tissue, body fluids, skin, and fine-needle aspirates of masses.[4] In addition, leukapheresis products may be used to evaluate CD34 stem cell harvests.

Establishment of optimal handling and storage conditions for patient specimens is necessary to maintain specimen integrity. One way of assessing the adequacy of these procedures (specimen handling, transport, etc) is to monitor the cellular viability of specimens. In this way, it may be possible to detect a recurring problem, such as contamination of the transport media with bacteria or fungi, which causes poor tissue viability. This is not meant to exclude samples with marginal viability, because it must be recognized that many of these specimens are obtained by invasive procedures, and every attempt should be made to provide useful information within the guidelines for sound medical practice. However, for peripheral blood IP where *quantitation* of lymphocyte subsets is the objective, analysis of low-viability specimens may produce inaccurate data. For fresh blood specimens, viability assessment probably does not offer useful information. However, with more aged specimens (> 24 hours), laboratories are encouraged to document acceptability of the specimen viability, which should be > 85%.[7] A recent survey by McCoy and Keren[8] indicated that 92.6% of laboratories participating in the survey stain specimens within 24 hours. They also found that the proportion of laboratories that routinely assess viability was quite varied, as was the definition of acceptability. There should be written laboratory policies that address acceptable levels of viability for blood and tissues and exceptions based on medical judgment. Even when a marginal sample is examined, a notation should be made of the specimen's appearance as part of the data interpretation in the report.

It is more important to assess specimen viability in the area of leukemia/lymphoma IP than with peripheral blood, since such tissues may be more variable in terms of viability. Data from the College of American Pathologists (CAP) FL3-A 1999 survey indicated that laboratories that tested for viability mainly used trypan blue (67%) or propidium iodide (20%), with the remaining 13% using other methods.

In some situations, cell concentration plays a significant role in quality control. Commercially supplied MoAbs normally have recommended amounts of blood (or cells) for which the reagents are acceptable. However, if a blood or bone marrow specimen from a patient with leukemia and a high cell count is processed by an erythrolytic method without any adjustment in cell concentration, it is possible that a very dim (or negative) pattern will be produced due to the very low ratio of MoAb to cells. Limits for when and how to adjust cell concentrations should be determined in the laboratory. In particular, there may not be specific directions on the use of MoAbs that have been classified as analyte-specific reagents (ASRs). Therefore, the laboratory is responsible for assuring adequacy of the reagents for their intended purpose (see the discussion of ASRs below).

Policies and procedures should be written for the handling of all these specimen types, along with rejection criteria and documentation of actual specimen rejections. These include the types of anticoagulants and transport media that are acceptable. Monitoring these rejection criteria can help to identify problems with transport media and potential personnel training issues.

Wright-stained cytocentrifuge preparations and morphologic examination can also be an important QC/QA tool in IP of malignancies.[9] It is important to first ascertain that malignancy is present in order to fully interpret the data.

Process Controls

In order to monitor the quality of the IP process, cellular materials are needed. Cellular targets for testing have historically depended on the availability of viable cells. Therefore, many laboratories use fresh blood, cell lines, or preserved cells. Recently, other types of cells have become commercially available that may offer alternatives in some instances.

Sources of Cells

Normal Whole Blood Controls

Quality control is intended to monitor all components in an assay system that might affect the end result. One method for monitoring the total process in clinical flow cytometry is analysis of a "normal" peripheral blood specimen with each test specimen or group of test specimens. In many laboratories, the normal specimen is from one of the laboratory personnel or some other person believed to be healthy. The specimen is processed just as a test specimen using the same MoAb panel. The primary information provided by immunostaining control blood is the adequacy of erythrolysis (for whole blood methods) and the quality or stability of the MoAb reagents in daily use.

This procedure is intended to document the adequacy of the immuno-staining and analysis procedures. However, there are potential pitfalls with this method that should be recognized. First, the addition of MoAb to a control specimen does not necessarily ensure the addition to test specimens. Second, the fresh control specimen may not be of the same age or handled in the same way as a test specimen. Third, the biological variability achieved by using many donors may actually exceed the method variability to such an extent that it is of limited use in detecting analytical problems. This method does, however, test the overall process of immunostaining, lysis, and evaluation and is the most common procedure used in clinical laboratories.

The parameter typically recorded for QC is the percentage of positive cells for each cluster designation (CD) MoAb tested. Percentages of cellular subsets are relatively reproducible in some individuals, but wide fluctuations occur in others, and there is also a diurnal pattern and a seasonal change in lymphocyte subsets, with as much as a 2-fold lower value during the summer.[10] These are issues that need to be considered when evaluating controls and test specimens.

Cultured Cell Lines

Cultured lymphohematopoietic cell lines are an alternative type of specimen used by some laboratories for regular quality control of immunostaining. This allows detection of antigens on a relatively consistent and stable target and avoids the biological variability inherent in the use of normal donor blood. Maintaining cell lines, however, is relatively expensive and technically beyond the expertise of some laboratories.

Cryopreserved Cells

Cryopreservation of cells in liquid nitrogen or ultra-low-temperature freezers offers an additional method of preparing large pools of consistent target cells. Following density gradient separation of a large volume of blood from a single donor, cells can then be aliquoted, frozen, and recovered when needed for use as cellular targets. This method facilitates MoAb comparisons between different lots of cells prior to routine use of that lot. While a good source of cells, it is somewhat laborious and requires the purchase or availability of cryopreservation equipment and freezers. However, the QC data produced from either cell lines or frozen cells are quite useful for longitudinal monitoring of immunostaining. **Figure 5-3** illustrates a typical month of data obtained from the use of frozen cells. Use of frozen cells does not lend itself well to the process of monitoring the complete process including erythrolysis.

Using a cryopreserved cell pool, **Figure 5-4** shows the effect of using a single lot of CD4 MoAb over the course of 110 days using cells from 3 donors. The first donor was used from day 1 to day 38, donor 2 from day 39 to 61, and donor 3 from day 62 to 110.

Lyophilized Cells

Another form of preserved cell targets is commercially produced by lyophilization of human peripheral blood cells (CytoTrol; Beckman Coulter, Miami, FL). Similar to cell lines and cryopreserved cells, lyophilized cells still provide good light scatter and FI signals and are a source of identical cell pools that may be used longitudinally for good MoAb QC. One disadvantage is their lability with erythrolytic methods. However, newer methods of cellular stabilization allow for use with lytic methods.

Chemically Preserved Cells

Chemically preserved cells are now commercially available and offer certain advantages over the other types of cells and cell lines mentioned above. **Table 5-2** (p 128) includes representative vendors of these types of preparations that have been approved for in vitro diagnostic use.

Figures 5-5 (p 128) **and 5-6** (p 129) show representative light scatter plots of one such control. As shown in **Figure 5-5,** the cells provide good light scatter patterns whether used with a commercial erythrolytic agent or with ammonium chloride. **Figure 5-6** shows a comparison between the cell control and a normal peripheral blood specimen. The use of these commercial control cells is a simple method of QC. However, before being placed into routine use, these

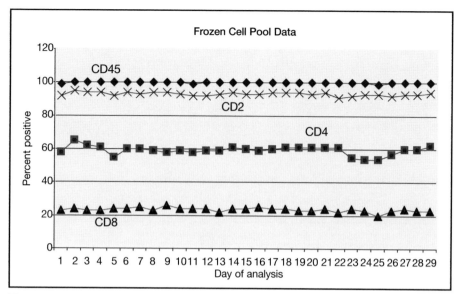

Figure 5-3
Representative illustration of the use of cryopreserved cells for longitudinal monitoring of 4 different MoAbs.

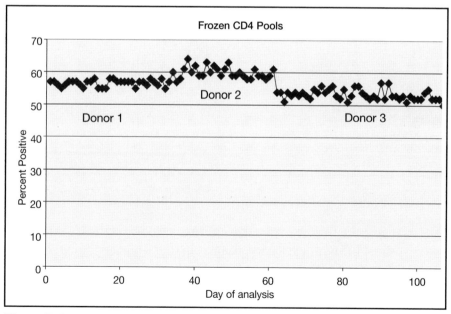

Figure 5-4
Cryopreserved cells from 3 donors using a single lot of CD4 MoAb.

Table 5-2

Commercial Suppliers of Cellular Controls

Product	Supplier	Location
Immuno-Trol; Stem-Trol	Beckman Coulter	Miami, Florida
StatusFlow	R+D Systems	Minneapolis, Minnesota
CD-Chex Plus	Streck Laboratories	Omaha, Nebraska
FluoTrol	BioErgonomics, Inc.	St. Paul, Minnesota

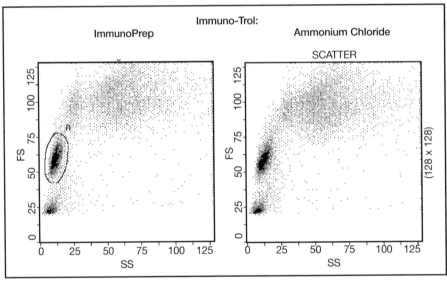

Figure 5-5

Examples of the light scatter profiles of a chemically-preserved whole blood control after treatment with a commercial erythrolytic (ImmunoPrep) or ammonium chloride. (This figure is courtesy of Beckman Coulter, Miami, FL. ImmunoPrep is a trademark of Beckman Coulter.)

products should all be tested for acceptability in your laboratory using your specific methods.

The keys to the successful use of daily (or regular) target cells in QC are: (1) selecting the type of target cells; (2) processing and analyzing the cells using standard patient testing protocols; (3) monitoring the measured parameters (percentage positive, FI, etc); and (4) determining acceptable value ranges and corrective actions upon failure.

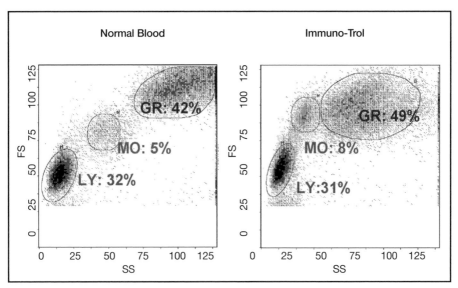

Figure 5-6
Examples of light scatter profiles from a normal peripheral blood sample (left panel) and a commercially available cellular control; Immuno-Trol (right panel). Both were treated with the erythrolytic ImmunoPrep.

Abbreviations: LY = lymphocytes, MO = monocytes, GR = granulocytes. (This figure is courtesy of Beckman Coulter, Miami, FL. ImmunoPrep and Immuno-Trol are trademarks of Beckman Coulter.)

Correction of Results for CD45/CD14 Staining (Red Cell and Monocyte Contamination)

When peripheral blood is examined by flow cytometry, it is common to use an erythrolytic method to remove red cells from the light scatter gate of the lymphocytes, such that percentages of positive cells in this gate really represent data from lymphocytes only. A common method of correcting data involves the use of a CD45 MoAb paired with a CD14 MoAb. Within the lymphocyte gate, contaminating monocytes may be identified by CD14 positivity, and all leukocytes will be CD45$^+$, thus detecting red cell contamination. The formula used to correct immunophenotypic data is as follows:

(Raw % Positive/% Bright CD45$^+$CD14$^-$) $\times$ 100

For example, if the CD4 value was 45%, with a bright CD45$^+$CD14$^-$ value of 92%, then the corrected CD4 percentage would be 49%.

Most clinical laboratories perform this type of correction, but many have determined that only levels of bright CD45$^+$CD14$^-$ of < 95% will trigger such a calculation. For most clinical purposes, this is acceptable. There have been no good studies published that show whether there is a level of contamination that must be reached before this calculation is invalid.

Data from the CAP surveys indicate this correction is probably useful down to a level of only 50% CD45$^+$ cells in the gate. Therefore, laboratories should establish some internal policy about when and how to correct sample data for incomplete erythrolysis.

Lymphosum and Backgating

A *lymphosum* may be thought of as a mathematical check on the relationships expected biologically between various lymphoid subsets. For instance, a lymphosum may be calculated as the sum of the percentage of CD2$^+$ and CD19$^+$ (or CD20$^+$) cells, which should be > 95%, or the sum of the percentage of CD3$^+$, CD19$^+$ (or CD20$^+$), and CD16$^+$ cells. For 2-color MoAb combinations, the sum of dual-positive CD3/CD4 cells and dual-positive CD3/CD8 cells should approximate the percentage of CD3$^+$ cells.

While this method is useful for peripheral blood QC, it does not pertain to IP examination of leukemias and lymphomas, where the actual percentage of positive cells is less important than the determination of the composite immunophenotype of the malignancy. However, it does pertain to nonmalignant cells in lymph nodes or bone marrow.

Additionally, a variation of the lymphosum might be a *cell sum*, whereby in a bone marrow sample, the sum of CD2$^+$, CD19$^+$, and CD13$^+$ (or CD33$^+$) cells should approximate the percentage of CD45$^+$ cells, and the sum of CD45 and anti-glycophorin A should approximate 100%. The point is that any specimen under analysis likely has cells present with mutually exclusive subsets, such that addition of these subsets should closely account for the percentage of CD45$^+$ cells.

Backgating is the process of using the CD45/CD14 fluorescence signals to then generate a side scatter/forward scatter plot from the bright CD45$^+$CD14$^-$ cell population and thus identify the region of the light scatter histogram occupied by the lymphoid cells. This will then allow adjustments, if necessary, to account for the highest proportion of lymphoid cells in the region to be analyzed.

Accuracy and Imprecision

As with most laboratory tests, both accuracy and variability (imprecision) of measurements within or between runs is a significant concern. Each laboratory should determine analytical performance and establish acceptable operational limits based on analytical and biological variations.

Accuracy and Bias

Accuracy of results in flow cytometry is somewhat difficult to assess within a single laboratory, and this issue is best handled through peer comparisons and group means.

Lack of accuracy may be secondary to analytical bias, whereby a method, reagent, or instrument provides results with good precision, but they are systematically low or high compared with appropriate peer groups. As an example, the use of one CD8 clone versus another leads to a statistical (but not clinically important) bias.[11]

Imprecision

Allowable imprecision in IP continues to be a disputed area of investigation. For quantitative testing (CD4, CD34) it takes on a significant meaning, whereas for IP of leukemias/lymphomas it is not of great importance. Some guidance comes from the 1997 revised guidelines of the Centers for Disease Control and Prevention (CDC),[12] which indicate that replicate measurements of percentage of $CD3^{\pm}$ cells within an individual dual-color panel containing multiple instances of the CD3 MoAb paired with a second MoAb should produce variances of < 3% among all 4 tubes. In the case of 3-color analysis where 2 tubes each contain CD3 MoAb, the variance should be < 2%. Intuitively, the 3% figure would produce different CVs, dependent on the actual target value of the CD under analysis. For instance, a 3% difference about a target of 70% CD3 positivity would yield a lower CV than a 3% difference about a target of 20% CD8 positivity. The actual determination of the CV is by the formula $CV = (SD/X) \times 100$, where X is the mean value and SD is the calculated standard deviation.

Recent data from the CAP flow cytometry surveys provide additional insight into imprecision. The Diagnostic Immunology Resource Committee examined replication of results on a broad scale. The strength of this approach is that a large number of results were examined over 3 separate surveys, with more than 500 laboratories participating. This facilitated a more robust statistical analysis, and, perhaps more importantly, sensitized laboratorians to the issue of reproducibility and confidence limits for analytes that have significant biological variability in addition to analytical variability. Summarized results indicated that approximately 80% of participants replicated at the ± 3% level, and > 90% at the ± 4% level. This was true for CD3, CD4, and CD8, even though the absolute percentages of each were different in the specimens. Thus, each had a different CV.

Interestingly, the CAP data also showed a correlation between variability in replication and accuracy, as determined by distance from the group mean. Those laboratories reporting the greatest variation also reported results furthest from the group means.

For comparison, results of replication were generated in one laboratory using a single blood sample on each of 5 consecutive days (**Table 5-3**). In each case, the sample was aliquoted into 10 individual tubes and immunostained individually. Results for CD4 showed that there was little difference in CV between 2 FITC-labeled MoAbs and 2 PE-labeled MoAbs. Results for CD8 in the same study produced CVs approximately 2 times those of CD4 (range, 2.61 to 3.39). The patterns of daily change were similar.

Historically, maximum allowable *analytical* imprecision has been defined based on reference ranges,[13] medical significance,[14] the state of the art,[15] and biological variation.[16,17] The landmark 1976 Aspen Conference of the CAP[17] resulted in recommendations including the following: (1) Analytical goals can only be defined in terms of the need of care of patients. (2) For individual single and multipoint testing, the analytical goal is that the CV should be equal to or less than half the within-subject variation, and this should be the goal for short-term laboratory imprecision. An international Subcommittee on Analytical Goals in Clinical Chemistry of the World Association of Societies of Pathology, sponsored by the CIBA Foundation, firmly supported the Aspen recommendations. Similarly, the European Group for the Evaluation of Reagents and Analytical Systems in Clinical Chemistry agreed that total imprecision should be less than half the within-subject biological variation or less than the state of the art achieved by the best 20% of laboratories when data on biological variation do not exist.[15]

Table 5-3
Replication Data for CD4 Using 2 MoAbs and 2 Fluorochromes

	CD4 #1 FITC			CD4 #2 FITC			CD4 #1 PE			CD4 #2 PE		
	Mean	SD	CV	Mean	SD	CV	Mean	SD	CV	Mean	SD	CV
1	53.44	0.80	1.49	54.31	0.65	1.19	56.30	1.08	1.92	56.77	1.09	1.93
2	54.55	0.62	1.14	55.08	0.53	0.97	57.78	0.34	0.56	58.66	1.06	1.81
3	46.77	0.88	1.89	47.49	0.53	1.12	47.82	0.35	0.74	48.12	0.52	1.08
4	56.96	1.00	1.76	57.98	1.07	1.84	58.48	1.42	2.42	59.05	0.99	1.68
5	54.15	0.62	1.14	54.00	1.33	2.46	54.64	0.78	1.43	54.99	0.94	1.71
	53.17	0.78	1.48	53.77	0.82	1.52	55.00	0.79	1.41	55.52	0.92	1.64

There have been no large, systematic studies of biological variability in flow cytometry, but data from 2 longitudinal studies provide some insight into intraindividual variations in peripheral blood lymphocyte subsets. Giorgi et al[18] reported on a 4-center study using the same instruments and monoclonal antibodies, but different specimen processing methods. The researchers obtained intraperson standard deviations for CD3, CD4, and CD8 percentages in homosexual HIV-seronegative subjects of 4.5 to 7.9, with CVs of 6% to 24%. The heterosexual control group from one center had SDs of only 3.3 to 4, which correlate with an estimated CV of 5%, 9%, and 14%, respectively. Edwards et al[10] reported data from a panel of 15 individual healthy longitudinal donors, using a single instrument and reagent set. They obtained intraindividual median CVs of 4.1%, 4.5%, and 3.9% for CD3, CD4, and CD8, respectively, with ranges of 2.7% to 7.4% for CD3, 3.2% to 7.8% for CD4, and 1.8% to 6.8% for CD8. Therefore, differences in the level of homeostatic control probably exist among individuals. These values from Edwards et al are close to those of the heterosexual control group reported by Giorgi et al. For all 3 CDs in the Giorgi study, the difference in intraindividual variation between homosexual and heterosexual groups was significant (P ranging from < .001 to < .004), thus illustrating the need for more longitudinal studies in healthy individuals, as well as in patient groups.

Such data on intraindividual biological variations then allow an approximation of analytic precision goals,[17] where $CV_a \leq {}^{1}\!/_{42}CV_b$, or the analytic precision is $\leq 50\%$ of the biologic variation. The specimens used in the CAP surveys were obtained from healthy individuals. Thus, for comparative purposes, assume that, based on averaging of results from the studies above, the average biologic variation for CD3 is 4.6%, CD4 is 6.8%, and CD8 is 9.0%. Then the respective analytic CVs would be < 2.3%, < 3.4%, and < 4.5%. Within a single laboratory, this is clearly achievable, based on the CAP survey data discussed above.

Doumas[19] advocates that although improvement of accuracy for some tests may be warranted, for most tests the improvement is irrelevant to patient care, and that if more accuracy is desirable, then it must also be affordable and the benefits must outweigh the costs. The major use of flow cytometry in peripheral blood IP is not in diagnosis, but in monitoring therapy of HIV-positive individuals. In fact, recent work has documented the strength of measuring HIV messenger RNA (mRNA) and the further strengthening of $CD4^+$ T cell measurements in management of such patients.[20] The intraindividual biologic variation in HIV-positive individuals is much greater than in healthy controls.[10,18] Clearly, better analytical accuracy and precision are relevant in this circumstance, which leads to a need for more stringent, rather than less stringent, application of technology to improve analytical measurements.

Generally, within the laboratory, 2 types of reproducibility of quantitative results should be addressed: (1) within-sample and (2) between-sample reproducibility. Replicate measurements of an individual immunostained and prepared sample on a single flow cytometer sets the basis for establishing that instrument's imprecision. Replicate measurements of this sample should therefore be unaffected by the sample preparation method, because it is a single-sample preparation, and instead focus on instrumental analysis. The major cause of imprecision under these conditions is the instrument itself. A reasonable target for the SD of this method is 1%. That means that if a lymphocyte subset value is 40%, then any additional measurement should vary within the range of 38% to 42%, assuming a 95% confidence limit (± 2 SD).

To assess the effects of sample preparation on imprecision, a single blood sample should be aliquoted into several tubes (at least 10) and each tube individually immunostained and analyzed. This procedure was used to produce the data in **Table 5-4.** The results obtained from this procedure included the effects of variation in sample preparation in addition to those related to the instrument itself. Therefore, the SD obtained from the first could be subtracted from that of the second procedure to obtain an estimate of variability from preparation alone. This procedure now introduces an additional layer of complexity to variability: the immunostaining and erythrolytic procedures. In this case, an SD of 3% might be acceptable.[12]

Knowledge of a laboratory's imprecision (SD) allows determination of analytic confidence limits that may then be applied to the interpretation of potential changes in quantitative CD levels such as CD4 or CD34 for an individual patient. Thus, it is not enough to be accurate. Results must be reproducibly accurate.

Table 5-4
Comparison of Standard Deviation Within-Sample and Between Samples.

Tube #	Within-Sample	Between Samples
1	40	42
2	41	36
3	40	40
4	39	43
5	40	38
6	40	39
7	41	41
8	39	42
9	41	37
10	38	41
Mean	39.9	39.9
Std. Dev.	0.99	2.33

Reference Ranges

For quantitative IP analyses, reference ranges related to the population under study are clinically useful. Only with knowledge of the experimental variation can an acceptable reference range be established within a laboratory.

Ideally, laboratories should have age-adjusted reference ranges established for peripheral blood IP. Obtaining blood from normal, healthy infants and young children may be problematic for many laboratories. Based on published studies and a conspectus of such studies,[21] it may be reasonable for laboratories to perform limited in-house studies of certain populations and compare the results with published studies for verification while additional data are being accumulated. In a recent survey, it was found that aside from adult peripheral blood, most laboratories do not have reference ranges established in-house, but rather rely on published ranges and/or manufacturer's recommended ranges.[8]

Reference ranges for other tissues such as bone marrow and lymph nodes are problematic in that most institutions do not acquire samples from healthy individuals, but only from those requiring diagnostic evaluations. Flow cytometric examination of these tissues is usually for the purpose of detecting/characterizing leukemias or lymphomas. Therefore, reference ranges are essentially meaningless in this setting.[4] Additional quality assurance methods come into play when immunophenotyping these malignancies and include the addition of morphology/histology and pattern recognition based on a panel of MoAbs.[9]

Reagent or Monoclonal Antibody QC

Isotype Negative Control MoAbs

MoAbs of the same isotype (and fluorochrome conjugate) that do not react with the target cells have been used for determining the combination of non-specific reagent binding and cellular autofluorescence. In an era of cost-consciousness, persuasive arguments have been presented against the use of isotypic control MoAbs in flow cytometric analysis of nonmalignant peripheral blood T cells.[22] The 1997 revision of the Flow Cytometry Checklist of the CAP Laboratory Accreditation Program (LAP) addressed this issue by removing the requirement for use of isotype controls in enumerating peripheral blood lymphocytes.[23] Because this issue is not as clear in the analysis of hematologic malignancies,[4] it has been left to the discretion of laboratory directors.[23] While some advocate the use of isotypic controls when evaluating leukemic samples,[24] others prefer to use nonreactive MoAbs in the panel as internal isotypic controls, similar to the approach used with peripheral blood immunophenotyping.[4] Examination of histograms and results from the CAP FL3 Leukemia/Lymphoma survey indicates that the majority of laboratories still use these control reagents. This points out the fact that isotype controls may be useful in some settings, while less so in other settings.

Whereas nonmalignant cells from peripheral blood labeled with fluorescent MoAbs tend to produce little background fluorescence and reasonably bright, consistent signals for light scatter and FI, the same is not always true of malignant cells. It is common to experience "excessive background" when analyzing certain acute myeloid leukemias of French-American-British (FAB) M4 and M5 subtypes by flow cytometry. This is generally due to cellular autofluorescence or cytophilic binding of MoAbs in a nonspecific manner, or via functional receptors for the Fc region of immunoglobulins (FcR).

Clues to recognition of nonspecific antibody binding include the following: (1) Under standard conditions, the isotypic control fluorescence appears too high. (2) Certain other CD MoAbs in the panel appear significantly dimmer than the isotypic controls. The CAP Laboratory Accreditation Program Flow Cytometry Checklist[23] asks: "Are methods established to ensure that immunoglobulin staining is intrinsic and not extrinsic (cytophilic)?" and "Is there a procedure to distinguish fluorescence-negative and fluorescence-positive cell populations?" This second question also contains commentary: "This does not imply that a separate negative control sample must be run. It is possible to coordinate panels of monoclonal antibodies to compare the binding of monoclonal antibodies of the same subclass that typically have mutually exclusive patterns of reactivity of subsets of hematopoietic cells, provided the reagents under comparison are similar in protein content and fluorochrome:protein ratio. In this way, test antibodies may also double as control reagents." Clearly, the intent of these questions, and of good laboratory practice, is to adequately control for potential artifacts during flow cytometric analysis of malignancies.

CD MoAbs

Over the years in research laboratories, huge numbers of different MoAb clones have been produced, many of which were quite similar in their reactivity/specificity. The First International Workshop on Leukocyte Differentiation Antigens[25] examined various different clones, and MoAb specificities determined to be the same were grouped into what became known as clusters of differentiation (CD). The aim was to standardize nomenclature and establish a form of equivalency. These workshops, which now number 5 and span over 15 years, played an exceedingly important role in characterizing the performance of these biological reagents through detailed chemical and physical studies and, more importantly, their cellular patterns of reactivity on both normal and malignant cells.

Most clinically useful MoAbs are classified into CDs, with a few exceptions. One of the purposes of the international workshops was to examine many MoAb clones from many laboratories around the world and to determine those that reacted similarly with the same target antigens. In this way, it was hoped that MoAb clones that were the same (or very similar) could be used interchangeably and the terminology could be simplified to CD nomenclature. For the most part, this has been a very successful approach. However, in the case of clinical diagnosis, it should be noted that not all MoAb clones from the same CD have exactly the same reactivity. In fact, the results obtained with specific clones from the same CD are known to be slightly (statistically but not clinically) different. An example is CD8, where the Leu 2 clone produced slightly higher results than the CCT8 clone.[11] This information should be used when making decisions to change reagents within a laboratory. That is, if reference intervals have been determined with one clone, they may need to be reexamined with another clone. However, published data show that these differences should not be clinically important.

Stability/Variability of Fluorochromes

The sudden deterioration of MoAbs is extremely uncommon; deterioration occurs gradually. Therefore, there is little to be gained from repetitively examining a control specimen throughout the day. MoAbs do deteriorate over time, and measurement or monitoring of FI is an earlier and more sensitive indicator of MoAb instability or degradation than the percentage of positive cells. By the time alterations in the percentage of MoAb positivity are seen, a very significant loss of quantitative MoAb reactivity may already have occurred. The FI of cells is stable for at least 24 hours at ambient temperature when stored as whole blood. In addition, because the "normal" controls are usually obtained from different individuals each day, the biological variation in percent positivity may mask any meaningful determination of MoAb deterioration in a timely fashion. As shown in **Figure 5-7,** for CD4 on normal controls, FI varies less between individuals than does percent positivity.

It is important to compare existing and new MoAb lot numbers for similar reactivity and FI prior to using the new lot number for clinical analysis. This is not only a practical issue, but is also addressed by the CAP in its LAP Laboratory General Inspection Checklist.[26] This may be done by simply examining a small number of specimens using both reagents and comparing them for any clinically important differences in FI or percentage of positive cells. As shown by Davis et al,[27] various clones of CD4 MoAbs have variable binding to human cells, and a switch between clones should be carefully examined prior to implementation.

Aliquoting/Dilution of MoAbs

Many MoAb reagents that are used in the clinical laboratory are approved by the US Food and Drug Administration (FDA) for in vitro diagnostic use. These reagents should not be further diluted beyond the manufacturers' recommendations or they will no longer be considered in compliance with their approved uses. Any alterations need to be validated by the laboratory as an in-house or "home-brewed" test. Dilution and aliquoting of other MoAbs, whether developed in-house or labeled as ASRs (see discussion below), creates a potential variable that must be documented. That is, the reagent may be diluted too far for the number of cells under analysis and therefore produce a very weak signal, or may be too concentrated and result in excessive background. In any case, these reagents need to be validated for their intended use in the laboratory and

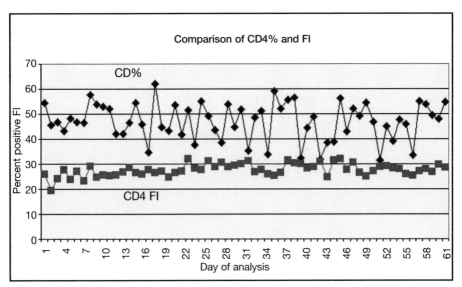

Figure 5-7
Graphic representation of percent positivity (upper line/diamonds) and FI (lower line/squares) of 18 different healthy adult controls over a 2-month time frame. The y-axis represents percent positivity, as well as relative mean fluorescence intensity.

documentation of this process provided (see Validation of Analyte Specific Reagents below).

Purvis and Stelzer[28] have addressed an extensive reagent standardization and internal validation program in a commercial laboratory environment. While their program is robust and technically of a high standard, it is beyond the reach of most clinical laboratories. Nevertheless, the information contained in their program provides a sound basis for considerations of internal QC/QA programs.

Preparation Controls, Lysing, and Other Reagents

One of the assumptions made in flow cytometry is that for a given blood sample, the degree of erythrolysis between tubes within the MoAb panel is similar. This assumption is one of the bases for the CD45/CD14 correction of data described previously. Therefore, the reliability of the lysing process is important. Automated methods of erythrolysis have improved the consistency, although the problem with instrument malfunction whereby too little reagent is introduced into the tube for adequate lysis remains. Visual inspection sometimes detects this problem, but not always. Routine use of lymphosum-type calculations may also help detect aberrant results.

Buffers and/or tissue culture media used to wash or dilute cells may become contaminated with bacteria or fungi over time. Many laboratories include antimicrobials in such buffers, but bacterial contamination should be checked for by visual inspection (cloudy) and by appearance of bacteria on Wright-stained cytocentrifuge cell preparations. Bacterial contamination of MoAbs can cause proteolysis and may create artifactual results. Contamination can also alter light scatter properties and create excessive "debris."

Some laboratories prepare specimens using density gradient separations. The CAP surveys show that fewer than 5% of laboratories use this method for IP of peripheral blood lymphocyte subsets. However, this method is more common for IP of leukemias/lymphomas. These media are also susceptible to contamination and should be checked regularly. The centrifuge speed/time for optimal separation should be determined, and the centrifuge speed monitored regularly by use of a tachometer.

Validation of Analyte-Specific Reagents

One of the more recent issues affecting QC/QA and the practice of clinical flow cytometry is the need for validation of MoAbs that are classified as analyte-specific reagents, or ASRs.[29] This is particularly relevant in the immunophenotypic evaluation of leukemias and lymphomas. Though there is clear guidance regarding the validation of laboratory tests of certain types, a number of questions remain unanswered with respect to validation of MoAbs (ASRs) in diagnosis of these diseases, in part due to the biologically variable nature of the analytes in question: cellular proteins. While many laboratories have used MoAbs for this purpose for years, recent actions by the FDA have led to the requirement for laboratories to address the validation process specifically in this area.[29]

The FDA holds authority over commercialization of diagnostic products as they pertain to health care. Commercial providers of reagents such as MoAbs typically perform clinical trials to provide evidence of equivalence for new versus existing products under the 510(k) premarket notification process. When deemed equivalent and otherwise appropriate, the FDA allows manufacturers to market these reagents for in vitro diagnostic (IVD) use. In some cases, such as leukemia and lymphoma immunophenotyping, no IVD MoAbs were available for the intended use. Laboratories then used "unapproved" MoAbs for medical diagnosis, or used IVD MoAbs in combinations or in methods that rendered them no longer IVD-approved.

The Immunology Devices Panel proposed rules to regulate ASRs, and following a comment period, the FDA published the final rule for ASRs on November 21, 1997, which became effective on November 23, 1998.[29] The FDA regards ASRs as laboratory reagents comprising chemicals or antibodies that are "active ingredients" of tests used to identify one specific disease or condition.

Specific issues need to be addressed when using MoAbs labeled as ASRs by manufacturers. Sale of ASRs is now restricted to laboratories designated under the Clinical Laboratory Improvement Amendments (CLIA) of 1988 as qualified to perform high-complexity testing. Only physicians and other health care practitioners authorized by applicable state law can order the use of in-house developed tests using ASRs.

The rule specifically requires that laboratories provide a disclaimer with results obtained through the use of tests incorporating ASRs. The disclaimer must read as follows: "This test was developed and its performance characteristics determined by [Laboratory Name]. It has not been cleared or approved by the U.S. Food and Drug Administration."

The FDA has no objection to the inclusion of additional clarifying language in the report, as long as the required disclaimer is present. Clarifying language suggested by the CAP might include: "The FDA has determined that such clearance or approval is not necessary. This test is used for clinical purposes. It should not be regarded as investigational or for research."

To be in compliance with the final rule, flow cytometry laboratories should have policies and procedures to document the validation of individual, or combinations (panels) of, ASRs (MoAbs) for use in characterizing leukemias and lymphomas or other appropriate applications prior to their use in patient testing.

One of the first issues to address in validation is determination of the flow cytometric "test" to be validated. The FDA states that ASRs are "used to identify one specific disease or condition." Because individual MoAbs are of limited use in this regard, and the standard of practice is to use panels of reagents,[9,30] one approach might be to make the "test" (ASR) the composite panel of reagents and then validate the combinations, or panels, of MoAbs used in the laboratory for their intended purpose.

Potential components of a validation protocol might include:

- Peer-reviewed literature to support use of specific ASRs or combinations of ASRs
- CLIA requirements, as applicable, for test validation
- Results of flow cytometry proficiency surveys
- Correlative morphologic information from cytology/histology
- Ancillary testing results such as cytochemical staining or molecular diagnostics

Pertinent peer-reviewed literature might include journal articles that reference the clones used for clinical testing, potentially with outcomes of their use. Additionally, pertinent clinical reviews might include that of Jennings and Foon[31] on immunophenotypic evaluation of leukemias and lymphomas and papers comprising the US-Canadian Consensus Conference Recommendations,[32] and, for those clones that have been examined through the international workshops, the appropriate volume of the proceedings of the workshops.[25]

The CLIA document[1] addresses validation of test procedures using non-IVD reagents developed after September 1, 1992. There are stated requirements to verify or establish laboratory methods. Similar items are covered in the CAP Laboratory General Inspection Checklist[26] and the Flow Cytometry Inspection Checklist.[23]

Pertinent to the validation process, Sub-Part K, 493.1213 of CLIA ("Establishment and verification of method performance specifications"), states that "prior to reporting patient test results," the laboratory should "verify or establish for each method the performance specifications for the following performance characteristics, as applicable."

This paragraph specifies the attributes of validation of general laboratory tests, but not all are necessarily applicable to all tests, such as leukemia and lymphoma immunophenotyping. Included in the validation process are:

- Accuracy
- Precision
- Analytical sensitivity
- Analytical specificity (to include interferences)
- Reportable range of results
- Reference range
- Any other performance characteristic required for test performance

The main issue pertaining to implementing this approach in flow cytometry is determination of what is applicable. As an example, validation of ASRs for immunophenotyping leukemia/lymphoma might be viewed in the following manner:

- Accuracy (applicable, if the test is a panel and the purpose is lineage identification)
- Precision (not applicable)
- Analytical sensitivity (applicable, if sensitivity is defined as detection of dimly expressed antigens necessary for a composite immunophenotypic characterization)
- Analytical specificity (applicable, if specificity is defined as specific lineage identification)
- Reportable range of results (not applicable)
- Reference range (not applicable)
- Any other performance characteristic required for test performance (applicable, discussed below)

Sub-Part H specifies that "All laboratories must enroll in a proficiency testing (PT) program that has been approved by HHS (Health and Human Services). The laboratory must test PT samples just as patient samples." This may be addressed by participation in the CAP Flow Cytometry Survey Sets (FL) and Leukemia/Lymphoma Survey FL3, or equivalent approved programs. Successful participation is another element to document in a prospective fashion the validity of an individual laboratory's ASRs (panels) compared with other laboratories using similar or dissimilar methods.

Correlation of flow cytometric data with cytology/histology is particularly important in the validation of ASRs used in immunophenotyping malignancies such as leukemias and lymphomas.[9] Morphology and histology observations will determine if a malignancy is present (at diagnosis). Morphology of cytocentrifuge-prepared cell samples will also determine if representative malignant cells are present if a density gradient separation method is employed. As a validation tool, the morphology may be used to support the interpretation of the flow cytometric data.

Because the validation process is being initiated after the fact, and these MoAbs have been used clinically for some time, what is the role of retrospective data? Most laboratories now have historical data and comparisons are available for cytology/histology results, the FAB classification of acute leukemias, and lymphoma classifications that can help in validation and even in clinical outcome assessments. Therefore, building case files, particularly in the area of leukemia and lymphoma, can help validate the methods and reagents retrospectively, provided the panels (ASRs) have not changed.

One example of validation might involve something named "Acute Leukemia Panel #1" (**Table 5-5**).

Guidance and Consensus Documents for Quality Control/ Quality Assurance

Certain groups have put forth guidelines and recommendations that are helpful in the flow cytometry laboratory.

The College of American Pathologists (CAP) addresses many issues, including QC/QA, through its Laboratory Accreditation Program (LAP) and the Flow Cytometry Proficiency Surveys Programs (FL1,2,3).

The National Committee for Clinical Laboratory Standards (NCCLS) has published the following series of guidelines pertinent to flow cytometry and quality assurance. These offer consensus-derived guidelines for many aspects of flow cytometry.

H42-A: *Clinical Applications of Flow Cytometry: Quality Assurance and Immunophenotyping of Lymphocytes; Approved Guideline (1998)*

This document provides guidance for the immunophenotypic analysis of non-neoplastic lymphocytes by immunofluorescence-based flow cytometry; sample and instrument quality control; and precautions for acquisition of data from lymphocytes. ISBN 1-56238-364-7

H43-A: *Clinical Applications of Flow Cytometry: Immunophenotyping of Leukemic Cells; Approved Guideline (1998)*

Guidelines for immunophenotypic analysis of leukemic and lymphoma cells using immunofluorescence-based flow cytometry; sample and instrument quality control; and precautions for acquisition of data from leukemic cells. ISBN 1-56238-351-5

H44-A: *Methods for Reticulocyte Counting (Flow Cytometry and Supravital Dyes); Approved Guideline (1997)*

Provides guidance for the performance of reticulocyte counting by flow cytometry. It includes methods for determining the accuracy and precision of

Table 5-5
ASR Name: Acute Leukemia Panel #1

Intended Use: Identification and assignment of cell lineage in acute leukemias.
Date of Implementation: November 23, 1998.
Composition of the ASR (panel):

CD	Conjugate	MoAb	CD	Conjugate	MoAb
CD2	FITC	CCT11 (1)	CD1a	RD1	CCT1 (1)
CD3	FITC	CCT3 (1)	CD19	RD1	B4 (1)
CD4	FITC	CCT4 (1)	CD8	RD1	CCT8 (1)
CD19	FITC	Leu 12 (2)	CD10	PE	CALLA (2)
CD19	FITC	B4 (1)	CD20	RD1	B1 (1)

Manufacturers:
1. Beckman-Coulter, Miami, FL
2. BD Immunocytometry, Mountain View, CA

Accuracy: This panel (ASR) accurately determined the cell lineage in 74/75 cases of acute leukemias.

Precision: Not applicable.

Analytical Sensitivity: Not applicable. This test is used only to identify cell lineage of morphologically defined acute leukemias.

Analytical Specificity:
- B-cell precursor Acute Lymphocytic Leukemia (ALL), as defined by morphology and ancillary testing, shows 25/25 cases correct.
- T-cell ALL, as defined by morphology and ancillary testing, shows 25/25 cases correct.
- Acute Monocytic Leukemia (AML), as defined by morphology and ancillary testing, shows 24/25 cases positive (see "Corrective Action" for explanation).

Reportable Range: Not applicable.

Reference Range: Not applicable.

Any Other Performance Characteristic Required for Test Performance:
- Correlation with cytology/morphology/histochemistry (74/75 cases agreed).
- Correlation with outside referrals (agreed with 15/15 Cancer and Leukemia, Group B [CALGB] referrals).

Proficiency Surveys (CAP):
This panel correctly assigned the cell lineage to:
    B-cell precursor ALL (FL3-01, 1998)
    AML (FL3-02, 1997)
    T-cell ALL (FL3-01, 1997)
This panel incorrectly assigned lineage to:
    AML (FL3-02, 1998)

Corrective Action:
The CAP sample (FL3-02, 1998) was not examined in a timely fashion, and the viability was too low for accurate interpretation.

Pertinent Literature:
1. Jennings CD, Foon KA. Recent advances in flow cytometry: application to the diagnosis of hematologic malignancy. *Blood.* 1997;90:2863-2892. (Discusses immunophenotypes of specific acute leukemias.)
2. Stewart CC, Behm FG, Carey JL, et al. U.S.-Canadian consensus recommendations on the immunophenotypic analysis of hematologic neoplasia by flow cytometry: selection of antibody combinations. *Cytometry (Comm Clin Cytometry).* 1997;30:231-235. (Addresses composition of panels for acute leukemias.)
3. Specific workshop citations regarding MoAb clone reactivity.

Data to support these statements should be stored for retrieval when needed. The validation document(s) will likely be dynamic, and updated periodically to reflect additional cases and supportive data. Validation will also need to be updated as components of the panel (ASR) are changed.

the reticulocyte flow cytometry instrument and a recommended reference procedure. ISBN 1-56238-302-7

The Centers for Disease Control and Prevention (CDC) published the *1997 Revised Guidelines for Performing CD4⁺ T-Cell Determinations in Persons Infected with Human Immunodeficiency Virus (HIV) Recommendations*. Morbidity and Mortality Weekly Report. January 10, 1997. The CDC also administers the T-Lymphocyte Immunophenotyping (TLI) Program, a peer quality assurance program.

Additional sources of consensus-derived recommendations and guidelines include national and international programs from the US-Canadian[32] and European[24] conferences.

The American Society for Histocompatibility and Immunogenetics (ASHI) *Standards for Histocompatibility Testing: Section Q (Flow Cytometry)*. Copyright © 1995, 1995, 1996, 1997, 1998 American Society for Histocompatibility and Immunogenetics.

Peer Comparison Surveys

Participation in peer comparison surveys is a very useful way for laboratories to compare their performance with other laboratories using the same (or similar) instrumentation, reagents, and preparation methods. A number of international organizations have reported studies of peer comparison data:

- The United Kingdom National External Quality Assessment Scheme (UK NEQUAS)[33]
- The Dutch Cooperative Study Group on Immunophenotyping of Haematological Malignancies (SIHON)[34]
- The Gruppo Italiano di Citometria (GIC)[35]
- The Central European Immunophenotyping Quality Control Program (CEQUAL)[36]
- The French Etalonorme National Quality Control Program[37]
- The Canadian Quality Assurance Program (CQAP)[38]

These groups have all worked toward improvements in clinical flow cytometry through large peer comparison groups. These documents offer considerable insight into the international state of the art in flow cytometric QC/QA.

In the US, the CAP offers proficiency surveys for peripheral blood immunophenotyping, leukemia/lymphoma immunophenotyping, CD34 stem cell analysis, and DNA analysis. Results from some of these surveys have been previously reported.[39,40] Tholen et al[41] reported that participation in CAP proficiency testing led to significant improvements in clinical laboratory areas.

CAP surveys have addressed a number of pertinent issues related to laboratory performance in immunophenotypic evaluation of leukemias and lymphomas through the surveys program. One important element of such an approach is that laboratories may be able to help document validation of ASRs used in evaluation of these diseases through peer comparisons of specific MoAb panels and test systems.

The CDC administers the T-Lymphocyte Immunophenotyping (TLI) Program, a peer quality assurance program for IP peripheral blood lymphocyte subsets.

Commercially available peer surveys include STATS (Becton Dickinson Immunocytometry, Mountain View, CA, and Streck Laboratories, Omaha, NE), SplashBack (R+D Systems, Minneapolis, MN), and IQAP (Beckman-Coulter, Miami, FL). Of these, the most complete system, including alignment and standardization particles, lysable cellular controls, and QC monitoring software, is currently available from Beckman-Coulter.

Special Consideration Analysis

Leukemia and Lymphoma Immunophenotyping

Immunophenotypic analysis of leukemias and lymphomas has become a valuable clinical tool in the diagnosis and management of patients. As evidenced by multiple reviews, textbooks, consensus conferences, and proficiency surveys, the procedure of immunophenotyping certain neoplasms has become a mainstay of medical diagnostics.[24,31,32] Considerable worldwide debate has ensued over the proper manner to use these reagents to classify malignancies. This debate is based on the wide variation that exists in clinical laboratories in the use of MoAbs and flow cytometry. Such concerns by the medical community resulted in performance guidelines for immunophenotyping leukemic cells[42] and recent European[24] and US-Canadian[32] consensus conferences on immunophenotypic analysis of leukemias and lymphomas.

The thrust of flow cytometric analysis of lymphohematopoietic neoplasms is identification and characterization of the cell lineage. Thus, many of the quantitative issues discussed with respect to analysis of non-neoplastic peripheral blood do not pertain. Similarly, QC and QA issues are somewhat different. For instance, one of the major controls is morphologic determination of the presence of malignancy. The exception to this might be in detection of minimal residual disease, but this is then based on a previously defined aberrant immunophenotype of the malignancy. The US-Canadian consensus recommendations for QC/QA in leukemia/lymphoma IP can be found in Stelzer et al.[4]

CD34+ Cells

The analysis of CD34+ stem cells represents an area that has many of the same QC issues as other quantitative IP studies, but others that are unique. For instance, there are multiple gating and analysis strategies that have been described, not all of which give the same results, even though any one of these is reproducible. Gratama et al[43] have recently reviewed this area and reported a summary of interlaboratory studies of CD34 enumeration that demonstrated marked variation in the interlaboratory CVs, ranging from approximately 5% to 15% (including percentage and absolute number) with a single method to as high as 35% to 285% using varied methods. When the Nordic Stem Cell Laboratory Group allowed participants to use the guidelines of their method locally within each laboratory, the interlaboratory CV was 27% to 156%, but upon convening a workshop and applying their standard method, this dropped to 9% to 12%, similar to the single-method study above. Standardization clearly improves interlaboratory variation.

QC of CD34 testing also presents special challenges that are only now being met. One of the most difficult issues is the low frequency with which these cells appear clinically (as low as 0.1%, or 5 cells/microliter). Proficiency surveys will need to make special provisions for this low level of positivity, with inherently high CVs. The UK NEQUAS study uses a stabilized cell suspension of CD34+ cells that has significantly improved upon interlaboratory CVs,[33] which indicates that technology is finally now catching up with some of the clinical needs in this area.

Reticulocytes

Another area of special consideration is that of reticulocyte analysis by flow cytometry. This issue has been addressed by the NCCLS in its document H44-A: *Methods for Reticulocyte Counting (Flow Cytometry and Supravital Dyes); Approved Guideline (1997).* Many of the issues addressed for analysis of leukocytes do not pertain to reticulocyte analysis. However, the need for QC/QA in reticulocyte analysis is as strong as for any other application.

Tissue Cross-matching

HLA cross-matching is performed by flow cytometry in some laboratories. These standards apply to histocompatibility testing and leukocyte phenotyping by flow cytometry:

Standards for Histocompatibility Testing: Section Q (Flow Cytometry)
Copyright © 1995, 1995, 1996, 1997, 1998 American Society for Histocompatibility and Immunogenetics.

Pattern Recognition as Quality Assurance

When flow cytometers are operated under standardized conditions each day, quantitative or semiquantitative measures become more reliable. One of the parameters that has been found useful is that of using the FI of immunostained cells for identification of histogram patterns that may aid in diagnosis or in quality assurance.

Pathologists and other laboratory scientists are familiar with the concept of pattern recognition in other disciplines such as clinical chemistry, in which electrolytes are usually present in a consistent pattern, and this can be used for internal quality assurance. An example of pattern recognition in flow cytometry is the use of the lymphosum based on percentages of positivity for peripheral blood subsets, in which the percentage of lymphocytes measured as $CD3^+$ T cells, $CD20^+$ B cells, and $CD16/56^+$ NK (natural killer) cells should approximate 100% in each patient specimen. Quantitative analysis of FI lends itself well to pattern recognition. Therefore, it may be possible, and in fact desirable, to use pattern recognition of each patient sample as its own QC. In such a process, consideration should be given to both the lymphosum, as a measure of percent positivity, and the relative FI, as a measure of the quality of the immunostained cells by the MoAb. Laboratorians are familiar with the typical placement and pattern of specific reagent combinations such as CD3/CD4, and consciously or subconsciously use pattern recognition on the histogram pattern to detect problems. Visual examination of histograms from flow cytometry can be very helpful in the context of detecting problems. These can run the gamut from light scatter alterations (potentially poor samples) to alterations in fluorescence intensity that may signal reagent problems.

To properly use pattern recognition, it is necessary to standardize sample preparation and instrument setup. Under standardized conditions, the light scatter of normal peripheral blood cells (or other cells) should be relatively consistent. If there is a sudden change in the light scatter pattern, it may signal a partial obstruction or a problem with specimen integrity. Fluorescence intensity of immunostained cells provides a reasonably consistent pattern on normal cells over time and between subjects (**Figure 5-7**, p 139). For this reason, it is possible to set limits of FI that should accompany a specific CD combination and monitor this parameter on Levy-Jennings charts. When the signal falls below (or above) this designated level, it should suggest that either the reagent is faulty (occurs slowly) or the wrong reagent has been added to the tube.

When immunophenotyping leukemias and lymphomas, FI can play an adjunctive role in histogram analysis. It has been shown that FI of malignancies can suggest possible diagnoses.[44] Therefore, it is important to standardize these measurements in order to use this parameter effectively.

Pattern recognition in CD34 testing is also important and must be standardized. For instance, these cells typically express low levels of CD45 (as opposed to bright), low side scatter, and commonly a dual population of dim and bright CD34+ cells. Therefore, reliance on FI is important in this type of analysis.

Laboratory Reports for Quality Assurance

The main purpose of clinical and surgical pathology reports is to convey meaningful information in a timely fashion to those caring for patients. Report content and report standardization issues have been a popular topic in the surgical pathology literature and have had their importance recognized. Flow cytometry has undergone an evolution into clinical use, but is still in an early stage of standardizing certain elements, such as reporting, that are important for good medical management.

Through the LAP Laboratory General Inspection Checklist,[26] the CAP addresses certain issues common to all laboratory reports but not to flow cytometry specifically. A European group[24] provided certain guidelines for flow cytometry reporting in its consensus document which have merit. Report content for leukemia/lymphoma immunophenotyping was also addressed by a US-Canadian consensus panel in the form of recommendations on data reporting.[45] Using a questionnaire format, Hassett and Parker[46] collected information from a number of laboratories describing their reporting practices.

Participants in the CAP 1997 FL3 Leukemia/Lymphoma Survey were requested to submit copies of clinical flow cytometry reports for the survey specimens as if they represented patient reports. These were examined to determine the presence or absence of certain data elements considered important in recent consensus panel recommendations, and in previous survey results.

The reports involved cases of chronic lymphocytic leukemia of B-cell type (FL3-01), acute lymphoblastic leukemia of B-cell precursor type (FL3-02), acute myeloid leukemia (FL3-03), and acute lymphoblastic leukemia of T-cell type (FL3-04). Therefore, the laboratory reports from participants included a typical cross section of specimen and disease types.

Of 574 evaluable submissions from 287 laboratories, certain items were present in > 90% of clinical reports. These included the name or identification of the patient (98.5%), source of specimen (96.2%), date of the report (92.5%), use of CD nomenclature (100%), percent positive staining (92.5%), identification of a specific disease (94.3%), and the identity of the laboratory director (94.3%). A number of additional data elements were present in > 80% of reports: patient age (84.9%), ordering physician (88.7%), a specimen identification number (86.4%), the main cellular reactivity of each CD (83.0%), and the name/address of the laboratory (81.1%). The composite immunophenotype of the cells was identified in 75.5% of reports. For most of the data elements thought to be important by consensus groups, the CAP participants met or exceeded these recommendations.

Examination of laboratory reports is useful for determining clerical errors, but also for longitudinal comparisons of patient data. For instance, if a patient was originally diagnosed with a small non-cleaved cell lymphoma expressing CD19, CD20, and kappa immunoglobulin light chains, but returns 2 years later with a mass that also expresses CD19, CD20, and lambda immunoglobulin light chains, this should be cause for more intensive investigation. It is certainly possible for a patient to have a second malignancy such as this, but it is extremely uncommon.

Comparisons with Cytology and Histology as Quality Assurance Tools

Routine comparison of the flow cytometric analysis to that of cytology or histology is quite useful in the context of lymphoid and hematologic malignancies.[9] This is particularly useful with lymphoid tissues, where the clinical differential diagnosis is typically reactive hyperplasia versus lymphoma. Comparisons can help determine if sampling bias may have occurred, or, in some cases, if specimen mix-ups occurred. It gives an indication of how well the laboratory can detect the pertinent disease processes. Morphology is particularly useful when using density gradient separations for leukemia evaluation of bone marrow. It is important to know that the neoplastic cells are still present in the specimen. It is also very useful for specimens of soft tissue masses or lymph nodes obtained by needle aspiration, again to ascertain the presence of the cells of interest.

In a laboratory survey of practices, McCoy and Keren[8] found that 52.7% of those performing leukemia/lymphoma immunophenotyping do not perform morphologic examinations, but in almost all cases, the morphology is correlated with the flow cytometry data at some point. Consensus groups advocate inclusion of morphology as an integral part of the diagnostic process.[9]

Acknowledgement

I would like to express my gratitude for the assistance of colleagues at the College of American Pathologists, Patricia Styer, Ph.D., and Dina Rappette, MT(ASCP), as well as the members of the Diagnostic Immunology Resource Committee, who were very helpful in collecting and analyzing data from the Flow Cytometry Proficiency Surveys. This information was used by kind permission of the CAP.

References

1. Medicare, Medicaid and CLIA programs: regulations implementing the Clinical Laboratory Improvement Amendments of 1988 (CLIA), 42 CFR Parts 405 et al. Federal Register 7002–7243 (1992).

2. Pinckus MR. Interpreting laboratory results: reference values and decision making. In: Henry JB, ed. *Clinical Diagnosis and Management by Laboratory Methods*, 19th ed. Philadelphia, Pa: WB Saunders Co; 1996:74–91.

3. McCoy JP Jr, Carey JL, Krause JR. Quality control in flow cytometry for diagnostic pathology, I: cell surface phenotyping and general laboratory procedures. *Am J Clin Pathol*. 1990;93(suppl 1):S27–S37.

4. Stelzer GT, Marti G, Hurley A, et al. U.S.-Canadian consensus recommendations on the immunophenotypic analysis of hematologic neoplasia by flow cytometry: standardization and validation of laboratory procedures. *Cytometry (Comm Clin Cytometry)*. 1997;30:214–230.

5. Chase ES, Hoffman RA. Resolution of dimly fluorescent particles: a practical measure of fluorescence sensitivity. *Cytometry*. 1998;33:267–279.

6. Wood JCS, Hoffman RA. Evaluating fluorescence sensitivity on flow cytometers: an overview. *Cytometry*. 1998;33:256–259.

7. National Committee for Clinical Laboratory Standards. Clinical applications of flow cytometry: quality assurance and immunophenotyping of peripheral blood lymphocytes. Approved Guideline. NCCLS document H42-A. Villanova, Pa: NCCLS; 1998.

8. McCoy JP Jr, Keren DF. Current practices in clinical flow cytometry: a practice survey by the American Society of Clinical Pathologists. *Am J Clin Pathol*. 1999;111(2):161–168.

9. Borowitz MJ, Bray R, Gascoyne R, et al. U.S.-Canadian consensus recommendations on the immunophenotypic analysis of hematologic neoplasia by flow cytometry: data analysis and interpretation. *Cytometry (Comm Clin Cytometry)*. 1997;30:236–244.

10. Edwards BS, Altobelli KK, Nolla HA, et al. Comprehensive quality assessment approach for flow cytometric immunophenotyping of human lymphocytes. *Cytometry*. 1989;10:433–441.

11. Gelman R, Cheng S-C, Kidd P, et al. Assessment of the effects of instrumentation, monoclonal antibody, and fluorochrome on flow cytometric immunophenotyping: a report based on 2 years of the NIAID DAIDS flow cytometry quality assessment program. *Clin Immunol Immunopathol*. 1993;66:150–162.

12. Centers for Disease Control and Prevention. 1997 revised guidelines for performing CD4+ T-cell determinations in persons infected with human immunodeficiency virus (HIV). Morbidity and Mortality Weekly Report. 1997;46(No. RR-2):1–29.

13. Tonks DB. A study of the accuracy and precision of clinical chemistry determinations in 170 Canadian laboratories. *Clin Chem*. 1963;9:217–233.

14. Barnett RN. Medical significance of laboratory results. *Am J Clin Pathol.* 1968;50:671–676.

15. Fraser CG, Hyltoft Petersen P. Desirable standards for laboratory tests if they are to fulfill medical needs. *Clin Chem.* 1993;39:1447–1455.

16. Cotlove E, Harris EK, Williams GZ. Biological and analytic components of variation in long-term studies of serum constituents in normal subjects, III: physiological and medical implications. *Clin Chem.* 1970;16:1028–1032.

17. Elevitch FR, ed. College of American Pathologists Conference Report. Conference on analytical goals in clinical chemistry, at Aspen, Colo. Skokie, Ill: College of American Pathologists; 1976.

18. Giorgi JV, Cheng H-L, Margolick JB, et al, and the Multicenter AIDS Cohort Study Group. Quality control in the flow cytometric measurement of T-lymphocyte subsets: the Multicenter AIDS Cohort Study experience. *Clin Immunol Immunopathol.* 1990;55:173–186.

19. Doumas BT. The evolution and limitations of accuracy and precision standards. *Clin Chim Acta.* 1997;260:145–162.

20. Mellors JW, Munoz A, Giorgi J, et al. Plasma viral load and CD4+ lymphocytes as prognostic markers of HIV-1 infection. *Ann Intern Med.* 1997;126:946–954.

21. McCoy JP, Overton WR. Quality control in flow cytometry for diagnostic pathology, II: a conspectus of reference ranges for lymphocyte immunophenotyping. *Cytometry (Comm Clin Cytometry).* 1994;18:129–139.

22. Sreenan JJ, Tbakhi A, Edinger MG, et al. The use of isotypic control antibodies in the analysis of CD3+ and CD3+, CD4+ lymphocyte subsets by flow cytometry: are they really necessary? *Arch Pathol Lab Med.* 1997;121:118–121.

23. College of American Pathologists, Commission of Laboratory Accreditation. Flow Cytometry Inspection Checklist, 1997.0. Northfield, Ill: College of American Pathologists; 1997.

24. Rothe G, Schmitz G. Consensus protocol for the flow cytometric immunophenotyping of hematopoietic malignancies: working group on flow cytometry and image analysis. *Leukemia.* 1996;10:877–895.

25. Bernard A, Boumsell L, Dausett J, et al, eds. *Leukocyte Typing.* Berlin: Springer-Verlag; 1984.

26. College of American Pathologists, Commission of Laboratory Accreditation. Laboratory General Inspection Checklist, 1996.2. Northfield, Ill: College of American Pathologists; 1996.

27. Davis KA, Abrams B, Iyer SB, et al. Determination of CD4 antigen density on cells: role of antibody valency, avidity, clones, and conjugation. *Cytometry.* 1998;33:197–205.

28. Purvis N, Stelzer G. Multi-platform, multi-site instrumentation and reagent standardization. *Cytometry.* 1998;33:156–65.

29. Medical Devices; Classification/Reclassification; Restricted Devices; Analyte Specific Reagents. 21 CFR 809. Final rule. Federal Register 62:62243–62260 (1997).

30. Stewart CC, Behm FG, Carey JL, et al. U.S.-Canadian consensus recommendations on the immunophenotypic analysis of hematologic neoplasia by flow cytometry: selection of antibody combinations. *Cytometry (Comm Clin Cytometry)*. 1997;30:231-235.

31. Jennings CD, Foon KA. Recent advances in flow cytometry: application to the diagnosis of hematologic malignancy. *Blood*. 1997;90:2863-2892.

32. Braylan RC, Borowitz MJ, Davis BH, et al. U.S.-Canadian consensus recommendations on the immunophenotypic analysis of hematologic neoplasia by flow cytometry. *Cytometry (Comm Clin Cytometry)*. 1997;30:245-248.

33. Barnett D, Granger V, Storie I, et al. Quality assessment of CD34+ stem cell enumeration: experience of the United Kingdom National External Quality Assessment Scheme (UK NEQUAS) using a unique stable whole blood preparation. *Br J Haematol*. 1998;102:553-565.

34. Kluin-Nelemans JC, van Wering ER, van'T Veer MB, et al. Pitfalls in the immunophenotyping of leukemia and leukaemic lymphomas: survey of 9 years of quality control in the Netherlands. Dutch Cooperative Study Group on Immunophenotyping of Haematological Malignancies (SIHON). *Br J Haematol*. 1996;95:692-696.

35. Brando B, Sommaruga E. Nationwide quality control trial on lymphocyte immunophenotyping and flow cytometer performance in Italy. *Cytometry*. 1993;14:294-306.

36. Vesely R, Barths J, Vanlangendonck F, et al. Initial results of Central European Immunophenotyping Quality Control Program (CEQUAL). *Cytometry*. 1996;26:108-112.

37. Goguel AF, Crainic K, Ducailar A, et al. Interlaboratory quality assessment of lymphocyte phenotyping: Etalonorme 1990-1992 surveys. *Biol Cell*. 1993;78:79-84.

38. Bergeron M, Faucher S, Minkus T, et al. Impact of unified procedures as implemented in the Canadian Quality Assurance Program for T lymphocyte subset enumeration. *Cytometry*. 1998;33:146-155.

39. Homburger HA, McCarthy R, Deodhar S. Assessment of interlaboratory variability in analytical cytology. *Arch Pathol Lab Med*. 1989;113:667-672.

40. Homburger HA, Rosenstock W, Paxton H, et al. Assessment of interlaboratory variability of immunophenotyping. In: Landay AL, Ault KA, Bauer KD, et al, eds. *Annals of the New York Academy of Sciences, Clinical Flow Cytometry*. Vol 677. New York, NY: The New York Academy of Sciences; 1993:43-49.

41. Tholen D, Lawson NS, Cohen T, et al. Proficiency test performance and experience with College of American Pathologists' programs. *Arch Pathol Lab Med*. 1995;119:307-311.

42. National Committee for Clinical Laboratory Standards. Clinical applications of flow cytometry: immunophenotyping of leukemic cells. Approved Guideline. NCCLS document H43-A. Villanova, Pa: NCCLS; 1998.

43. Gratama JW, Orfao A, Barnett D, et al. Flow cytometric enumeration of CD34+ hematopoietic stem and progenitor cells. *Cytometry (Comm Clin Cytometry)*. 1998;34:128-142.

44. Caldwell CW, Patterson WP. Relationship between CD45 antigen expression and putative stages of differentiation in B-cell malignancies. *Am J Clin Pathol.* 1991;36:111–115.

45. Braylan RC, Atwater SK, Diamond L, et al. U.S.-Canadian consensus recommendations on the immunophenotypic analysis of hematologic neoplasia by flow cytometry: data reporting. *Cytometry (Comm Clin Cytometry).* 1997;30:245–248.

46. Hassett J, Parker J. Laboratory practices in reporting flow cytometry phenotyping results for leukemia/lymphoma specimens: results of a survey. *Cytometry (Comm Clin Cytometry).* 1995;22:264–281.

6

Development of a Relational Flow Cytometry Database Application

Charles W. Caldwell
Adam L. Asare
Harpreet K. Monga

Overview

Databases, repositories of accurate and easily accessible data, are integral to laboratory decision support. A database management system (DBMS) is software that helps users manage a database by providing storage and retrieval operations, granting of access privileges, automation of repetitive tasks, and logging of transactions. One popular DBMS application is Microsoft Access®, which is part of the professional edition of the Microsoft Office® Suite. The sample applications and much of the database design theory described in this chapter are explained using Access. For this reason, it will be helpful for readers to create some of the sample tables in this chapter using Access for a better understanding of the concepts presented.

One may wonder how databases differ from spreadsheets, which are much more commonly used for generating reports and summarizing data. Typically these data are entered into a gridlike entry screen. Database applications, however, offer added functionality over spreadsheets by allowing searches, or *queries,* across a large number of data elements that would typically be found in separate spreadsheet files. At first glance, entering data into a database table resembles entering data into a spreadsheet. However, the underlying mechanism for generating reports and charts is far more powerful in relational databases than in spreadsheets.

The drawback to databases is that there is somewhat of a learning curve for designing the underlying data storage model and the forms that will be used for inserting data into this structure. For this reason, this chapter begins with an introduction to relational database design theory, followed by a brief tutorial for building a flow cytometry laboratory database application. Applying the design concepts presented in the first part of the chapter to the tutorial in the second part will provide the reader with a hands-on approach to developing a DBMS for a clinical flow cytometry laboratory.

Relational Database Design Concepts

The Relational Model

When designing a database, one must figure out an effective data storage model that best represents a laboratory's activities. Decisions are made on the number of tables to build, the columns they will contain, and the relationships among data elements across different tables. While a well-designed database takes time and effort, some of the benefits of using a database application that makes use of a relational model include:

- Data entry, with efficient updating and deletion of prior data
- Data retrieval, with efficient summarization and reporting
- Predictable behavior, by following a well-thought-out model
- Modifiable architecture, whereby changes to the database schema are easy to make

The following discussion on relational design is by no means comprehensive; this chapter is meant as an informal introduction to database design theory for laboratory personnel. While the examples in this chapter use Access, the concepts presented also apply to database development using tools such as the Microsoft SQL Server™ or Oracle DBMS.

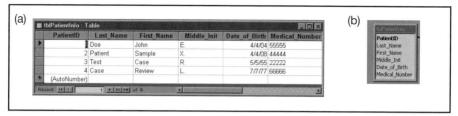

Figure 6-1
In this case, the best choice for primary key for the Patient Info table is Patient ID.
*Note: The naming of the application's tables, queries, and forms are prefixed with "tbl,"
"qry," and "frm," respectively.*

Tables and Uniqueness

Each table in the relational model is used to represent "things" or objects in the real world. These objects can also be called *entities,* hence the term *entity-relationship diagram* for showing the objects and the relationships they have with one another.

A real-world object can be a patient, a specimen, or a report. An event can be patient visits, orders, or results reported. **Figure 6-1(a)** shows a patient table that represents multiple patient objects. **Figure 6-1(b)** shows the same table in design mode, where the names of the column headings of the patient table are listed vertically. The user should be comfortable with switching between the design and data-entry modes for each table before continuing. First-time database users are occasionally confused between data stored in database tables and the column headings being used to describe the stored data.

The relational model requires that the data in each row of a table be unique. If duplicate rows are allowed in a table, there is no way to uniquely address a given row programmatically. Uniqueness for a row occurs through the designation of a *primary key*—a column in the table that contains values that uniquely identify each data row. Each table should have only 1 primary key, which can be simple or composite. A *simple key* is a key made up of 1 unique column, whereas a *composite key* is made up of 2 or more columns whose combination of values is unique.

The decision as to what data element to assign as the primary key is subjective—there is no absolute rule as to what constitutes the best primary key. The decision should be based upon the principles of minimality (choose what leads to the use of the fewest number of columns), stability (choose a key that will not change), and simplicity/familiarity (choose a key that is both simple and familiar to users). For example, a database might have a table of patients called Patient Info, which appears in **Figure 6-1**.

Candidate keys for the patient information table might include Last Name + First Name, Date of Birth, Hospital Medical Record Number or a system-generated number (Patient ID). Following minimalist guidelines, the name composite (Last Name + First Name) should be ruled out because of its potential instability—names can change—and because more than 1 patient may have the same first and last names. Date of Birth should also be ruled out because a number of patients could have the same date of birth. In a single institution, a hospital medical record number may be considered unique; however, if specimens are received from multiple sites with different numbering systems, duplications are possible. One should favor numeric primary keys because names do sometimes change and because searches and sorts of numeric columns are more efficient than of text columns in most database programming environments.

Patient ID does not allow manual entry of data into the field. Instead, Patient ID has been configured as an "AutoNumber" column that automatically generates an integer value through an internal counter. Autogenerated integer columns make good primary keys, especially when there is difficulty in coming up with good candidates for a primary key and when no existing arbitrary identification number is already in place. One should not use a counter column if there will be a need to renumber the values (this is not possible with autogenerated numeric columns) or if an alphanumeric ID is required (Microsoft Access supports only numeric counter values).

Foreign Keys and Domains

If databases were created that consisted of only independent and unrelated tables, there would be little need for primary keys, and we'd be just as well off entering data into a spreadsheet. Primary keys become essential, however, when creating relationships that join multiple tables in a database. A *foreign key* is a column in a table used to reference a primary key in another table. Continuing with the example, Patient ID was selected as the primary key for the Patient Info table. Now a second table is defined, the Request table shown in **Figure 6-2**.

The values in the Patient ID column are called foreign keys in the Request table because those values can be used to refer to a specific patient (ie, a row in the Patient Info table). It is important that both foreign keys and the primary keys used to reference data from various tables share a common meaning and draw their values from the same *domain*. Domains are simply pools of values from which the data are drawn. For example, Patient ID is of the domain of valid tblRequest : Table

Request_ID	Patient_ID	Date_Received
2	1	1/5/99
3	3	1/15/99
4	1	1/31/99
5	2	2/12/99
6	1	2/27/99
7	2	3/14/99
(AutoNumber)	0	

Record: 1 of 6

Figure 6-2
Patient ID is a foreign key in the Request table that can be used to reference a patient stored in the Patient Info table.

patient ID numbers, which in this case might be numbers ranging between 1 and 50,000. Similarly, a column named Sex might be based on a 1-letter domain equaling "M" or "F."

Relationships

Foreign keys in a database are defined to model relationships in the real world. Such relationships between real-world entities can be complex, involving numerous entities each having multiple relationships with one another. For example, a family has multiple relationships among multiple individuals—all at the same time. In a relational database, however, we'll consider relationships between pairs of tables. These tables can be related in 1 of 3 different ways: *one-to-one, one-to-many,* or *many-to-many.*

One-to-One Relationships

Two tables are related in a one-to-one (1-1) relationship if for every row in the first table, there is at most 1 row in the second table. True one-to-one relationships seldom occur in the real world. This type of relationship is often created to circumvent some limitation of the database management software rather than to model a real-world situation. One-to-one relationships may be necessary in a database when it is necessary to split a table into 2 or more other tables because of security or performance concerns. For example, most patient information might be kept in the Patient Info table, but especially sensitive information (eg, patient name, social security number, and address) might reside in the Confidential table. **Figure 6-3** shows an entity-relationship diagram presented in Access between the Patient Info and Confidential tables, where the "1" on both sides of the relationship designates the relationship as one-to-one. When

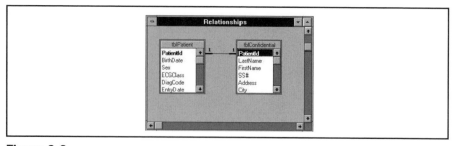

Figure 6-3
The Patient Info and Confidential tables are related in a one-to-one relationship. The primary key of both tables is Patient ID.

showing entity relationships, the tables are presented in design mode, with the column heading appearing in a vertical list. Data stored within tables are neither visible nor relevant when analyzing entity relationships. In **Figure 6-3,** access to data in the Confidential table could be more restricted than that in the Patient Info table. As a second example, there may be a need to transfer only a portion of a large table to some other application on a regular basis for archival storage. In this instance, a table can be split into the transferred and the nontransferred table and then rejoined in a one-to-one relationship. Tables that are related in a one-to-one relationship *should always have the same primary key* that serves as the join column.

One-to-Many Relationships

Two tables are related in a one-to-many (1-M or 1-) relationship if for every row in the first table, there are 0, 1, or many rows in the second table, but for every row in the second table there is exactly 1 row in the first table. For example, each patient can have multiple test requests over time, but each test request can only be related to only 1 patient. The one-to-many relationship is also referred to as a parent-child or master-detail relationship. One-to-many relationships are the most commonly modeled relationship type. **Figure 6-4** shows this type of relationship, where the Patient Info table has a "1" on its side of the relationship while the Request table has an "•" symbol designating the 0, 1, or many instances of the patient ID found in the Patient Info table.

One-to-many relationships are also used to link base tables to information stored in *lookup tables.* A lookup table contains detailed information about columns in a primary table and is created primarily to preserve the uniqueness and simplicity of the primary table. For example, the Patient Info table might have an integer code or ID for physicians that is linked to a lookup table, Physician, which stores more thorough physician data. In this case, the Physician

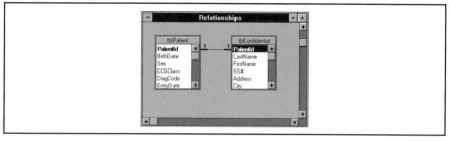

Figure 6-4
There can be many test requests for each patient, so tblPatient Info and the Request table are related in a one-to-many relationship.

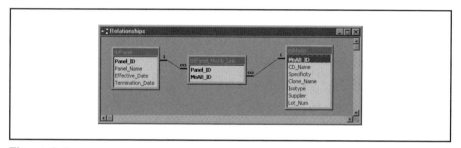

Figure 6-5
A linking table, Panel MoAb Link, is used to model the many-to-many relationship between the Panel and MoAb tables.

table is related to the Patient Info table in a one-to-many relationship. Once again, by the one-to-many definition, 1 row in the Physician lookup table is used in 0 or more rows in the Patient Info table.

Many-to-Many Relationships

Two tables are related in a many-to-many (M-M) relationship when for every row in the first table, there can be many rows in the second table, and for every row in the second table, there can be many rows in the first table. Many-to-many relationships can't be directly modeled in relational database programs. These types of relationships must be broken into multiple one-to-many relationships as shown in **Figure 6-5**. For example, an antibody panel may have many monoclonal antibodies (MoAbs), and each MoAb may be used in many different panels. In this case, a Panel table would be related to the MoAb table in a many-to-many relationship. To model this relationship effectively, it is recommended that one create a third, linking table, called a Panel MoAb Link table.

This table would contain a row for each unique combination of Panel ID and MoAb ID. By the way, the 2 fields (Panel ID and MoAb ID) together in **Figure 6-5** form a compound key for this table, and both appear in bold text. Neither value, in and of itself, can uniquely identify the column; both values need to be used together to define uniqueness for each row in the Link table. The many-to-many relationship between the Panel and MoAb tables can now be broken into 2 one-to-many relationships; the Panel table is related to the Panel MoAb Link table and the MoAb table is related to the Panel MoAb Link table in one-to-many relationships.

Normalization

As mentioned earlier, database design involves a series of choices to be made in designing the tables and relationships for storing data within the database. These include:

- How many tables will there be and what will they represent?
- Which columns will go in which tables?
- What will the relationships between the tables be?

The answers to each of these questions derive from a term called *normalization*, which is the process of constructing and linking tables correctly so that they are essentially "normal." Typically, the process for large information systems such as those designed for hospitals results from deep insights into the information used in health care systems and how the various elements of that information are related to one another. In the limited scope of this chapter, we will only briefly touch upon the normalization theory; however, one should be aware that the use of *normal forms* in database design is critical in achieving an optimal table structure. The use of normal forms leads to minimal data redundancy and increased data accuracy. Normal forms are a linear progression of rules that are applied to a database, with each higher normal form achieving a better, more efficient design. The most commonly used normal forms are First Normal Form, Second Normal Form, and Third Normal Form.

Tables in normal form have the following attributes:

- The table has no duplicate rows; hence there is always a primary key.
- The columns in the table are unordered.
- The rows in the table are unordered.

Figure 6-6
The Request1 table violates First Normal Form because the data stored in the Results column are not atomic.

Microsoft Access does not require definition of a primary key for each and every table, but it is strongly recommended. Needless to say, the relational model makes this an absolute requirement. In addition, tables in Microsoft Access automatically meet the second and third attributes listed above for normal forms since the manipulation of tables in Access doesn't depend upon a specific ordering of columns or rows.

First Normal Form

First Normal Form (1NF) requires that all column values be atomic. In other words, for every row-by-column position in a given table, there exists only 1 value, not an array or list of values. If lists of values are stored in a single column, there is no simple way to manipulate those values, as shown in **Figure 6-6**. Retrieval of data from the Results column becomes difficult. So in this example, the table shown in **Figure 6-6** violates First Normal Form.

First Normal Form also prohibits the presence of repeating groups, even if they are stored in multiple columns. For example, the same table from **Figure 6-6** could be redesigned as shown in **Figure 6-7**, where , the Results column has been replaced with 6 columns: MoAb1, Value1, MoAb2, Value2, MoAb3, and Value3.

While this design has divided the information into multiple fields, it is still problematic. For example, how would the values of CD4 be determined for all patients during a particular month? Any type of query of this table would have to search all 3 MoAb columns (MoAb1, MoAb2, MoAb3) to determine if a CD4 was reported and then compute a summation over the 3 Value columns. Even worse, what if a patient had more than 3 MoAbs used in a single panel? Additional columns could be added, but where would this stop? MoAb10, MoAb20? If it were decided that a physician would never order more than

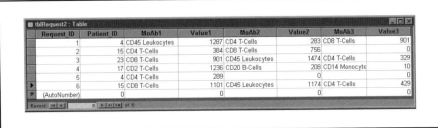

Figure 6-7
A better, but still flawed, version of the Request table, Request2. The repeating groups of information violate First Normal Form.

Request ID	Patient ID	MoAb1	Value1	MoAb2	Value2	MoAb3	Value3
1	4	CD45 Leukocytes	1287	CD4 T-Cells	283	CD8 T-Cells	901
2	15	CD4 T-Cells	384	CD8 T-Cells	756		0
3	23	CD8 T-Cells	901	CD45 Leukocytes	1474	CD4 T-Cells	329
4	17	CD2 T-Cells	1236	CD20 B-Cells	208	CD14 Monocyte	10
5	4	CD4 T-Cells	289		0		0
6	15	CD8 T-Cells	1101	CD45 Leukocytes	1174	CD4 T-Cells	429
(AutoNumber)	0		0		0		0

Request ID	Patient ID	MoAb#	MoAb	Value
1	4	1	CD45 Leukocytes	1287
1	4	2	CD4 T-Cells	283
1	4	3	CD8 T-Cells	901
2	15	1	CD4 T-Cells	384
2	15	2	CD8 T-Cells	756
3	23	1	CD8 T-Cells	901
3	23	2	CD45 Leukocytes	1474
3	23	3	CD4 T-Cells	329
4	17	1	CD2 T-Cells	1236
4	17	2	CD20 B-Cells	208
4	17	3	CD14 Monocytes	10
5	4	1	CD4 T-Cells	289
6	15	1	CD8 T-Cells	1101
6	15	2	CD45 Leukocytes	1174
6	15	3	CD4 T-Cells	429
0	0	0		0

Figure 6-8
The Request3 table is in First Normal Form.

25 MoAbs in any one panel, the table could be designed accordingly. In this case, the application would use 50 columns to store the MoAb and Value information per patient test record, even for orders that involved only 2 or 3 MoAbs. Clearly this is a waste of space. Furthermore, it is likely that someone would eventually want to order more than 25 MoAbs.

The table in **Figure 6-8** is in First Normal Form because each column contains 1 value and there are no repeating groups of columns. In order to attain First Normal Form, the column MoAb# was added. The primary key of this table is a composite key made up of the Request ID and the MoAb#. A query tblRequest4 : Table

Request_ID	Patient_ID	Order_Date	MoAb#	MoAb_ID	MoAb	Value
1	4	1/5/99	1	67	CD45 Leukocytes	1287
1	4	1/5/99	2	119	CD4 T-Cells	283
1	4	1/5/99	3	23	CD8 T-Cells	901
2	15	1/24/99	1	119	CD4 T-Cells	384
2	15	1/24/99	2	23	CD8 T-Cells	756
3	23	1/30/99	1	23	CD8 T-Cells	901
3	23	1/30/99	2	67	CD45 Leukocytes	1474
3	23	1/30/99	3	119	CD4 T-Cells	329
4	17	2/7/99	1	12	CD2 T-Cells	1236
4	17	2/7/99	2	71	CD20 B-Cells	208
4	17	2/7/99	3	5	CD14 Monocytes	10
5	4	2/15/99	1	119	CD4 T-Cells	289
6	15	3/12/99	1	23	CD8 T-Cells	1101
6	15	3/12/99	2	67	CD45 Leukocytes	1174
6	15	3/12/99	3	119	CD4 T-Cells	429
0	0		0	0		0

Record: 15 of 15

Figure 6-9

The Request4 table is in First Normal Form. Its primary key is a composite of Request ID and MoAb#.

could now easily be constructed to calculate the number of panels ordered that included CD4.

Second Normal Form

A table is said to be in Second Normal Form (2NF) if it is in First Normal Form and every non-key column is fully dependent on the (entire) primary key. Put another way, tables should only store data relating to one thing (or entity), and that entity should be described by the primary key.

Figure 6-9 shows a slightly modified version of the Request table that is in First Normal Form. Each column is atomic, and there are no repeating groups. To determine if this table meets Second Normal Form, one first notes the primary key, which is a composite of Request ID and MoAb#. For the table to be Second Normal Form, each non-key column in the table (every column other than Request ID and MoAb#) needs to be fully dependent on the primary key.

One should systematically ask, "For each record, does the value of Request ID and MoAb# for a given record imply the value of every column in the table?" The answer to this question is no. Given the Request ID, the Patient ID and Order Date of the test can be determined, without having to know the MoAb#. Therefore, Order Date and Patient ID are not dependent on the entire primary key composed of both Request ID and MoAb#. For this reason the table in **Figure 6-9** is not in Second Normal Form.

Second Normal Form can be achieved by breaking this table into 2 tables. The process of breaking a non-normalized table into its normalized parts is

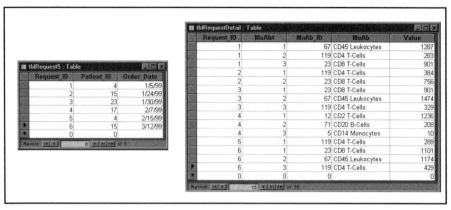

Figure 6-10
The Request5 and Request Detail tables satisfy Second Normal Form. Request ID is a foreign key in Request Detail that one can use to rejoin the tables.

---

called *decomposition*. Because the table in **Figure 6-9** has a composite primary key, the decomposition process is straightforward. Simply put everything that applies to each order in 1 table and everything that applies to each order item in a second table. The 2 decomposed tables are shown in **Figure 6-10**.

Two points are worth noting here. When normalizing, there is no loss of information, and the tables are decomposed in such a way as to allow them to be put back together again using queries. Therefore, it is important to make sure that the Request Detail table contains a foreign key to the Request table. The foreign key in this case is Request ID, which appears in both tables shown in **Figure 6-10**.

Third Normal Form

A table is said to be in Third Normal Form (3NF) if it is in Second Normal Form and if all non-key columns are mutually independent. The Request Detail table from **Figure 6-10**, for example, was said to be in Second Normal Form because all of its non-key columns (MoAb ID, MoAb, Value) are fully dependent on the primary key. That is, given a Request ID and a MoAb#, the values of MoAb ID, MoAb, and Value are known. Unfortunately, the Request Detail table contains a dependency between 2 of its non-key columns, MoAb ID and MoAb.

Such dependencies cause problems when records are added, updated, or deleted. For example, if the description of the item for MoAb ID 119 in **Figure 6-10** was changed from "CD4 T Cells" to "CD4⁺ T Cells" at some later time, all records with MoAb ID 119 would need to be updated. Another problem arises when deleting a set of records. If one were to inadvertently delete all instances of a particular MoAb ID when deleting a set of records, it would be difficult to know what that MoAb ID represented since the descriptor for the MoAb IDs was part of the deleted records. Such a problem, called a *deletion anomaly,* can be remedied by further normalizing the database to achieve Third Normal Form.

An anomaly is an error or inconsistency in the database. A poorly designed database runs the risk of introducing numerous anomalies. There are 3 types of anomalies:

- **Insertion**—an anomaly that occurs during the insertion of a record. For example, the insertion of a new row causes a calculated total field stored in another table to report the wrong total.
- **Deletion**—an anomaly that occurs during the deletion of a record. For example, the deletion of a row in the database deletes more information than one wished to delete.
- **Update**—an anomaly that occurs during the updating of a record. For example, updating a description column for a single MoAb in a database requires making a change to thousands of rows.

In **Figure 6-11**, the table is now further decomposed to achieve Third Normal Form by breaking out of the MoAb ID–MoAb dependency by using a lookup table. This provides a revised Request Detail table. When decomposing the Request Detail table shown in **Figure 6-11**, one should be careful to put a copy of the linking column, in this case MoAb ID, in both tables. In this case,

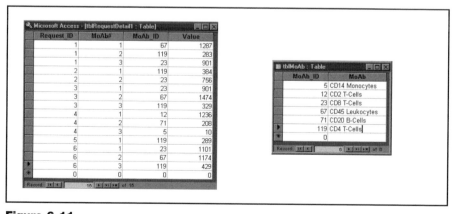

Figure 6-11
The Request Detail1 and MoAb tables are in Third Normal Form. The MoAb ID column in Request Detail1 is a foreign key referencing MoAb.

MoAb ID becomes the primary key of the new MoAb table and it also becomes a foreign key column in the Request Detail table. This allows for rejoining of the 2 tables using a query.

Integrity Rules

The relational model defines several integrity rules that are a necessary part of any relational database. There are 2 types of integrity rules: general and database-specific.

General Integrity Rules

The relational model specifies 2 *general integrity rules* that apply to all databases: the *entity integrity rule* and the *referential integrity rule*.

The entity integrity rule states that primary keys cannot contain *null*, or missing, data. The reason for this is that it is impossible to uniquely identify or reference a row in a table if the primary key of that table is equal to null. This rule applies to both simple and composite keys. For composite keys, none of the individual columns can be equal to null. Fortunately, Microsoft Access automatically enforces the entity integrity rule. No component of a primary key in Access can be equal to null.

The referential integrity rule states that the database can not contain any unmatched foreign key values. This implies that: (1) A row may not be added to a table with a foreign key unless the referenced value exists in the referenced (parent) table. (2) If the value in a table that is referenced by a foreign key is changed or the entire row in the referenced table is deleted, the rows in the table with the foreign key should not be "orphaned." In general, there are 3 options available when a referenced primary key value changes or a row is deleted. The options are:

- Disallow: The change is completely disallowed.
- Cascade update: For updates, the change is cascaded to all dependent tables.
- Cascade delete: For deletions, the rows in all dependent tables are deleted.

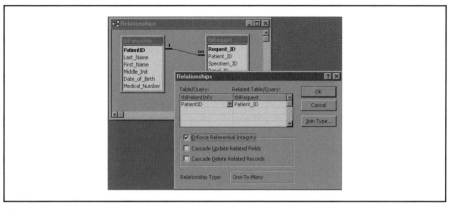

Figure 6-12
Specifying a relationship with referential integrity between the Patient Info and Request tables using the Edit\Relationships command. Updates of Patient ID in the Patient Info table will be cascaded to the Request table. Deletions of rows in Patient Info will be disallowed if rows in the Request table would be orphaned.

As shown in **Figure 6-12**, Microsoft Access has a form that accepts *disallow* or *cascade* referential integrity updates and deletions using the Edit\Relationships command.

Database-Specific Integrity Rules

Integrity constraints that do not fall under entity integrity or referential integrity are termed *database-specific rules,* or *business rules.* These rules are specific to each database and come from the rules of the laboratory being modeled by the database. It is important to note that the enforcement of business rules is as important as the enforcement of the general integrity rules discussed earlier.

Without the specification and enforcement of business rules, bad data will get in the database. For example, a laboratory might have the following rules that would need to be modeled in the database:

- A test order date should always be between the date the database was implemented and the current date (both dates inclusive).
- The order time and date can be only be in the form of a 24-hour clock (eg, 13:15) and a 4-digit year (eg, 2000).
- A reporting date must be greater than or equal to the ordering date.
- A patient medical record number must be within a certain range—dependent on the organization.

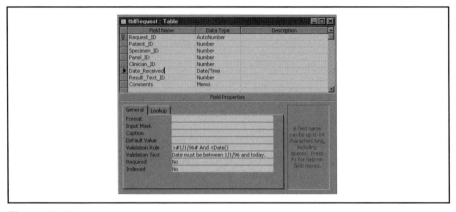

Figure 6-13
A column validation rule has been created to limit all order dates to some time between the database installation (1/1/96) and the current date.

Microsoft Access supports the specification of validation rules for each column in a table. For example, the first business rule from the above list has been specified in **Figure 6-13**.

Although business-rule support in Microsoft Access is better than in most other desktop DBMS programs, it is still limited. Additional business-rule logic will typically be built into applications/data-entry forms for insertion of data into tables. The logic in these forms is layered on top of any table-based rules, as shown in **Figure 6-13**. A way of enforcing constraints upon what is entered into a database table is to use drop-down list boxes. As shown in **Figure 6-19** (p 177), Panel Name is an example of a list box. When the down arrow of the box is clicked, there is an option of selecting only 1 panel. Behind the scenes, the primary key from a panel lookup table is being inserted into a reference table's foreign key column. This will be explained in greater detail in the next section. Such application/form-based rules, however, should be used only when the table-based rules cannot do the job. The more business rules that can be built in at the table level, the better, because these rules will always be enforced and will require less ongoing maintenance.

Prototype Flow Cytometry Application

A Practical Approach

As mentioned earlier in this chapter, database design is more art than science. While it is true that a properly designed database should follow normal forms and the relational model, the developer still has to come up with a design that reflects the business being modeled. Relational database design theory can usually dictate what *not* to do, but it won't determine where to start or how to manage a laboratory. This is where it helps to understand a business operation being modeled. Properly designing a database requires insight, time, and experience. Above all, it shouldn't be rushed.

Having a normalized table structure with integrity rules is not enough for one to start using a database within a laboratory. End-users expect screens with some aesthetic appeal, not tables, for data entry. Furthermore, the manipulation of primary and foreign keys among tables should appear transparent to end-users as data are added, edited, or deleted by laboratory personnel.

The database application presented in this section allows users to:

- Search for patients—to determine if a patient has previous results in the system
- Search for clinicians—to either look up or enter new physician information
- Create panels—using a library of predefined monoclonal antibodies
- Define reference ranges—using age-related reference range data
- Enter request information—where the test ordering process begins
- Write reports—where results are entered and final reports are generated

In this section, we begin the application development process by designing *forms* and *queries*. A form allows one to enter and retrieve data in a customized format. **Figure 6-14** (p 174) and **Figure 6-18** (p 176) show 2 different types of forms. The form in **Figure 6-14** represents the main screen of the demo application.

The application allows the user, by clicking on various command buttons, to proceed to a particular screen to insert, retrieve, update, or delete data. Aside from the Main Menu screen, most forms allow for the selective display of certain fields within a given table. **Figure 6-18** shows a form for data entry of MoAb information. This is an example of a *data-entry form*. Data-entry forms help users insert data into tables rapidly and accurately.

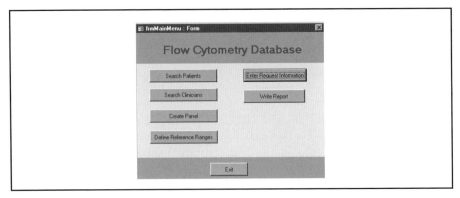

Figure 6-14
The Main Menu screen, or *switchboard,* provides an overview of the navigation to various areas of the application.

Queries are methods of manipulating and presenting stored data in a more user-friendly, understandable format. Queries function by extracting data from selected columns within tables. The columns can be from individual tables, or they can be from multiple tables where one selects specific fields, defines sort orders, creates calculated expressions, and enters selection criteria. Query results can be displayed in a data sheet that appears to the end user as a "virtual" table. The results from queries can also be displayed in forms or reports. The query in **Figure 6-15** is shown in design mode, where it is programmed to retrieve all records with the designation "CD4 T Cells" from the Request3 table. This query can be further modified to include tests sorted by a physician's name or for those tests ordered during a certain time period.

The database application described in the following sections is not intended to be complete—it is used to demonstrate how to move from the principles presented in the first section toward building a laboratory information system. In this case, we're assuming that all the hard work of normalizing table structures is complete, and it has led to the entity-relationship diagram shown in **Figure 6-16**. Note the primary key–foreign key relationships between the different tables. The goal of our application will be to insert and retrieve data from these various tables.

Data Entry of Lookup Data

Before using the application, certain reference, or lookup, tables will need to have data entered into them. Lookup tables allow for rapid data entry by not

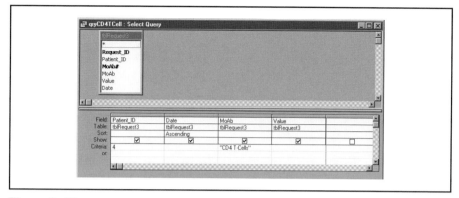

Figure 6-15
Because table Request3 (**Figure 6-8**, p 166) is in First Normal Form, one can easily construct a CD4 T Cell query to determine the total number of CD4s ordered by physicians.

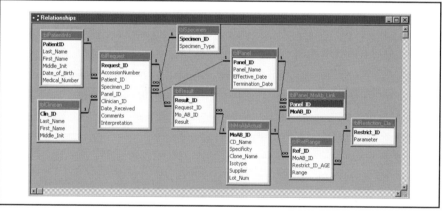

Figure 6-16
Entity-relationship (E-R) model for the flow cytometry laboratory application. Primary and foreign keys are identified for the relationships, as well as the tables and their field names.

requiring end users to retype data. Examples of data that could be stored in lookup tables include physician name, specimen types, and MoAbs that make up a panel.

Let's say we want to start entering data into the Clinician table (**Figure 6-17(b)**). This is also known as *populating* a table with data. **Figure 6-17** shows the New Clinician form that allows data entry directly into the Clinician table. One could say that the New Clinician form is *bound* to the Clinician table in terms of its data source. The form contains the same number of fields as the underlying data source table: it has fields for the first, middle, and last name, along with a Clinician ID field.

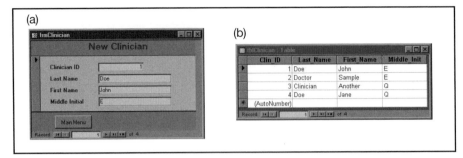

Figure 6-17
The form for entering new clinician data (a) and the associated table (b) illustrate the process of populating lookup tables.

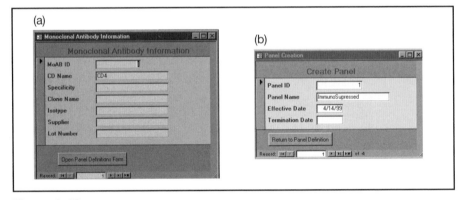

Figure 6-18
The Monoclonal Antibody Information form (a) and the Create Panel form (b) are used to populate lookup tables.

One can scroll through records in the Clinician table by using the Record Navigation button located at the bottom of the form. With each click, the fields in the form are altered to show data in subsequent rows in the table. Using the New Clinician form is more user-friendly than entering data directly into a table. Furthermore, the direct entry of data into tables by users not familiar with the underlying table architecture is inefficient, confusing, and error-prone.

Another example of a lookup table is the MoAb table that stores individual MoAbs or combinations of MoAbs, such as $CD3^+$ or $CD3^+CD4^+$. **Figure 6-18(a)** shows the Monoclonal Antibody Information form for populating the MoAb table, while **Figure 6-18(b)** shows the Create Panel form for populating the Panel table. The individual tables associated with these forms are shown in **Figure 6-20**.

Figure 6-19 shows the Panel MoAb Link form that automates copying of primary keys from both the MoAb table and the Panel table into the Panel MoAb

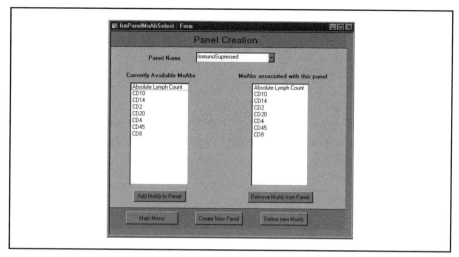

Figure 6-19

The Create Panel form allows the user to construct MoAb panels.

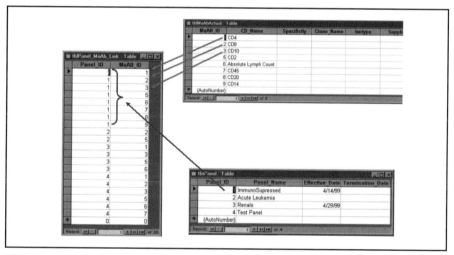

Figure 6-20

The tables and relationships underlying the Create Panel form.

Link table (**Figure 6-20**). The MoAb and Panel tables have a many-to-many relationship, as described in Part I. This relationship is broken down into 2 one-to-many relationships by using the Panel MoAb Link table. Refer to **Figure 6-16** (p 175) to verify this relationship.

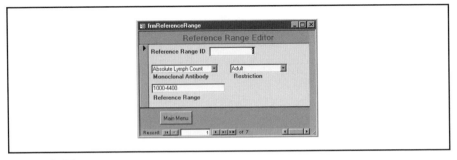

Figure 6-21
Data-entry form for setting reference ranges of each parameter based on age.

The Panel MoAb Link form in **Figure 6-19** has a drop-down box at the top titled Panel Name that references panel names and their corresponding primary keys from the Panel table. The keys are kept hidden from the end user. A list box on the form's left side titled Currently Available MoAbs references MoAbs and their keys from the MoAb table. In order to link the individual MoAbs with the panel name selected at the top of the form, the end-user selects a panel name along with any number of MoAbs from the Currently Available MoAbs list box. When the Add MoAb to Panel button is clicked, the individual keys of the selected MoAbs from the MoAb table and the single key of the selected panel from the Panel table are inserted into the Panel MoAb Link table. The list box titled "MoAbs Associated With this Panel" is bound to the Panel MoAb Link table and shows the end result of the automated insertion.

There is a fair bit of coding and querying of the database that take place for this form to function and it is not expected that the end user be able to construct such a form at first pass. Microsoft Access includes a number of "wizards" to automate some of the coding. For example, a List Box Wizard is used to bind the Currently Available MoAbs list box to the MoAb table, where it programmatically "hides" the key but displays the name. Clicking on the command button labeled Add MoAb to Panel activates the procedure for the copying of the MoAb key into the Panel MoAb Link table.

The final lookup table requiring data is the Reference Range table. The Reference Range form in **Figure 6-21** allows end users to enter absolute numbers or percentages for each MoAb or MoAb combination. Looking back at the entity-relationship diagram for the application (**Figure 6-16**, p 175), one could have done away with the Reference Range table by placing the table's Range column in the MoAb table. If this had been done, we could have included a field for entering the reference range into the Monoclonal Antibody Information form shown in (**Figure 6-18**, p 176). We are not doing this, however, because this would allow only 1 reference range per MoAb subset. To allow greater flexibility, reference

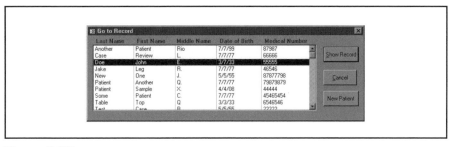

Figure 6-22
The Previous Patient screen with all patients in the Patient table sorted by Last Name.
Clicking the Show Record button causes the Patient ID associated with that record to
appear in the Patient Information form.

range data have been moved into their own table with a one-to-many relationship with the MoAb table. By doing this, a number of different reference ranges
can be presented for each MoAb based on age or other conditions.

Entry of a Request

Clicking the Enter Request Information button from the Main Menu
(**Figure 6-15**, p 175) opens a *pop-up form,* shown in **Figure 6-22,** that displays
all prior patient records stored within the Patient table. If the patient for whom
a test is being ordered appears within the list box, the name can be double-
clicked, which in turn activates the Show Record button. This leads to the copying of the highlighted record's Patient ID into a new row or in the Request table.
This form allows one to do away with having to retype a patient's name and
medical number each time a test is ordered on a previous patient. The creation
of a new row and copying of the key into the Request table is followed by display of the Request Data Entry form (**Figure 6-23(b)**) that is set for entering data
into the Request table. The form's fields will insert data specifically into the new
row that was just created in the Request table, with the correct Patient ID pasted
into the Patient ID column.

Had a test been ordered on a patient not listed in the Previous Patient form
shown in **Figure 6-22,** the end user could click the New Patient button. This
would lead to the insertion of a new row in the Patient table and the display of
the New Patient Data Entry form (**Figure 6-23(a)**).

By clicking the Enter Request Information button at the bottom of the form,
the data are saved to the Patient table and the Patient ID is autogenerated by the
table. The Patient ID is then copied and inserted into a new row in the Request

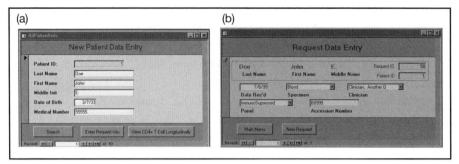

Figure 6-23
This New Patient Data Entry form (a) is displayed when the New Patient button is activated from **Figure 6-8** (p 166). The form allows entry of new patient demographic information. The Request Data Entry form (b) is activated when a name is double-clicked or the Show Record button is activated from **Figure 6-22**.

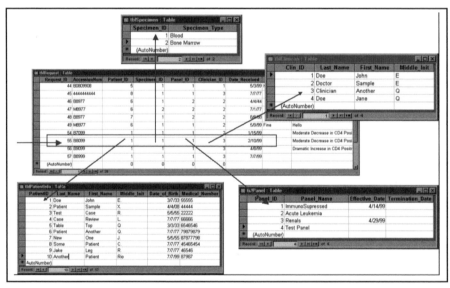

Figure 6-24
Illustration of the tables and data elements needed to comprise a request entry.

table, as discussed earlier for patients who had previously existed in the system. The Request Data Entry form is subsequently displayed, awaiting data for other columns in the Request table.

As shown in **Figure 6-24,** the Request table has 4 foreign keys that are referenced to lookup tables. The Request table automatically generates a unique Request ID each time a test is entered. The Request ID is displayed in the upper

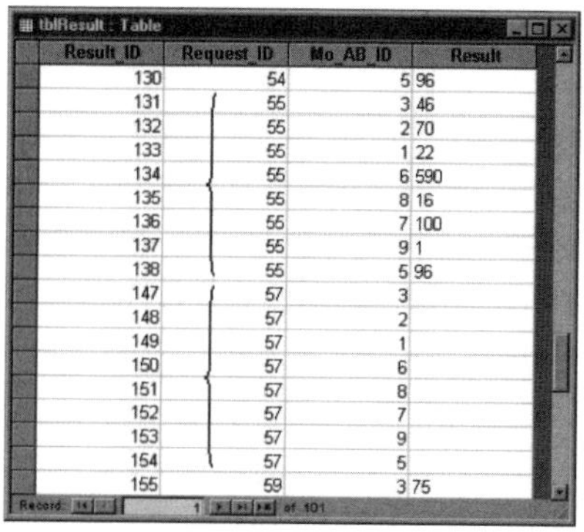

Result_ID	Request_ID	Mo_AB_ID	Result
130	54	5	96
131	55	3	46
132	55	2	70
133	55	1	22
134	55	6	590
135	55	8	16
136	55	7	100
137	55	9	1
138	55	5	96
147	57	3	
148	57	2	
149	57	1	
150	57	6	
151	57	8	
152	57	7	
153	57	9	
154	57	5	
155	59	3	75

Figure 6-25
The Result table, showing the rows inserted upon closing of the Request Data Entry form. The Request record with an ID of 55 is bracketed in blue. Based on the MoAbs associated with the panel selected (not shown), the corresponding MoAb IDs from the Panel MoAb Link table are selected and inserted. Request 55 has already had results entered, while request 57 is pending data entry.

right corner next to the Patient ID (**Figure 6-23(b)**). While the form shows the patient's last, first, and middle names, these fields are not referenced by any underlying table. The patient name fields are programmatically copied over from the either the New Patient or Previous Patient forms. While the application could function perfectly well without displaying the patient's name, it would be confusing to users. Therefore, the patient name is presented throughout the data-entry process.

Entering Results

Entering data into the Result table shown in **Figure 6-25** is somewhat more complicated than the data insertions discussed so far. Up to now, various Wizards included within Microsoft Access automated the insertion of ID values once selections were made from reference tables. The design of the Result table, however, requires that the application insert a *variable* number of rows into the table to accommodate the MoAbs associated with a selected panel.

To provide this type of dynamic row insertion, once an end user completes data entry using the Request Data Entry form, either button at the bottom of the Request Data Entry form executes a series of queries prior to the form's closing.

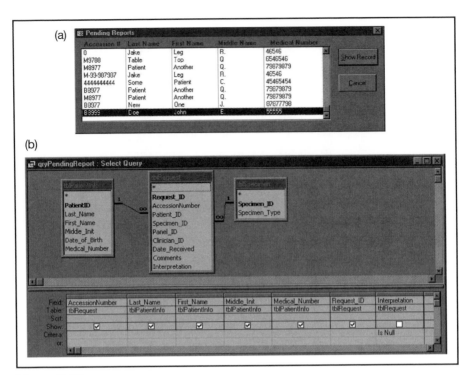

Figure 6-26
The Pending Reports form (a) and the query to select the data for this form (b).

The first query is on the Panel MoAb Link table to determine the set of MoAb keys associated with the panel selected by the end user. A second type of query, called an *insert query,* inserts the set of records from the first query into the Result table. The procedural code written to accomplish this is beyond the scope of this chapter. However, for those interested, the code to the application is readily viewable through the Microsoft Access Visual Basic for Applications (VBA) code editor.

Figure 6-25 shows a series of MoAb IDs that have been inserted after selecting the Immunosuppressed panel in the Request form (**Figure 6-22(b)**). The table's MoAb ID column stores foreign key values that reference the MoAb ID primary keys found in the MoAb table. The MoAb Result column for Request ID 55 has already been populated with data, while those for Request ID 57 are pending entry. While copying sets of keys from 1 table to another may appear complicated, this database design allows for great flexibility in terms of having panels designed with varying numbers of test elements. Once the block of MoAb IDs is inserted, the Report form for result entry opens. The form displays the correct labels and fields for each of the MoAbs that are part of the

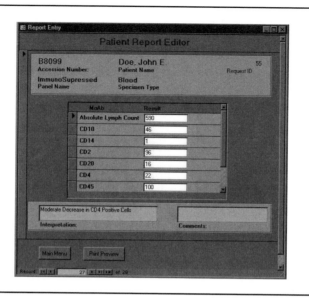

Figure 6-27
The Patient Report Editor shows the data elements that will be incorporated into the final report. From here the report may be previewed prior to printing from the Print Preview button, or the user may return to the main menu.

ordered panel (**Figure 6-27**). These fields are displayed as part of a subform whose record source is the Result table. Only those rows in the Request table that have a Request ID that matches the Request ID shown in the upper right corner of the Report form are displayed (**Figure 6-27**).

An alternative to using this design is to have a different Result table for each panel, or to have a single Result table that has a column for all possible MoAbs. In the second case, there would be a number of blank fields, or null values, inserted into the table, because panels rarely include all possible MoAbs. In either case, one would have produced an inefficient application that would have been difficult to maintain and query.

Writing a Patient Report

A Pending Reports form allows end users to view tests that have been ordered but are pending results (**Figure 6-26**). The set of records shown in the Pending Report's list box is obtained through a query of the Request table that

Flow Cytometry Report

B8099	*Doe*	*John*	*E.*
AccessionNumber	**Last Name**	**First Name**	**Middle Name**
3/7/33	*55555*		
Date of Birth	**Medical Number**		
2/10/99			
Date Received			

Absolute Lymph Count 590 ***Normal Range*** 1000-4400

Monoclonal AB	*Percent Positive*	*Absolute Number*	*Normal Range*
CD14	1	6	30-528
CD2	96	566	720-3830
CD20	16	94	30-528
CD4	22	130	350-2420
CD45	100	590	1000-4400
CD8	70	413	200-1630

Comments

Interpretation *Moderate Decrease in CD4 Positive Cells*

Thursday, May 13, 1999 *Page 1 of 1*

Figure 6-28
Partial representation of the patient report. By clicking on the Print Preview button on the Report Entry form (**Figure 6-27**), the end user views the report that will be printed and archived.

selects rows that have had no data entered for the Interpretation field. Below the form is the query design panel used to construct this query. The query is essentially performing the following action: Find all records within the Patient, Request, and Specimen tables that have linked records by way of their Patient ID and Specimen ID and have no data entered in the Request table's Interpretation field.

Clicking on an entry in the Pending Reports form opens the Report Entry screen shown in **Figure 6-27**. The end user can enter data in the MoAb result fields and also enter an interpretation or any additional comments in the appropriate fields. Clicking on the Print Preview button in **Figure 6-27** displays a preview of the printed report for this panel (**Figure 6-28**).

The reporting of individual laboratory test results without reference to prior values is commonly done in many institutions. This is not optimal, because it is difficult to monitor changes in laboratory values over a period of time. However, one of the advantages of designing an application with highly normalized data is that it allows rapid customization of reports, which can improve decision support. For example, clinicians monitoring immunosuppressed patients can receive longitudinal plots of $CD4^+$ T cells for their patients (**Figure 6-29**). A graphical presentation of the data not only makes the report more informative to clinicians,

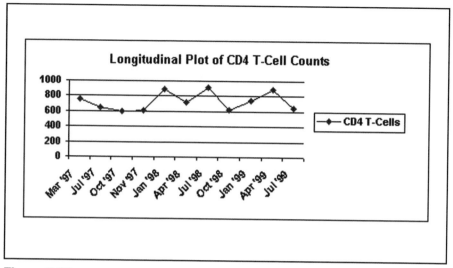

Figure 6-29
Longitudinal plot of CD4+ T cell counts for an individual patient. The graph can be embedded as part of the report.

but also assists the laboratory director in writing the clinical impression or interpretation. In certain laboratories, quantitative HIV viral load measurements might be included as part of the graphical plot of CD4 results, giving an even greater overall picture of how a patient is responding to antiretroviral therapy.

Summary

This prototype application's functionality, along with a sound understanding of its underlying relational data model, will serve as the basis for the reader to design his or her flow cytometry database application. Clearly, parts of this application are designed for demonstration purposes and will have to be modified prior to implementation within a laboratory. Using the functions described and a little imagination, it is possible to build a complete and customized application suitable for most laboratories. For downloads of the software described, tips for improving the application, and other inquiries, e-mail the authors: caldwellc@health.missouri.edu.

7

Economics of Flow Cytometry

Dennis Grimaud

Flow Cytometry Cost Analysis

The utility of flow cytometry in the laboratory industry has been well defined over the past 10 years. The technology has continued to expand, providing services primarily for patients with cancer and human immunodeficiency virus (HIV) infection. This chapter will not address flow cytometry research and development, which is driven by different motivational and economic forces than the clinical laboratory and physician markets. The expansion of the market for flow cytometry is largely due to education, which is providing an understanding of the use of flow cytometry as a prognostic and diagnostic tool in both HIV and cancer. Furthermore, specialists in hematology, oncology, and infectious diseases have placed demands on providers to provide this technology as a value-added service in patient care, which has opened the market for the equipment and reagent manufacturers to sell their products to the entire industry. Soon it became apparent that the market for flow cytometric evaluation of patients with HIV infection would be dominated by the large national reference laboratories because it was high volume and price sensitive. Hospitals and regional reference laboratories, on the other hand, saw the lymphoma and leukemia market for both inpatients and outpatients as an opportunity to increase testing volume and revenue.

As the market continued to evolve between 1988 and 1992, flow cytometry generated not only revenues but also profits for those laboratories that understood the rules and regulations relating to reimbursement. But all that changed, starting in 1992 with the implementation of the resource-based relative value scale (RBRVS), or physician fee schedule. This fee schedule changed the economics of flow cytometry over a 4-year period, becoming fully implemented in 1996. This meant that Medicare paid 75% less in 1996 than in 1992 for the same service. This single event, RBRVS, influenced hospital administrations, and finance departments in particular, to analyze the cost-benefit ratio for flow cytometry services provided to patients within their institutions.

A major factor affecting the economics of flow cytometry, especially in hospitals, is the diagnosis-related group (DRG), a system that reimburses hospitals a set amount for a specific diagnosis which includes all services performed on a patient. Enacted as part of the prospective payment system in 1984 under the Tax Equity Fiscal Responsibility Act (TEFRA), the DRG system changed laboratories within hospitals from profit to cost centers. Following TEFRA, if a hospital purchased the flow cytometry equipment, and the services were performed by hospital employees, then the service was included in the DRG rate, or hospital inpatient services. This means there is no reimbursement for Medicare inpatients or Medicare nonpatients receiving flow cytometry services within the hospital. With approximately 50% of hospital patients qualifying for Medicare, it does not take long to see the financial pressure that is inevitably being placed on this service by hospital administrations.

To help you evaluate your own situation, whether you currently own a flow cytometer or are considering acquiring one, **Table 7-1** is a financial pro forma that can assist you in calculating your current or proposed profit or loss in flow cytometry. Provided is an example of a 634-bed hospital (hospital A) and a 230-bed hospital (hospital B) and the analysis necessary to calculate revenue to cost.

Though the table depicts a set charge per test for AIDS testing, DNA analysis, and lymphoma/leukemia immunophenotyping reimbursement, Medicare, Medicaid, and private insurance is based on a fee per cell surface marker. If the calculations were performed in that manner, the net revenue would be lower than shown. (Note: Net revenue is best case for illustration purposes.) As you work through **Table 7-1**, be aware of patient categories, since this will determine whether payment is made under Part A, hospital services or Part B, physician services. There are 3 classifications of patients:

(1) Inpatients: patients who remain in the hospital longer than 24 hours.
(2) Outpatients: patients who are referred to the hospital, sign in, and register. Services are provided by hospital personnel.
(3) Nonpatients: patients whose specimens are referred to the laboratory without their registering as outpatients.

Table 7-1

Cost Analysis—Flow Cytometry Testing

	Hospital A	Hospital B	Your Facility
Hospital vs Reference Laboratory			

Assumptions	Hospital A	Hospital B	Your Facility
1. Hospital bed size	634	230	
2. Census percentage	71	66	
3. Medicare to private patient as a %	38	65	
4. Hospital owns flow cytometer and performs testing	Part A*	Part A*	Part A*
5. Hospital orders flow cytometry testing and sends to reference laboratory	Part B*	Part B*	Part B*

*Part A refers to services performed within the hospital that are considered part of the DRG.
*Part B refers to services sent to an outside reference laboratory not part of the hospital and considered physician services reimbursed through the physician fee schedule (RBRVS).

Number of Procedures Performed Monthly		
1. Lymphoma/leukemia Immunophenotyping	8	3
2. DNA content assay (ploidy S-phase)	10	2
3. Helper/suppressor ratios (CD4/CD8) AIDS	16	10

Hospital Owns Equipment		
	Dollar Amount Spent per Year	
1. FTEs	1	1
2. Laboratory supplies as percent of revenue	12	12
3. Proficiency testing (CAP) per year	$1500	$1500
4. Training/education 1st year	$5000	$5000

Table 7-1 (continued)

Hospital Sets Up Outpatient Services

---

1. Outpatient is defined as a patient referred to the hospital who signs in and registers. Services are provided by hospital personnel.
2. Non-patients are those patients whose specimens are referred to the laboratory without their registration as an outpatient.

Hospital Purchases a Flow Cytometer

	Hospital A	Hospital B	Your Facility
1. Equipment purchase price	$100,000	$100,000	
2. FTE(s) salary	$42,000	$42,000	
3. Revenue			
a. Occupied beds	450	152	
b. Occupied beds times Medicare %*	241	99	
c. Number of samples times Medicare %			
—Lymphoma/leukemia	3	1	
—DNA content analysis	4	1	
—CD4/CD8 ratios	0	0	

Because the hospital performing flow services cannot bill Medicare for testing performed, you must know the number of Medicare-occupied beds in order to calculate revenue accurately for non-Medicare services.

Immunophenotyping

Lymphoma/Leukemia	Hospital A	Hospital B	Your Facility
Total tests	8	3	
Charge/test	$495	$495	
Gross revenue	$3960	$1485	
DRG patients Part A	3	1	
Lost revenue DRG patients	–$1485	–$495	
Gross revenue	$2475	$990	

DNA Analysis			
Total tests	10	2	
Charge/test	$120	$120	
Gross revenue	$1200	$240	
DRG patients Part A	4	1	
Lost revenue DRG patients	–$480	–$120	
Gross revenue	$720	$120	

Table 7-1 (continued)

	Hospital A	Hospital B	Your Facility
AIDS Testing			
Total tests	16	10	
Charge/test	$100	$100	
Gross revenue	$1600	$1000	
DRG patients Part A	0	0	
Gross revenue	$1600	$1000	

	Totals		
Monthly Revenue	$4795	$2110	
Allowance for bad debt/			
Non-allowed 12%	$575	$253	
Net revenue	$4220	$1857	
1. Equipment depreciation Projected @ 60 mos.	$1667	$1667	
2. Salary cost	$3500	$3500	
3. Benefits @ 20%	$875	$875	
4. Laboratory supplies @ 12% of Gross Revenue	$811	$327	
5. Proficiency testing	$125	$125	
6. Training/education	$417	$417	

(NOTE: There are no costs included in this pro forma for space, administration, medical director fee, or other related expenses that may be pertinent to your institution.)

Total Expenses Per Month	**$7395**	**$6911**	
Monthly			
Net revenue	$4220	$1857	
Total expense	$7395	$6911	
Pre-tax	–$3175	–$5054	
Annual			
Net revenue	$50,640	$22,284	
Total expense	$88,740	$82,932	
Pre-tax	–$38,100	–$60,648	

Reimbursement and CPT Coding

It is critical to understand that flow cytometry is a physician service and therefore not subject to the same reimbursement guidelines as clinical laboratory testing. Clinical laboratory procedures are found in *Current Procedural Terminology (CPT)* (3)codes 80000 to 87999 and are subject to the national laboratory fee schedule as published annually by each Medicare carrier. Physician services are *CPT* (3)codes 88000 to 83999, except cytogenetics, which is subject to the clinical laboratory fee schedule. Physician services or Part B, are subject to the RBRVS, which includes flow cytometry. Clinical laboratory services are global billed whereas physician services are component billed. In other words, when you bill clinical laboratory tests you are paid one fee. When you bill physician services there are 3 components that can be billed: technical, professional, and global services.

Currently, when considering flow cytometry and the economics of this service, be aware that reference laboratories can accept billing assignment for the Professional component only and must bill the hospital for the Technical component. This billing provision changed in August 2000 as part of the Balanced Budget Amendment (BBA), whereby the technical component became part of the DRG, or Part A under Medicare. This is true for inpatients, outpatients, and nonpatients. However, if a hospital owns the flow cytometer and it is part of the hospital laboratory service, then all inpatients and nonpatients are considered Part A under Medicare and, therefore, fall under the DRG and are part of the hospital's cost report.

To accurately assess the economics of flow cytometry you must track not just your gross billables but also your net receivables (collections). Net receivables could be as little as 15%, or as much as 60%, of gross billables, so make sure you develop a good working relationship with the billing department and the finance department (collections) at your institution in order to accurately track your billables and receivables. In this way, you will be proactive in justifying your flow cytometry service instead of waiting for financial cost reduction pressures from your institution's administration.

An area to be considered when assessing the economics of flow cytometry is managed care. Managed care organizations (MCOs) negotiate payment for flow cytometry services through one of the following mechanisms. The first method is a capitated fee (a negotiated rate for each service performed vs a per marker fee, aka, "cap"), usually part of a negotiated contract with the hospital for pathology services. This is the least desirable method since reimbursement is based not on cost but rather on overall services provided to managed-care patients within the hospital. There is no provision for the anatomic pathology department to recover lost revenues since payment is capped under contract for services provided for the managed care patient. In most cases, these cap rates are on a per member per month basis and, therefore, not related to any one patient. This eliminates any balanced bill to the patient for service not covered by the provider. A balanced bill is any unpaid portion of the bill that would be the patient's responsibility for payment. Under the managed care contract, the balanced bill provision is eliminated and the provider of the service has no right to bill the patient.

The second method is a negotiated contract based on a preset price per case. In this plan you negotiate a price based on your cost to perform the case. This method assures you of recovering your cost, assuming you know your cost per analysis, by charging a rate above your cost with an ability to sustain this price over the term of the contract. This is considered a "carve-out," whereby the service is not part of any other contract and is negotiated separately, assuring 100% remuneration at the agreed-upon contract price.

A third method is to negotiate a set fee per cell surface marker, allowing billing per case based on the number of markers performed. In this method of negotiation you can recover cost on the sample type (eg, fine needle biopsies, effusions, and pleural fluids), because payment is based on actual markers performed. Because reimbursement is based on the number of reported markers, it is the preferred method of payment for providing flow cytometry services to MCOs.

A major factor today is reduction of payments for services by private insurers. However, the economic effect of private insurance is decreasing annually as patients convert to health maintenance organizations (HMOs) and MCOs. As this trend continues, specialty laboratories will find it increasingly difficult to compete on price with the large reference laboratories. On the other hand, the specialty laboratory can provide a level of service unsurpassed by large reference laboratories and, therefore, have an opportunity to bid on contracts for carve-out services to the MCOs and HMOs. The driving forces in this sector of health care are patient satisfaction, turnaround time, result accuracy, and cost control. In many cases, it is not whether you can reduce the cost per test but whether you can reduce the cost of patient care while providing a positive patient outcome. These are the true economics of health care in a managed care environment.

Billing for flow cytometry services has been well defined by the Health Care Financing Administration (HCFA) since April 1988, when the services were approved for reimbursement. Flow cytometry was placed in the physician services rather than the clinical laboratory services category. This was significant because it provided for component billing (technical, professional, and/or global), allowing payment to the laboratory providing the technical service, the physician providing the professional service, or the independent laboratory pro-

Table 7-2
Reimbursable Flow Cytometry Procedures

CPT-4 Code	Application	Approved ICD-9-CM Codes(4)	
88180	Immunophenotyping (per cell surface marker)	Leukemia	200.0-208.91
		Lymphoma	200.0-208.91
		AIDS and ARC	042.0
		Transplant	996.81-996.83
88182	DNA content/cell cycle analysis	Breast	174.0-174.9
		Bladder	188.0-188.9
		Ovarian	183.0
		Carcinoma in situ	233.7
85045	Reticulocyte analysis	Same as for other reticulocyte methods	

Modifiers: TC – Technical component; 26 – Professional component.

viding both or the global service. It is important to understand the appropriate billing or procedure codes (*CPT*) in order to receive the appropriate reimbursement and to not violate the compliance rules and regulations. **Table 7-2** identifies the appropriate *CPT* codes for flow cytometry as well as the modifier required for appropriate payment.

Diagnosis Codes

Another important factor to understand in billing flow cytometry services is the area of diagnosis codes (*International Classification of Diseases, Ninth Revision, Clinical Modification*, or *ICD-9-CM* codes). Payment for flow cytometry is dependent upon the accuracy of the *CPT* code in conjunction with the approved diagnosis code. Without these 2 codes, claims will be rejected (see **Table 7-2**). Also, only certain diagnosis codes are approved for reimbursement and, therefore, familiarity with these codes is vital if you expect to receive proper payment. Remember that not all anatomic specimen sites are approved for payment, especially if the performance of the service does not change the treatment of the patient. This is considered medical necessity and can only be assessed by the ordering or attending physician. If the physician deems it medically necessary for appropriate patient care, be sure that if the service is not covered (because the diagnosis code is not authorized for payment) you obtain an advance beneficiary notice (ABN). An ABN notifies the patient that Medicare may not cover this service and, therefore, the patient accepts responsibility for payment of the service. It is essential that the ABN be obtained from the patient at the time the physician orders the procedure, because if the patient is not informed at the time of the order, the laboratory will have no recourse in going back to the patient for payment. Furthermore, billing Medicare patients without an ABN or a properly signed notice can expose the laboratory to fraud liability. The Office of the Inspector General's revised compliance plan published in August 1998 included ABN in a new section, suggesting that the government considers the proper signing of ABNs an important compliance issue. Become familiar with this procedure to ensure proper payment when providing services to Medicare patients. Check with your local Medicare carrier for instructions and a copy of the policy. In this way, you will be able to instruct and inform your client (physician, hospital, clinic or laboratory) of this policy in order for patients to be aware of their financial responsibilities at the time of service.

Flow cytometry has made a significant impact on the laboratory industry by providing information that is used for diagnosis, prognosis, and monitoring therapy. Use of this technology continues to increase because it provides information necessary to properly manage disease. As technological advances in flow cytometry expand in the future, the laboratory industry's ability to be adequately compensated will be critical. Understanding the rules and regulations of this discipline, especially as they relate to the HCFA, the Office of the Inspector General, and the state guidelines, is vital to ensure receiving proper payment for services rendered. The economics of flow cytometry are closely aligned with the ordering physician and medical necessity, the diagnosis with its associated diagnosis code, and the use of the proper procedure codes. If the established guidelines are not followed, you will soon understand the economics of flow cytometry.

8

Clinical Molecular Cytometry: Merging Flow Cytometry with Molecular Biology in Laboratory Medicine

J. Philip McCoy, Jr.
Charles Goolsby

Introduction

Since the publication of the first edition of this text in 1994, rapid advances have been made in the application of molecular techniques to diagnostic pathology. Today, virtually every pathology department has at least one division or laboratory using molecular biology to assist in diagnosis, with the term "molecular pathology" frequently used to describe these applications. Scientific societies centered on molecular pathology have been formed (such as the Association for Molecular Pathology) and professional certification is offered in this area by several organizations (such as the American Board of Medical Genetics and the American Board of Bioanalysis). Molecular techniques have been applied to numerous aspects of pathology including, but not limited to, the diagnosis of infectious disease, neoplasia, and genetic disorders. For a more detailed description of the general application of these techniques to diagnostic pathology the reader is referred to several recent reviews.[1-6]

The application of molecular biological techniques to diagnostic pathology has flourished because of the exquisite sensitivity of these techniques as well as their ability to acquire information at the genomic level as well as the phenotypic level. In broad terms, assays used in molecular pathology fall into 3 categories:

(1) detection of specific gene products; (2) detection of specific sequences of nucleic acids; and (3) detection of specific rearrangements of germline DNA. These assays may involve immunochemical staining, nucleic acid amplification, blotting techniques, in situ hybridizations, or assorted combinations of the above. While each approach has much to offer the pathologist, these molecular techniques are not without shortcomings. Molecular biological techniques are often time-consuming and require extraction of nucleic acids from homogenates of a group of cells or of tissues (thus becoming population analyses, not analyses of individual cells). Although it is possible with fluorescence in situ hybridization, rarely are multiple features of intact cells examined using molecular biological techniques.

In contrast, flow cytometry traditionally has not involved analysis of nucleic acids, other than gross quantitation of DNA or chromosomes. However, flow cytometry does permit rapid interrogation of many individual cells for multiple features. It is readily apparent that the major weaknesses of flow cytometry are addressed by molecular biological techniques and vice versa. Therefore, a merger of these 2 technologies stands to provide an aid to diagnostic pathology far greater than the sum of the 2 approaches individually. Rather than being viewed as technologies that must compete for funding and specimens, molecular biology and flow cytometry should be considered 2 complementary cornerstones of 21st-century diagnostic pathology.

Combining flow cytometry with molecular biological techniques offers the opportunity to study heterogeneous populations of cells with varying phenotypic or genotypic characteristics. This may be of extreme importance when examining heterogeneous tumors, identifying an infectious process, or detecting minimal residual disease—all situations where potentially only a minority of cells in a population may be affected. This combining of molecular techniques with flow cytometry is only just beginning and the field of clinical molecular cytometry should be considered in its infancy. Described below are a few of the molecular cytometric approaches to detecting gene products and nucleic acids that may have a role in diagnostic pathology.

Gene Product Analysis

The flow cytometric analysis of specific gene products has numerous applications in the clinical laboratory, including detection of gene rearrangements and oncogene products, detection of products of genes transfected into cells in vitro, and assessment of the relationship of specific gene products to the cell cycle. Detection of gene products is most often accomplished through the use of monoclonal or polyclonal antibodies, although fluorochrome-labeled ligands or lectins may also be used to detect the expression of specific receptors. In the strict sense, assays of surface markers, as practiced routinely in the clinical laboratory, are for the detection of the products of genes or combinations of genes. Here discussion will be limited to more nontraditional products that have in most instances been defined on the genomic level.

Detection of TCR Gene Rearrangements

A potentially very useful application of flow cytometry for the detection of gene rearrangements is the use of monoclonal antibodies directed against variable regions of the T-cell receptor (TCR) to detect clonal excesses of T lymphocytes. The TCR is the surface structure pivotal for specific antigen binding on T lymphocytes. The specificity of antigen binding is associated with rearrangements at the genomic level that result in the construction of corresponding variable regions of the TCR. Two chains of the TCR, the alpha and beta chains, both vary as the result of genomic rearrangements. There are approximately 20 "families" of rearrangements for each chain. Monoclonal antibodies have been produced which recognize families of many of these variable regions (particularly the beta chain) and which are well suited for use in flow cytometry. A panel consisting of some of these antibodies to the TCR beta-chain families has been used to immunophenotype normal peripheral blood, yielding at least a partial reference range for these reagents on both CD4[+] helper T cells and CD8[+] suppressor T cells[7] (**Figures 8-1 and 8-2**).

These reagents are useful indicators of possible clonal expansions of T cells in a variety of diseases such as T-cell neoplasms where no other markers of clonal expansion are currently available. In cutaneous T-cell lymphoma (CTCL), for example, delineation of the abnormal cells is difficult using standard surface marker analysis, as the abnormal cells are generally CD4[+] and are not necessarily distinguishable from normal CD4[+] lymphocytes on the basis of phenotype, morphology, or DNA content.[8] In CTCL, the neoplastic CD4[+] lymphocytes often demonstrate a predominant variable segment rearrangement, whereas the CD4[+] lymphocytes from a normal individual reveal a heterogeneity of rearrangements distributed among the 20 families of rearrangements. It should be noted that not all CTCLs are associated with a single variable-chain

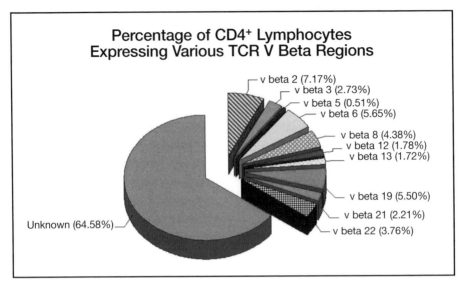

Figure 8-1

A summary of expression of T-cell receptor variable-chain expression on normal adult peripheral blood CD4+ T cells. Each TCR V chain was detected using 3-color flow cytometric analysis with monoclonal antibodies specific for the respective family or subfamily of the chain.

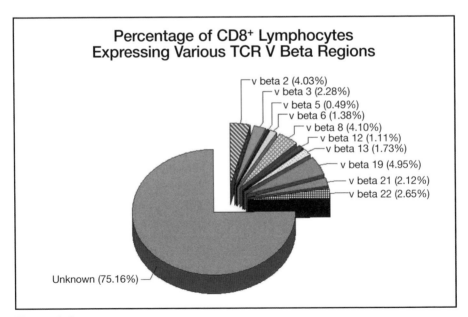

Figure 8-2

A summary of expression of T-cell receptor variable-chain expression on normal adult peripheral blood CD8+ T cells. Each TCR V chain was detected using 3-color flow cytometric analysis with monoclonal antibodies specific for the respective family or subfamily of the chain.

rearrangement, rather each patient, if CD3$^+$, may express a predominance of any 1 of the 20 possibilities. The finding of an excess of 1 family of TCR beta-chain rearrangements not only can assist in the diagnosis of a clonal lesion, but also can be used to monitor the efficacy of therapy against this clone.

Analysis of TCR beta-chains is also of potential use in other diseases, such as human immunodeficiency virus (HIV) disease.[9] Here these reagents may be used to assess specific deletions or expansions in the repertoires of CD4$^+$ and CD8$^+$ subsets. Specific alterations within these subsets may prove to be of more prognostic significance than total CD4$^+$ cell counts or CD4/CD8 ratios. Similar applications may be possible in other infectious or autoimmune diseases.

A limitation on the use of these reagents is the relatively large panel of monoclonal antibodies that is necessary to encompass the entire TCR repertoire; however, once a clonal excess or deletion is found, it is not necessary to use the entire panel for repeated monitoring of the specific defect. Thus, in high-volume laboratories, these reagents might prove practical as well as useful.

Steroid Hormone (Estrogen and Progesterone) Receptors

The detection of estrogen receptors (ERs) and progesterone receptors (PgRs) is of considerable diagnostic and prognostic value in breast cancer, as well as cancers of the endometrium, vulva, and cervix. Determination of receptor status is a useful predictor of response to endocrine therapy and systemic adjuvant therapies such as tamoxifen.[10,11] Historically, detection of estrogen and progesterone receptors has been accomplished by ligand-binding assays; however, the development of high-quality monoclonal antibodies to these receptors has led to the widespread use of immunohistochemical methods.[12-14] Flow cytometric assays for ER/PgR detection have been recently developed,[15-19] but have not yet become commonplace in the clinical laboratory. Flow cytometry offers advantages over the other methods in that the receptors of individual cells may be analyzed, thus providing an indication of tumor heterogeneity. Additionally, ER and PgR expression may be measured simultaneously on the same cell or together with an additional parameter such as DNA content/cell cycle or cytokeratin.[15,16]

ERs and PgRs are located in the nuclei of cells;[20,21] thus flow cytometric assays to detect these receptors must be performed on permeabilized cells or on nuclei stripped free of cytoplasm. This adds somewhat to the technical complexity of these assays compared with the detection of cell surface receptors, although the presence of ERs and PgRs in the nucleus permits analysis of these receptors on paraffin-embedded tissue. Redkar and Krishan[15] have demonstrated the feasibility of using paraffin-embedded tissue for the multiparametric analysis of ERs and PgRs or DNA content. For fresh tissue, permeabilizing agents such as saponin have been demonstrated to be suitable for the detection of ERs/PgRs.[16] Finally, it has been demonstrated that flow cytometry may be used to quantitate steroid hormone receptors on individual cells,[16] thus further dissecting tumor heterogeneity.

Multidrug Resistance Gene Products

Expression of a multidrug resistance phenotype has been associated with resistance of neoplasms to a variety of chemotherapeutic agents, such as antimitotics, anthracyclines, and certain antibiotics, among others.[22-26] A transmembrane glycoprotein, referred to as p-glycoprotein (Pgp) or the *MDR1* gene product, functions as a pump that actively transports chemotherapeutic agents out of the cell. The expression of this glycoprotein is associated with activation of the *MDR1* gene and elevated levels of *MDR1* messenger RNA (mRNA).[22] Flow cytometric detection of the *MDR1* gene product is possible using any one of several commercially available antibodies to *MDR1* (such as MRK16, UIC2, and 4E3.16). *MDR1* may then be detected by flow cytometry either alone or in conjunction with other cellular features such as DNA content. The feasibility of the flow cytometric assays has been demonstrated in cell lines and patient-derived material from a variety of solid tumors and leukemias and has illustrated the potential utility of detection of the *MDR1* gene product.[27-36] *MDR1* has also been functionally demonstrated by measuring efflux of fluorescent compounds from cells,[37,38] and these functional efflux studies have been combined with detection of *MDR1* by monoclonal antibodies to establish a 2-color method for detection of multidrug resistance on both a phenotypic and functional basis.[40] Given the broad numbers and types of flow cytometric assays possible for *MDR1*/Pgp, at least one group, the French Drug Resistance Network, has published guidelines for the cytometric detection of Pgp.[36]

In the past few years, other drug resistance genes (and corresponding proteins) have been described, such as the multidrug resistance protein (MRP) and the lung resistance-related protein (LRP).[41-43] These have functions distinct from the *MDR1* gene/Pgp pump and are encoded by different genes. MRP[44-46] transports drugs conjugated with glutathione (GSH) and has been demonstrated to be associated with poor prognosis in a variety of human cancers. LRP, which maps proximal to MRP on chromosome 16, has similarly been demonstrated to be associated with multidrug resistance in Pgp-negative cell lines and patient specimens.[47] Flow cytometric assays for the detection of MRP and LRP have been described and employed to study a number of different human tumors.[42,48,49] Furthermore, a flow cytometric assay has been developed which simultaneously, but distinctly, detects Pgp, MRP, and LRP.[50] Assays such these permit a better dissection of the mechanism of multidrug resistance and may, in the future, contribute to the application of agents to reverse the mechanism of multidrug resistance.

Oncogene Products

Oncogenes are involved in the control of cell growth; their mutation or activation can lead to alterations in the expression and function of their gene products. A large number of monoclonal antibodies have been developed that recognize many of the normal or activated oncogene products. Flow cytometry for the detection of oncogene products offers certain advantages over other methods: information concerning the oncogene product may be gathered on individual cells and in the context of additional features or markers of each cell (reviewed in part by Stewart[51]). Flow cytometric techniques have been developed to detect and quantitate many oncogene products expressed on the cell surface, in the cytoplasm, or in the nucleus of the cell.[52-64] The vast majority of these flow cytometric assays have not become part of the routine diagnosis of most cancers, although some oncogene products are examined by immunohistochemical methods as an adjunctive component of diagnosis.[65,66] In solid tumors much of the attention has focused on examining multiple oncogenes simultaneously, as their expression has been postulated to reflect tumor heterogeneity and clonal evolution (see **Figure 8-3**).[67,68] This scenario may only apply to a group or subset of tumors in which oncogenes are expressed or overexpressed in a defined sequence that correlates with tumor aggressiveness and metastatic capacity. It is conceivable that this approach to studying multiple oncogenes on a cell-by-cell basis may yield prognostic information concerning each tumor and may ultimately culminate in a clinically useful laboratory test.

The application of oncogenes to the initial diagnosis of hematologic malignancies has yet to become a widespread standard, although, as with solid tumors, some may be used adjunctively to help distinguish malignant from benign specimens. Detection of oncogenes or elevated expression of oncogene products has also been applied to the study of minimal residual disease, particularly among hematologic neoplasms. A flow cytometric application related to

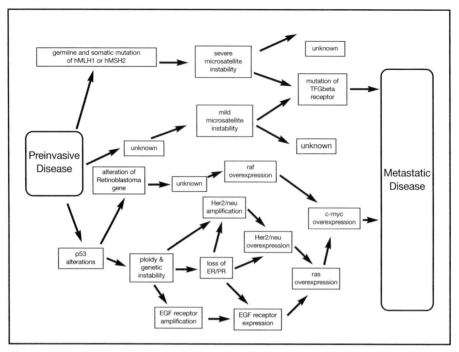

Figure 8-3

A summary of genetic evolutionary sequences that occur in human solid tumors. Modified from Shackney and Shankey[56]

Abbreviations: hMLH1 = human homologue of the yeast DNA mismatch repair gene MLH1; hMLH2 = a second human DNA mismatch repair gene; EGF receptor = receptor for the epidermal growth factor, associated with aggressive tumor characteristics; raf = a 74 kDa serine/threonine kinase product of the raf oncogene which plays a role in signal processes that regulate cell growth and proliferation and is part of the raf kinase family that is thought to play an important role in the development of some solid tumors; TGF beta receptor = receptor for transforming growth factor beta, a factor which affects cellular proliferation and differentiation and is conventionally regarded as having growth-inhibitory activity.

this endeavor includes the detection of the *bcr/abl* transcript using fluorescence in situ hybridization (FISH) followed by cytometric analysis in chronic myeloid leukemia.[69]

The 2 distinct advantages of flow cytometry over other techniques for the detection of oncogene products are its ability to interrogate individual cells and to examine multiple features of the individual cells. Given the generally accepted concept of tumor heterogeneity, these multivariate flow cytometric analyses will facilitate better identification of subpopulations, or clones, within a neoplastic lesion, which may have prognostic significance.

Gene Product Markers of Apoptosis

Gene expression has been increasingly examined, by flow cytometry as well as other methods, in relationship to apoptosis in both solid tumors and hematologic neoplasms. Apoptosis, or programmed cell death, appears to be a key factor in regulating cell survival and in removing specified cells from the body. Genes have been identified which are involved in the regulation of apoptosis, and the upregulation, downregulation, or mutation of the products of these genes alters the normal sequence of cell survival. Gene products involved in regulation of apoptosis that may be of clinical interest include the bcl-2 family of proteins, as well as the p53 and Fas proteins. The bcl-2 protein, for example, is an anti-apoptotic gene product whose overexpression inhibits apoptosis by blocking the release of cytochrome c.[70] This overexpression, either on the cellular or mitochondrial level,[71] may readily be measured by flow cytometric methods, including multiparametric methods.[72]

The *p53* gene product also plays a role in apoptosis and cell survival, albeit through a different mechanism of action. Wild-type *p53* is pro-apoptotic and functions to remove cells that have suffered DNA damage from a variety of causes.[73,74] Mutation or alteration of the *p53* gene can lead to proliferation by damaged cells and is thus associated with neoplasia. Numerous investigators have reported flow cytometric assays for the detection of *p53* gene product in human malignancies.[74-78] Because it has been implicated in control of cell growth and is a nuclear antigen, *p53* is quite often analyzed in conjunction with cellular DNA content. The examination of *p53* is more of an attempt to define a prognostic marker of tumor progression or response to therapy rather than to develop a new diagnostic modality. Although this effort remains in the experimental phase, in the future, detection of *p53* expression or mutation may translate into clinical assays.

Flow Cytometry and Gene Therapy

Among of the most significant accomplishments of molecular biologists has been the development of techniques to implant (or *transfect*) specific functional genes into foreign host cells. The new host cell is often capable of transcribing the implanted gene and thus expressing the novel gene product. DNA transfer techniques are being adapted to devise potential new therapies for a number of diseases, including cystic fibrosis, adenosine deaminase defects, Gaucher disease, chronic granulomatous disease, and various forms of cancer, to name a few.[79-83] In gene therapy, genes may be transferred into a variety of cell types, although transfer into pluripotent stem cells is often of therapeutic advantage since these cells will contribute to hematopoietic reconstitution for the duration of the life of the recipient.

Gene therapy involves several stages that benefit from the use of flow cytometric techniques. These potential uses include isolation of the cells to receive the gene (eg, stem cells), monitoring of the efficiency of DNA transfer, assessment of expression of the transferred gene, selection of clones of recipient cells with high expression of the gene, determination of proliferation of genetically altered cells in the host, and assessment of the maintenance of expression in recipients. These potential applications will be briefly discussed below.

As mentioned previously, pluripotent stem cells are often desirable for use in gene therapy. Flow cytometry can be used to sort these cells on the basis of CD34 expression or, if larger numbers of cells are needed—and obtained by other methods—to determine the purity and viability of the stem cells.

Flow cytometry has been used to assess the efficiency of transfection. Rice and Pennica[84] used flow cytometry to measure protoplast fusion-mediated transfer and expression of a plasmid containing the gene coding for the CD4 antigen. By prelabeling the protoplasts with fluorescein prior to transfection and quenching extracellular fluorescence after transfection, it was possible to demonstrate by flow cytometry that intracellular fluorescence immediately after fusion showed a strong correlation with transient CD4 transfection efficiencies. In an intriguing approach, Erlich and coworkers[85] described a method for assessing gene transfer based on enzymatic reduction of fluorescent-conjugated ligand in acid sphingomyelinase-deficient mice, which might be adaptable to certain human disease processes.

Fiering and coworkers[86] devised a method for the detection of a reporter gene and selection of viable transfected cells based on the gene's expression. The reporter gene (a gene used to "report" that transfer of DNA has occurred) used in this method is the *Escherichia coli lacZ* gene, which encodes a beta-galactosidase. Thus this method has been termed FACS-Gal. In simplest terms, this method is based on the ability of cells with beta-galactosidase activity to break down the nonfluorogenic substrate fluorescein di-B-D-galactoside (FDG) to the fluorescent product, fluorescein. Transfected cells are loaded with FDG, appropriately incubated, and analyzed by flow cytometry. Transfected cells may be sorted if desired, thus avoiding the tedious procedure of selecting transfectants using a drug resistance marker. More recently, green fluorescent protein (GFP) has been used as a reporter gene to monitor gene expression.[87-90] As its name implies, this *GFP* gene encodes a fluorescent protein which can be detected by flow cytometry if the gene is successfully transfected and expressed.

GFP is generally considered to be a better reporter system than the FACS-Gal method[89,90] and is being used with increasing frequency.

In some instances it is possible to directly detect the product of the transferred gene, using the appropriate fluorescent assay. This may involve antibodies to the gene product, a fluorescent ligand for a novel receptor, or a substrate with a fluorescent product for a new enzyme (as detailed above). Not only is this useful in pretherapy stages, it may also be useful in periodic monitoring of the patient to ensure the stable expression of the gene and the continuing survival of the transfected cells in the recipient.

Nucleic Acid Analysis

The previous section described the detection of gene products and the coupling of those measurements in multiparameter assays examining other cellular characteristics. Certainly, development of flow cytometric assays to detect specific nucleic acid sequences (DNA and mRNA) coding for those proteins and to detect genetic aberrations associated with human disease in individual cells, which can be coupled with examination of other cellular characteristics, will be of significant advantage in both basic and clinical research. These approaches will potentially foster a number of clinical applications.

Clearly, detection of specific genetic aberrations is becoming increasingly important in diagnosis and patient management in a number of human diseases. In a large number of hematologic malignancies, specific chromosomal abnormalities are strongly associated with specific leukemias or lymphomas.[91-106] In some cases, chronic myelogenous leukemia (CML) and acute promyelocytic leukemia (APL) being the classic examples,[98,99] the chromosomal abnormalities are helpful in defining the disease with, in general, documentation of the specific translocation being required to confirm the diagnosis. These classic examples of the t(9;22) translocation in CML[91,99,101,103] and the t(15;17) translocation in APL[98,100] have now been joined by a fairly lengthy list of chromosomal abnormalities which are strongly associated with specific leukemias[92-96,102,105,106] and lymphomas.[94,97,104,105] In fact, the increasing importance of chromosomal aberrations and immunophenotype for diagnosis of hematologic malignancies is reflected in the most recent acute leukemia diagnostic classifications proposed by the World Health Organization.

Although the increasing diagnostic importance of genetic aberrations is clear, the prognostic information that specific genetic changes may carry is equally important in terms of patient management and counseling. For example, B-lineage acute lymphoblastic leukemia (B-ALL) patients harboring the t(1;19) translocation have a significantly poorer prognosis[107,108] than patients lacking this translocation. It should be noted that immunophenotypic features, such as cytoplasmic mu expression, also correlate with a poorer prognosis. Interestingly, the significance of a group of translocations involving the core binding transcription factor has come to light following the application of classical molecular techniques to the detection of these abnormalities. Associations have been reported for several translocations involving the alpha and beta chains of the core binding factor, including t(12;21) in childhood B-ALL,[92,95] t(8;21) in acute myelogenous leukemia (AML),[96,102] and inv(16) in AML-M4 with eosinophilia.[93] Although a diverse group of acute leukemias, all of them have a good prognosis, and further, in aggregate, account for approximately 15%-20% of all acute leukemias. Thus, for both diagnostic and prognostic information, the feasibility of adding detection of specific genetic aberrations to routine immunophenotypic analyses is appealing.

In the arena of solid tissue malignancies, enticing correlations between the patterns of alteration in expression of a number of cell-cycle and apoptosis-regulatory molecules and the nature of the underlying genetic instability driving the malignant process have been pointed out.[68] This heterogeneity in dysregulation of cell cycle and/or apoptosis, reflected either in the genetic abnormalities or the resultant altered protein expression, clearly defines tumors with distinctly different biology. Thus, the ability to differentiate these biologically different tumors may be fundamental to understanding and predicting tumor progression and tumor response to therapy. Additionally, understanding heterogeneity at the cellular level in the dysregulation of cell cycle and apoptosis within a tumor will be equally important. Ultimately, this understanding will lead to the ability to select more effective, potentially patient-specific, therapies and to the development of new therapeutic approaches.

Furthermore, in many diseases, it is clear that a better understanding of minimum residual disease is required to predict which patients with residual disease are to experience recurrence. Although in some malignancies, such as APL,[100] any level of residual disease indicates a poor prognosis, in other malignancies, such as CML,[99,109] a significant number of patients with detectable residual disease do not have recurrences. It has been suggested in CML that it is the number of residual cells, not their simple presence as determined by polymerase chain reaction (PCR) or reverse transcriptase-polymerase chain reaction (RT-PCR) techniques, which is the best predictor of recurrence.[110] However, molecular cytometry measurements on individual cells will not only provide additional information on the actual numbers of residual cells in treated patients but will allow the simultaneous determination of other cellular characteristics of these residual disease cells. For example, knowing not only the number of residual cells but their proliferation and apoptosis status will clearly be important. In addition, understanding the heterogeneity within the residual disease cells of growth potential will be critical in predicting which patients will experience recurrence and which will not. This will allow a patient-specific determination of the requirement for more intensive follow-up therapy.

Application of cellular-based molecular cytometry techniques in infectious disease is also of interest. In HIV, flow cytometric assays employing in situ PCR and RT-PCR coupled with immunophenotyping permitted determination of which cell populations were actively and latently infected[111] and how cellular characteristics were altered in response to the expression of viral genes.[112] Biologically, it is obviously important to understand how the cellular reservoirs of viral infection are affected by drug therapy and how they change with disease progression. In fact, enticing preliminary data from a study employing direct hybridization detection of HIV RNA coupled with immunophenotypic analyses indicated that in situ, or cellular-based, measures of viral load as opposed to plasma viral load measures may provide additional prognostic information.[113] Similar potential obviously exists for in situ detection of other viruses such as cytomegalovirus (CMV), human papillomavirus (HPV), and Epstein-Barr virus (EBV).[114-118] Successful application of fluorescence in situ hybridization detection of EBV RNA coupled with cellular immunophenotyping has been done in both cell lines[119] and patient samples.[120] Application of these approaches in viral diseases where informative surrogate markers are not available, such as CMV, for example, may be particularly fruitful.

Flow Karyotyping

Cellular DNA content, a gross measure of karyotypic alteration, is not the subject of this chapter and is discussed elsewhere in this volume. Techniques to isolate and identify chromosomes in suspension have been developed by a number of groups.[121-123] For these techniques, chromosomes are isolated from a mitotically enriched cell population using a hypotonic solution containing 1 or more agents to stabilize the chromosome. The chromosomes are either stained with a single DNA binding dye for univariate analyses[124-126] or with 2 DNA binding dyes for bivariate analyses.[121,123,124,126] In the case of bivariate analyses,

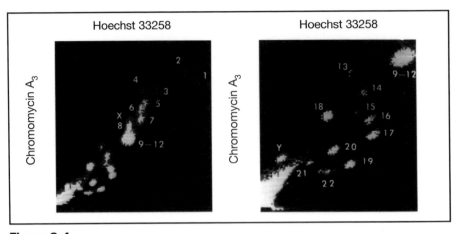

Figure 8-4

Bivariate histogram of Hoechst 33258 versus chromomycin A_3 fluorescence for chromosomes isolated from the human transformed cell line, HSF4-T12 (118), at an early passage following transformation. The chromosomes were prepared using a slightly modified procedure of Silar and Young (see Goolsby et al[118]). Although some alterations in the relative number of individual chromosomes are seen in this transformed cell line, all of the human chromosomes except 9-12 are resolved and are labeled with the appropriate number on the figure.

the 2 dyes used, such as Hoechst 33258 and chromomycin A_3, have different affinities for GC-rich and AT-rich regions of DNA. Separation of the chromosomes is then based on either total DNA content in univariate analyses or both total DNA content and variation in the GC/AT ratio of individual chromosomes in bivariate analyses. The variability in Hoechst 33258 and chromomycin A_3 staining reflected in the spread about the diagonal in these 2 parameter histograms reflects the variability in GC/AT ratio between the individual types of chromosomes. Employing bivariate analyses, all of the human chromosomes except the 9-12 group can be resolved[121] **(Figure 8-4)**, and with special staining techniques,[127] one can resolve chromosome 9 from this group, although resolution of other chromosomes is lost. With careful preparation and analysis, chromosomal number anomalies, reciprocal translocations, and other aberrant chromosomes can be detected.[128,129] Although information on the chromosome constitution of individual cells is lost, in studies of karyotype instability in cancer, flow karyotyping is a particularly useful approach when coupled with traditional G-banded analyses to monitor the evolution and population frequency of specific chromosomal alterations.[125,130] However, probably due to the complexity of the techniques and susceptibility to preferential loss of specific chromosomes, particularly the larger ones, these techniques have not seen general use in a clinical setting. Nonetheless, sorting of individual chromosomes based on these techniques was instrumental to the generation of chromosome-specific libraries in the Human Genome Project.[131]

Sorting of individual chromosomes onto nitrocellulose filters followed by hybridization with gene-specific probes, in a technique termed *spot blot analyses,* has proved useful in the chromosomal localization of specific genes.[132] Another application reported in a clinical or clinical research setting has been as an aid in the characterization of complex marker chromosomes[133] which could not be fully identified by banding techniques. Marker chromosomes are sorted, followed by isolation of DNA from the sorted chromosomes and PCR generation of labeled probes from the isolated DNA. These labeled probes are then used in multicolor, slide-based FISH analyses coupled with other chromosome-specific probes to identify the chromosome constitution of the marker or aberrant chromosome.

Cellular-based Fluorescence In Situ Hybridization

Detection of both specific DNA and RNA sequences in individual cells by flow cytometry employing FISH techniques has been reported.[113-115,117,119,120,134-149] In these approaches, fluorescently labeled nucleic acid probes with homology to specific DNA or RNA sequences within the cell are used. Both direct and indirect fluorescent labeling techniques can be used. Additionally, FISH detection can be coupled with simultaneous immunophenotypic characterization of cells,[113,119,120] enhancing the ability to characterize cells positive for a specific RNA or DNA sequence. Several studies have also demonstrated the ability of these assays to quantitate both target RNA and DNA levels within individual cells.[113,137,140,143,147,148] Readers are referred to Goolsby et al[150] and Mosiman et al[151] for detailed discussion of the technical aspects of these approaches.

FISH Detection of Specific DNA Sequences

Although sorting of specific cell populations followed by hybridization for specific DNA sequences has been reported,[152] the first report of the cellular FISH detection of specific DNA sequences in flow cytometry was by Trask et al,[146] employing a labeled total genomic probe. Improvements in these FISH techniques soon led to the detection of chromosome-specific probes (with a target size of several hundred kilobases) with coefficients of variation (CV) adequate to resolve chromosome number alterations.[143,147,148] Reproducibly obtaining this level of resolution was difficult, resulting in limited use of these techniques for that purpose following initial reports. However, recently, utilization in a clinical transplant setting to detect successful allogeneic engraftment and chimerism in sex-mismatched bone marrow transplants has been reported.[134,153] Flow cytometric detection of viral DNA using FISH techniques has also been reported. Lizard et al have detected approximately 600 copies of the HPV genome in CaSki cells by FISH in a flow cytometry assay.[117] In these same studies, 20-50 copies of HPV present in HeLa cells could not be detected by the flow cytometry assay but could be in parallel confocal analyses. The limit to sensitivity in the flow cytometry assays with fluorescein isothiocyanate (FITC)-labeled probes was autofluorescence,[117] as has been seen by others.[149,154]

FISH Detection of RNA Sequences

Successful FISH detection of specific cellular RNA sequences by flow cytometry was first demonstrated by Bauman et al[135] in detection of ribosomal RNA (rRNA). Using similar methods, Pajor et al[141] monitored rRNA levels in differentiating cells; quantitative measurements of poly(A)+ RNA have also been demonstrated.[137] FISH detection of a number of specific high-abundance mRNAs has been reported,[113,119,120,136,140,142,144] including cytokine mRNAs[145] and actin mRNA.[143] Lower-copy-number target RNAs have also been detected. Lalli et al reported detection of 1200 copies of glyceraldehyde-3-phosphate dehydrogenase (GAPDH) mRNA,[140] and Yu et al reported detection of 1800 copies of H4, 18S, and 28S mRNAs.[149] Additionally, 500 copies of beta-globin mRNA have been detected,[136] as have as few as 150-300 copies of immunoglobulin V_H mRNA.[144] More recent work, employing large pools of oligonucleotide probes having homogeneous hybridization and nonspecific binding characteristics directed at detection of HIV viral RNA, has detected as few as 30 copies of RNA per cell in an activated ACH-2 cell line model system.[113] However, detection of positive cells in a heterogeneous population was at a somewhat higher cellular target copy number. Other viral studies, using flow cytometric approaches employing FISH, have been reported in HIV,[138] HPV,[117] and EBV.[119,120] Interestingly, enticing preliminary data point to the potential additional prognostic information that cellular viral load measurements may provide above that given by more classic viral load measurements.[113]

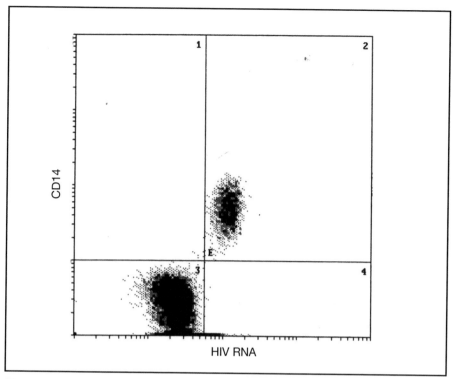

Figure 8-5

Bivariate histogram of CD14 staining intensity versus bound HIV RNA probe intensity for peripheral blood mononuclear cells isolated from a HIV+ patient. Cells were stained with a phycoerythrin-labeled anti-CD14 antibody and hybridized with a cocktail of 5(6)-carboxy-fluoroscein-labeled oligonucleotide probes directed against HIV RNA.

In a study of 39 HIV-infected patients, for 6 of 7 patients who showed a significant increase in their plasma viral load levels, the increase in plasma viral load was preceded by an increase in the cellular viral load levels as reflected in numbers of monocytes positive for HIV RNA.[113] An example of detection of HIV RNA in peripheral blood monocytes isolated from an HIV-positive patient is shown in **Figure 8-5.**

In Situ PCR and In Situ RT-PCR Approaches

To improve the sensitivity of detection of specific nucleic acid sequences in individual cells, a number of groups have employed either in situ PCR or in situ RT-PCR techniques adapted for cells in suspension.[69,111,112,155-157] In this approach, a target sequence of interest within the cell is amplified to a very high copy number using primers that span the sequence of interest. This amplified target is then detected either by incorporating a labeled nucleotide into the amplified product[155-157] or by using a labeled probe having homology for the amplified product in a subsequent FISH step.[69,111,112] Some improvement in signal-to-noise has been reported for the in situ PCR (RT-PCR) and FISH combination compared with incorporation of the label into the amplified product for direct detection.[112,157-159] Indeed, these approaches can be very sensitive, with detection of a single copy HIV DNA sequence per cell being reported.[111] As shown in **Figure 8-6,** cellular-based in situ PCR can be coupled with cellular immunophenotyping, allowing characterization of positive cells[112] and increasing sensitivity by examining nucleic acid expression, or presence, in only a subpopulation of cells within a heterogeneous sample. At least at present, greater than 3%-5% positive cells within the selected population is necessary for reliable detection.[111,112] Nonetheless, with the appropriate choice of immunophenotypic marker, this can be a sensitive technique detecting less than 1% positive cells within a sample.

Cellular-based in situ PCR in flow cytometry has been used in the study of HIV disease[111,112] as well as to detect higher copy number genomic targets.[157] Studies of the technique coupled with simultaneous CD4 detection using multiple anti-CD4 antibodies demonstrated that the reduced CD4 staining seen in HIV DNA–positive helper cells (**Figure 8-6**) was due to either epitope alteration/deletion or masking and not to down-regulation of the CD4 antigen.[112] In situ RT-PCR techniques for cells in suspension with flow cytometric detection of positive cells have also been developed.[69,111,155,156] Parallel coupling of the in situ RT-PCR and PCR approaches permitted determination of latent and active infection in HIV-positive patients, demonstrating that the majority of circulating peripheral blood mononuclear cells were latently infected.[111] In situ RT-PCR approaches have also been used to detect the *bcr/abl* translocation mRNA resultant from the t(9;22) translocation in both cell lines[156] and in chronic myelogenous leukemia patients.[69]

At present, successful coupling of simultaneous immunophenotyping and in situ RT-PCR in flow cytometric analyses has not been reported. The successful reports of in situ RT-PCR with cells in suspension have all involved a digestion of cellular protein, generally with proteinase K.[69,111,150] This digestion step has precluded the ability to do simultaneous antigen detection, pointing to the need for a more specific destruction, or elimination, of the cellular proteins that inhibit reverse transcription while leaving other cellular markers intact.[150] At least at present, these flow cytometry-based assays offer no sensitivity advantage over more robust-slide based approaches, and therefore, without the ability

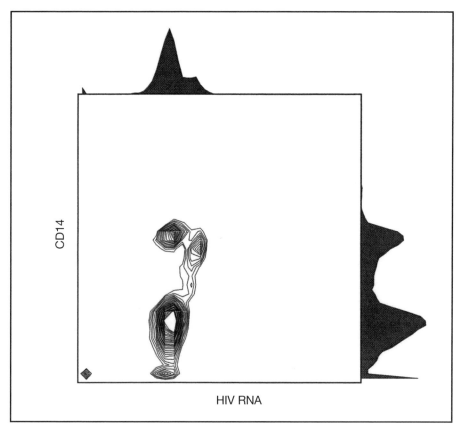

Figure 8-6

Bivariate histogram of CD4 staining intensity versus bound HIV DNA probe intensity for peripheral blood lymphocytes isolated from an HIV+ patient. Peripheral blood mononuclear cells were depleted of monocytes using an anti-CD14 magnetic bead system. Cell suspensions were then stained with a biotinylated anti-CD4 antibody and in situ PCR for HIV DNA was performed. The intracellular amplified PCR product was detected in a hybridization reaction employing a single 5(6)-carboxyfluorescein-labeled oligonucleotide probe directed against the HIV DNA PCR-amplified product. The biotinylated antibody was detected using a phycoerythrin-labeled streptavidin.

to more completely characterize the positive cells, lose most of their attractiveness. However, increases in their sensitivity, or more importantly, development of techniques to permit coupling with the detection of other cellular characteristics, could still prove beneficial. Successful in situ RT-PCR with suspension cells has been achieved using an acidic extraction of cellular protein rather than wholesale digestion.[150]

Summary and Comments

A conscious effort to integrate flow cytometry and molecular biology in the clinical laboratory is only just beginning. To date, the majority of the clinically relevant applications of this integration involve the use of antibodies to specific gene products in straightforward immunofluorescence assays. Returning to the example of flow cytometric detection of specific variable regions of the T-cell receptor, these analyses, although involving immunofluorescence staining with antibodies, would not be possible or meaningful without an understanding of the molecular biology of the T-cell receptor. This same statement can be made about the detection of oncogene products, *MDR1* and other specific gene products by flow cytometry.

Perhaps the greatest potential integration of flow cytometry with molecular biology lies in the possibility of "genotyping" individual cells; in other words, adapting the exquisite specificity of molecular biological techniques for providing genomic information to the approach that is commonly used to phenotype cell populations. This has the potential of genotypically discriminating between normal and neoplastic cells, activated and resting cells, cells of different lineages or levels of maturation, and so forth. Fluorescence in situ hybridization (FISH) techniques demonstrate great promise for detecting specific sequences of nucleic acids by flow cytometry, particularly in instances where multiple copies of the nucleic acid sequence are present (such as detection of mRNA sequences). The examples given in this text are from preliminary work in this field and as of yet have only limited application in today's clinical laboratory. Almost certainly, many of these prototype methods—or derivatives of them—will become common clinical assays in the near future. Few question the potential of multiparameter, flow cytometry-based cellular measurements of nucleic acid sequences. However, in general, it has been difficult for individual laboratories to implement these assays and to reproduce the work of others. In many or most instances, these problems can be traced to a lack of adequate quality reagents for performing the techniques[73,74] or to a lack of appreciation of potential artifacts and background problems as well as critical details in the protocols. Nonetheless, an increasing number of laboratories have successfully repeated the work of others and successfully utilized these techniques in their studies. An exciting future lies ahead for the incorporation of these measurements into more and more sophisticated, multiparametric molecular cytometry techniques. Given the rapid technical developments in both molecular biology and flow cytometry, developments in clinical molecular cytometry will be limited only by the boundaries of creativity.

References

1. Fletcher JA. DNA in situ hybridization as an adjunct in tumor diagnosis. *Am J Clin Pathol.* 1999;112(1suppl 1):S11-S18.

2. Vnencak-Jones CL. Molecular testing for inherited diseases. *Am J Clin Pathol.* 1999;112(1suppl 1):S19-S32.

3. Bagg A, Kallakury BVS. Molecular pathology of leukemia and lymphoma. *Am J Clin Pathol.* 1999;112(1suppl 1):S76-S92.

4. Tsongalis GJ, Wu AHB, Silver H, et al. Applications of forensic testing in the clinical laboratory. *Am J Clin Pathol.* 1999;112(1suppl 1):S93-S103.

5. Association for Molecular Pathology: Association for Molecular Pathology Statement: Recommendations for in-house development and operation of molecular diagnostic tests. *Am J Clin Pathol.* 1999;111:449-463.

6. Kiechle FL. Diagnostic molecular pathology in the twenty-first century. *Clin Lab Med.* 1996;16:213-222.

7. McCoy JP, Overton WR, Schroeder K, et al. Immunophenotypic analysis of the T cell receptor Vβ repertoire in normal peripheral blood: survey of expression in CD4+ and CD8+ lymphocytes. *Cytometry.* 1996;26:148-153.

8. Charley MR, McCoy JP, Deng JS, et al. Anti-V region antibodies as "almost clonotypic" reagents for the study of cutaneous T cell lymphomas and leukemias. *J Invest Dermatol.* 1990;95:614-617.

9. McCoy JP, Overton WR, Blumstein L, et al. Alterations of T cell receptor variable region expression in the progression of HIV disease. *Cytometry.* 1995;22:1-9.

10. Jordan VC. Studies on the estrogen receptor in breast cancer: 20 years as a target for the treatment and prevention of cancer. *Breast Cancer Res Treatment.* 1995;36:267-285.

11. Buzdar AU, Hortobagyi GN. Recent advances in adjuvant therapy of breast cancer. *Semin Oncol.* 1999;26(4 suppl 12):21-27.

12. Nichols GE, Frierson HF, Boyd JC, et al. Automated immunohistochemical assay for estrogen receptor status in breast cancer using monoclonal antibody CC4-5 on the Ventana ES. *Am J Clin Pathol.* 1996;106:332-338.

13. Tesch M, Shawwa A, Henderson R. Immunohistochemical determination of estrogen and progesterone receptor status in breast cancer. *Am J Clin Pathol.* 1993;99:8-12.

14. Harvey JM, Clark GM, Osborne CK, et al. Estrogen receptor status by immunohistochemistry is superior to the ligand-binding assay for predicting response to adjuvant endocrine therapy in breast cancer. *J Clin Oncol.* 1999;17:1474-1481.

15. Redkar AA, Krishan A. Flow cytometric analysis of estrogen, progesterone receptor expression and DNA content in formalin-fixed, paraffin-embedded human breast tumors. *Cytometry.* 1999;38:61-69.

16. Brotherick I, Lennard TWJ, Cook S, et al. Use of the biotinylated antibody DAKO-ER 1D5 to measure oestrogen receptor on cytokeratin positive cells obtained from primary breast cancer cells. *Cytometry.* 1995;20:74-80.

17. Remvikos Y, VuHai M, Laine-Bidron DE, et al. Progesterone receptor detection and quantification in breast tumors by bivariate immunofluoresecnce/DNA flow cytometry. *Cytometry.* 1991;24:260-267.

18. Schutte B, Scheres HME, De Goij AFPM, et al. Flow cytometric steroid receptor analysis. *Prog Histochem Cytochem.* 1992;26:68-76.

19. Van NT, Raber M, Barrows GH, et al. Estrogen receptor analysis by flow cytometry. *Science.* 1984;224:876-879.

20. Green S, Gronemeyer H, Chambon P. Structure and function of steroid hormone receptors. In: Sluyser M, ed. *Growth Factors and Oncogenes in Breast Cancer.* Hemel Hempstead, Hertfordshire, UK: Ellis Horwood; 1987:7-28.

21. King WJ, Green GL. Monoclonal antibodies localize estrogen receptor in the nuclei of target cells. *Nature.* 1984;307:745-747.

22. Riordan JR, Deuchars K, Kartner N, et al. Amplification of P-glycoprotein genes in multidrug-resistant mammalian cell lines. *Nature.* 1985;316:817-820.

23. Kartner N, Riordan JR, Ling V. Cell surface P-glycoprotein associated with multidrug resistance in mammalian cell lines. *Science.* 1983;221:1285-1288.

24. Zaman GJR, Borst P. MRP: mode of action and role in MDR. In: Gupta S, Tsuruo T, eds. *Multidrug Resistance in Cancer Cells.* New York, NY: Wiley-Liss Inc; 1996:95-107.

25. Gottesman MM, Pastan I. Biochemistry of multidrug resistance mediated by the multidrug transporter. *Ann Rev Biochem.* 1993;62:385-427.

26. Germann UA. P-glycoprotein: a mediator of multidrug resistance in tumour cells. *Eur J Cancer.* 1996;32A:927-944.

27. Krishan A, Singh SV, Nair S, et al. Flow cytometric monitoring of drug resistant related markers in human tumor cells. *Cytometry.* 1990;Suppl 4:10.

28. Epstein J, Xiao H, Oba BK. P-glycoprotein expression in plasma cell myeloma is associated with resistance to VAD. *Blood.* 1989;74:913-917.

29. Bell DR, Gerlach JH, Kartner N, et al. Detection of P-glycoprotein in ovarian cancer: a molecular marker associated with multidrug resistance. *J Clin Oncol.* 1985;3:311-315.

30. Salmon SE, Grogan TM, Miller T, et al. Prediction of doxorubicin resistance in vitro in myeloma, lymphoma, and breast cancer by p-glycoprotein staining. *J Natl Cancer Inst.* 1989;81:696-701.

31. Pallis M, Turzanski J, Harrison G, et al. Use of standardized flow cytometric determinants of multidrug resistance to analyse response to remission induction chemotherapy in patients with acute myeloblastic leukaemia. *Br J Haematol.* 1999;104:307-312.

32. Labroille G, Belloc F, Bihou-Nabera C, et al. Cytometric study of intracellular P-gp expression and reversal of drug resistance. *Cytometry.* 1998;32:86-94.

33. Den Boer ML, Zwaan CM, Pieters R, et al. Optimal immunocytochemical and flow cytometric detection of P-gp, MRP, and LRP in childhood acute lymphoblastic leukemia. *Leukemia.* 1997;11:1078-1085.

34. Brotherick I, Shenton BK, Egan M, et al. Examination of multidrug resistance in cell lines and primary breast tumors by flow cytometry. *Eur J Cancer.* 1996;32A:2334-2341.

35. Ferrand VL, Montero FA, Chauvet MM, et al. Quantitative determination of the MDR-related P-glycoprotein, Pgp 170, by a rapid flow cytometric technique. *Cytometry.* 1996;23:120-125.

36. Huet S, Marie JP, Gualde N, et al. Reference method for detection of Pgp mediated multidrug resistance in human hematological malignancies: a method validated by the laboratories of the French Drug Resistance Network. *Cytometry.* 1998;34:248-256.

37. Krishan A, Ganapathi R. Laser flow cytometric studies on the intracellular fluorescence of anthracyclines. *Cancer Res.* 1980;40:3895-3900.

38. Ross DD, Thompson BW, Ordonez JV, et al. Improvement of flow cytometric detection of multidrug-resistant cells by cell-volume normalization of intracellular daunorubicin content. *Cytometry.* 1989;10:185-191.

39. Legrand O, Simonin G, Perrot JY, et al. Pgp and MRP activities using calcein-AM are prognostic factors in adult acute myeloid leukemia patients. *Blood.* 1998;91:4480-4488.

40. Gheuens EEO, van Bockstaele DR, van der Keur M, et al. Flow cytometric double labeling technique for screening of multidrug resistance. *Cytometry.* 1991;12:636-644.

41. Leith C. Multidrug resistance in leukemia. *Curr Opinion Hematol.* 1998;5:287-291.

42. Den Boer ML, Pieters R, Kazemier KM, et al. Relationship between major vault protein/lung resistance protein, multidrug resistance-associated protein, P-glycoprotein expression, and drug resistance in childhood leukemia. *Blood.* 1998;91:2092-2098.

43. Hart SM, Ganeshaguru K, Scheper RJ, et al. Expression of the human major vault protein LRP in acute myeloid leukemia. *Exp Hematol.* 1997;25:1227-1232.

44. Krishnamachary N, Center MS. The MRP gene associated with a non-p glycoprotein multidrug resistance encodes a 190 k-Da membrane-bound glycoprotein. *Cancer Res.* 1993;53:3658-3661.

45. Loe DW, Deeley RG, Cole SPC. Biology of the multidrug resistance-associated protein, MRP. *Eur J Cancer.* 1996;32A:945-957.

46. Zaman GJ, Lankelma J, van Tellingen O, et al. Role of glutathione in the export of compounds from cells by the multidrug-resistance-associated protein. *Proc Natl Acad Sci U S A.* 1995;92:7690-7694.

47. Slovak ML, Ho JP, Cole SPC, et al. The LRP gene encoding a major vault protein associated with drug resistance maps proximal to MRP on chromosome 16: evidence that chromosome breakage plays a key role in MRP or LRP gene amplification. *Cancer Res.* 1995;55:4214-4219.

48. Webb M, Brun M, McNiven M, et al. MDR1 and MRP expression in chronic B-cell lymphoproliferative disorders. *Br J Haematol.* 1998;102:710-717.

49. Den Boer ML, Zwaan CM, Pieters R, et al. Optimal immunocytochemical and flow cytometric detection of P-gp, MRP, and LRP in childhood acute lymphoblastic leukemia. *Leukemia.* 1997;11:1078-1085.

50. Boutonnat J, Bonnefoix T, Mousseau M, et al. Coexpression of multidrug resistances involve proteins: a flow cytometric analysis. *Anticancer Res.* 1998;18:2993-2999.

51. Stewart CC. Flow cytometric analysis of oncogene expression in human neoplasias. *Arch Pathol Lab Med.* 1989;113:634-640.

52. Freedman D, Auersperg N. Detection of an intracellular transforming protein (v-Ki-ras p21) using the flow activated cell sorter (FACS). *In Vitro Cell Dev Biol.* 1986;22:621.

53. Takeda T, Krause JR, Carey JL, et al. Detection of the ras p21 gene product in human leukemias by flow cytometry. *J Clin Lab Analysis.* 1989;3:108-115.

54. Watson JV, Sikora K, Evan GI. A simultaneous flow cytometric assay for c-myc oncoprotein and DNA in nuclei from paraffin embedded material. *J Immunol Methods.* 1985;83:179-192.

55. Giardina SL, Evans SW, Gandino L, et al. Generation of a murine monoclonal antibody that detects the fos oncogene product. *Analytical Biochem.* 1987;161:109-116.

56. Andreeff M, Slater DE, Bressler J, et al. Cellular *ras* oncogene expression and cell cycle measured by flow cytometry in hematopoietic cell lines. *Blood.* 1986;67:676-681.

57. McCoy JP, Takeda T, Hanley K, et al. Multiple parameter (three-color) flow cytometric analysis of surface marker, oncogene product, and DNA content in human leukemias. *Federal Proc.* 1989;3:A614.

58. Watson, JV, Curling OM, Munn CF, et al. Oncogene expression in ovarian cancer: a pilot study of c-myc oncoprotein in serous papillary ovarian cancer. *Gynecol Oncol.* 1987;28:137-150.

59. Watson, JV, Stewart J, Evan GI, et al. The clinical significance of flow cytometric c-myc oncoprotein quantitation in testicular cancer. *Br J Cancer.* 1986;53:331-337.

60. Bains MA, Hoy TG, Baines P, et al. Nuclear c-myc protein, naturation and cell-cycle status of human haemopoietic cells. *Br J Haematol.* 1987;67:293-300.

61. Holte H, Stokke T, Smeland E, et al. Levels of myc protein, as analyzed by flow cytometry, correlate with cell growth potential in malignant B-cell lymphomas. *Int J Cancer.* 1989;43:164-170.

62. Hughes RG, Neill WA, Norval M. Papillomavirus and c-myc antigen expression in normal and neoplastic cervical epithelium. *J Clin Pathol.* 1989;42:46-51.

63. Watson JV, Munn CF, Cox H, et al. A simultaneous assay for c-myc and c-fos nuclear oncoproteins plus DNA in human archival cancer biopsies. *Cytometry.* 1987; (Suppl 1):2.

64. Kelsten ML, Berger M, Chianese D. Analysis of c-erb B-2 protein expression in conjunction with DNA content using multiparameter flow cytometry. *Cytometry.* 1990;11:522-532.

65. Swanson PE, Fitzpatrick MM, Ritter JH, et al. Immunohistologic differential diagnosis of basal cell carcinoma, squamous cell carcinoma, and trichoepithelioma in small cutaneous biopsy specimens. *J Cutaneous Pathol.* 1998;25:153-159.

66. Falini B, Flenghi L, Fagioli M, et al. Immunocytochemical diagnosis of acute promyelocytic leukemia (M3) with the monoclonal antibody PG-M3 (anti-PML). *Blood.* 1997;90:4046-4053.

67. Shackney SE, Pollice A, Smith CA, et al. A genetic staging system for human solid tumors. *Cytometry* 1991; (Suppl 5):28.

68. Shackney SE, Shankey TV. Common patterns of genetic evolution in human solid tumors. *Cytometry.* 1997;29:1-27.

69. Testoni N, Martinelli L, Farabegoli P, et al. A new method of "in-cell reverse transcriptase-polymerase chain reaction" for the detection of BCR/ABL transcript in chronic myeloid leukemia patients. *Blood.* 1996;87:3822-3827.

70. Yang J, Liu X, Bhalla K, et al. Prevention of apoptosis by Bcl-2: release of cytochrome c from mitochondria blocked. *Science.* 1997;275:1129.

71. Jia L, Macey MG, Yin Y, et al. Subcellular distribution and redistribution of bcl-2 family proteins in human leukemia cells undergoing apoptosis. *Blood.* 1999;93:2353-2359.

72. DiGiuseppe JA, LeBeau P, Augenbraun J, et al. Multiparametric flow-cytometric analysis of bcl-2 and Fas expression in normal and neoplastic hematopoiesis. *Am J Clin Pathol.* 1996;106:345-351.

73. Finlay CA, Hinds PW, Levine AJ. The p53 proto-oncogene can act as a suppressor of transformation. *Cell.* 1989;57:1083-1093.

74. Brown JM, Wouters BG. Apoptosis, p53, and tumor cell sensitivity to anticancer agents. *Cancer Res.* 1999;59:1391-1399.

75. Danova M, Giordano M, Mazzini G, et al. Expression of p53 protein during the cell cycle measured by flow cytometry in human leukemia. *Leukemia Res.* 1990;14:417-422.

76. Remvikos Y, Laurent-Puig P, Salmon RJ, et al. Simultaneous monitoring of p53 protein and DNA content of colorectal adenocarcinomas by flow cytometry. *Int J Cancer.* 1990;45:450-456.

77. Blount PL, Ramel S, Raskind WH, et al. 17p allelic deletions and p53 protein overexpression in Barrett's adenocarcinoma. *Cancer Res.* 1991;51:5482-5486.

78. Filippini G, Griffin S, Uhr M, et al. A novel flow cytometric method for the quantification of p53 gene expression. *Cytometry.* 1998;31:180-186.

79. Weinberg KI, Kohn DB. Gene therapy for congenital lymphoid immunodeficiency diseases. *Semin Hematol.* 1998;35:354-366.

80. Roskrow MA, Gansbacher B. Recent developments in gene therapy for oncology and hematology. *Crit Rev Oncol-Hematol.* 1998;28:139-151.

81. Cusack JC Jr, Tanabe KK. Cancer gene therapy. *Surg Oncol Clin North Am.* 1998;7:421-469.

82. Karpati G, Pari G, Molnar MJ. Molecular therapy for genetic muscle diseases—status 1999. *Clin Genetics.* 1999;55:1-8.

83. Boucher RC. Status of gene therapy for cystic fibrosis lung disease. *J. Clin. Invest.* 1999;103:441-445.

84. Rice GC, Pennica D. Detection by flow cytometry of protoplast fusion and transient expression of transferred heterologous CD4 sequence in COS-7 cells. *Cytometry.* 1989;10:103-107.

85. Erlich S, Miranda SR, Visser JW, et al. Fluorescence-based selection of gene-corrected hematopoietic stem and progenitor cells from acid sphingomyelinase-deficient mice: implications for Niemann-Pick disease and the development of improved stem cell gene transfer procedures. *Blood.* 1999;93:80-86.

86. Fiering SN, Roederer M, Nolan GP, et al. Improved FACS-Gal: flow cytometric analysis and sorting of viable eukaryotic cells expressing reporter gene constructs. *Cytometry.* 1991;12:291-301.

87. Mazurier F, Moreau-Gaudry F, Maguer-Satta V, et al. Rapid analysis and efficient selection of human transduced primitive hematopoietic cells using the humanized S65T green fluorescent protein. *Gene Ther.* 1998;5:556-562.

88. Wiechen K, Zimmer C, Dietel M. Selection of a high activity c-erbB-2 ribozyme using a fusion gene of c-erbB-2 and the enhanced green fluorescent protein. *Cancer Gene Ther.* 1998;5:45-51.

89. Klein D, Indraccolo S, von Rombs K, et al. Rapid identification of viable retrovirus-transduced cells using the green fluorescent protein as a marker. *Gene Ther.* 1997;4:1256-1260.

90. Misteli T, Spector DL. Applications of the green fluorescent protein in cell biology and biotechnology. *Nat Biotechnol.* 1997;15:961-964.

91. Blennerhasset GT, Furth M, Anderson A, et al. Clinical evaluation of a DNA probe assay for the Philadelphia (Ph1) translocation in chronic myelogenous leukemia. *Leukemia.* 1988;2:648-657.

92. Borkhardt A, Cazzaniga G, Viehmann S, et al. Incidence and clinical relevance of TEL/AML1 fusion genes in children with acute lymphoblastic leukemia enrolled in the German and Italian multicenter therapy trials. *Blood.* 1997;90:571-577.

93. Claxton DF, Liu P, Hsu HB, et al. Detection of fusion transcripts generated by the inversion 16 chromosome in acute myelogenous leukemia. *Blood.* 1994;83:1750-1756.

94. Gauwerky CE, Croce CM. Chromosomal translocations in leukemia. *Semin Cancer Biol.* 1993;4:333-340.

95. Harbott J, Viehmann S, Borkhardt A, et al. Incidence of TEL/AML1 fusion gene analyzed consecutively in children with acute lymphoblastic leukemia in relapse. *Blood.* 1997;90:4933-4937.

96. Kita K, Shirakawa S, Kamada N, and the Japanese Cooperative Group of Leukemia/Lymphoma. Cellular characteristics of acute myeloblastic leukemia associated with t(8;21)(q22;q22). *Leukemia Lymphoma.* 1994;13:158-165.

97. Lambrechts AC, Hupkes PE, Dorssers LCJ, et al. Translocation (14;18)-positive cells are present in the circulation of the majority of patients with localized (stage I and II) follicular non-Hodgkin's lymphoma. *Blood.* 1993;82:2510-2516.

98. Larson RA, Kondo K, Vardiman JM, et al. Evidence for a 15;17 translocation in every patient with acute promyelocytic leukemia. *Am J Med.* 1984;65:673-677.

99. Lee M-S, Kantarjian HM, Talpaz M, et al. Detection of minimal residual disease by polymerase chain reaction in Philadelphia chromosome positive chronic myelogenous leukemia following interferon therapy. *Blood.* 1992;79:1920-1923.

100. LoCoco F, Diverio D, Pandolfi PP, et al. Molecular evaluation of residual disease as a predictor of relapse in acute promyelocytic leukemia. *Lancet.* 1992;340:1437-1438.

101. Nowell PC, Hungerford DA. A minute chromosome in human chronic granulocytic leukemia. *Science.* 1960;132:1497.

102. Nucifora G, Rowley JD. The AML1 and ETO genes in acute myeloid leukemia with a t(8;21). *Leukemia Lymphoma.* 1994;14:353-362.

103. Rowley JD. A new consistent chromosomal abnormality in chronic myelogenous leukemia identified by quinacrine fluorescence and Giemsa staining. *Nature.* 1973;243:290-293.

104. Soubeyran P, Cabanillas F, Lee MS. Analysis of the expression of the hybrid gene bcl-2/IgH in follicular lymphoma. *Blood.* 1993;81:122-127.

105. Taub R, Krisch L, Morton C, et al. Translocation of the c-myc gene into the immunoglobulin heavy chain locus in human Burkitt lymphoma and murine plasmacytoma cells. *Proc Natl Acad Sci USA.* 1982;79:7837-7841.

106. Thirman MJ, Gill HJ, Burnett RC, et al. Rearrangement of the MLL gene in acute lymphoblastic and acute myeloid leukemias with 11q23 chromosomal translocations. *N Engl J Med.* 1993;329:909-914.

107. Hunger SP, Galili N, Carroll AJ, et al. The t(1;19)(q23;p13) results in consistent fusion of E2A and PBX1 coding sequences in acute lymphoblastic leukemias. *Blood.* 1991;77:687-693.

108. Izraeli S, Janssen JWG, Haas OA, et al. Detection and clinical relevance of genetic abnormalities in pediatric acute lymphoblastic leukemia: a comparison between cytogenetic and polymerase chain reaction analyses. *Leukemia.* 1993;7:671-678.

109. Zhao L, Kantarhian HM, Oort JV, et al. Detection of residual proliferating leukemic cells by fluorescence in situ hybridization in CML patients in complete remission after interferon treatment. *Leukemia.* 1993;7:168-171.

110. Westbrook CA. The role of molecular techniques in the clinical management of leukemia: lessons from the Philadelphia chromosome. *Cancer.* 1992;70:1695-1700.

111. Patterson BK, Till M, Otto P, et al. Detection of HIV-1 DNA and messenger RNA in individual cells by PCR-driven in situ hybridization and flow cytometry. *Science.* 1993;260:976-979.

112. Patterson BK, Goolsby CL, Hodara V, et al. Detection of decreased CD4 expression in CD4 positive HIV-1 DNA positive cells by dual immunophenotyping and fluorescence in situ polymerase chain reaction. *J Virol.* 1995;69:4316-4322.

113. Patterson BK, Mosiman VL, Cantarero L, et al. Detection of persistently productive infection of monocytes in the peripheral blood of HIV positive patients using a flow cytometry based FISH assay. *Cytometry.* 1998;31:265-274.

114. Imbert-Marcille BM, Robillard N, Poirier AS, et al. Development of a method for direct quantification of cytomegalovirus anitgenemia by flow cytometry. *J Clin Microbiol.* 1997;35:2665-2669.

115. Just T, Burgwald H, Broe MK. Flow cytometric detection of EBV (EBER snRNA) using peptide nucleic acid probes. *J Virol Methods.* 1998;73:163-174.

116. Komminoth P, Adams V, Long AA, et al. Evaluation of methods for hepatitis C virus detection in archival liver biopsies. *Pathol Res Pract.* 1994;190:1017-1025.

117. Lizard G, Chignol MC, Chardonnet Y, et al. Detection of human papillomavirus DNA in CaSki and HeLa cells by fluorescent in situ hybridization. *J Immunol Methods.* 1993;157:31-38.

118. Montone KT, Lizky LA, Wurster A, et al. Analysis of Epstein-Barr virus associated posttransplantation lymphoproliferative disorder after lung transplantation. *Surgery.* 1996;119:544-551.

119. Crouch J, Leitenberg D, Smith BR, et al. Epstein-Barr virus suspension cell assay using in situ hybridization and flow cytometry. *Cytometry.* 1997;29:50-57.

120. Stowe RP, Cubbage ML, Sams CF, et al. Detection and quantification of Epstein-Barr virus EBER1 in EBV-infected cells by fluorescent in situ hybridization and flow cytometry. *J Virol Methods.*1998;75:83-91.

121. Gray JW, Lucas J, Peters D, et al. Flow karyotyping and sorting of human chromosomes. *Cold Spring Harbor Symp Quant Biol.* 1986;LI:141-149.

122. Jensen RH, Langlois RG, Mayall BH. Strategies for choosing a deoxyribonucleic acid stain for flow cytometry of metaphase chromosomes. *J Histochem Cytochem.* 1977;25:954.

123. Langlois RG, Yu L-C, Gray JW, et al. Quantitative karyotyping of human chromosomes by dual beam flow cytometry. *Proc Natl Acad Sci U S A.* 1982;79:7876-7880.

124. Bartholdi M, Meyne J, Albright K, et al. Chromosome sorting by flow cytometry. *Methods Enzymol.* 1987;151:252-267.

125. Bartholdi MF, Ray FA, Cram LS, et al. Karyotype instability of Chinese hamster cells during tumor progression. *Somatic Cell Mol Genetics.* 1987;13:1-10.

126. Cram LS. Flow cytogenetics and chromosome sorting. *Hum Cell.* 1990;3:99-106.

127. Meyne J, Bartholdi MF, Travis GL, et al. Counterstaining human chromosomes for flow karyology. *Cytometry.* 1984;5:580-583.

128. Gray JW, Trask B, van den Engh G, et al. Application of flow karyotyping in prenatal detection of chromosome aberrations. *Am J Hum Genetics.* 1988;42:49-59.

129. Lebo RV, Golbus MS, Cheung MC. Detecting abnormal human chromosome constitutions by dual laser flow cytogenetics. *Am J Med Genetics.* 1986;25:519-529.

130. Goolsby CL, Wiley JE, Steiner M, et al. Karyotype evolution in a simian virus 40-transformed tumorigenic human cell line. *Can Genet Cytogenet.* 1990;50:231-248.

131. Deaven LL, van Dilla MA, Bartholdi MF, et al. Construction of human chromosome-specific DNA libraries from flow-sorted chromosomes. *Cold Spring Harbor Symp Quant Biol.* 1986;LI:159-167.

132. Lebo RV, Tolan DR, Bruce BD, et al. Spot blot analysis of sorted chromosomes assigns a fructose intolerance gene locus to chromosome 9. *Cytometry.* 1985;6:478-483.

133. Blennow E, Telenius H, Larsson C, et al. Complete characterization of a large marker chromosome by reverse and forward chromosome painting. *Hum Genetics.* 1992;90:371-374.

134. Arkesteijn GJ, Erpelinck SL, Martens AC, et al. Chromosome specific DNA hybridization in suspension for flow cytometric detection of chimaerism in bone marrow transplantation and leukemia. *Cytometry.* 1995;19:353-360.

135. Bauman JGJ, Bentvelzen P. Flow cytometric detection of ribosomal RNA in suspended cells by fluorescent in situ hybridization. *Cytometry.* 1988;9:517-524.

136. Bayer JA, Bauman JGJ. Flow cytometric detection of beta-globin mRNA in murine haemopoietic tissues using fluorescent in situ hybridization. *Cytometry.* 1990;11:132-143.

137. Belloc F, Lacombe F, Dumain P, et al. Flow cytometric estimation of Poly(A)+ RNA by fluorescent in situ hybridization. *Cytometry.* 1993;14:339-343.

138. Borzi RM, Piacentini A, Monaco MC, et al. A fluorescent in situ hybridization method in flow cytometry to detect HIV-1 specific RNA. *J Immunol Methods.* 1996;193:167-176.

139. Donovan JA, Simmons FA, Esrason KT, et al. Donor origin of a posttransplant liver allograft malignancy identified by fluorescence in situ hybridization for the Y chromosome and DNA genotyping. *Transplantation.* 1997;63:80-84.

140. Lalli E, Gibellini D, Santi S, et al. In situ hybridization in suspension and flow cytometry as a tool for the study of gene expression. *Analyt Biochem.* 1992;207:298-303.

141. Pajor L, Bauman JGJ. Flow cytometric measurement of rRNA levels detected by fluorescent in situ hybridization in differentiating K-562 cells. *Histochemistry.* 1991;96:73-81.

142. Pennline KJ, Pellerito-Bessette F, Umland, SP, et al. Detection of in vivo-induced IL-1 mRNA in murine cells by flow cytometry (FC) and fluorescent in situ hybridization (FISH). *Lymph Cyto Res.* 1992;11:65-71.

143. Pinkel D, Gray JW, Trask B, et al. Cytogenetic analysis by in situ hybridization with fluorescently labeled nucleic acid probes. In: *Cold Spring Harbor Symp Quant Biol.* 1986;LI:151-157.

144. Ravichandran KS, Semproni AR, Goldsby RA, et al. Immunoglobulin VH usage analysis by fluorescent in situ hybridization and flow cytometry. *J Immunol Methods.* 1992;153:249-259.

145. Timm Jr, EA, Stewart CC. Fluorescent in situ hybridization en suspension (FISHES) using digoxigenin-labeled probes and flow cytometry. *BioTechniques.* 1992;12:363-366.

146. Trask B, van den Engh G, Landegent J, et al. Detection of DNA sequences in nuclei in suspension by in situ hybridization and dual beam flow cytometry. *Science.* 1985;230:1401-1403.

147. Trask B, van den Engh G, Pinkel D, et al. Fluorescence in situ hybridization to interphase cell nuclei in suspension allows flow cytometric analysis of chromosome content and microscopic analysis of nuclear organization. *Human Genetics.* 1988;78:251-259.

148. van Dekken H, Arkesteijn GJA, Visser JWM, et al. Flow cytometric quantification of human chromosome specific repetitive DNA sequences by single and bicolor fluorescent in situ hybridization to lymphocyte interphase nuclei. *Cytometry.* 1990;11:153-164.

149. Yu H, Ernst L, Wagner M, et al. Sensitive detection of RNAs in single cells by flow cytometry. *Nucleic Acids Res.* 1992;20:83-88.

150. Goolsby CL, Thompson E, Mosiman V. Combined immunophenotyping and molecular phenotyping. In: Stewart C, Nicholson J, eds. *Immunophenotyping.* New York, NY: John Wiley & Sons Inc. In press.

151. Mosiman VL, Goolsby CL. In situ hybridization in flow cytometry. In: Faguet G, ed. *Hematologic Malignancies.* Cleveland, Ohio: CRC Press. In press.

152. Bianchi DW, Harris P, Flint A, et al. Direct hybridization to DNA from small numbers of flow-sorted nucleated newborn cells. *Cytometry.* 1987;8:197-202.

153. van Tol MJ, Langlois van den Bergh W, Mesker W, et al. Simultaneous detection of X and Y chromosomes by two-color fluorescence in situ hybridization in combination with immunophenotyping of single cells to document chimaerism after sex-mismatched bone marrow transplantation. *Bone Marrow Transplantation.* 1998;21:497-503.

154. Mosiman VL, Patterson BK, Canterero L. Reducing cellular autofluorescence in flow cytometry: an in situ method. *Cytometry.* 1997;30:151-156.

155. Bains MA, Agarwal R, Pringle JH, et al. Flow cytometric quantitation of sequence-specific mRNA in hemopoietic cell suspensions by primer-induced in situ (PRINS) fluorescent nucleotide labeling. *Exp Cell Res.* 1993;208:321-326.

156. Embleton MJ, Gorochov G, Jones PT, et al. In-cell PCR from mRNA: amplifying and linking the rearranged immunoglobulin heavy and light chain V-genes within single cells. *Nucl Acids Res.* 1992;20:3831-3837.

157. Timm EA Jr, Podniesinske E, Duckett L, et al. Amplification and detection of a Y-chromosome DNA sequence by fluorescence in situ polymerase chain reaction and flow cytometry using cells in suspension. *Cytometry.* 1995;22:250-255.

158. Komminoth P, Adams V, Long AA, et al. Evaluation of methods for hepatitis C virus detection in archival liver biopsies. *Pathol Res Pract.* 1994;190:1017-1025.

159. Long AA, Komminoth P, Lee E, et al. Comparison of indirect and direct in-situ polymerase chain reaction in cell preparations and tissue sections: detection of viral DNA, gene rearrangements and chromosomal translocations. *Histochemistry.* 1993;99:151-162.

9

Immunophenotyping in Diagnosis and Prognosis of Mature Lymphoid Leukemias and Lymphomas

John L. Carey

General Concepts

This chapter discusses the use of immunophenotyping in the diagnosis and prognosis of mature lymphoid leukemias and lymphomas. The author takes the viewpoint of a general pathologist encountering the prevalence of disease expected in such a practice, using the diagnostic modalities commonly available, and defining what will be relevant to oncologists. Although this chapter will obviously emphasize flow cytometric immunophenotyping, it will also cover the alternative use of immunohistochemical techniques.

Specimen Collection

Optimal tissue collection and transport is essential for flow cytometric immunophenotyping, given that the tissue must usually be in an unfixed state during this time. If such procedures are not used, there is an increased risk of loss of diagnostic cells, degradation of antigen expression, and increases in autofluorescence. Marrow and blood must be collected in an anticoagulant, typically 1 of

Table 9-1

Anticoagulant Characteristics of Marrow and Blood Specimens

Agent of Preservation	ACD	Heparin	EDTA
Preservation of cell viability*	Greatest (3 days)	Intermediate (2 days)	Least (1–2 days)
Availability			
in vacutainers	Least	Greatest	Greatest
as liquid **	Least	Greatest	Intermediate
Utility in hematology analyzers	Limited to none	Limited	Greatest

*Viability may be extended by storage at 4° C and/or diluting 1:1 with cell media; samples older than indicated expiration date may still retain sufficient viability for diagnostic analysis.
**Marrow aspiration kits usually require (and are optimally used with) an anticoagulant that is available in a liquid form that can be aspirated into the syringe.

3 major types (acid citrate dextrose [ACD], ethylenediaminetetraacetic acid [EDTA], or heparin). Any of these will adequately maintain marrow or blood cell viability and relevant antigenicity for at least 24 and probably up to 48 hours at room temperature. The exact choice depends on the specimen type, method of obtaining the sample, and/or availability of anticoagulant (**Table 9-1**).

Solid tissue specimens must be transported in an unfixed and nonfrozen condition until a cell suspension can be prepared. The key issue for the caregiver is the likely time until the flow laboratory will be able to process the specimen. Several approaches are used to ensure representative fresh and fixed tissue for diagnostic exam by routine histology and flow cytometry (**Figure 9-1**). Once received, the solid tissue should be processed as soon as possible to generate a cell suspension.

The most common approach is the mince/scrape method, with or without the use of a wire mesh. The minimum quantity of tissue needed to yield sufficient cells for flow analysis varies according to the extracellular matrix and density of lymphoid infiltrate. The former is probably more important, as it is quite difficult to obtain adequate cell yields from skin samples and other densely fibrotic tissue. On the other hand, delicate tissues, such as gastric mucosa, with dense lymphoid infiltrates and lymph nodes can yield diagnostic material for flow cytometry from small biopsies.[1]

Even if cellularity appears quite sparse ($< 1 \times 10^5$ cells), in the author's experience, a single tube with 3 or 4 color reagents is often able to answer clinically significant questions (eg, B-cell clonality, presence of terminal deoxynucleotidyl transferase [TdT$^+$] blasts). As a corollary, the laboratorian should

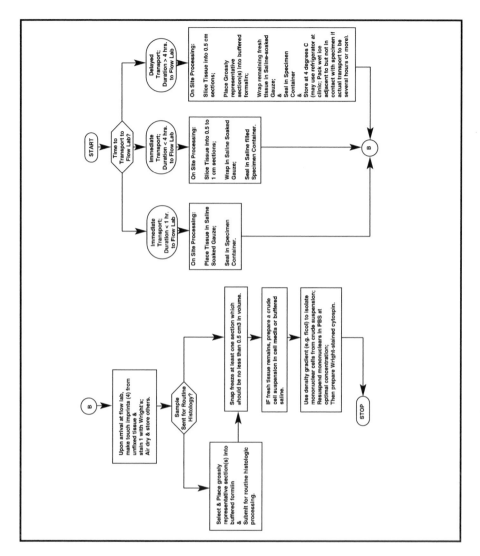

Figure 9-1
Transport and Gross Processing Triage of Solid Tissue Samples for Flow Cytometry

This figure details potential approaches to the pre-analytic transport and gross processing of samples submitted for flow cytometry. For the sake of simplification, the scenario is divided between the site where the sample is obtained (eg, operating room, physician's office) and the flow cytometry lab. In reality, more complex scenarios are possible, where there is a tissue procurement site, primary lab receiving site (where some tissue processing may occur and/or the sample may be held pending morphologic review), and the flow laboratory (where the sample may either be directly analyzed or held pending morphologic review by the referring site). The key points are to (1) make sure that material is submitted for routine morphologic review, unless the biopsy was procured solely for the purpose of immunophenotyping; (2) assure a representative sample for potential immunohistochemical or genotypic analysis; and (3) prepare a representative cell suspension for flow cytometry.

always try to analyze a low-cellularity sample, choosing the markers that will answer the most medically significant questions. Lastly, it is important to keep in mind that any negative results may simply reflect an inadequate sample.

Cell suspensions derived from solid tissue or bone marrow almost always contain significant numbers of dead cells, cell clusters, cellular fragments, and/or acellular tissue clumps. These, along with a large fraction of mature red cells and neutrophils, can be removed by ficol density gradient centrifugation. Advantages of this approach include the following:

- It provides greater than 95% viability of isolated cells
- It enriches diagnostic cells (eg, lymphocytes, blasts)
- It allows resuspension in cell media, extending "shelf life" for up to 48 hours at 4°C, without significant loss of antigenicity[2]
- It washes the cells of serum that contains circulating immunoglobulin
- It allows for the precise adjustment of cell concentrations for immunostaining

It should be pointed out that most low-grade and non-large-cell intermediate-grade lymphomas yield representative suspensions with density gradient purification.

Some laboratories do not use ficol gradients, particularly with blood and marrow specimens. This approach minimizes the loss of diagnostic cells and avoids the additional time and labor involved in ficol purification. In reality, it is not always possible to maintain a "native" cell constitution by "whole blood" lysis, for the following reasons:

- The tube being stained with antibodies to immunoglobulins needs to first be "washed" (spun down, supernatant discarded, then cells resuspended in isotonic buffer) to eliminate free extracellular immunoglobulin.
- To avoid antigen excess, the technologist needs to dilute samples with high cell concentrations.

If the laboratorian does not wish to use density gradient centrifugation to "clean up" marrow or solid tissue suspensions, the use of a vital dye (eg, 7-aminoactinomycin D [7-AAD]) may be quite helpful in identifying nonviable cells, whereas forward light scatter gating may be useful in excluding cell fragments and cell clusters.

Medical Triage

Once the sample is received, the laboratorian must decide 2 crucial issues: (1) Will immunophenotyping be medically useful in the given clinical setting? (2) What antibody panel should be run if immunophenotyping is indicated? In a routine clinical setting, medical usefulness is often interpreted to mean that the test allows the clinician to alter clinical outcomes with well-established therapy and/or predict large differences in survival. It should be pointed out that medically useful tests might legitimately be defined differently:

- Institutions may wish to evaluate new therapeutic strategies for leukemias/lymphomas that would routinely require immunophenotyping (eg, diagnosis, presence of minimal residual disease, multidrug resistance phenotype).
- Medical urgency (eg, thoracic vascular compression by tumor) may dictate a more "shotgun" diagnostic approach to ensure rapid diagnosis and/or treatment.
- Reference/high-volume laboratories may need to do immunophenotypic analysis without waiting for morphologic review to ensure high throughput and rapid turnaround time.

The standard clinical and laboratory evaluations often supply sufficient diagnostic and prognostic information about benign and malignant mature lymphoid proliferations, obviating the need for immunophenotyping.[3,4] The most common questions that immunophenotyping must resolve in the setting of a hematolymphoid proliferation are:

- Is the lymphoid proliferation benign or neoplastic?
- What is the type or differentiation of leukemia or lymphoma?
- Is there a minimal amount of leukemia or lymphoma present, either at the time of diagnosis (staging) or posttherapeutic remission evaluation (minimal residual disease)?

These, along with issues involving cell gating, will define the antigen profiles, and thus the antibody panels, that must be determined.

While new classifications of leukemias and lymphomas include immunophenotypic features, the authors of these classifications readily concede that immunophenotypic and/or genotypic studies are not always needed for routine clinical care *if* the clinical and morphologic features are diagnostic.[5] Furthermore, the integration of newer tests or markers into the routine "first-tier" workup of neoplasias will depend heavily upon their wide acceptance by oncologists. Closely aligned with this will be the need for new therapies that effectively treat entities defined only by immunophenotyping or genotyping.

Lastly, one must ascertain whether to use immunohistochemistry (IHC) or flow cytometry. Usually, this is an issue only with solid tissue specimens, and a quick comparison of the routine tissue sections and cytospin preparation from the cell suspensions will reveal whether diagnostic material is present in the latter. Fortunately, most diagnostically relevant antigens can be detected in paraffin-embedded fixed tissue from hematolymphoid neoplasms.[6-14] Often, IHC is preferred in a small-to-intermediate sized pathology laboratory, because it allows one technique (IHC) to cover a broad spectrum of immunophenotyping needs for routine diagnostic pathology.

Flow Cytometric Identification of Leukocytes

A core issue in flow cytometry is the accurate identification of the cell type(s) whose phenotype(s) one wishes to determine (arbitrarily defined here as *gating*). Such gating strategies are essential for accurate immunophenotyping, particularly when there is a heterogeneous cell suspension and/or the target cell population is present in a low percentage. In the setting of leukemia and lymphoma assessment, the cell types that need to be definable by flow cytometry are usually mature lymphocytes, large lymphoid cells, blasts and plasma cells.

Careful correlation with the original specimen and/or cell suspension cytomorphology is a critical quality assurance function of the cytometer operator and/or the interpreter. This helps in identifying the small minority of cases where the standard gating protocols fail to detect the neoplastic cells (eg, large-cell lymphomas). If the flow laboratory is not able to review the original aspirate smear or tissue biopsy, a written statement should be added to the report to caution the ordering clinician or pathologist to do so. This guards against a false-negative result (due to marked reduction of neoplastic cells) or undergrading of a neoplastic result (eg, based on a loss of most large neoplastic cells, with only small malignant lymphocytes left).

Lymphocytes

The flow cytometric identification (gating) of lymphoid cells is often accomplished by light scatter gating (**Figure 9-2**).[15] This is most reliably done when dealing with lymphoid suspensions from solid tissue, where the benign and/or

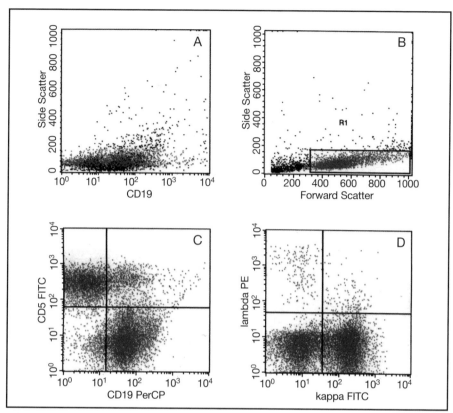

Figure 9-2
Light Scatter Gating of Mature Lymphocytes
The traditional method for identification of cells is shown here in a ficol-purified sample from a follicular center lymphoma. Bivariant plots A and B show CD19 PerCP vs linear side light scatter (SSC) and linear forward light scatter (FSC) vs SSC, respectively. A gate (R1) is drawn around the small-to-large lymphoid cells in Plot B. All cells in this R1 gate are shown as red-colored in all plots, and bivariant plots C and D show their expression of CD19 PerCP vs CD5 FITC and kappa FITC vs lambda PE, respectively.

An advantage of this approach and of CD45 antigen gating is that they include virtually all mature lymphoid cells. Hence, there are typically antigen-negative cells in all plots for one or both of the antigens. These are useful as intrinsic negative controls for adjusting the positive/negative immunofluorescence gates for subtle variations in background staining from one monoclonal antibody to another. A further advantage of having a mixed B and non-B cell population is assisting in defining dual staining patterns. In dot plot C, the dual-positive CD5+CD19+ cluster is probably T cells, because they are continuous with the major CD5+CD19- negative T cell cluster. Lastly, the presence of B and non-B cells gives the laboratorian an idea of the relative scale of a proliferation. Typically, neoplastic B lymphoproliferations tend to comprise the majority of cells, whereas reactive B lymphoproliferations are in the minority (and T cells are in the majority).

malignant lymphocytes usually comprise the vast majority of all cells. Difficulties with pure light scatter gating typically arise in other sample types (eg, blood, marrow) due to the low fraction of neoplastic cells. This may occur because of poor recovery (eg, large-cell lymphomas) and/or because there are a large number of benign cells (eg, erythroid cells in marrow specimens). In such instances, 1 or 2 immunofluorescence markers in each tube can be combined with light scatter characteristics to gate the desired cell population.

As an alternative, a single (surveillance) tube containing differentiation markers to general hematolymphoid cell lineages can be used to define light scatter gating that is the most sensitive or specific for the target population (eg, CD45/glycophorin A/CD14, CD45/CD71/CD33) (**Figure 9-3**). This tube can also be used to correct for contamination in subsequent tubes containing other analytic antibodies, much as is done with Centers for Disease Control and Prevention (CDC) recommendations for CD4 T-cell quantitation in human immunodeficiency virus (HIV)-infected individuals.[16]

The most useful antigens to direct gating are CD45, CD19 (CD20), and CD3 (**Figures 9-4**, p 236 and **9-5**, p 237). Anti-CD45 immunofluorescence is quite strong in mature lymphoid cells.[17,18] Therefore, gating upon the brightly CD45[+]/low-side-light-scatter cluster is highly specific for mature T, B, and natural killer (NK) lymphoid cells (**Figure 9-4**).[16,19] The primary exceptions are some large-cell lymphomas (with dim-to-negative CD45 and/or higher side light scatter), and plasma cell proliferations (with CD45[-] and/or higher side light scatter; see plasma cell gating). Gating upon CD45 is also usually more variable for hairy cell leukemias (with slightly higher side light scatter than normal lymphocytes) and B-chronic lymphocytic leukemia (with slightly dimmer CD45 than normal lymphocytes). As an alternative, pan B antigen (CD19; **Figure 9-5**),[20,21] and pan T antigen expression (eg, CD3) can usually be relied upon to identify mature B and T lymphoid cells, respectively.

Plasma Cells

The identification of plasma cells by flow cytometry is more difficult, because plasma cells lack the membrane antigens seen on less mature B lymphoid cells (eg, CD19, CD20, CD22, CD45, surface immunoglobulin [sIg]). Simply using light scatter gating for plasma cells is not specific, because plasma-cell light scatter overlaps with the often more frequent large lymphoid or monocytoid cells.[20,22] Therefore, it is difficult to identify plasma cells by light scatter alone in a complex multilineage cell suspension.

As a result, immunophenotypic gating, with or without concomitant light scatter, is usually essential for the accurate identification of plasma cells. It should be pointed out that, in the author's experience, plasma cells appear to be somewhat more fragile than lymphocytes. As with large lymphoid cells, the

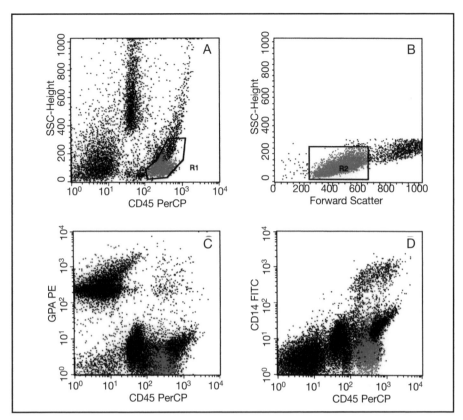

Figure 9-3
CD45/Glycophorin A/CD14 Surveillance Tube
This is a demonstration of the CD45/glycophorin A (GPA)/CD14 used as a surveillance tube to define a complex mixture of cells from a ficol-purified spleen sample of splenic marginal zone lymphoma. CD45-PerCP log immunofluorescence vs linear side light scatter is shown in plot A. The polygonal gate (R1) is drawn around the CD45 bright-positive/low side light scatter cluster of cells. The bivariant plot B shows the linear forward vs linear side light scatter of the cells in the R1 gate in plot A. The rectangular gate R2 is drawn around the cells with small-to-intermediate size lymphoid light scatter. Cells in both R1 and R2 are shown in fuchsia. Bivariant plots C and D show the sample populations defined by CD45 PerCP vs GPA PE and CD45 PerCP vs CD14 FITC, respectively. Virtually all the CD45-negative/low side light scatter cells seen in plot A are brightly GPA-positive in plot C, defining them as erythroid cells. In marrow samples, these could also include nucleated erythroid precursors. There is a small fraction of CD45 negative cells that also lack GPA expression, and these are most likely plasma cells, platelets, and/or very primitive blasts. The dimmer CD45+ cells with high side light scatter seen in plot A (neutrophils and related mature myeloid cells and eosinophils) show no significant reaction with either GPA (plot C) or CD14 (plot D). In plot D, CD45+CD14+ monocytes are seen in the upper right hand area. There is a minor population of very bright CD45+CD14- cells in plot D (just to the right of the fuchsia lymphoid cells). These are probably larger lymphoid cells, which appear as large cells in plot B. While these are admixed with the monocytes in plot B, it would be worthwhile to adjust the initial R2 gate to assess this population.

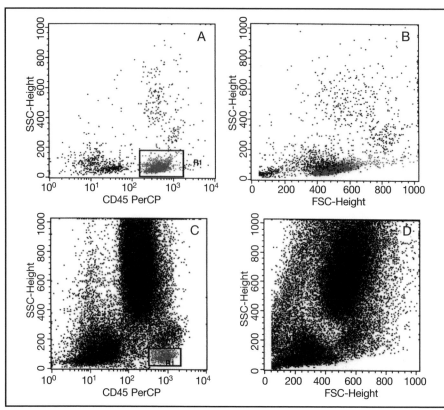

Figure 9-4
CD45 Antigen Gating of Mature Lymphocytes

The approach to and advantages of CD45/SSC gating are shown in ficol-purified samples from a B-chronic lymphocytic leukemia (plots A and B) and mantle-cell lymphoma (plots C and D). Bivariant plot A is CD45-FITC log immunofluorescence vs SSC. A polygonal gate (R1) is drawn around the CD45 bright-positive/low side light scatter cluster, and these cells are colored red in all dot plots. The bivariant plot B shows the FSC vs SSC of the same population as in A. The vast majority of the mature lymphoid cells in gate R1 have typical lymphocyte light scatter in B. Note the minimal overlap between the bright CD45+ lymphoid cells (red) and the negative CD45 cells (black). This is not a problem in this case, but with greater erythroid cell or debris contamination, it can be difficult to identify the mature lymphocytes by light scatter.

An example of this is seen in the bone marrow sample from a case of mantle-cell lymphoma (MCL). Bivariant plot C is CD45-FITC log immunofluorescence vs linear side light scatter. A polygonal gate (R1) is drawn around the small number of CD45 bright-positive/low side light scatter cluster. The bivariant plot D shows the linear forward vs linear side light scatter of the same sample as in C. The vast majority of the mature lymphoid cells in gate R1 (red) have typical lymphocyte light scatter in B. However, note the extensive overlap of the light scatter of the bright CD45+ lymphoid cells (red) and the negative CD45 cells (black). The latter almost certainly are mature and immature erythroid cells. In this instance, it is virtually impossible to specifically identify mature lymphocytes by light scatter. Even if the gate is drawn around the light scatter likely to contain the lymphocytes, the much more abundant erythroid cells will result in a dramatic reduction in the number of lymphoid events collected. This may result in difficulty in defining clonality and/or differentiation of the B lymphocytes.

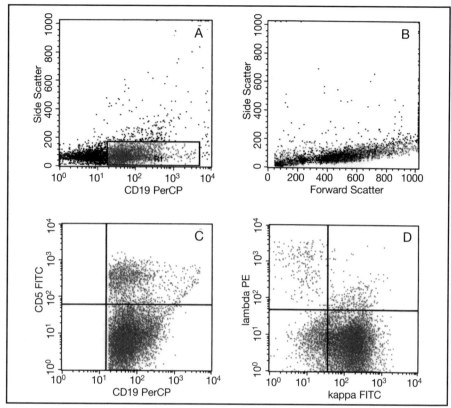

Figure 9-5
CD19 Antigen Gating of Mature Lymphocytes

An alternative method for identification of B cells is shown here using the same samples as in Figure 9-3. Bivariant plots A and B show CD19 PerCP vs linear side light scatter (SSC) and linear forward light scatter (FSC) vs SSC, respectively. A gate (R1) is drawn around the CD19+/low SSC cells in plot A. All cells in this R1 gate are shown as red-colored in all plots, and bivariant plots C and D show the expression of CD19 PerCP vs CD5 FITC and kappa FITC vs lambda PE, respectively.

An advantage of this approach is that only B cell immunofluorescence is seen. This may aid in more precisely defining the expression of B differentiation antigens. The author does not usually use this as a primary method, relying instead on light scatter or CD45/SSC gating. CD19 gating is used as a backup, particularly when non-B cells have high levels of background immunofluorescence and/or predominate.

The primary drawback to this approach is that intrinsic negative controls are not present in every tube. This limits the ability to adjust the positive/negative immunofluorescence gates for subtle variations in background staining from one monoclonal antibody to another. This may be overcome with large panels, where there are typically one or more non-reactive test antibodies in different tubes.

Another disadvantage of lineage-specific antigen gating like CD19/SSC is a degree of ambiguity in assigning dual staining patterns. In dot plot C, the dual-positive CD5+CD19+ cluster is probably T cells, as shown in Figure 9-3C. However, this is not as readily apparent when only CD19+ cells are included. Lastly, the presence of B and non-B cells gives the laboratorian an idea of the relative scale of a proliferation. Typically, neoplastic B lymphoproliferations tend to comprise the majority of cells, whereas reactive B lymphoproliferations are in the minority (and T cells are in the majority).

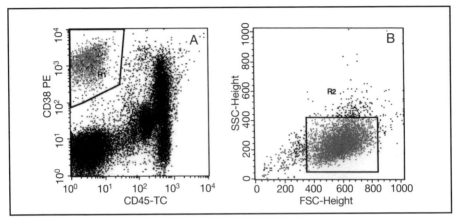

Figure 9-6
CD45/CD38 Appearance of Plasma Cells
This figure illustrates a ficol-purified sample from a case of plasma cell leukemia. Bivariant plot A is CD45-FITC log immunofluorescence vs CD38 PE log immunofluorescence. A polygonal gate (R1) is drawn around the CD45⁻CD38^bright+ cluster. Those cells in R1 which are also in R2 are colored red. The bivariant plot B consists of only those cells in R1, and shows the linear forward vs linear side light scatter of the R1 population. The majority of the cells have a "monocytoid" or "large blast" light scatter, which is typical but not specific for plasma cells. Only those cells in both R1 and R2 are colored red.

laboratorian may see a dramatic reduction or total absence of plasma cells in the flow cytometer, as compared with the native sample. Therefore, careful correlation with routine morphology is necessary so as not to render a false-negative result. As a related issue, plasma-cell percentages derived from flow cytometry should not be used in place of morphologically calculated fractions for diagnostic purposes.

The 3 most common antigens used in plasma cell gating are CD38, CD45, and CD138.[23-25] CD38 is a very sensitive yet nonspecific marker.[17,18,20,22,26] As such, its expression must be combined with other antigens and/or light scatter to yield accurate plasma cell gates. The best-established combination is CD45 and CD38.[23] Typically, plasma cells are CD45⁻ to dimly CD45⁺, but have very bright coexpression of CD38 (**Figure 9-6**). Because such a gate in a complex specimen (eg, bone marrow) may also include cellular debris, more specific identification of plasma cells may be done by combining a CD45⁻CD38⁺ population with cells with light scatter of large lymphoid cells. When cells gated by this 2-step method are sorted for morphologic analysis, a very pure population of plasma cells is seen.[27]

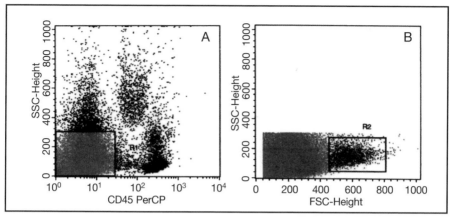

Figure 9-7
CD45 & Light Scatter Appearance of Plasma Cells
Ficol-purified sample from the same case of plasma cell leukemia as in Figure 9-6. Bivariant plot A is CD45-FITC log immunofluorescence vs linear side light scatter. A rectangular gate (R1) is drawn around the CD45⁻SSC^low+ cluster, which is colored red. This includes erythroid cells, platelets, debris, and plasma cells. The bivariant plot B includes only those cells in R1 and shows the linear forward vs linear side light scatter of the R1 population. Only a minority of the cells have a "monocytoid" or "large blast" light scatter, and a rectangular gate (R2) is drawn around these, which are colored green.

Alternative gating methods use only 1 immunophenotypic marker for gating, leaving 2 (or 3, depending upon instrument capability) for profiling the plasma cells. One would gate upon the CD45⁻/low-to-intermediate side light scatter population first, then gate upon the cells from this cluster that had monocytoid light scatter (intermediate-to-large forward light scatter with intermediate side light scatter; **Figure 9-7**). Another approach is to gate upon cells with large lymphoid to monocytoid light scatter, then define plasma cells in each tube by virtue of their being brightly CD38- or CD138-positive.

The CD138 antigen has been advocated as a marker for malignant plasma cells, usually in place of CD38.[24] However, CD138 is not always present on malignant plasma cells or is expressed dimly on only a fraction of these cells. This limits its effectiveness as a stand-alone gating antigen. CD138 is also detectable in fixed paraffin-embedded tissue, where it appears to be quite specific for the IHC definition of plasma cells.[28,29] Lastly and historically, the PCA-1 and PC-1 antigens were advocated as useful markers of plasma cell differentiation.[20,30] However, neither is commercially available, and the PCA-1 antigen lacks sensitivity.[22]

Table 9-2
Laboratory, Morphologic, and Clinical Features Associated with Mature T Lymphoid Neoplasms[5,33]

	Feature	Comment
Laboratory	Hypercalcemia	• Classically seen with ATCL. • Nonspecific – can be seen with myeloma or other metastatic cancers.
	Neutropenia	• Classically seen in T-LGL. • Nonspecific
Morphologic	Marked nuclear irregularity	• Classically seen with ATCL (polylobate nuclei) or Sézary syndrome/ leukemias (cerebriform nuclei in small cells). • Be cautious of interpreting nuclear contours from cytospin preparations.
	Cytoplasmic granules	• Classically seen with T- or NK-LGL. • Be cautious of making a diagnosis based on this indication because benign T- or NK-large granular lymphoproliferations may be seen in isolation or in the setting of other hematolymphoid neoplasias (eg, PCL).
Clinical	Skin infiltrates or rashes	• ATCL and CTCL • Nonspecific
	Prior history of T-cell lymphoma	
	Unusually aggressive clinical course	• Rapid increase in WBC or organomegaly or profound cytopenias unlikely to be seen in morphologically corresponding B lymphoid neoplasias.

Immunophenotyping Panels: General Concepts

B- and T-Cell Lineage

The choice of diagnostic antibodies is based on the antigen profile required to resolve the question(s) of differentiation and/or clonality, along with antigens required for gating. It is reasonable to assume that most mature lymphoid leukemias and lymphomas are of B lineage, particularly in North America and Europe.[31,32] This is particularly valid in the absence of features of T-cell differentiation (**Table 9-2**).[5,33] Therefore, when B-cell neoplasia is the primary differential, T versus B lineage can be reliably determined in a single tube that contains a reasonably specific pan T antigen (eg, CD3 or CD5) along with a reliable B-lineage marker (eg, CD19 or CD20), as follows: a T-lineage cell is CD3$^+$, or CD5$^+$ and CD19$^-$; a B-lineage cell is CD19$^+$, or CD20$^+$ and CD3$^-$.

Of these 2 B-lineage antigens, the author prefers to use CD19, particularly when a pan-B antigen is to be used for gating. The CD19 antigen is distinctly present on virtually all B-cell leukemias and lymphomas and is extremely specific when dealing with mature lymphoid neoplasms.[20,21,34] In contrast, the CD20 antigen has a lesser degree of sensitivity and specificity. It is found to be dimly expressed on a variable minority of T cells in both blood and marrow,[35,36] and, rarely, on T-cell neoplasias.[36,37] This lack of specificity may be important when there is a significant population of benign T lymphocytes admixed with the neoplastic B cells, particularly when one is assessing CD5 expression on the latter.

More importantly, CD20 is often dimly expressed on B-chronic lymphocytic leukemia/small lymphocytic lymphoma (B-CLL/SLL) cells.[5,20] This may limit its ability to clearly define a B cell in some instances. Similarly, the expression of CD22, CD79 beta, and sIg may be dim to absent in B-CLL/SLL.[20,38] Lastly, B neoplastic cells may be rendered CD20$^-$ with treatment with anti-CD20. Taking this and the prevalence of B-CLL/SLL[31,32] into account eliminates CD20, CD22, CD79 beta, or sIg as an ideal membrane B-cell marker for routine B-cell identification.

The definition of mature T cells revolves around 2 antigens. The choice of CD5 as a T-cell marker is appropriate only when it is combined with a specific B-cell antigen. This is due to the frequent presence of CD5$^+$ B-cell neoplasms such as B-CLL/SLL and mantle cell lymphoma. Therefore, CD19$^+$CD5$^+$ cells are presumed to be of B lineage, while CD19$^-$CD5$^+$ cells are presumed to be of T lineage. While CD3 is an effective stand-alone marker of T lineage (it has greater specificity), it does not aid in the differentiation of mature B-lymphoid neoplasias (eg, CD5$^+$ vs CD5$^-$). Furthermore, in the author's experience, a significant discrepancy between the percentage of CD3$^+$CD19$^-$ and CD5$^+$CD19 cells is very rare. The use of CD2 and CD7 antigens is not recommended, as NK cells distinctly express these antigens.

Kappa and Lambda Light Chains

The surface or cytoplasmic light chain expression (sIg, cIg) is critical in the assessment of B-cell clonality. Reactivity with anti-kappa and -lambda must be assessed by a multicolor method in order to establish that it is only B cells that are being evaluated and that the light chain is not present on other cells due to Fc-receptor binding or by some other nonspecific adherence.[39] Such "Ig$^+$" cells include lymphocytes (typically NK or a small set of T cells) and monocytes.

Because of this, flow cytometry laboratories accredited by the College of American Pathologists (CAP) are required to use techniques to differentiate between specific (membrane-bound sIg) and nonspecific (eg, Fc-receptor-mediated) immunoglobulin binding. As a corollary of the above, single-antigen analysis (1-color) of sIg light chain is neither analytically reliable nor acceptable for laboratory certification (in the US). The primary methods to measure light chains are:

- kappa/lambda in a single tube (2-color) (**Figure 9-8**)
- a pan-B antigen (eg, CD19) in a tube with either kappa or lambda (2-color) (**Figure 9-9**)
- a pan-B antigen in a tube with both kappa and lambda (3- or 4-color)

The first method arbitrarily defines true B cells as either kappa *or* lambda positive. Any cell with *both* kappa and lambda reactivity is assumed to be a non–B cell. In the author's experience, this method gives clearer separation of the kappa$^+$ and lambda$^+$ B cell clusters than does the pan B/light chain method. The difficulty with the single-tube kappa/lambda approach is that some true clonal B cells may lack detectable sIg and/or have such dim expression that a clear assessment of clonality is not possible based upon kappa/lambda staining.

The inclusion of a pan-B antigen with the light chain(s) allows positive identification of true B cells via the pan-B antigen. Thus, sIg$^-$ or partially dim sIg$^+$ B-cell populations can be clearly identified. There are 2 primary problems with the 2-color pan-B/light-chain approach: (1) It requires 2 tubes to complete the analysis. When there is a limited amount of cells to work with (eg, cerebrospinal fluid lymphocytosis), this may result in an insufficient number of cells to clearly define clonality. (2) Sometimes there is no clear separation between the light chain-positive and -negative B cells (eg, no clear delineation between CD19$^+$ kappa$^+$ and CD19$^+$ kappa$^-$ clusters; **Figure 9-9**). In the author's experience, this is the most common difficulty with this method. It may be resolved by seeing if the other tube has a monoclonal or polyclonal ratio of CD19$^+$Ig$^+$ to CD19$^+$Ig$^-$ cells.

Ultimately, no one approach for light chain analysis works for all instances of B-cell leukemia/lymphoma, and a combined approach with kappa/lambda/pan-B antigen, using light scatter and/or pan-B immunophenotype for identification, is probably the most effective method.[39] Obviously, if the third fluorescence marker is used for CD45 gating, then this is not possible. However, with instruments capable of 4-color analysis, the limitation is not relevant.

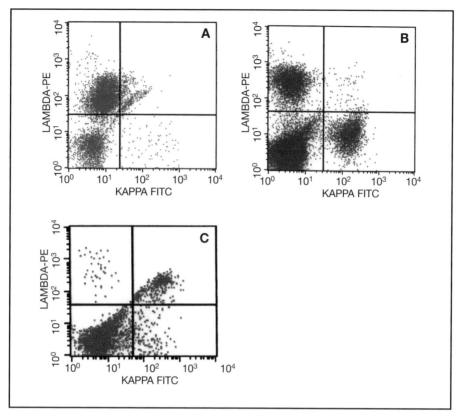

Figure 9-8
Kappa and Lambda Profile of Mature Lymphoid Cells

This is a demonstration of the CD45 PerCP/lambda PE/kappa FITC to define B cell clonality from complex mixture of cells in a single tube. The cases are a ficol-purified spleen sample of splenic marginal zone lymphoma (plot A; same sample as in Figure 9-9), polyclonal B-cell hyperplasia (plot B), and normal peripheral blood B cells (plot C). Four cell populations are seen in all plots. Most non-B cells lack expression of either kappa or lambda and are in the dual-negative cluster in the lower left quadrant. In the upper left quadrant are the B cells, which are lambda+/ kappa-, while the kappa+/lambda- cells are in the right lower quadrant. Both of these populations are arbitrarily defined as B lineage based upon their expression of one or the other immunoglobulin light chain. The somewhat linear cluster of cells that express BOTH kappa and lambda (kappa+lambda+ ; upper right quadrant) are by definition *not* B cells. The immunoglobulin detected on these non-B cells is usually derived by membrane Fc-receptors binding circulating immunoglobulin.

The advantage to this approach is that the kappa+ and lambda+ B cell clusters are usually clearly defined. This may not always be the case with CD19/ kappa and CD19/lambda definition (see Figure 9-9). The only real reservation to this approach is that a minority of B cell neoplasms will not express detectable light chains. This can be demonstrated by the fact that there are a significant number of B cells detected by CD19 or CD20 in other tubes, yet none are noted by immunoglobulin light chain analysis. Cases with large monoclonal proteinemias (eg, myeloma) will result in Fc-mediated binding of monoclonal immunoglobulins on non-B cells. In the author's experience, this problem only rarely occurs in the usual workup of leukemias and lymphomas, but is a variant that the laboratorian should be aware of.

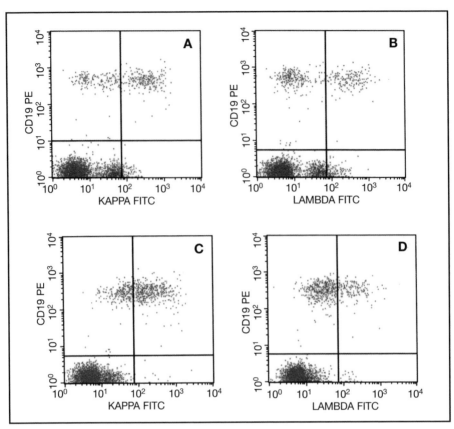

Figure 9-9
CD19/kappa and CD19/lambda Profile of Mature Lymphoid Cells
This is a demonstration of the CD45 PerCP/CD19 PE/kappa FITC and CD45
PerCP/CD19 PE/lambda FITC assay, which is used to define B cell clonality from complex
mixtures of cells from a ficol-purified blood sample from normal peripheral blood (plots A
through D) and B CLL/SLL (plots E through J). The major advantage to this approach is a
clear immunophenotypic identification of B cells by a non-immunoglobulin antigen (CD19).
This clearly excludes any non-B cells that are dimly positive for immunoglobulin due to
Fc-mediated binding. Furthermore, it directly defines B cell neoplasms that lack
immunoglobulin expression. A drawback is the need for 2 tubes if the third antigen is
CD45 (this assumes a 3-color cytometer; with 4 colors, this is not an issue). Another issue
is the variable separation of the CD19+light chain+ cluster from the CD19+light chain- population. This variability tends to happen when there are lower counts of B cells, as is often
the case with reactive lymphoproliferations.

The classic appearance is seen in each plot from the first polyclonal sample (plots A
through B). In blood and marrow, 4 populations are seen; 2 are CD19+ and 2 are CD19-.
The CD19+Ig$^{dim+ or negative}$ cluster is presumed to be truly negative. The most reliable way
to set the Ig positive/negative gate is to place it between the kappa+CD19+ and kappa-
CD19+ clusters. Typically, the kappa+CD19+ fraction (upper right quadrant, plot A) is quan-
titatively approximate to the lambda-CD19+ fraction (upper left quadrant, plot B), and vice-
versa. This is a good QC check on the gating. The CD19- populations are Ig- (furthest to
the lower left) and Ig^{dim+}, the latter straddling the positive/negative gate. The CD19-Ig^{dim+}

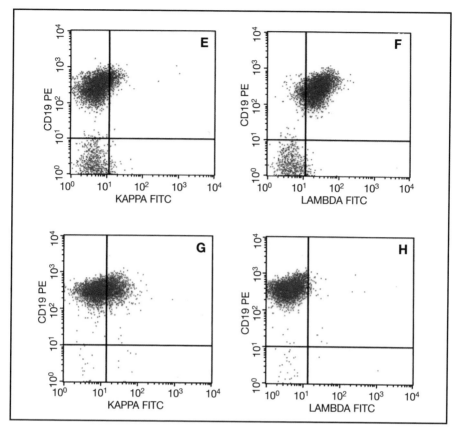

Figure 9-9 (continued)

is due to both kappa⁺ and lambda⁺ Ig binding, usually via Fc receptors. These appear in the kappa vs lambda dot plots as a relatively linear cluster in the dual-positive quadrant (see Figures 9-8A and 9-8C).

A not unusual variant appearance of polyclonal B cells is shown in plot C and D. Here, there is not a distinct "trough" or break between the Ig⁺ and Ig⁻ B cells in the upper left and upper right quadrants (CD19⁺ group). This is particularly likely to happen in polyclonal samples, where the B cells are usually in a distinct minority. The limited number of B cell events may make identification of the appropriate positive/negative gate quite difficult. The best approach is to set the kappa positive/negative gate, then replicate it with the lambda/CD19 sample. If the sample is polyclonal, the kappa⁺ events should approximate the lambda⁻ events, and vice-versa. This fact, and the absence of other immunopheno-typic abnormalities (eg, a lack of CD5 or CD10 coexpression), should allow a diagnosis of polyclonal B cells.

The next 3 cases are from B CLL/SLL (plots E through J). These slides have been chosen because this is one of the most common B-cell neoplasms and because of the frequency of dim-to-absent sIg staining on them, as opposed to virtually every other B lymphoid malignancy. In all cases predominant B cells are clearly defined by CD19, whereas non-B cells are CD19⁻. In plot E, the B cells clearly lack kappa expression, while in plot F, they are dimly yet distinctly lambda⁺. In the next case, there is very dim expression of monoclonal kappa on a minority of cells (plot G; upper right quadrant), while no lambda reactivity is seen (plot H). In the last B CLL/SLL case, both plots I and J fail to

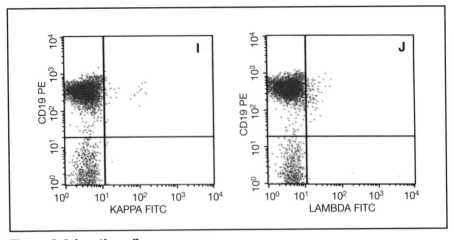

Figure 9-9 (continued)

demonstrate any kappa or lambda light chain expression. These can usually be recognized as clonal by the absence of sIg on a predominant population of B cells *in the presence of* other antigen abnormalities (eg, CD5 expression), persistent lymphocytosis, and/or atypical biopsy morphology.

Other Differentiation Antigens

The above antigens, along with any other markers indicated by the initial clinical and morphologic differentials, are usually all that are needed for diagnosis and typing of mature B-cell leukemias and lymphomas (**Tables 9-3** and **9-4**, p 248). Typically, the latter include antibodies to CD5, CD10, CD23, and either CD11c or CD103. For efficiency (particularly in laboratories with a high volume and/or limited ability to review clinical and morphologic details), one may also include FMC7 and/or CD25 in the primary panels, particularly if using a 3- or 4-color setup. While CD20, CD22, and CD79 beta are not favored for primary B-cell identification, the inclusion of at least one of these is deemed optimal for accurate differentiation of B-chronic lymphoid neoplasia, principally B-CLL/SLL from other mature B lymphoproliferations.

A more extensive T-cell panel is not indicated, unless T lineage is suggested (**Table 9-2**, p 240). In such instances, a panel directed at T-cell neoplasias is appropriate (**Tables 9-5**, p 248 and **9-6**, p 249). Usually, this includes all major pan T antigens (CD2, CD3, CD5, CD7), CD4, and CD8. Depending upon the degree of prior clinical and morphologic evaluation, NK antigens (CD16, CD56, CD57) and/or CD25 may be included. As discussed more extensively in the sections on T cell neoplasias, once the general lineage of mature T-cell leukemias and lymphomas are established, the addition of other differentiation antigens has a much more limited value in defining specific entities than in B-lineage neoplasms.

Table 9-3

B Chronic Lymphoid Neoplasms: Diagnostically Useful Antigens and Antigen Combinations

	Useful in the Differential Diagnosis?		
	CLL/SLL, MCL, FCL, MZL, PLL	HCL, vHCL, SLVL	PCL/ WM/ SLLP
CD5/CD19	Yes	Yes	Yes
kappa/lambda/pan-B or kappa/pan-B and lambda/pan-B	Yes	Yes	Yes
CD10/pan-B	Yes		
CD11c/pan-B	±	Yes	
CD20	Yes	±	±
CD22	±	Yes	
CD23/pan-B	Yes		
CD38/pan-B	±		Yes
CD103/pan-B		Yes	
FMC7/pan-B	±	±	
Others:	M/D (±); CD79 beta (±); CD43 (±)	CD25 /pan-B (Yes)	cyt. kappa; cyt. lambda (Yes); CD45/38 (Yes); CD138 (±), CD56 (±)

CD138 (±), CD56 (±) _Abbreviations: pan-B = an antibody to an antigen relatively sensitive and specific for the broad range of mature B cells (eg, CD19, CD20); CLL/SLL = chronic lymphocytic leukemia (leukemic phase of small lymphocytic lymphoma /SLL); MCL = mantle cell lymphoma;[52] MZL = marginal cell lymphoma (both nodal & MALT);[5] SCCL = small cleaved cell leukemia (leukemic phase of follicular NHL);[96] FCL = follicular center lymphoma; B-PLL = B-lineage prolymphocytic leukemia;[102] CLL/PL = prolymphocytic transformation of CLL or CLL/PLL hybrid;[43,102] HCL = hairy-cell leukemia;[112] vHCL = variant HCL; SLVL = splenic lymphoma with veiled lymphocytes;[106] PCL = plasma cell leukemia;[122] WM = Waldenström's macroglobulinemia; SLLP = small lymphocytic lymphoma with plasmacytoid differentiation; YES = essential; ± = desirable but not essential; cyt. = cytoplasmic.

Diagnostic Interpretation

The modern diagnosis of hematolymphoid neoplasia optimally includes multiple methods, *beginning* with morphologic evaluation by the clinician, pathologist, and/or cytometrist. Indeed, the combination of clinical, immunophenotypic, and other laboratory data is probably essential to accurately diagnose T- and B-cell leukemias/lymphomas. From the standpoint of flow cytometry, the laboratorian interpreting data should begin with a careful review of the cell identification gate(s), the resultant immunofluorescence plots, and the cutoffs used to define the percentages of antigen-positive and -negative cells (eg,

Table 9-4
3-Color Flow Cytometric Immunophenotyping Panels for Mature B Lymphoid Leukemias and Related NHLs

Tube (Well) #	Gating Method	
	Light Scatter (FITC/PE/PerCP)	CD45 / SSC (FITC/PE/PerCP)
1	Cont./Cont./Cont.	Cont./Cont./CD45
2	CD5/CD23 /CD19	CD5/CD19/CD45
3	FMC7/CD10/CD19	CD19/CD23/CD45
4	CD103/CD22/CD19 or CD22/CD11c/CD19	CD103/CD22/CD45 or CD22/CD11c/CD45
5	CD3/CD20/CD19	FMC7/CD19/CD45
6	kappa/lambda/CD19	CD19/CD10/CD45
7	(CD25/CD11c/CD19)	CD19/CD20/CD45
8		kappa/lambda/CD45
9		(CD25/CD19/CD45)
10		(CD19/CD11c/CD45)

Table 9-5
T/NK Chronic Lymphoid Leukemias and Related Lymphomas: Diagnostically Useful Antigens

	T/NK LGL; T/NK NHLs	Mycosis Fungoides/ Sézary Syndrome	ATCL; PTCL; T CLL; T PLL
CD5/19	Yes	Yes	Yes
kappa/lambda	Yes	Yes	Yes
CD7/3	Yes	Yes	Yes
CD2, 4, 8	Yes	Yes	Yes
CD16, 56, 57	Yes		
CD25	±		Yes
TCR alpha-beta/ TCR gamma-delta	±	±	±

Abbreviations: LGL = large granular cell leukemia (NK & T gamma lymphoproliferative disease);[148,149] Sézary = leukemic phase of cutaneous T cell lymphoma (mycosis fungoides);[181] T- CLL & PLL = T-lineage chronic lymphocytic & prolymphocytic leukemias;[161,182] PTCL = peripheral T-cell leukemia/lymphoma; ATCL = adult T-cell leukemia/lymphoma;[183,184] Yes = always included in panel; ± = desirable but not essential; cyt. = cytoplasmic.

Table 9-6

Flow Cytometry Immunophenotyping Panels for T/NK Lymphoid Leukemias and Related NHLs

Tube (Well) #	Gating Method	
	Light Scatter (FITC/PE/PerCP)	CD45 / SSC (FITC/PE/PerCP)
1	Cont./Cont./Cont.	Cont./Cont./CD45
2	CD7/CD4/CD3	CD7/CD3 /CD45
3	CD5/CD16/CD3	CD57/CD8/CD45
4	CD57/CD8/CD3	CD5/CD56/CD45
5	CD2/CD56/CD3	CD2/CD16/CD45
6	CD25/ - /CD3	CD25/CD4/CD45
7	kappa/lambda/CD19	kappa/lambda/CD45
8	(TCR alpha-beta/ TCR gamma-delta/CD3)	(TCR alpha-beta/ TCR gamma-delta/CD45)

quadrants). The subjective nature of gating for cell identification and variation in background immunofluorescence staining from one monoclone to another can lead to subtle errors on the part of the cytometrist.

Each plot's numerical data should also be checked for evidence of defective staining and/or changes in a given tube's identification gate. These would include marked changes in (1) the number of cells analyzed; (2) the time taken to acquire a given number of cells; and (3) the background immunofluorescence. If questionable data or fluorescence is seen, the identification gate for each tube should be examined, the tube reacquired, and/or a fresh aliquot newly stained.

If there is evidence of neoplasia, the antigen should be given a "positive" or "negative" assignment for the neoplastic cells. There is no consensus on the threshold fraction of antigen positive cells for making such a designation. Most reports in the peer-reviewed literature require at least 10% to 30% of the neoplastic cells to express an antigen for the neoplasm to be considered "positive." The quantitation of the fraction of antigen-positive cells becomes more difficult if the fluorescence peaks of the specific and nonspecific populations are overlapping due to dim specific staining or high nonspecific staining. Such interpretation of such "dim-positive" staining is controversial and not standardized.[19] In the author's opinion, dim staining is more likely to be negative or nonspecific if the positive peak:

- is less than 0.5 log more fluorescent than the negative control peak, and
- extensively overlaps the negative peak (33% to 50% or more), and/or
- lacks any "trough" area between it and the negative peak.

Such minor increases in fluorescence may simply reflect variation in non-specific staining among reagent antibodies.[40,41]

Careful consideration of the immunophenotypic profile can aid in the interpretation of dim immunofluorescence staining. One should expect to see a pattern of both positive and negative immunoreactivities that is appropriate to the final interpretation. If a series of antibodies considered negative in the profile exhibit similar dim shifts from the negative control, then the dim reactivity is probably best considered negative.

Reporting

Flow cytometric immunophenotyping reports should include:

- Patient, physician, and sample demographics. This is essential.
- Basic description of methodology. This is optional, particularly if included in diagnostic comments. The major exception is the analyte-specific reagent (ASR) disclaimer (see below).
- Quantitative immunophenotyping results (percentage of antigen-positive cells). There is controversy over whether such data are needed, particularly if the diagnostic comments include the antigen profile of any neoplastic cells or the normal immunophenotypes if the diagnosis is benign. However, many knowledgeable customers do like to see these data.
- Diagnostic comments. This is essential, and should include 3 distinct subsections, each of which can range from 1 sentence to a few paragraphs. The first should be a description of the cytomorphology of the major cell population(s). This should be more detailed with a neoplastic diagnosis, particularly if it is of a mature lymphoid leukemia. The second section should begin with a sentence or phrase detailing the cell gating. Next, if the flow diagnosis is of a neoplasia, a profile of pertinent positive and negative antigens should be given. If one does not include a quantitative section (see above), then one may need to include more antigens in the description. Lastly, there should be a summary diagnosis tying together the cytomorphology and referencing any complementary laboratory studies (eg, surgical pathology report). One can include at this point any suggestions to the referring physicians for additional studies or procedures (eg, biopsy, protein electrophoresis, nucleic acid studies).

The vast majority of antibodies to leukocyte antigens were defined and their clinical utility determined in the less-regulated 1980s and early 1990s. As a corollary, most of the antibody reagents used in flow cytometric analysis of leukemias and lymphomas have not been formally submitted to the US Food and Drug Administration (FDA) for approval for such use. In many instances, this was because there simply was no such requirement, and the vendors are understandably loath to seek such approval, particularly when there is extensive independent data on the clinical utility of these reagents. The FDA recently created a category of reagents that have not been formally cleared by the organization.[42] These are known as analyte specific reagents (ASRs) and are used in "home-brew" tests (eg, flow cytometric immunoanalysis of leukemias/lymphomas). An FDA panel recommended that most ASRs be classified as class I devices (governed by lowest level of regulatory controls needed to protect the US public health). The significance to the laboratory is that if an ASR is used, the following disclaimer must be given somewhere in the report: "This test was developed and its performance characteristics determined by [Laboratory Name]. It has not been cleared or approved by the U.S. Food and Drug Administration."[42] One may include additional explanatory comments to the customer about this disclaimer.

Mature Leukemias and Related Lymphomas of B Lineage

The optimum differential diagnosis of any mature lymphoid leukemia or lymphoma begins with a careful correlation of cytomorphology, complete blood cell (CBC) count, and any clinical evidence and location(s) of organomegaly. One should also adjust for a variation of the prevalence of various diagnostic entities based upon location and/or ethnic origin (eg, East Asia vs North America). Questionable cases will remain after immunophenotyping, particularly with leukemias. These will benefit from biopsy of a tissue mass (with or without IHC), serum protein electrophoresis, and/or genotypic studies, depending on the individual circumstances.

"Lymphocytic" Leukemias/Lymphomas

These B-lineage leukemias and lymphomas are among the most frequently seen, particularly in North America and Europe.[5,31,32] The author arbitrarily includes in the B "lymphocytic" neoplasias the following entities: B-chronic lymphocytic leukemia/small lymphocytic lymphoma (B-CLL/SLL); follicular center lymphomas (FCLs) and their leukemic counterpart, the disease sometimes called small-cleaved-cell leukemia (SCCL); mantle-cell lymphoma (MCL); and marginal zone lymphomas (MZLs), including mucosal-associated (MALT) and nodal-based forms.

These neoplasias have a variable combination of "mature" morphologic features: small-to-intermediate size, relatively high nuclear/cytoplasmic (N/C) ratio, sharp cellular borders, chromatin that is uniformly dense or clumped ("mature"), and absent or very small nucleoli. As a clinical correlate, most are usually rather indolent, but incurable, with the major exception of MCL.[5] While these neoplasias are often readily diagnosed when presenting as lymphomas (due to the contribution of the architecture), the leukemic forms can be difficult to diagnose as malignant. It can also be difficult to distinguish among specific leukemic types. As a result, flow cytometric immunophenotyping is often performed on the leukemic phases.

B-Chronic Lymphocytic Leukemia/Small Lymphocytic Lymphoma

Clinical and Morphologic Features

The most common lymphoid leukemia in adults in North America and Europe is B chronic lymphocytic leukemia/small lymphocytic lymphoma (B-CLL/SLL),[31,32,43-45] and its nodal presentation is a very common type of non-Hodgkin's lymphoma (NHL).[5] Its frequency is lower in East Asia, where most chronic lymphoproliferative disorders are other mature B NHLs.[46] B-CLL/SLL is most often seen in individuals older than 50, and is quite rare in those under 30 years of age.[43,47] It is an indolent but incurable neoplasm, with median survivals of greater than 10 years for those patients presenting with low-stage disease.[48] A significant minority of cases are associated with humoral immunodeficiency and/or autoimmune problems. Prognosis is stage-dependent and is often strongly correlated with the doubling time of the blood lymphocytes. Other adverse features include prolymphocytoid cytomorphology, trisomy 12, deletion of chromosome arm 17p, and *p53* gene mutations.[49-51]

More common cytogenetic abnormalities (deletion of 13q14 and 11q22-23) do not correlate with more aggressive disease.[51]

The classic cytomorphology of a B-CLL/SLL lymphocyte is that of a small lymphoid cell, with sharp cellular borders, high N/C ratio, lightly basophilic undifferentiated cytoplasm, essentially round nuclear contours, and a "blocky" chromatin pattern. However, more pleomorphic cytomorphologies (eg, intermediate size Downy or prolymphocytoid with, rarely, a minor fraction of clefted nuclei) are not unusual and can comprise a striking fraction of the neoplastic cells.[5,48] This is paralleled in nodal presentations by the so-called "pseudofollicular" pattern. It is ironic that while the presence of prolymphocytoid forms as pseudofollicles in SLL is essentially diagnostic based solely on morphology,[5,52] the presence of a significant fraction of prolymphocytoid forms in CLL raises legitimate diagnostic confusion with other mature lymphoid leukemias (eg, B prolymphocytic leukemia [B-PLL], MCL), hence indicating the need for flow cytometric immunophenotyping.

Immunophenotypic Features

Like most mature B-lymphoid neoplasms, B-CLL/SLL is brightly CD45[+], although it may show somewhat dimmer CD45 intensity than that seen on benign lymphocytes or other types of mature B-lymphoid neoplasms (**Figures 9-10**, p 254 and **9-11**, p 255). As a corollary, if CD45 is being used as a gating parameter, the cytometrist may have to use a wider range of CD45 immunofluorescence to be sure of including all lymphoid cells. B-CLL/SLL usually has a distinct profile of differentiation antigens, clearly expressing CD5, CD21, CD23, and CD43 antigens, while lacking CD10 and CD103.[5,20,53,54]

Among the mature lymphocytic leukemias/lymphomas, B-CLL/SLL is relatively unique in that the concentration of sIg is usually low. This dim immunofluorescence intensity is best defined as the median channel of the sIg[+] peak being no more than 1 log more immunofluorescent than the negative control. As a minority of B-CLL/SLLs are either sIg[-] or brightly sIg[+], it is not feasible to use intensity alone as a reliable discriminator of CLL/SLL from other mature B-lymphoid neoplasias.[55] When detectable, the sIg has an IgM and/or IgD isotype.[5]

Other major B-cell antigens have reduced expression in B-CLL/SLL (**Figure 9-12**, p 256). Although CD22 was originally reported as absent,[20,56] later researchers have noted that in B-CLL/SLL it has a more variable expression but is still dimmer than when seen in other mature B-cell leukemias and lymphomas.[38,57] In the author's experience, when using a phycoerythrin (PE) - conjugated CD22 antibody, most B-CLL/SLLs are CD22[+], but only dimly so. The CD20 antigen expression is also typically dimmer in B-CLL/SLLs than in

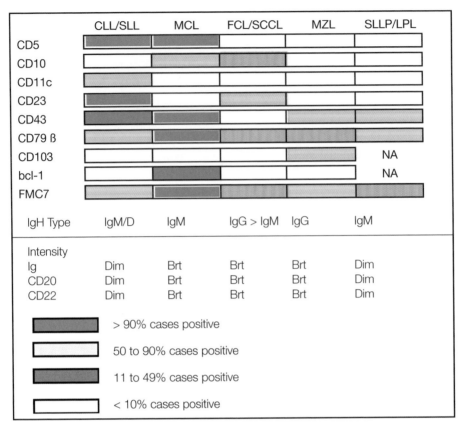

Figure 9-10
Antigen Profiles of Chronic B "Lymphocytic" Leukemias and Related Lymphomas
Intensity of immunofluorescence (assumes a 4 log immunofluorescence scale):
Brt (bright) = Median of antigen+ immunofluorescence is ≥ to 1 log more than negative control median, with no significant overlap with the negative control.
Dim = Median of antigen+ population's immunofluorescence is < 1 log than the negative control median, with no significant overlap with the negative control (< 50% overlap).

normal B or other mature neoplastic B cells.[20,58] Indeed, when one is using less sensitive immunocytochemical techniques, B-CLL/SLLs appear to lack the CD20 antigen in some series,[31] although more modern immunohistochemical methods reveal CD20 in most cases.[59] This change is best appreciated using the immunofluorescence intensity seen on normal B lymphocytes. Lastly, this dimmer CD20 seen in B-CLL/SLL appears more broadly distributed, probably due to the log scale.

Some investigators have noted that most cases of B-CLL/SLL also lack detectable membrane CD79 alpha and CD79 beta antigens, which are closely

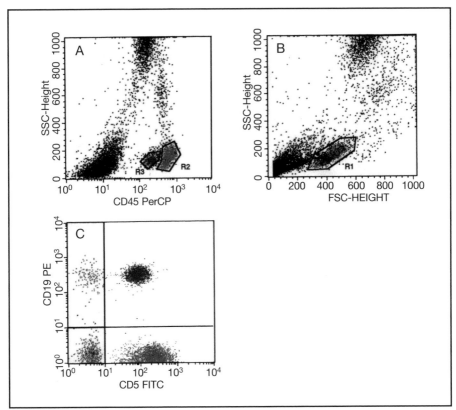

Figure 9-11
Variant CD45 Expression of B CLL/SLL
This is a whole blood sample from a case of B-CLL/SLL that is stained with CD5 FITC/CD19PE/CD45PerCP. In bivariant plot A, 2 bright CD45+ populations with low angle side light scatter are present (R2/red; R3/green). As seen in the corresponding forward and side light scatter bivariant plot (B), these populations are intimately admixed in the small lymphoid cluster (R1/green and red). However, as seen in bivariant plot C, the slightly dimmer CD45+ population (R3/green) comprises virtually all of the CD5+CD19+ B-CLL cells. The brighter CD45+ lymphoid cells (R2/red), are predominantly mature T and NK cells. When such a bimodal set of "bright" CD45+ lymphoid cells are seen, both should be analyzed, because exclusion of one or the other may result in a falsely negative result.

linked to sIg physically and functionally.[57,60-64] It should be pointed out that distinct expression of CD79 alpha by tissue immunohistochemistry (IHC) has been reported in most cases of B-SLL.[59] This difference with flow cytometric immunophenotyping probably reflects detection of only membrane antigen versus cytoplasmic expression by IHC. It has been shown that the lack of CD79 antigens in some cases reflects a variation in messenger RNA (mRNA)

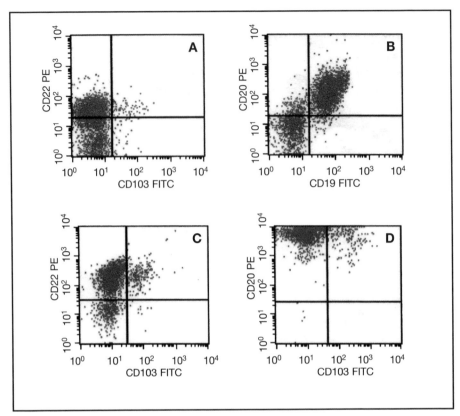

Figure 9-12
CD20 and CD22 Expression in B CLL/SLL vs Other Mature B Lymphoid Neoplasms

The bivariant plots A and B are from a case of B CLL/SLL, while plots C and D are from a case of variant HCL. The median fluorescence of the CD22$^+$ B CLL/SLL cells (plot A; upper left quadrant) is slightly less than 1 log brighter than the negative control and over-laps the positive/negative cursor for the PE channel. Compare this to the vHCL cells (plot C; upper left quadrant), where there is essentially no overlap, and a greater than 1 log shift in median fluorescence intensity. This is more dramatic for CD20 (plots B and D). Typically, the expression in B CLL/SLL (plot B, upper right quadrant) is dimmer than normal and appears more broadly distributed. The latter is probably due to the expression being lower in value on a log scale. In contrast, the vHCL cells actually have an abnormally bright CD20 expression (plot D; upper right quadrant); normal B cells have an arbitrary median fluorescence of around 10^3.

processing of transcripts for CD79 alpha and CD79 beta in CLL/SLL, result-ing in deletion of the membrane components of these antigens.[63,64]

The use of CD79 beta expression in the differential diagnosis and prog-nostication of B-CLL/SLL is controversial. Membrane CD79 beta was initially reported to be absent in 95% of 298 B-CLL/SLL cases.[60] However, other investigators have reported CD79 beta expression in 35% (total cases = 40), 50% (total cases = 40), and 77% (total cases = 27) of B-CLL patients.[62-64] In most CD79 beta$^+$ cases, the intensity of CD79 beta was judged to be dimmer than that seen in normal or other neoplastic mature B cells, and in proportion to sIg intensity. In some but not all studies, the CD79 beta$^+$ B-CLLs tended to be disproportionately associated with other adverse prognostic features (eg, CLL/PL [CLL with prolymphocytoid features], bright sIg intensity, advanced clinical stage).[60,62,64]

A variety of other antigens are present in a limited fraction of B-CLL/SLL cases. Expression in individual cases may range from distinct positivity on most cells to, more typically, dim expression on a minority of neoplastic lymphocytes. The best known examples of the latter are FMC7 and/or CD11c antigens, which are dimly expressed on a minority of B-CLL/SLLs [56,65-68,69,70] although not all researchers agree.[7] The controversy appears to revolve around (1) the definition of true dim immunofluorescence; (2) the sensitivity of the staining method and cytometer; and (3) the fraction of antigen-positive cells required to call the case "positive."

A similar fraction of cases also express CD25 and CD38.[47] The cCLL antigen (cCLLa) has been reported in most B-CLL cases.[71] While cCLL is not found on polyclonal B and T cells, it is expressed on a fraction of neoplastic cells from most cases of B-PLL and hairy-cell leukemia, as well as a few cases of myeloma and Sézary syndrome. In the setting of previously diagnosed B-CLL/SLL, the cCLL expression may be used to quantitate residual disease. The absence of commercial monoclonal reagents to cCLLa has limited its application severely. Lastly, a very small minority of B-CLLs coexpress the CD8 antigen.[72]

Not all cases of B-CLL/SLL are clinically indolent, even when corrected for stage. As such, there has been a great deal of interest in trying to define those cases that act more aggressively. This has included cytogenetic, nucleic acid, and immunophenotypic analysis, along with morphology and advancement of stage.[44,49,50] Several groups have found that white blood cell (WBC) count, lymphocyte doubling times, and Binet clinical stages have often proved to be the best prognostic markers in multivariant studies.[50,73]

The independent prognostic utility of antigen phenotype for B-CLL/SLL is controversial (in terms of best defining positive vs negative and the intensity of positives).[44,48,55,70,73] While initial reports suggested that sIg intensity was prognostic,[48] more recent investigations have not confirmed this.[44,55,73] Significant correlations do exist between markers of more aggressive clinical course (trisomy 12) and atypical immunophenotype in B-CLL/SLL (bright CD20$^+$ or sIg$^+$; CD22$^+$; and/or CD23$^-$).[55,74]

The presence of the CD38 antigen (> 30% B-CLL cells positive) has been shown in one study to be associated with (1) a poorer prognosis and (2) a germline DNA sequence for the variable segment of the Ig gene.[75] The latter is also associated with poorer prognosis for B-CLL.[75,76] It remains to be seen if subsequent studies confirm this. If so, morphology and/or immunophenotype might be useful in screening for cases of B-CLL/SLL that require cytogenetic analysis and/or nucleic acid sequence analysis. Obviously, the definition of effective therapeutic alternatives for such cases would advance the need for this kind of immunophenotyping.

Differential Diagnosis in General

Based upon frequency and morphology, the differential diagnosis for B-CLL/SLL is primarily the leukemic phase of MCL and plasmacytoid SLLs (SLLP). The leukemic phase of an MZL is distinctly less common than B-CLL/SLL. While the site and heterogeneous morphology of MZL usually allow clear distinction from B-SLL, its leukemic phase at times can mimic more pleomorphic B-CLL. Follicular center lymphomas and their leukemic presentations are usually morphologically quite distinct from B-CLL/SLL.

The immunophenotypic differentiation of B-CLL/SLL begins with the evaluation of CD5, CD10, and CD23 expression. In paraffin section immunohistochemistry, CD43 is often added to enhance or replace CD5's role in the definition of B-CLL/SLL and MCL. In reasonably good-sized sections, the pattern (follicular vs diffuse) will be apparent, so that the inclusion of CD10 may not be necessary with immunohistochemical analysis. The $CD5^+CD10^-CD23^+$ profile in a mature monoclonal B lymphoproliferation is virtually diagnostic of B-CLL/SLL. In such an instance, the diagnosis is made if the expected range of B-CLL/SLL cytomorphology is present.

It should be pointed out that the differential diagnosis of $CD5^+$ mature B-cell neoplasms is not limited. Among the small-to-intermediate-sized lymphoid leukemias/lymphomas, CD5 is expressed in B-CLL/SLLs, in both typical and "blastoid" MCLs, and in a minority of SLLPs and MALT NHLs.[5,77] With "large" B-lymphoid morphology, generic large-cell NHLs, intravascular large-cell NHL,[78] Burkitt's lymphoma/leukemia,[79] the blastoid variant of MCL, and B-PLL express CD5 in a variable proportion of cases. Clearly, careful correlation of immunophenotypic results with cytomorphology, clinical history, and, in some cases, cytogenetics and/or nucleic acid studies is necessary for the accurate diagnosis of $CD5^+$ B-cell neoplasia.

Differential Diagnosis of Mantle-Cell Lymphoma

The tissue/immunohistochemical distinction of B-CLL/SLL from MCL is best defined by the CD23[+]/bcl1[-] profile for the former and CD23[-]/bcl1[+] for the latter.[80,81] The differential value of CD23 relies critically upon the expression of CD5, as many FCLs and some MZLs are CD23[+]. The flow cytometric CD5[+]CD23[+] profile is quite reliable in distinguishing B-CLL/SLL from MCL, whereas immunohistochemistry accomplishes the same with bcl1[-]/CD23[+] combined with CD5[+] and/or CD43[+] expression for tissue sections. Lastly, CD20, CD22, and sIg are usually of dim intensity, as opposed to their bright expression in MCL, FCL, and MZL and very bright expression in HCL and splenic lymphoma with veiled lymphocytes (SLVLs).

To a lesser extent, the absence or presence of FMC7 and/or CD11c, respectively, may be used in the differential diagnosis of B-CLL/SLL and MCL. Their primary value appears to be to *rule out* MCL in the setting of a CD5[+] B-lymphoid leukemia. Specifically, the FMC7/CD11c profiles are useful if either (1) CD5 or CD23 has a dim partial expression on the neoplastic B lymphocytes that are morphologically typical for B-CLL/SLL; and/or (2) the cytomorphology is more variable than that typically seen with B-CLL/SLL. Usually, the intensity of FMC7 and CD11c expression on B-SLL/CLL and MCL is dim, and only a limited fraction of neoplastic cells may be positive in a given case. Because of this and a lack of standardization of flow immunofluorescence analysis, not all investigators find similar percentages of reactive cases. From multiple studies, it appears as if more than 95% of MCLs are FMC7[+]CD11c[-].[7,57,69,70,82] Therefore, the presence of CD11c and/or the absence of FMC7 would tend to weigh against MCL. While the FMC7[-]CD11c[+] phenotype in a CD5[+] B lymphoproliferation is significantly associated with B-CLL/SLL, all 4 combinations are seen frequently enough in B-CLL/SLL to preclude the use of FMC7/CD11c status as a tool to either rule in or rule out B-CLL/SLL.

Differential Diagnosis of Other B-cell Leukemias/Lymphomas

While B-CLL/SLLs and MCLs are CD5[+] and CD43[+], only a very small fraction of MZLs and plasmacytoid SLLs express either of these antigens.[6,7,59,77,81,83] Furthermore, virtually all FCLs are CD5[-]CD43[-], and most are dimly CD10[+]. The HCLs, their variants, and SLVLs are also typically CD5[-] and CD43[-], although they are not usually in the morphologic differential of B-CLL/SLL.

Differential Diagnosis of "Atypical" B-CLL/SLL

Unusual cases of CD5⁻ B-CLL/SLL do exist.[48,84,85] Such cases should not be lumped together with standard CD5⁺ B-CLL/SLL; rather, the designation CD5⁻ or variant B-CLL/SLL is advised. This is due to the presence of more significant cytopenias, higher stage, and adverse cytogenetic features with this CLL variant.[85] To render a diagnosis of CD5⁻ B-CLL/SLL, most investigators insist upon (1) small lymphocytic or CLL/PL morphology[43]; and (2) the absence of antigenic, cytogenetic, or nucleic acid markers of MCL or FSL (eg, CD10⁺, bcl1⁺, t:[11;14], t[14;18]) or a significant serum proteinemia (eg, <10g/L). The presence of CD23 strengthens the initial designation of CD5⁻ B-CLL, because unusual cases of CD5⁻CD23⁻ MCL have been reported.[85] However, because many other mature B-lymphoid leukemias are CD5⁻CD23⁺, this alone is not sufficient for diagnosis of CD5⁻ B-CLL/SLL.

Profiles and Scoring Systems

Given the known case-to-case variability of antigen expression, the use of a combined immunomorphologic profile is critical in defining mature B-lymphoid neoplasms. In particular, scoring systems have been designed to assure the laboratorian that a chronic B-lymphoid neoplasm is B-CLL/SLL and define those other cases where further studies are needed.[38,57] Matutes et al defined 6 critical antigens, assigning 1 point each for either expression or absence (**Table 9-7**).[38,57] Scores of 4 to 5 were highly correlated with B-CLL/SLL, whereas scores of 0 to 2 virtually excluded it (**Figure 9-13**).

There are 2 drawbacks to this proposal. First is the equal scoring given to all antigens. In practice, CD5 and CD23 expression are much more sensitive and (together) specific for B-CLL/SLL than is expression of FMC7. Second, scoring intensity (eg, dim sIg) is fraught with interlaboratory variation, making its use as an interinstitutional standard dubious at this time. This author uses a limited number of major parameters (cytomorphology, CD5, CD10, CD23) to rule in or rule out B-CLL/SLL (**Table 9-8**, p 262). If it is ruled out, other studies (eg, biopsy, cytogenetics) may be required to render the definitive diagnosis.

Mantle Cell Lymphoma

Clinical and Morphologic Features

Mantle cell lymphoma (MCL) has only recently been formally defined as a distinct entity.[52] MCL is characterized by the t(11;14) translocation, involving

Table 9-7

Immunophenotypic Differential of B-CLL/SLL vs Mature B Lymphoid Neoplasias (adapted from Moreau, et al[57])

Antigen	Expression	Score
CD5	Present	+1
CD23	Present	+1
CD79 beta	Absent	+1
FMC7	Absent	+1
sIg	Weakly present/absent	+1

Score	Sensitivity for CLL/SLL	Specificity for Non-CLL/SLL
4 to 5 points	89 %	< 1 %
3 points	9 %	5 %
1 to 2 points	2 %	76 %
0 points	0 %	19 %

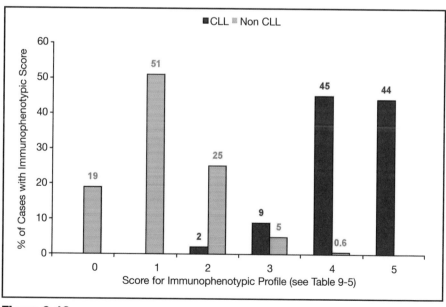

Figure 9-13

Immunophenotypic Scoring of B-CLL/SLL vs Other Mature B Lymphoid Neoplasms (Moreau, et al[57])

Table 9-8
Critical Features in the Immunomorphologic Diagnosis of B-CLL/SLL

Feature	Does Feature "Rule In" B-CLL/SLL?	Does Feature "Rule Out" B-CLL/SLL?
Morphology	Yes, if: Pseudofollicles seen in tissue sections.	Yes (presence), if: Marked nuclear irregularity; markedly irregular cellular borders; ≥ 55% prolymphocytes; cytoplasmic granules
CD5	No—presence is sensitive but not specific for B-CLL/SLL.	Yes – Absence excludes diagnosis of standard B-CLL/SLL; if all other features support CLL, consider diagnosis of CD5-negative CLL vs plasmacytoid CLL or Waldenström's.
CD10	No	Yes – Presence of CD10 effectively rules out B-CLL/SLL; dim expression seen in follicular center NHLs and Burkitt's-like/small cell noncleaved NHLs; bright expression seen in Precursor B acute lymphoblastic leukemias.
CD23	No—presence is sensitive but not specific by itself for B-CLL/SLL. However, in the setting of a CD5+ monoclonal B lymphoproliferation with appropriate morphology, the presence of CD23 is quite capable of "ruling in" B-CLL/SLL.	Yes (absence) – however, the absence does not exclude B-CLL/SLL IF all other features of B-CLL/SLL are present AND additional studies have ruled out MCL and MZL.

the *bcl-1* (cyclin D1) and *IgH* genes.[86] This is detected in approximately 66% of patients by standard cytogenetic exam and in virtually all patients by fluorescence in situ hybridization (FISH) methods.[86] This translocation is fairly specific for MCL, although it has been reported in unusual cases of B-CLL/SLL and myeloma and approximately 33% of B-PLLs.[86] Many of the latter may indeed actually be MCLs with more blastoid leukemic presentation.

The cyclin D1 protein is a key molecule in the control of cellular proliferation, and its translocation, along with other genetic alterations (eg, *p53* gene), may explain MCL's aggressive nature. The prognosis for this neoplasm is distinctly worse than FCL or B-CLL/SLL and more like untreated B large-cell lymphomas (patients have a median survival of 2-3 years).[87,88] And unlike most

B large-cell NHLs, no effective therapeutic approaches are currently known for MCL. Presentation in lymph nodes, blood, and marrow is typical.[87-89]

The cellular proliferation is usually composed of small-to-intermediate-sized lymphocytes, typically very similar in size to CLL/SLL cells.[86] These have a high N/C ratio, with sharp cellular borders and a scant amount of undifferentiated cytoplasm. The nuclear contours are irregular and variable, ranging from mildly indented (typical) to distinctly clefted (rare). The chromatin is dense and smooth. In tissue sections, epithelioid histiocytes are often widely interspersed among the neoplastic cells. The growth patterns are variable, ranging from diffuse to vaguely nodular to a mantle zone. While these patterns appear to define statistically significant differences in survival, these differences are quite small, particularly at 10 years from diagnosis.[88] Lastly, pseudofollicles are not seen, although residual benign germinal centers may be present.

A blastoid variant of MCL can mimic lymphoblastic and Burkitt's lymphomas.[5,86,90] These comprise a minority of cases of MCL. The blastoid cells are of intermediate size, with a high N/C ratio, mildly irregular nuclei, and a finely dispersed chromatin without nucleoli. The overall growth pattern is diffuse, and the mitotic rate high. Residual benign germinal centers and/or interspersed macrophages may be seen. This variant is often associated with *p53* mutations.[86]

The leukemic cytomorphology of MCL is quite variable, probably reflecting that seen in the node. It ranges from mildly pleomorphic mature lymphocytes to cells closely resembling prolymphocytes or acute leukemia blasts. It is in the leukemic setting, particularly with the more blastic morphology, that immunophenotyping plays a particularly important role.

Immunophenotypic Features

The diagnosis of MCL may be strongly suspected from the initial morphologic review. However, given MCL's aggressive behavior, additional immunophenotyping and/or genotyping are used by most laboratorians to make the definitive diagnosis.[5,91] Most MCLs express CD45 brightly, with a typical mature lymphoid cluster in a CD45 versus SSC plot. The antigen profile is fairly characteristic, being distinctly sIg+ (IgD+ > IgM+IgD+; lambda+ > kappa+), CD5+, CD43+, and FMC7+ (variable intensity), while lacking CD11c, CD23, CD34, and TdT (**Figure 9-10**, p 254).[7,70,80,86,92] The pan-B antigens are usually strongly expressed (CD19, CD20, CD22, CD79 alpha, CD79 beta).[7,57,58] Furthermore, most MCLs lack CD10, although some studies have indicated a small minority are CD10-positive.[80,83,87,93] Using immunohistochemical analysis, one can demonstrate strong expression of the bcl-1 protein in virtually all neoplastic cells.[5,8,59,90]

Differential Diagnosis in General

The diagnosis of MCL begins with its morphology and location. Because of the absence of architectural features in blood, marrow, and fine-needle aspirates, the morphologic differential usually includes B-CLL/SLL, MZL, and FCL. In tissue biopsies, the FCLs are usually not included due to the strong diagnostic impact of a follicular growth pattern. Because MCL can present in gastric mucosa, location in this instance is not useful in differentiating from MALT lymphomas.

Differential Diagnosis from B-CLL/SLL

The immunophenotypic triage starts with CD5 (and CD43 with immunohistochemistry). Both MCL and B-CLL/SLL are distinctly CD5$^+$ and CD43$^+$. The most effective profile to differentiate these 2 entities is CD23 and bcl1. MCLs are usually CD23$^-$ bcl1$^+$, whereas B-CLL/SLLs have the opposite phenotype.[80-82,87,92,94] Since the bcl1 antigen is not often measured by flow cytometry, additional markers are sometimes deemed helpful when using this method. Most MCL cases are dimly FMC7$^+$CD11c$^-$, whereas only a minority of B-CLL/SLLs have this profile.[7,70,82] The principal utility of FMC7$^-$ and/or CD11c$^+$ profiles is to rule out MCL, particularly in the leukemic phase. However, in the author's opinion, these antigens are less definitive than CD5, CD10, CD23, and bcl1. The presence or intensities of pan-B antigens on MCL are also different from B-CLL/SLL. The CD79 alpha, CD79 beta, CD19, CD20, and CD22 antigens are clearly present in MCL. In contrast, B-CLL/SLLs usually lack detectable membrane CD79 antigens, may or may not express CD22 (and if so, only dimly), and have dimmer expression of CD19 and CD20.[20,38,57,58,61] If the diagnosis of MCL is still in question after the initial morphologic and immunophenotypic exams, then definitive cytogenetic/molecular studies would probably be more effective in confirming the diagnosis than additional immunophenotypic markers.

Differential Diagnosis from Follicular Center and Marginal Zone Lymphomas

The presence of the CD5$^+$CD43$^+$ profile strongly favors the diagnosis of MCL, while the CD5$^-$CD10$^+$ and CD5$^-$CD10$^-$ phenotypes support FCL and MZL, respectively. Because FMC7 and CD10 can be found in both FCLs and MCLs, the usefulness of their presence alone in distinguishing between these 2 entities is limited. In addition, because a small minority of MZLs are CD5$^+$, the CD5$^+$CD10$^-$CD23$^-$ profile in a mucosal B lymphoproliferation is not always definitive for MCL. By immunohistochemical analysis, MCL would be expected to be diffusely bcl1+, while FCL would be bcl-1-. Unfortunately, bcl-2 expression is not useful in the differential diagnosis of mature B-lymphoid NHLs and leukemias, because a significant majority of each type of neoplasm are bcl2+.[95] Ultimately, either excisional biopsy and/or cytogenetic/ polymerase chain reaction (PCR) studies are needed to distinguish among these entities.

Differential Diagnosis for Blastoid Variant of MCL (MCL-BV)

The differential diagnosis for this variant of MCL includes lymphoblastic and Burkitt's lymphomas in tissue. When evaluating blood and marrow samples, acute leukemias and B-PLLs are also a consideration. The B-lineage lymphoblastic NHLs can be most clearly distinguished from MCL-BV because they are typically TdT+ and lack CD5, bcl1, and sIg, in marked contradistinction to MCL-BV.[90] In addition, the presence of CD34 strongly favors lymphoblastic NHL. Burkitt's lymphoma and MCL both have bright sIg and pan-B antigen expression and lack CD34 and TdT. However, MCL-BVs should be CD5+, whereas Burkitt's lymphomas are not. A distinct minority to outright majority of SCNCs are dimly CD10+. While a small fraction of MCLs have also been reported to be CD10+, this is controversial; hence, CD10 expression probably favors a diagnosis of Burkitt's over MCL-BV.

Other specific methods of confirming the diagnosis of MCL are cytogenetic or PCR assays for the t(11;14)/*bcl1* translocation. If FCL is in the differential, then assessing t(14;18) translocation via cytogenetics, FISH, and/or PCR is helpful. However, these assays are employed only when morphologic and immunophenotypic studies have failed to unequivocally diagnose a case.

Follicular Center Lymphomas

Clinical and Morphologic Features

The follicular center lymphomas (FCLs) are common NHLs in North America and Europe. However, they occur less frequently in East Asian populations.[46] Most FCLs are, for the most part, low-grade/indolent neoplasms, with median survivals between 5 and 10 years.[5] Typically, patients with FCL present with advanced-stage disease, and they are usually not curable by standard therapy. The morphologic diagnosis of FCL is typically made from an excisional biopsy of tissue and is usually definitive by itself. True *de novo* presentation as an

SCCL is rare.[96,97] However, FCL's presentation in a leukemic phase is not infrequent, particularly in the later phases of the disease. As a corollary, most of these leukemias are associated with prominent lymphadenopathy. In many instances, the oncologist will go ahead with a biopsy regardless of the immunophenotype results from the leukemia. Therefore, one may wish to have a conversation with the clinician to ascertain the most efficient route to diagnosis.

Cytologically, the cells are of small to intermediate size, with a high N/C ratio, sharp cellular borders, and undifferentiated cytoplasm. The nuclear contours are quite irregular, ranging from twisted to frankly cleaved. The chromatin is condensed, although usually not on the scale of a B-CLL/SLL or MCL. While tissue sections reveal variable fractions of large round neoplastic cells (grade I-III), the small cleaved lymphocytes tend to predominate in blood and marrow specimens.

Immunophenotypic Features

FCL and SCCL cells have the usual mature lymphoid pattern on CD45 versus SSC plots. They also strongly express the major pan B antigens and sIg (**Figure 9-10**, p 254). Furthermore, they often coexpress CD10 dimly (in 70% to 96% of cases); most researchers find that approximately 66% of cases are CD10+. A distinct minority dimly-to-moderately express CD23 and/or FMC7.[20,98] Virtually all FCL/SCCL cases lack CD5, CD11c, CD103, and bcl1. Although the bcl2 protein is often strongly expressed in FCL, it is not specific because it is seen in many other B-cell leukemias and lymphomas.[95]

Differential Diagnosis

FCLs are antigenically and morphologically distinct from B-CLL/SLL and MCL. The most compelling profile is the absence of CD5 and/or CD43 on FCL/SCCL cells, and their presence on CLL/SLL and MCL cells. Furthermore, FCL cells have a significantly stronger expression of monoclonal sIg, CD20, and CD22 than is seen with B-CLL/SLL cells. Although the dim presence of CD10 in many cases of FCL allows one to exclude B-CLL/SLL from the diagnosis, some investigators have found CD10 expression in a minority of MCL cases. However, the presence of bcl1, along with CD5, should allow one to confidently separate MCL from FCL. A significant minority of FCLs have a CD5⁻CD10⁻ CD23± profile that overlaps with both MZL and Waldenström's macroglobulinemia cases with CLL morphology. If the morphology is not sufficient to distinguish between these latter 2 entities, then cytogenetic/PCR analysis (t[14;18]), *bcl2-IgH*) and/or serum protein electrophoresis should allow the diagnosis.

Marginal Zone Lymphomas

Clinical and Morphologic Features

The marginal zone lymphomas (MZL) share a presumed common origin from B lymphoid cells in the marginal zones of lymph nodes, spleen, and MALT.[5] MZL include monocytoid B-cell lymphoma (MBCL) and splenic marginal zone lymphoma. For the sake of simplicity, the following discussion will focus on only the MALT and nodal MZL. Splenic MZL and lymphomas with villous lymphocytes will be discussed later, with the prolymphocytic and hairy-cell leukemias. MALT lymphomas are typically rather indolent, and tend to relapse in mucosal sites, whereas MBCLs are typically more aggressive.

MALT lymphomas are cytologically heterogeneous and usually contain reactive B-cell germinal centers and/or lymphoplasmacytic cells at the mucosal surface. The intensity of the infiltrate and the presence of lymphoepithelial lesions serve as useful diagnostic features. The neoplastic lymphoid cells are a mixture of small-to-intermediate-sized lymphocytes. Many of the latter may have "monocytoid" features. The cell borders are typically sharp, with a moderate N/C ratio and pale, undifferentiated cytoplasm. The chromatin is mature and densely reticular. Nucleoli, if present, are small. The mitotic rate is slow to absent. MBCL is a relatively rare entity.[5,99] The histologic appearance is fairly specific, combined with the clinical presentation of a low-stage, node-based NHL, usually without splenomegaly or marrow involvement.[99]

Immunophenotypic Features

MZL cells have the usual mature lymphoid pattern on CD45 versus SSC plots. The neoplastic lymphoid cells distinctly express the membrane pan-B antigens (CD19, CD20, CD22, CD79 alpha, CD79 beta) and sIg. In more than 90% of cases, the CD5, CD10, CD23, and CD43 antigens are absent, as is bcl1 (**Figure 9-10**, p 254).[6,8,34,59,77,95] It should be pointed out that a very minor fraction of MALTs have been reported to be CD5⁺ or CD103⁺.[77]

Differential Diagnosis

The diagnosis of MZL is primarily based on morphology and is aided by immunophenotypic evidence of monoclonality. This is most true with solid tissue samples, where the architectural features are most helpful. However, with blood or marrow samples, the combined immunomorphologic appearance, while clearly that of a monoclonal B-cell proliferation, is not specific for MZL. The CD5⁻CD10⁻CD23⁻ profile in mature B-cell neoplasms is most commonly seen in

MZLs and CLL associated with Waldenström macroglobulinemia (WM) and, to a lesser extent, FCL. The diagnosis of WM may be supported by serum protein electrophoresis revealing a large IgM monoclonal proteinemia, while the demonstration of the t(14;18) translocation or *bcl1-IgH* by PCR supports an FCL. As MCL may present in the gastrointestinal tract, this must be in the morphologic consideration of MALT NHLs. The presence or absence of a CD5⁺CD23⁻ profile is definitive in most cases in ruling MCL in or out, respectively.

MBCL is cytologically and architecturally distinct from B-CLL/SLL and MCL and does not express CD5, CD43, or bcl1. MBCL does share some immunophenotypic and cytologic features with HCL. In particular, most cases of MBCL, like most cases of HCL, are CD11c⁺. However, in virtually all MBCL cases: (1) there is a lack of significant splenomegaly,[99] (2) the cells have sharp cellular borders, and (3) the cells express only 2 or fewer of the "hairy-cell" antigens (CD11c, CD22, CD25, CD103).[38] Furthermore, the latter antigens, if present, are usually only dimly expressed.

Lastly, MBCL may require immunophenotyping to distinguish it from monocytoid B-cell hyperplasia (MBCH). Usually, the focal nature of MBCH will allow its distinction from MBCL.[5] In borderline cases, the demonstration of light-chain clonality is usually all that is needed. MBCL is typically bcl2⁺, while MBCH is bcl2⁻.[95] This latter profile is particularly useful in cases where only paraffin-embedded fixed tissue is available.

"Splenic" Leukemias/Lymphomas

The "splenic" B-cell neoplasms are those entities that are not in the lymphocytic group and that have a significant splenomegaly. These include prolymphocytic leukemia (B-PLL), hairy-cell leukemia (HCL), variant hairy-cell leukemia (vHCL), and splenic lymphoma with veiled lymphocytes (SLVL)/splenic marginal zone lymphoma (SMZL). Most of these neoplasms also share the cytologic characteristics of having intermediate-sized cells with a more moderate N/C ratio than that seen in most "lymphocytic" B-cell neoplasms, and having irregular cellular projections or borders. With the exception of HCL, these splenic lymphomas do not have characteristic immunophenotypes or cytogenetic or genotypic features. Most are rare, particularly in general practice. What is needed to render the diagnosis accurately is a clinicopathologic "profile" approach. This almost always includes the CBC count, morphology, and clinical exam along with the composite immunophenotype.

Prolymphocytic Leukemia

Clinical and Morphologic Features

B-lineage prolymphocytic leukemia (B-PLL) is a rare, aggressive neoplasm that most commonly presents in men between 50 and 70 years of age.[100,101] Most patients with B-PLL present with both a high WBC count and marked splenomegaly. However, peripheral lymphadenopathy is typically not present or is fairly minimal. Prolonged survival is not typical. Approximately 30% of cases have been shown to have the t(11;14) translocation, raising the possibility that these are really MCLs.[86]

Cytologically, the B-PLL cell is of intermediate-to-large size, with a high N/C ratio, sharp cellular borders, and undifferentiated cytoplasm. The nuclei are typically round or have only mild irregularities. The chromatin is open or reticular, usually with condensation around the single macronucleolus. In splenic tissue sections, the neoplastic cells tend to involve the white pulp. Rare examples of nodal involvement exhibit a diffuse effacement of the normal architecture.

Immunophenotypic Features

The immunophenotype of B-PLL is first and foremost that of a mature B-cell neoplasm and is strongly positive for sIg (M or G), CD19, CD20, and CD22 (**Figure 9-14**, p 270). While nonspecific, FMC7 is a sensitive marker and is typically brightly expressed. The B-PLL cells also express cCLLa, but usually lack CD10, CD11c, and CD23.[65,100,102] A significant proportion (approximately 50%) are dimly CD5+.[100,103] A caveat here is that many of the CD5+ PLLs were defined in the period prior to the recognition of MCL. It is very possible that some of these may have represented leukemic phases of MCL, which can express FMC7 and have distinct nuclei. Lastly, 50% to 66% express CD9, CD21, CD23, and CD25.

Differential Diagnosis

B-PLL is a true rarity, and both inclusionary and exclusionary criteria should be applied for diagnosis. Although some cases of B-CLL/SLL, prolym-

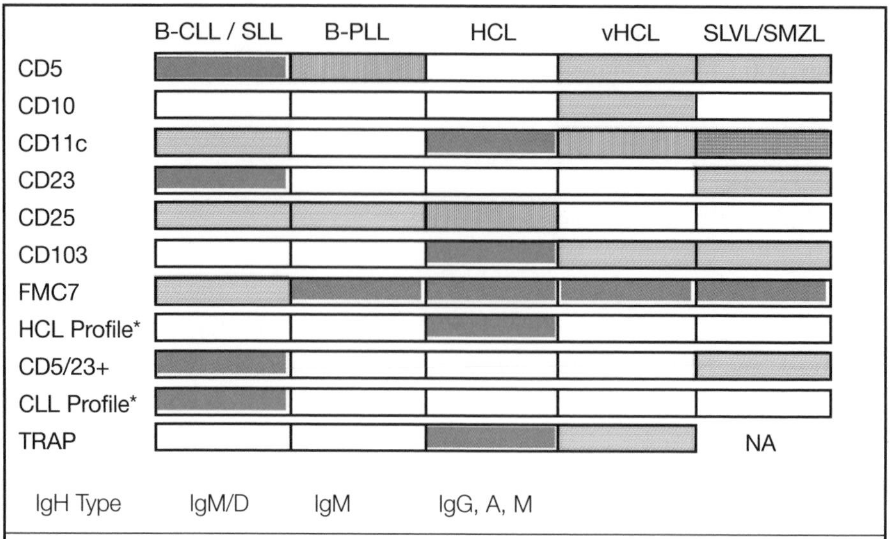

Figure 9-14

	B-CLL / SLL	B-PLL	HCL	vHCL	SLVL/SMZL
CD5					
CD10					
CD11c					
CD23					
CD25					
CD103					
FMC7					
HCL Profile*					
CD5/23+					
CLL Profile*					
TRAP					NA
IgH Type	IgM/D	IgM	IgG, A, M		

Antigen Intensity					
sIg	Dim	Brt	Brt	Brt	Brt
CD11c	Dim		Brt	Dim	Dim to Brt
CD25	Dim	Dim	Dim	Dim	Dim
FMC7	Dim	Brt	Brt		Dim to Brt

Figure 9-14
Antigen Profiles of Hairy Cell Leukemias and Related Entities
* HCL Profile = CD11c+ (brt) & CD22+ (brt), CD25+ & CD103+ (mod to brt).
* CLL Profile = CD5+, CD23+, dim sIg+, dim CD20+, absent to dim CD22+

phocytoid transformation of CLL (CLL/PL), and other mature B-lymphoid neoplasias do have small, distinct nucleoli and/or increased amounts of cytoplasm, typically they do not have the uniform cellular size and presence of true macronucleoli seen with B-PLL.[43,65,100,101,104] As a corollary, the definitions of B-PLL, CLL/PL, and the prolymphocytoid transformation of B-CLL/SLL are primarily morphologically-based.[43,102,105]

Unfortunately, the immunophenotypic profile of B-PLL is neither characteristic on a "positive/negative" basis, nor in qualitative features of intensity. As mentioned above, B-PLLs should be distinctly (brightly) FMC7+, and the lack of FMC7 should stimulate a search for other diagnoses. When B-CLL/SLL is in the differential diagnosis, B-PLL is favored based upon the strong expression of sIg, CD20, CD22, and FMC7, along with the lack of CD5 in at least 50% of cases. Typically, the FMC7 expression seen in a minority of B-CLL/SLLs is dim, not bright as seen in PLL. For B-CLL/PL or prolymphocytoid transformation of B-CLL/SLL, the cells show qualitative and quantitative antigen profiles varying from typical B-CLL/SLL to B-PLL. The diagnosis of CLL/PL or prolymphocytoid transformation of B-CLL/SLL is based upon clinical history and morphologic exam.

The leukemic phase of MCL can be difficult to distinguish morphologically from B-PLL. While most MCLs are FMC7$^+$, the intensity of this positivity is distinctly dimmer than that seen with B-PLL. However, it is often difficult to distinguish bright from dim in standard flow cytometry. The absence of CD5 for B-PLL is very helpful in this differential. A significant fraction of B-PLLs were reported to be CD5$^+$ prior to the recognition of MCL. We now know that many of these CD5$^+$ "PLLs" are probably MCLs with more blastoid morphology. Therefore, cytogenetic examination for t(11;14), PCR analysis for the *bcl1-IgH* fusion gene, and/or determination of bcl1 protein overexpression by immunocytochemistry are helpful in confirming or refuting this differential diagnosis.

Other mature B-lymphoid neoplasias (eg, HCL, FCL) can be separated from B-PLL primarily on morphologic grounds. HCLs and splenic MZLs typically have reduced or only modestly elevated WBC counts and variably irregular cell borders. These features, and the absence of "hairy-cell" antigens (CD11c, CD103), should allow for a clear diagnosis.[38,106,107]

Lastly, the morphologic differential of B-PLL includes acute leukemia (especially undifferentiated acute myelogenous leukemia [AML]) and, rarely, mature large-cell leukemia. Fortunately, membrane immunophenotyping is almost always able to separate acute leukemias (particularly AML) from a mature B-cell leukemia. The absence of sIg and CD20 and the presence of membrane CD13, CD33, and/or intracellular myeloperoxidase antigen are typical for AML. Although B-lineage acute lymphoblastic leukemias (ALL) are CD19$^+$, they are variably and dimly CD20$^+$ and lack the expression of sIg and the uniform bright expression of CD20 and CD22 that are seen with B-PLL. Lastly, the presence of CD34 and/or intracellular TdT should direct the diagnosis to B-lineage ALL over B-PLL.

Hairy-Cell Leukemia

Clinical and Morphologic Features

Hairy-cell leukemia (HCL) is rarely seen in general practice.[31,32,43] It predominates in middle-aged males, although the age range is broad.[108,109] HCL has a moderate-to-indolent clinical course, even without treatment.[108] A majority of deaths are due to infectious processes that are typically associated with granulocytopenia. The median survival is 5 years, with granulocytopenia predicting the group at highest risk for death. Those without neutropenia often survive for more than 10 years. Treatment with interferon alfa, nucleoside analogs, and/or pentostatin has been able to induce a durable remission in a large proportion of patients.[110]

Typically, patients with HCL present with pancytopenia associated with splenomegaly.[108] Only a minority have hepatomegaly (19%) or lymphadenopathy (11%); the latter is typically small and localized.[108] Modern therapy can quickly and durably induce a complete remission. However, residual HCL can often be found in the marrow of patients in clinical remission, though it does not portend imminent clinical relapse.[111] If relapse occurs, reinduction is usually easily produced.

The concentration of HCL cells in the blood is typically low, although it tends to increase over time in untreated patients.[111] In a small minority of cases, no hairy cells may be seen in the blood.[108] Cytologically, HCL is characterized by intermediate-sized lymphoid cells (10 to 25 micrometers) with irregular cellular borders.[111] The latter include the classic "hairy" projections, although some forms have only mildly irregular borders. The N/C ratio is moderate and the cytoplasm often appears very finely blue-gray and granular with Giemsa or Wright staining. The nuclear contours typically range from oval to reniform, with densely reticular chromatin. Nucleoli are almost always absent.

In the bone marrow, dry taps are not infrequent due to reticulin fibrosis. In untreated patients, the cellularity is normal or elevated with diffuse involvement by HCL.[111] In HCL patients given interferon or pentostatin treatment, the residual hairy cells may be quite difficult to identify and may require immunohistochemical and/or flow cytometric analysis. In the spleen, HCL typically involves the red pulp. Dense aggregates of hairy cells are often interspersed with blood "lakes."

Prior to modern immunophenotyping, the diagnosis of HCL could be confirmed by strong diffuse tartrate-resistant acid phosphatase reactivity in the neoplastic cells (TRAP),[109] with more than 99% of cases being positive. It should be pointed out that weak-to-moderate TRAP reactivity may also be observed in benign lymphocytes seen in Epstein-Barr virus (EBV) infections and in the neoplastic cells of Sézary syndrome, B-PLL, and B-CLL/SLL.[109]

Immunophenotypic Profile

HCL cells usually have bright CD45 expression, identical to most other mature B-lymphoid leukemias. However, the forward and side light scatter are increased (particularly the forward). Given this increase, light scatter plots of HCL cells typically resemble those of large lymphoid cells or monocytes. This effect is not as dramatic with a CD45/side-light-scatter plot, although the HCL cells are usually a distinct cluster that is closely opposed to the small lymphoid cluster. Therefore, the laboratorian will require some clinical history so as not to use just a standard "lymphocyte" gate and analyze the wrong population. This is particularly likely to happen with marrow aspirates, with their complex populations.

HCL, along with B-CLL/SLL, is one of the few types of leukemia whose immunophenotypic profile may be considered diagnostic by itself (**Figure 9-14**, p 270). First, HCL is a mature B-cell neoplasm, with strong expression of major B-cell antigens (CD19, CD20, CD22), including sIg. In a significant fraction of cases, the latter are composed of multiple, atypical combinations of the heavy-chain isotypes IgG, IgA, IgM, and IgD (eg, IgA⁺IgG⁺IgD⁺).[112,113] The latter finding may be explained by the results of functional studies, which have suggested that HCL represents leukemia "frozen" at a postproliferative, pre-plasmacytic stage of normal B-cell maturation.[30] At this stage, immunoglobulin isotype switching will occur.

Most HCLs fail to express CD5 or CD10.[112] A relatively unique feature of the hairy cells is the bright expression of CD11c, CD22, CD103, and FMC7.[38,53,112] This concomitant bright expression of CD11c and CD103 is very specific for HCL in the setting of a monoclonal B lymphoproliferation.[30,53,112] However, not infrequently, dimmer expression of either can be seen in many mature B-cell neoplasms. The CD25 antigen is found in approximately 70% to 80% of cases and is only dim-to-moderate in intensity.[30] The HCL profile can be used to detect minimal residual disease in HCL.[110] However, it does not appear to predict the risk of relapse or disease-free survival.[110]

Differential Diagnosis

The mature B-lymphoid leukemias and lymphomas (B-CLL/SLL, MCL, FCL, MZL) can usually be distinguished from HCL on the basis of cytomorphology and/or biopsy architecture. Although a minority of B-CLL/SLLs are dimly CD11c⁺ or FMC7⁺, they are almost always CD5⁺ and CD103⁻. Furthermore, the intensity of CD20, CD22, and sIg on B-CLL/SLL cells is dim as compared with that seen with HCL. In fact, CD22 and/or sIg may not be detectable at all on B-CLL/SLL cells. The presence of CD5⁺CD10⁻ and CD5⁻CD10⁺ profiles immunophenotypically allows one to define MCL and FCLs, although some FCLs lack CD10, along with most MZLs. In such instances, cytomorphology and the lack of the HCL antigen profile will allow distinction from HCL.

The differential diagnosis of HCL versus vHCL and SLVL is more complex due to the overlapping cytomorphology of these neoplasms, but clear distinctions can be made on the basis of the combined immunomorphologic phenotype.[43] HCL usually brightly expresses at least 3 of the following antigens: CD11c, CD22, CD25, and CD103. In contrast, vHCL, SLVL, and MZL usually only weakly express 0 to 2 of these antigens.[38] The variant form of HCL (vHCL) may be TRAP-positive. However, vHCL tends to lack detectable expression of CD25 antigens, and some cases lack CD11c as well.[43] Lastly, splenic MZL and SLVL variably mimic HCL morphologically and clinically. However, MZL and SLVL cells do not express TRAP, CD11c, or CD25 and have a different pattern of splenic infiltration.[43]

Variant Hairy-Cell Leukemia

Clinical and Morphologic Features

The variant form of HCL (vHCL) is a rare entity with an indolent clinical course.[43,114,115] The median age of vHCL patients is 69 years. Most patients present with distinct splenomegaly. In contrast to HCL, there is typically a marked lymphocytosis (median WBC count of 116×10^9/L), and neutropenia is uncommon.[109] Most vHCL cases do not respond to standard HCL chemotherapy. Despite this, median survival has not been reached at 4 years.

The morphology of vHCL is similar to HCL in that both are intermediate-sized lymphoid cells with fine, hairy projections. These projections are irregularly distributed around the cell. Compared with HCL, vHCL cells have a higher N/C ratio, rounder nuclei, coarser chromatin, and a more prominent nucleolus. Additionally, most cases of vHCL demonstrate a minor fraction of binucleated lymphocytes. Marrow aspirates can easily be obtained, with a distinct interstitial infiltrate of vHCL. Reticulin fibers are reported to be mildly increased.[114] Splenic involvement is predominantly in the red pulp, with blood "lakes" seen in only isolated cases.

Immunophenotypic Features

The vHCL is a mature B-cell neoplasm that distinctly expresses CD19, CD20, CD22, and monoclonal sIg (**Figure 9-14**, p 270). While TRAP reactivity may occasionally be noted, strong diffuse expression is not seen. Most cases are CD11c+ and FMC7+, but CD25, CD23, and HC2 antigens are absent. Only a small minority (10% to 20%) of vHCLs coexpress CD5 or CD10. One report revealed that 40% (4/10) of vHCL cases express CD103.[114] However, individual cases of vHCL almost always have fewer than 3 of the major "hairy-cell" antigens (CD11c, CD25, CD103).

Differential Diagnosis

The major differential features of vHCL and HCL are the degree of lymphocytosis (which is greater in vHCL), the presence of nucleoli (distinctly present in vHCL), neutropenia (not present in vHCL), and TRAP and/or expression of the HCL antigen profile (absent in vHCL; see HCL section for further discussion). Other diagnostic considerations include B-PLL. However, vHCL has not been reported to have the strong FMC7 expression typically seen in B-PLL. This, combined with the smooth cellular borders and macronucleolus seen in B-PLL cells, should allow distinction from vHCL.

Splenic Lymphoma with Veiled Lymphocytes

Clinical and Morphologic Features

Splenic lymphoma with veiled lymphocytes (SLVL) is a somewhat controversial entity that is more widely recognized in Europe than the United States.[116] Its relationship to and distinction from splenic marginal zone lymphoma is unclear at this time. It is typically seen at a median age of 70 years and is slightly more prevalent in women. Massive splenomegaly is noted in 75% of patients and is typically unassociated with hepatomegaly or lymphadenopathy. Lymphocytosis is seen in approximately 75% of patients at presentation and 87% during the course of their disease. The degree of lymphocytosis is quite variable (lymphocyte counts can range from 4×10^9/L to 150×10^9/L), although counts in excess of 100×10^9/L are very unusual.[107] Marked anemia or thrombocytopenia is not uncommon.

The clinical course of SLVL is usually indolent, with median survivals often not being reached after 10 to 12 years. Patients with low WBC counts ($< 30 \times 10^9$/L) and lymphocytosis (lymphocyte counts $> 4 \times 10^9$/L) have a more favorable prognosis than those not in this group.[116] No treatment or treatment with splenectomy seems to produce better outcomes than does chemotherapy.

Cytologically, the classic SLVL cell is small-to-intermediate in size with a moderately high N/C ratio.[106] The basophilic agranular cytoplasm has irregular borders, with typically coarse projections spaced at 1 or 2 sites about the cell. The nuclei have dense chromatin and round contours, often with distinct nucleoli. Although all patients with SLVL typically have such cells, a wide range of morphology exists within the neoplastic lymphocytes in any given case.[116] In marrow, dry taps are unusual, reticulin fibrosis is absent, and marrow involvement sparse.[109] The splenic involvement is typically in the white pulp.

Immunophenotypic Features

The major B-cell antigens CD19, CD20, and CD22 are present in SLVL cells with moderate-to-strong intensity (**Figure 9-14**, p 270).[107,116] The sIg is monoclonal and also has moderate-to-strong intensity. FMC7 is found in most cases, as is CD11c in 50% to 75% of cases. Most (> 75%) cases lack expression of CD5, CD10, CD23, CD25, and CD103. More specifically, 19% to 25% of SLVLs are CD5$^+$, 15% CD103$^+$, 19% to 31% CD23$^+$, and 2% to 30% CD10$^+$. No SLVL cases coexpress all 3 "hairy-cell" antigens: CD11c, CD25, and CD103. Furthermore, only 25% of CD5$^+$ SLVLs are also CD23$^+$, and none have the classic B-CLL/SLL profile of CD5$^+$, CD23$^+$, dim sIg$^+$, CD22$^-$ or dim$^+$, and FMC7$^-$.[107]

Differential Diagnosis

The major differentials are HCL, B-PLL, and B-CLL/SLL with variable morphology. A diagnosis of SLVL is most reliably made upon the combined clinical, morphologic, and immunophenotypic features. The presence of distinct nucleoli, the absence of reticular fibrosis in the marrow, and (if a spleen sample is obtained) predominant splenic white pulp involvement point to SLVL rather than HCL. The CD11c$^+$CD25$^+$CD103$^+$ profile typical of HCL is not seen in SLVL, although individual antigens in the HCL group may be present. The smooth cytoplasmic borders and distinct macronucleoli of B-PLL are quite useful in distinguishing it from SLVL. Although both are FMC7$^+$ and a significant minority CD5$^+$, the presence of CD103 and/or CD11c should point toward SLVL. In a majority of cases of SLVL, CD5 and/or CD23 are absent, in distinction to B-CLL/SLL. Lastly, as mentioned above, the classic immunophenotypic profile of B-CLL/SLL is not seen in SLVL.

Secretory/Plasmacytoid Neoplasms

Secretory lymphomas and leukemias have as their common denominator a prominent monoclonal proteinemia and/or proteinuria (> 10 g/L and often > 30 g/L in serum and/or > 0.5 to 1.0 g/24 hr in urine). As a corollary, a significant fraction of these neoplastic cells have plasmacytoid features. The defined entities in secretory B-cell malignancies are plasma cell leukemia (PCL), multiple myeloma, solitary plasmacytoma, and lymphoplasmacytic lymphoma/small lymphocytic lymphoma with plasmacytoid features (often associated with the clinical syndrome of Waldenström macroglobulinemia [WM]).[117-120] Despite related morphology and differentiation, these neoplasms have variable prognoses.[121,122]

Although typical cases of these plasmacytoid neoplasms do not require immunophenotyping for diagnosis, anaplastic variants of PCL/myeloma and CLL-like variants of WM may not be easily recognizable.[123,124] Furthermore, the laboratorian may not be aware of the presence of proteinemia or proteinuria. Therefore, immunophenotypic analysis may result in a more definitive diagnosis.[125]

Myeloma/Plasma-Cell Leukemia

Clinical and Morphologic Features

Myeloma is typically seen in individuals between 50 and 70 years of age. However, approximately 10% and 2% of patients with myeloma present when they are between the ages of 40 to 49 and 30 to 39 years of age, respectively.[117] The clinical features at presentation can be protean, ranging from pathologic fractures or renal failure to back pain or fatigue, all the way to essentially asymptomatic presentations that are discovered by hyperproteinemias on routine biochemical profile screens. Approximately 99% of myeloma patients have a monoclonal protein (typically large) present in serum and/or urine protein electrophoresis. Despite the rather differentiated nature of the neoplasm, the clinical course is moderately aggressive. Many patients exhibit a leukemic phase (secondary PCL) in the terminal months of the disease.

Primary PCL is a distinctly rare but aggressive disorder.[122-124] The morphology is variable, from clearly plasmacytic to plasmablastic to plasmacytoid lymphocytes. The median survival of untreated patients is typically a few months or less, although treatment with aggressive chemotherapy has been reported to increase median survival to 18 months.[126] The median age at onset and gender of PCL patients are similar to those of myeloma patients, although PCL patients have a higher incidence of stage III disease, extramedullary involvement, and Bence Jones proteinuria.

Immunophenotypic Features

Myeloma and PCL are best defined by a mixture of positive and negative antigens associated with bright monoclonal cytoplasmic light chain staining. Membrane CD45 and sIg are often absent, or weakly present in a minority of cells.[20] Additionally, most pan-B antigens typically found on less mature B cells (CD19, CD20, CD22) are usually not detected on either the cell surface or cytoplasm of myeloma and PCL cells, although membrane CD24 and/or cytoplasmic CD79 alpha may be detectable.[20,54,125,127-129]

Both benign and malignant plasma cells strongly express surface CD38, CD138, PCA-1, and PC-1 antigens.[20,28,29] Of these 4 molecules, only PC-1 is restricted to plasma cells.[20,25,29] In the setting of mature T- and B-lineage neoplasms, CD138 is expressed only in myeloma, plasmacytoma, and a minority of plasmacytoid immunoblastic lymphomas and effusion B large-cell lymphomas in HIV-infected individuals.[25,28,29] The CD138 antigen also works well when testing fixed paraffin-embedded tissue.[28,29] The PCA-1 antigen lacks specificity for plasma cells because it is expressed in a significant majority of HCLs and is also found on normal neutrophils and activated T cells.[30] PCA-1 also appears to be only sporadically expressed on benign and malignant plasma cells[22] and is not commercially available.

The prognostic utility of immunophenotyping in the setting of myeloma is unproven. Some reports indicate a more adverse prognosis for CD10+ myeloma,[130] while others have not found such a correlation. Cases of myelomonocytic-antigen-positive myeloma have also been correlated with a poorer prognosis.[121,131] The above observations need to be confirmed in large prospective studies. However, they raise the possibility that routine immunophenotypic analysis may be used in the future for prognostic purposes. These findings also raise the intriguing possibility that myeloma is a stem cell malignancy, analogous to chronic granulocytic leukemia.[132]

A question that may arise is the about the malignant potential of monoclonal plasma cell proliferations. Although this question typically arises in the differential diagnosis of serum monoclonal gammopathies of undetermined significance (MGUS),[120] it may also arise with minor monoclonal plasmacellular proliferations. Antigens such as NCAM/CD56 and syndecan-1/CD138 are found on a significant majority of malignant plasma cells and may be of potential use in differential diagnosis.[24] However, CD138 expression is not restricted to myeloma. Other B-lineage neoplasias (B-CLL/SLL, lymphoplasmacytoid lymphoma, HIV-associated human herpesvirus-8 [HHV8]-associated primary effusion B-cell NHL, and HIV-associated B-immunoblastic plasmacytoid NHL) may be CD138+. Unfortunately, MGUS may also be variably CD138+.[24,25,133] More recent studies have indicated that non-neoplastic plasma cells are often CD19+CD56-, while myeloma cells are CD19-CD56+.[134]

Differential Diagnosis

The most common differential diagnostic dilemma facing the laboratorian is distinguishing plasmablastic/anaplastic myeloma from large-cell NHLs.

In this setting, strong cytoplasmic light chain and CD38 or CD138 expression along with a lack of pan B antigens (CD19, CD20, CD22) and CD45 are quite specific for myeloma.[125] While B-lineage immunoblastic NHLs may be Ig⁻ and CD45⁻ (particularly in fixed tissue), most will express either CD45 or CD20.[125] The PCA-1 antigen is only rarely expressed on large-cell and immunoblastic lymphomas. However, its lack of sensitivity for myeloma is a drawback.

Atypical antigen expression may be useful in the differential diagnosis with plasmacytic proliferations in MGUS. Expression of CD10 and CD56 has been reported frequently in myeloma, but not usually with MGUS plasma cell proliferations.[121,134-136] A recent review of the literature suggests that MGUS patients have a monoclonal subset of CD56⁺CD138⁺CD19⁻ plasma cells admixed with a polyclonal population of CD56⁻CD138⁻ cells.[24] It is the ratio between the clonal CD56⁺CD138⁺ subset and the polyclonal CD56⁻CD138⁻ subset that best defines whether the proliferation is multiple myeloma or MGUS.[24]

Waldenström Macroglobulinemia

Clinical and Morphologic Features

Waldenström macroglobulinemia (WM) is most common in older individuals, with a median patient age of 61 years.[137] It is an indolent neoplasm, with median survivals of 5 to 8 years. Much like myeloma, the symptoms may be vague. The diagnosis of Waldenström macroglobulinemia is primarily a clinical and morphologic one.[137] Most investigators require:

- A non-Hodgkin's lymphoma, most commonly the lymphoplasmacytic type, less commonly CLL/SLL-like with plasmacytoid differentiation (if in the marrow, > 30% of the nucleated cells should be monoclonal B cells)
- A significant (≥10 g/L) serum monoclonal gammopathy, almost always IgM
- Pathologic hyperviscosity, usually with the clinical signs and symptoms of the hyperviscosity syndrome[138,139]

The large monoclonal gammopathy can give rise to other signs and symptoms, including type 1 cryoglobulinemia, hemostatic defects due to IgM–clotting protein binding, polyneuropathies, cold agglutinin hemolytic anemia, and amyloid and nonamyloid deposition disorders.[137]

Immunophenotypic Features

Immunophenotyping is usually employed only if there is a need to confirm clonality. However, anaplastic myelomas may mimic the morphologic heterogeneity of WM and have a more aggressive clinical course than WM. Furthermore, cases of WM with CLL-like morphology need to be distinguished from true B-CLL/SLLs, as the latter usually have an even more indolent clinical course. In such an instance, immunophenotyping, along with review of other clinical and laboratory data, is needed for a more precise diagnosis.

The malignant cells of WM have a hybrid antigen phenotype, expressing plasma cell–associated antigens (eg, CD38) along with membrane CD19, CD20, CD22, CD45 (dim to brightly), sIg, and FMC7.[20,137,140] Cytoplasmic monoclonal Ig is usually more distinctly expressed than sIg in WM with plasmacytoid features.

Differential Diagnosis

The major differentials are typically IgM MGUS, B-CLL/SLL, plasmacytoid immunoblastic NHL, and anaplastic myeloma. The last is usually excluded by a combination of the immunophenotype (CD19+, CD20+, and sIg+ in WM and CD19-, CD20-, and sIg- in myeloma) and the proteinemia isotype (IgM in WM, IgG > IgA in myeloma). Those cases of WM with a CLL-like morphology usually lack both CD5 and CD23, although approximately 20% of cases express either one or the other. In contrast, B-CLL/SLL cases are almost always CD5+CD23+ and usually have only small IgM monoclonal gammopathies (<10 g/L). An IgM MGUS is usually differentiated from WM on the basis of the size of the serum IgM concentration, although there is often significant overlap of the two in the 10 to 20 g/L range. The absence of a significant marrow or tissue plasmacellular proliferation best distinguishes IgM MGUS from WM. Plasmacytoid immunoblastic lymphomas are also usually differentiated from WM on the basis of serum IgM concentration.

Other Mature B-Lineage Neoplasms

So far, the only lymphoid neoplasias that have been discussed are those readily amenable to flow cytometric immunoanalysis and for which flow cytometry usually offers resolution superior to immunohistochemical or immunocytochemical analysis. This leaves a substantial percentage of lymphomas whose antigen profile is best determined by immunohistochemistry. In part, this reflects the difficulty of obtaining a representative cell suspension for flow cytometry. This may be due to the fragility of the neoplastic cells or their overall paucity. Other factors include the sample being processed entirely as fixed tissue (eg, small biopsies and tissues often not associated with lymphoma) and fibrosis.

Fortunately, antigen retrieval techniques, along with monoclonal and polyclonal antisera reactive to a wide range of clinically useful leukocyte antigens in formalin-fixed tissue, have been made commercially available over the last 10 years (CD1, CD2, CD3, CD4, CD5, CD7, CD8, CD10, CD14, CD15, CD20, CD21, CD23, CD30, CD34, CD43, CD45, CD45RO, CD45RA, CD56, CD57, CD61, CD79 alpha, CD79 beta, granzyme B, myeloperoxidase, TCR beta, TCR delta, TdT, TIA-1). These not only allow diagnostically effective immunophenotyping of the neoplasms discussed below, but also offer significant competition to flow cytometry for the classification of the lymphomas reviewed above. These immunohistochemical techniques have also become essential for the accurate classification of Hodgkin's lymphoma, T-cell-rich B-cell lymphomas, and some rare cutaneous and intestinal T-cell lymphomas.

B Large Cell Lymphomas

The B large cell lymphomas are aggressive, yet a majority of cases can be put into remission with chemotherapy. Indeed, a large fraction may be cured if the disease is low-stage.[5] Immunophenotyping is most often used to define lineage (eg, carcinoma, lymphoma), because the large-cell proliferation is typically diagnostic for malignancy. This is fortunate, as many B-cell NHLs lack detectable immunoglobulin light chains. A morphologic variant of B large cell NHL is the so-called "T-cell-rich B-cell lymphoma" (TCRBCL).[141,142] With either form, the typical loss of the large cells during processing and the robust nature of IHC antibodies for defining lineage in paraffin-embedded tissue sections make IHC immunophenotyping preferred.

An antibody panel similar or identical to that for mature B-lymphoid leukemias would be appropriate (**Table 9-3**, p 247). It is quite important for both the interpreter and the flow cytometer operator to be informed that the large lymphoid cells are to be examined. This will allow for both accurate collection of data and data analysis. As discussed above, the large lymphoid cells may be markedly diminished in the cell suspension due to lack of viability and/or cell rupture. Furthermore, many B large cell NHLs have dim or absent surface CD45 intensity. Lastly, some large cells have such a high forward light scatter that they fall on the upper limit of the scale and may be hidden by the plot lines (the "picture frame" effect).

In the author's experience, no one approach is sensitive enough for neoplastic B large cells to reliably work by itself. Rather, an informed analysis using multiple gating techniques and a high index of suspicion is probably the most effective approach. As a corollary, if the small lymphoid cluster from a tissue specimen is benign or not clearly neoplastic, the technologists in the author's laboratory are instructed to routinely analyze the large lymphoid cells.

Burkitt's Lymphoma (Small Cell Noncleaved Lymphoma)

The Burkitt's lymphomas are very aggressive neoplasms, but respond well to modern chemotherapy.[5] Like the large cell lymphomas, their morphologies are almost always diagnostic for malignancy. Immunophenotyping is used to define differentiation (eg, lymphoblastic leukemia/lymphoma and morphologically similar non-hematolymphoid neoplasms). Typically, this immunophenotypic differential can be defined by IHC in paraffin section (eg, TdT, CD3, CD20, CD45, CD79 alpha). However, unlike large-cell lymphomas, it is usually fairly easy to get Burkitt's lymphoma cells into a cell suspension in representative numbers, and these typically have an unambiguous gating profile (bright CD45, intermediate-range forward and low-to-intermediate-range side light scatter). As a result, flow cytometric immunoanalysis is also quite capable of defining these malignancies.

The flow panel should include antibodies to membrane CD3, CD5, CD7, CD10, CD19, CD20, CD34, CD45, kappa, lambda, intracellular CD79 alpha, and TdT. The Burkitt's lymphoma cell has a typically uniform and bright expression of CD19, CD20, CD45, and immunoglobulin light chains. The majority of cases are also dim but distinctly CD10$^+$. This profile defines B lineage and strongly suggests mature germinal center stage maturation. The major differential with CD10$^+$ B-lineage lymphomas is between precursor B-lymphoblastic lymphoma and follicular center lymphoma. The presence of one or more of the "blast"-associated antigens (CD34 and TdT), along with the bright intensity of CD10 and absence of sIg, should confirm the diagnosis of precursor B-lymphoblastic lymphoma. However, the immunophenotypic profile of follicular center lymphoma is so similar to Burkitt's lymphoma that only morphology can readily distinguish between the two entities. Lastly, although rare CD5$^+$ cases have been reported, most Burkitt lymphomas are CD5$^-$.[79]

Mature Leukemias and Lymphomas of T Lineage

The mature T-cell neoplasias are far less frequent in North America and Europe than their B-cell counterparts. While certain clinical and morphologic features are suggestive of T lineage (**Table 9-2**), these are not specific, and therefore immunophenotyping must be performed. A closely related issue is the immunophenotypic definition of T malignancy. There are no direct clonal markers on T cells that are analogous to kappa and lambda in B lineage. The CD4/CD8 ratio should *not* be used as a clonal marker. The "loss" of pan-T antigens (ie, < 50% of all $CD3^+$ T cells express CD7) is strongly associated with T-cell clonality (**Figure 9-15F**, p 284). Atypical variations in intensity of pan-T antigens are also suggestive of clonality (**Figure 9-15C,D**, p 284). However, these changes are not definitively diagnostic, because reactive T lymphocytosis has been reported to display a temporary loss of 1 or more pan-T antigens.[143] If, in a T proliferation associated with the "loss" of a "pan-T" antigen, the clinical and morphologic features are not definitively diagnostic of leukemia/lymphoma, then PCR or southern blot analysis of the T-cell antigen receptor gene (TCR) should be performed to confirm or refute clonality.

T- and NK-Large Granular Lymphocytic Leukemias and Benign NK Lymphoproliferations

Clinical and Morphologic Profile

T-large granular lymphocytic leukemia (T-LGL) is 1 of the 2 most common mature T-cell leukemias in North America.[31,32] It is usually a very low-grade leukemia and has been associated with survivals of several decades after diagnosis. No clear etiology or cytogenetic lesions are known. However, a minority of T-LGLs are associated with Felty syndrome. Rarely, T-LGL has also been reported in an immunosuppressed solid organ transplant patient.[144,145] Aggressive therapy is not usually required for T-LGL, as long as there is careful follow-up. Patients with symptomatic neutropenia have been effectively treated with cyclosporine A.[146]

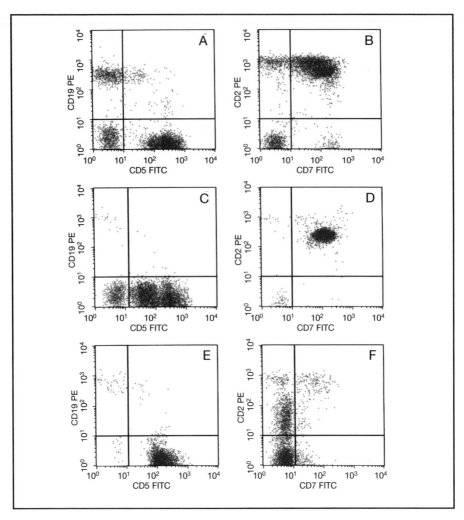

Figure 9-15
Pan-T Antigen Expression in Normal and Neoplastic T Cells.

The expression of CD5 and CD2 / CD7 on normal blood T and NK cells is shown in panels A and B, respectively. Note the moderate predominance of T lymphs (CD5+ CD19-) and the relatively broad unimodal distribution of CD5 and CD7. In contrast, a case of T-LGL in panel C reveals a distinctly bimodal distribution of CD5+ CD19- T cells (LR quadrant). The dimmer CD5+ T cells are neoplastic CD8+ T LGL lymphs, while the brighter CD5+ cells are residual benign CD4+ cells. In panel D and E, an abnormally tight distribution of CD7+ (UR quadrant; panel D) and CD5+ CD19- T cells (LR quadrant; panel E) is seen. These changes are not as readily appreciated in isolation. However, in both instances, the vast majority of cells are T lymphs, lymphocytosis. Further biopsy and genotypic studies confirmed the diagnosis. A case of Sezary syndrome is shown in panel F. This exhibits a marked loss of pan T antigens, most clearly CD7. Other tubes revealed that greater than 80% of the cells were CD3+. Such "loss" is distinctly associated with T cell neoplasia, although certain reactive conditions can result in similar profiles. Thus, clinical correlation, with or without genotypic and/or biopsy studies are necessary to confirm the diagnosis.

T-LGL is typically a proliferation of intermediate-sized lymphocytes with abundant cytoplasm containing a small number of red cytoplasmic granules and sharp cellular borders. The nuclei range from oval to reniform, with a smooth or densely reticular chromatin. Nucleoli are typically not seen.[144,145,147-150] Exceptions to each of these morphologic characteristics exist within the clinicopathologic spectrum of T-LGL.

A clonal NK-LGL variant exists that is morphologically identical to T-LGL.[149,151,152] This variant is usually much more aggressive than T-LGL itself; patients typically die within 1 year after diagnosis. Defining NK clonality is difficult, and requires methods outside of flow cytometric and standard nucleic acid analysis. This is unfortunate, because polyclonal/benign NK lymphoproliferations are much more frequent than malignant NK-LGLs. The former are morphologically and immunophenotypically identical to the latter. Therefore, differentiating benign NK- and T-LGLs from a malignant NK-LGL requires a retrospective or prospective "tincture of time". As a corollary, the diagnosis of a malignant NK leukemia is principally clinical: the patients are usually quite ill at presentation, with multiple cytopenias, weight loss, and fever. A prolonged history of an NK-large granular lymphoproliferation would be a significant factor arguing for a reactive process.

Immunophenotypic Features

Immunophenotyping will clearly define T-LGL as mature T lymphoproliferation. T-LGLs are mature T cells, usually expressing all major pan-T antigens (CD2, CD3, CD5, and CD7), with a CD8$^+$CD4$^-$ profile. Occasionally, there is a loss of a pan-T antigen, which would support a diagnosis of a clonal proliferation of T lymphocytes. Characteristically, 1 or more NK-associated antigens are present (CD11c, CD16, CD56, and/or CD57). Of these NK antigens, CD57 has been most commonly reported. It is not currently possible to define the very small minority of T-LGLs that will be clinically aggressive through immunophenotypic analysis.[147-149] However, CD56$^+$ T-LGL has been reported to be associated with a more aggressive clinical course.[144,145,150] The NK LGLs share the CD2$^+$CD7$^+$CD8$^+$NK-antigen$^+$ profile with T-LGLs. By definition, no T-specific antigens are present (CD3, CD5, TCR). No clear immunophenotypic features to separate NK-LGL from benign NK lymphoproliferations have been defined at this time.

Differential Diagnosis

The cytomorphology of LGL with a CD3$^+$CD8$^+$CD4$^-$NK-antigen(s)$^+$ profile is diagnostic. It should be pointed out that, as is the case with all T-cell neoplasias, the diagnosis requires careful correlation with clinical and other laboratory data. While a small minority of T-PLL and T-CLL patients may have a CD8$^+$CD4$^-$ profile, they usually lack the presence of NK-associated antigens found on T-LGL *and* the LGL cytomorphology. For similar reasons, adult T-cell lymphoma and mycosis fungoides/Sézary syndrome can be excluded.

Sézary Syndrome/Mycosis Fungoides

Clinical and Morphologic Profile

Mycosis fungoides (MF) is a malignant cutaneous T-cell lymphoma (CTCL) and Sézary syndrome (SS) is the peripheralized version of this CTCL.[153-156] MF/SS, along with T-LGL, make up the most prevalent forms of mature T-cell leukemia in North America.[31,32] MF is typically indolent, although the SS variant is associated with greater morbidity and mortality because of its higher stage.

The histologic appearance of MF is quite characteristic, with a direct extension of superficial lymphoproliferation into the epidermis (no "Grenz zone"). Classic features of the latter include Pautrier "microabscesses" of neoplastic T lymphocytes. Cytologically, the neoplastic T cells range from small to large in size. The Sézary cell is a smaller lymphocyte with deeply convoluted nuclear contours. Larger "Lutzner forms" of the neoplastic cells are not as characteristic of MF or SS.

Immunophenotypic Features

MF/SS cells have a CD4$^+$CD8$^-$ phenotype, although a small minority (< 10%) have been reported to be either CD4$^+$CD8$^+$ or CD4$^-$CD8$^+$. The CD2, CD3, CD5, and TCR alpha/beta antigens are almost always present, although some may show dimmer or brighter expression than that seen on reactive T cells. With the exception of very early stage MF, the neoplastic T cells lack expression of CD7 in most instances.[54,157-160] Caution should be shown in interpreting such a "loss" as neoplastic, because it is not definitively indicative of MF/SS nor of a clonal/neoplastic T-cell population. Reactive T lymphocytosis associated with viral infections (EBV, cytomegalovirus (CMV), hepatitis) can occasionally exhibit a temporary loss of one or more pan-T antigens.[143]

Differential Diagnosis

Once a diagnosis of a CD4$^+$ T-cell leukemia/lymphoma is established, the final diagnosis requires cytomorphology, clinical history, and/or human T-lymphotropic virus (HTLV)-1 and -2 serology. The presence or absence of other antigen markers (eg, CD25) is not sufficiently sensitive or specific to exclude or define type.

T-Prolymphocytic Leukemia

Clinical and Morphologic Features

T-prolymphocytic leukemia (T-PLL) is a rare neoplasm.[43,161] Two distinct presentations are noted. The first is usually quite aggressive, with an overall median survival of less than 12 months.[161] The second occurs in a minority of patients, who have an indolent phase of several years that usually ends in a terminal, clinically aggressive phase.[162] The aggressive cases of T-PLL have significant incidence of splenomegaly (81%), hepatomegaly (43%), and skin lesions (25%), whereas these features are absent or present to a limited degree in the initially indolent forms.[162]

A T-PLL cell is small- to intermediate-sized, with a sharp cellular border, undifferentiated cytoplasm, and a high N/C ratio. The nuclei range from subtly indented to frankly clefted. The chromatin is smooth to densely reticular. The nucleolus may be prominent or only appreciable upon electron microscopic exam. Because of its rather broadly defined morphologic features, T-PLL may be confused with a T-CLL, a leukemic phase of a lymphoma, adult and peripheral T-cell leukemias, Sézary syndrome, or a variant of B-CLL.[43,161,163,164]

Immunophenotypic Features

T-PLLs are mature T-cell neoplasias that express CD2, CD3, CD5, CD7, and TCR alpha/beta in almost all cases and lack expression of TdT and CD1.[161,162,165] Loss of pan-T antigens occurs infrequently.[43,161] Expression of CD4 and CD8 antigens is variable.[162] Approximately 60% are CD4$^+$CD8$^-$, while about 15% are either CD4$^-$CD8$^+$ or CD4$^+$CD8$^+$. Less than 10% lack both CD4 and CD8 antigens. The NK-associated antigens (CD11b, CD16, CD56, CD57) are only rarely reported to be present (< 5%), and CD25 is seen in only 18% of patients.[161,162,165]

Differentiation of T-PLL from T-LGL is fairly easy, based upon morphologic (absence of cytoplasmic granules) and immunophenotypic features (lack of NK-associated antigens, presence of CD4⁺CD8⁻ profile). However, differentiation from adult T-, peripheral T-, and cutaneous T-cell leukemias/lymphomas may be difficult, even with a combined immunomorphologic approach.[163] The extreme nuclear pleomorphism seen in adult T cell leukemia/lymphomas, along with hypercalcemia and a positive serology for the HTLV-1 retrovirus, will suffice to differentiate it from T-PLL.[43,166-168]

T-Chronic Lymphocytic Leukemia (T-CLL)

Clinical and Morphologic Features

T-CLL is a rare neoplasm. It is aggressive and refractory to chemotherapy, and patients with T-CLL usually have a median survival length of 13 months.[31,169,170] Patients typically have a moderate-to-marked lymphocytosis, but no neutropenia. No definitive association with viral or other etiologies has been established. Approximately half of T-CLL patients also have associated anemia or thrombocytopenia. Because of the rarity of this condition, it has not been possible to define effective protocols to evaluate therapy.

Morphologically, the dominant features of T-CLL are a small lymphocyte with undifferentiated cytoplasm, a high N/C ratio, and sharp cellular borders. The nuclear contours are essentially round, and the chromatin coarsely reticular. Few cells have anything more than small, inconspicuous nucleoli. A minor fraction of T-CLL cells are somewhat larger, more irregular lymphocytes.[170] In lymph node biopsy tissue, the appearance is most similar to a B-CLL/SLL. The cytomorphology of T-CLL may at times overlap with that of T-PLL, given the latter's broad morphologic parameters.[43,164,170]

Immunophenotypic Features

Most cases of T-CLL express all of the major pan-T antigens (CD2, CD3, CD5, CD7). Most cases have a CD4⁺CD8⁻NK-antigen⁻ profile.[170] There is insufficient data to define the incidence of CD25 expression.

Differential Diagnosis

Immunophenotyping and morphology will clearly distinguish T-CLL from T/NK-LGLs. Because the immunophenotype of T-CLL is indistinguishable from those of other mature T-cell neoplasms, morphology and serology are essential in distinguishing T-CLL from ATCL, peripheral T-cell lymphoma (PTCL), T-PLL, and MF/SS.[31,54,158,159,166-169,171-178] Because T-CLL and T-PLL are so rare and overlap in morphology and immunophenotype to such a large degree, the author tends to lump the cases together under the moniker "T-CLL/PLL" if there is not a clear-cut morphologic predominance. If the vast majority of neoplastic cells are distinctly small round lymphocytes without nucleoli, then the term "T-CLL" alone is used. Similarly, if most of the cells have distinct nucleoli, then T-PLL is the favored term.

Adult and Peripheral T-Cell Lymphomas

Clinical and Morphologic Features

The adult T-cell lymphomas (ATCLs) are characterized by their association with the HTLV-1 virus. By definition, peripheral T-cell lymphomas (PTCLs) are HTLV-1 negative. Both neoplasms are typically thought of as clinically aggressive and have a poor response to therapy and overall survival.[33,179,180] However, more indolent cases do exist. Classically, ATCL is associated with hypercalcemia and skin infiltrates, although neither symptom is specific. Angioimmunoblastic-like (AILD-like) T-cell lymphoma is a specific type of PTCL.[33] Clinically, AILD-like patients present with diffuse lymphadenopathy associated with weight loss and fever. A polyclonal hypergammaglobulinemia is also typically present.

Histologic examination is essential in the classification of all of these neoplasms. Both ATCL and PTCL have a wide range of morphologic presentations. Cytologically, the leukemic phase of ATCL is widely known for its very pleomorphic nuclei.[33,171,179,180] There is diffuse effacement of the normal node architecture by the neoplastic cells in ATCL and PTCL. With AILD-like T-cell NHL, there is a polymorphous lymphoplasmacytic proliferation. Intimately interspersed is an arborizing vascular network of venules. The neoplastic cells occur as clusters of "water-clear," atypical lymphoid cells.

ATCL and PTCL are mature TCR alpha/beta$^+$CD4$^+$ T-cell neoplasms. ATCL almost always coexpresses CD25 and has been reported to have atypically dim expression of membrane CD3.[168] In most cases, both ATCL and PTCL lack expression of CD7.[166,167] The immunophenotypic profiles of PTCL and ATCL overlap extensively with those of other mature T-cell neoplasias. Therefore, antigen profiles are not in and of themselves capable of diagnosing lymphoma in general or subclassifying it in particular. Usually, the combination of histologic exam with a demonstration of a clonal TCR gene rearrangement is all that is required to render the diagnosis.

Anaplastic Large-Cell and T/NK-Cell Lymphomas

These neoplasias are typically immunophenotyped by IHC. This reflects the difficulty in getting a representative cell suspension (due to the fragility of large cells and/or small biopsies). As a result of this difficulty, much of the specificity and sensitivity of various immunophenotypes has only been defined by immunohistochemistry in paraffin-embedded tissue sections. Therefore, although it is feasible to examine these cells with flow cytometry, it is difficult to make definitive statements about the utility of flow immunophenotyping in diagnosing these neoplasias.

Anaplastic large-cell lymphoma (ALCL) is a unique large-cell lymphoma associated with the t(2;5) cytogenetic abnormality.[33] Morphologically, classic cases have tightly clustered aggregates of neoplastic large cells, sometimes in a sinusoidal distribution. The classic ALCL cell has abundant cytoplasm with pleomorphic nuclei, often in a "horseshoe" configuration. Most cases are of T lineage, although a minority are "null" type. A typical antigen profile is CD2$^+$, CD4$^+$, CD15$^-$, CD25$^+$, CD30$^+$, CD45$^+$, TIA-1$^+$, perforin$^+$, and ALK1$^+$.[33] The T/NK-cell lymphomas are rare entities with very unique clinical/pathologic profiles.[33] Beyond defining T lineage, flow cytometry has little more to offer. Indeed, the neoplasms are best characterized by IHC.

Case Studies

Case 9-1

History

This sample is from a 40-year-old male with a history of a short-term (3 weeks) lymphocytosis, which was detected on a routine pre-employment exam. The individual is otherwise asymptomatic, and his physical exam is within normal limits for age and gender. The CBC count and peripheral smear reveal only a mild leukocytosis (WBC count = 12×10^9/L), associated with slightly elevated neutrophil and lymphocyte concentrations (lymphocytes: 4.5×10^9/L). The lymphoid cells are virtually all small, round lymphocytes, which are without morphologic atypia, as are the remaining leukocytes. No cytopenias are present. Viral serologies for EBV and CMV are negative for recent infection. The serum biochemical profile (electrolytes, alanine aminotransferase [ALT], aspartate aminotransferase [AST], bilirubin, glucose, albumin, total protein, blood urea nitrogen [BUN], and creatinine) is likewise normal for the patient's age.

Given the clinical symptoms and morphologic appearance of the cells, an antibody panel directed primarily at B chronic lymphoid neoplasia is run (**Figure 9-16, A through H**, p 292). The bright CD45$^+$ cells with lymphoid light scatter are analyzed (**Figure 9-16, A and B**). These are an unremarkable mixture of mature T (CD5$^+$CD19$^-$), NK (CD11c$^+$CD20$^-$), and B cells (CD19$^+$CD20$^{bright+}$) (**Figure 9-16, D and E**). The B cells have a polyclonal expression of surface immunoglobulin light chain (**Figure 9-16, G and H**), no atypical coexpression of CD5 or CD10 (**Figure 9-16, D and C**), and a normal intensity of CD20 (**Figure 9-16E**). The expression of CD2 and CD7 are unremarkable.

Interpretation

There is no immunophenotypic evidence of T- or B-cell neoplasia in this sample. The clinical history is consistent with either a normal individual whose WBC and lymphocyte counts fall just outside the reference range or an individual with an otherwise unexplained reactive lymphocytosis. On follow-up, the lymphocyte concentration dropped into high normal range, supporting the latter possibility. One may argue that considering the patient's relatively young age, very mild lymphocytosis of short duration could have been more effectively evaluated by a repeat CBC count and differential in a few months. Even if this was an early case of B-CLL/SLL, the patient would not have been jeopardized by this waiting period.

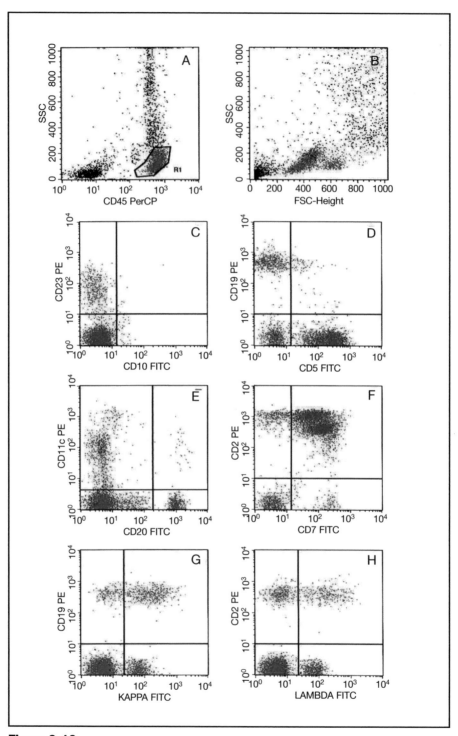

Figure 9-16

Case 9-2

History

This is a peripheral blood specimen from a 47-year-old female. She presents to her family physician with a complaint of increased fatigue of several months' duration. Her CBC count and differential are remarkable only for a moderate lymphocytosis (lymphocytes: 32.5×10^9/L). Morphologically, the lymphocytes are small to intermediate in size, with a high N/C ratio, undifferentiated cytoplasm, and sharp cellular borders. The nuclear contours are round to mildly irregular, but no frankly clefted or hyperlobated nuclei are seen. The chromatin is smooth and dense, and fewer than 5% of all lymphocytes have small indistinct nucleoli. No cytopenias are present. Her physical exam is unremarkable, with no lymphadenopathy, organomegaly, or skin lesions.

Given the clinical symptoms and morphologic appearance of the cells, an antibody panel directed primarily at B chronic lymphoid neoplasia is applied (**Figure 9-17, A through H**, p 294). The bright $CD45^+$ cells with lymphoid light scatter are analyzed (**Figure 9-17, A and B**). These are predominantly monoclonal B cells, with a composite antigen profile (> 20% B cells$^+$) of $CD19^+$, $CD20^+$ (dim), sIg$^+$ (lambda; dim), $CD5^+$, $CD10^-$, $CD11c^-$, and $CD23^+$.

Interpretation

The combined immunomorphologic profile is that of B-CLL/SLL. This is a fairly classic immunophenotype, both in terms of positive and negative antigen expression and of the dimmer intensities of the sIg and CD20 antigens. The percentage of $CD20^+$ cells that express CD11c dimly is less than the 20% threshold arbitrarily required to define expression (**Figure 9-17E**).

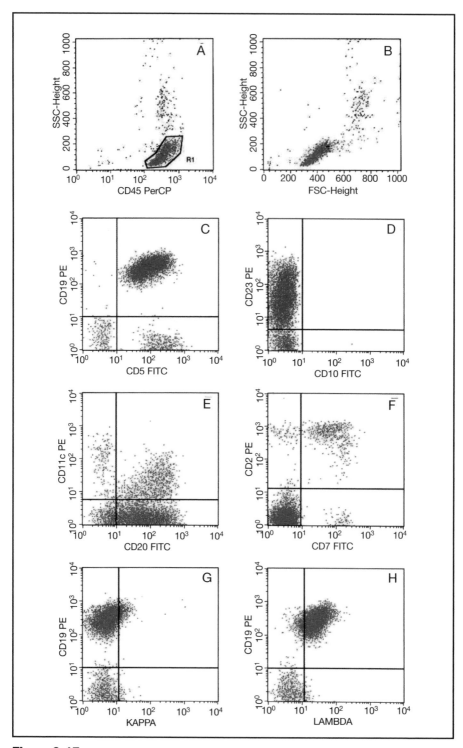

Figure 9-17

Case 9-3

History

This is a peripheral blood sample from a 68-year-old male. He has had a history of persistent lymphocytosis for approximately 18 months. While no lymphadenopathy is appreciated on physical exam, there is mild splenomegaly. A serum protein electrophoresis reveals a very small (0.2 g/dL) IgM kappa monoclonal gammopathy. Otherwise, beyond mild hypertension and hypercholesterolemia, there are no other pertinent clinical findings. The CBC count and differential reveal a moderate lymphocytosis (lymphocytes: 27.3×10^9/L). The lymphoid cells are small-to-intermediate in size, with a high N/C ratio, undifferentiated cytoplasm, and sharp cellular borders. The nuclear contours are essentially round, the chromatin is mature and blocky, and no nucleoli are seen.

Given the clinical symptoms and morphologic appearance of the cells, an antibody panel directed primarily at B chronic lymphoid neoplasia is conducted (**Figure 9-18, A through H**, p 297). The CD45 versus side light scatter plot (**Figure 9-18A**) reveals 2 predominant populations: bright CD45$^+$ cells with lymphoid light scatter (**Figure 9-18A;** R2 region, green color) and a population approximately 5 times dimmer (**Figure 9-18A;** R1 region, red color). These appear closely clustered together due to the log scale used. The forward light scatter is also different (**Figure 9-18B**) because the dimmer CD45$^+$ cells (R1 region, red color) have lesser forward light scatter, and hence a smaller cell size.

Both populations are analyzed and their immunophenotypes simultaneously examined (**Figure 9-18, C through H**). There is a predominant monoclonal B-cell population, which is almost entirely composed of the smaller CD45$^{\text{dimmer}+}$ cells (red). The slightly larger CD45$^{\text{bright}+}$ cells (green) are primarily composed of residual benign T and NK lymphocytes, with a very small number of polyclonal B lymphocytes. The monoclonal B cells have a composite antigen profile (> 20% B cells$^+$) of CD19$^+$, CD20$^+$ (dim), sIg$^+$ (kappa; dim), CD5$^+$, CD10$^-$, CD11c$^+$ (dim), and CD23$^+$.

This analysis could be approached in several ways. One is to separately analyze each of the major populations. This will clearly define the monoclonal B-cell population. The other is to simply define one gate around all of the lymphoid cells. This allows the use of the residual benign lymphocytes as intrinsic positive and negative controls. The major issue here is not to exclude slightly dimmer CD45$^+$ cells from a lymphocyte gate, because B-CLL/SLL tends to have dimmer CD45 expression than normal lymphocytes or other types of mature B-lymphoid leukemias and lymphomas.

Interpretation

This is a B-CLL/SLL, with a fairly classic profile. The expression of CD11c is seen in a distinct minority of B-CLL/SLLs. This is much dimmer than the intensity seen with HCLs and approximates what has been reported with vHCL and SLVLs. However, the latter would not have the CD5$^+$CD23$^+$ profile. In the differential of a CD5$^+$ B lymphoproliferation, the expression of CD11c would strongly tend to rule out MCL.

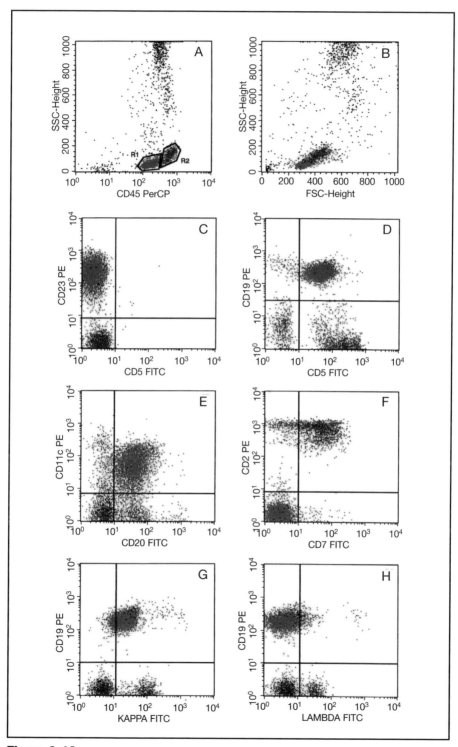

Figure 9-18

Case 9-4

History

This peripheral blood specimen is obtained from a 54-year-old male who has a 7-month history of a lymphocytosis. Physical exam is remarkable for a few small lymph nodes in the cervical region. No other lymphadenopathy or organomegaly is detected. The CBC and differential reveal a marked lymphocytosis (lymphocytes: 84×10^9/L) associated with a mild-to-moderate anemia. The lymphoid cells are a mixture of small-to-intermediate mature lymphocytes. All have undifferentiated cytoplasm, sharp cellular borders, and relatively high N/C ratios. The nuclear contours are round to mildly irregular. The smaller lymphocytes have smooth chromatin and lack nucleoli, while the larger lymphocytes have a somewhat more open chromatin and usually one small nucleolus. However, frank prolymphocytes comprise less than 10% of all lymphoid cells.

Given the clinical symptoms and morphologic appearance of the cells, an antibody panel directed primarily at B chronic lymphoid neoplasia is conducted (**Figure 9-19, A through H**, p 299). The bright CD45$^+$ cells with lymphoid light scatter are analyzed (**Figure 9-19, A and B**). These are predominantly atypical B cells, with a composite antigen profile (> 20% B cells+) of CD19$^+$, CD20$^+$ (bright), sIg$^-$, CD5$^+$, CD10$^-$, CD11c$^+$ (bright), and CD23$^+$.

Interpretation

The combined immunomorphologic profile is that of a B-CLL/SLL. A substantial fraction of these lack detectable sIg. However, this is an exceptionally strong marker of monoclonality, particularly when there is an absolute lymphocytosis comprising predominantly B cells. As mentioned above, the presence of both CD11c and CD23 effectively rule out an MCL, while the cytomorphology and presence of CD5 rule out an HCL or vHCL.

Some authors have reported a significant association of brighter CD20 and/or sIg expression with adverse cytogenetic features. The same association has also been seen with more pleomorphic cytomorphology. However, it is unclear if this is more relevant than clinical follow-up of lymphocyte doubling time, development of lymphadenopathy, or cytopenias. This is particularly true given the limited therapeutic options and older age range seen with B-CLL/SLL patients.

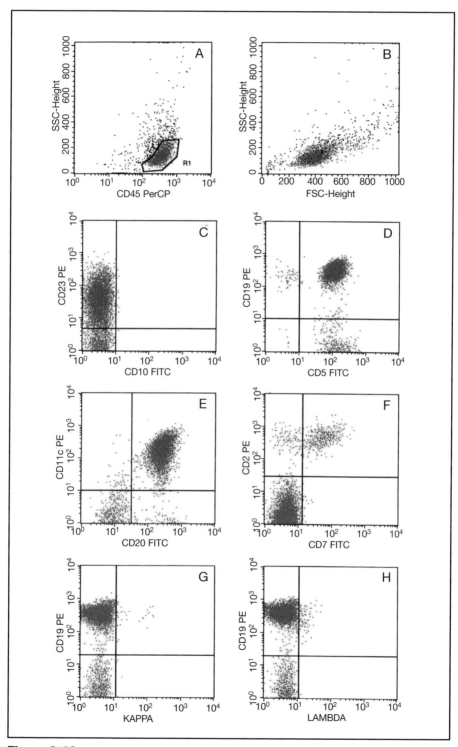

Figure 9-19

Case 9-5

History

A 57-year-old male presents with a history of MCL diagnosed 3 years previously and, until recently, who has been in remission after extensive chemotherapy. Now he has recurrent lymphadenopathy. Node biopsy sections show effacement of the lymph node architecture by a predominantly diffuse and focally vague nodular proliferation of malignant lymphoid cells. The lymphoid cells are composed of a fairly monotonous population of cells having round to oval irregular nuclei with occasionally prominent nucleoli. Frequent mitoses are observed.

Given the clinical symptoms and morphologic appearance of the cells, an antibody panel directed primarily at B chronic lymphoid neoplasia is conducted (**Figure 9-20, A through H**, p 301). The bright CD45$^+$ cells with lymphoid light scatter are analyzed (**Figure 9-20, A and B**). These are predominantly monoclonal B cells, with a composite antigen profile (> 20% B cells$^+$) of CD19$^+$, CD20$^+$ (bright), sIg$^+$ (lambda; bright), CD5$^+$, CD10$^-$, CD11c$^-$, and CD23$^-$.

Interpretation

This is a CD5$^+$CD23$^-$ mature B-lymphoid lymphoma. When combined with the architectural features, this is diagnostic of MCL. By itself, the immunophenotype is certainly diagnostic of a mature CD5$^+$ B-cell neoplasm. However, correlation with either biopsy morphology, intracellular protein expression, and/or molecular/cytogenetic studies to define the presence of the *bcl1-IgH* rearrangement/t(11;14) is essential to render a definitive diagnosis. In this instance, the morphology and prior history supply this need.

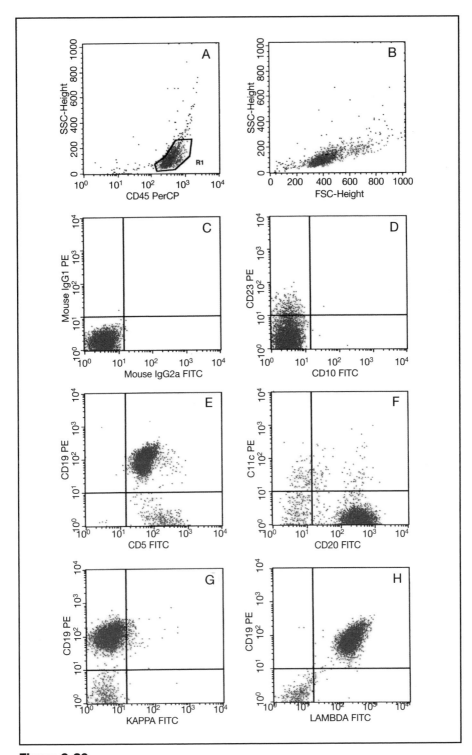

Figure 9-20

Case 9-6

History

The patient is a 59-year-old male with a prior diagnosis of a low-grade lymphocytic lymphoma not otherwise specified. He was treated with several cycles of chemotherapy, and now presents with marked splenomegaly but no lymphadenopathy or lymphocytosis. A bone marrow aspirate is performed. The marrow reveals predominantly intermediate-to-mature myeloid and erythroid precursors, admixed with a minor fraction of small mature lymphocytes. The latter have round to mildly irregular nuclear contours and mature chromatin, with occasional cells having small nucleoli. The N/C ratio is high, with undifferentiated cytoplasm and sharp cellular borders.

Given the clinical symptoms and morphologic features of the cells, an antibody panel directed primarily at B chronic lymphoid neoplasia is performed (**Figure 9-21, A through H**, p 303. The bright CD45$^+$ cells with lymphoid light scatter are analyzed (**Figure 9-21, A and B**). These are a roughly equal mixture of mature T and monoclonal B cells. The latter have a composite antigen profile (> 20% B cells$^+$) of CD19$^+$, CD20$^+$ (bright), sIg$^+$ (lambda; bright), CD5$^+$, CD10$^-$, CD23$^-$, and FMC7$^+$ (bright).

Interpretation

As discussed above, the CD5$^+$CD23$^-$ profile is fully consistent with MCL. The bright sIg and CD20 and presence of FMC7 strongly support this, although this trio of markers is not specific individually or together for MCL. Frankly, it is the absence of FMC7 that would be more significant in ruling against MCL, rather than FMC7's presence in ruling in MCL. In the author's opinion, blood or marrow presentations such as this should be followed with further confirmatory studies in order to render a definitive diagnosis. This reflects the very different clinical course expected with MCL compared with other mature B-lymphoid lymphomas. Such studies could include a biopsy of an enlarged lymph node, but this is not available in this case. A more likely alternative would be cytogenetics or PCR testing for the t(11;14) lesion. The former was done on the marrow sample and revealed the diagnostic t(11;14) translocation.

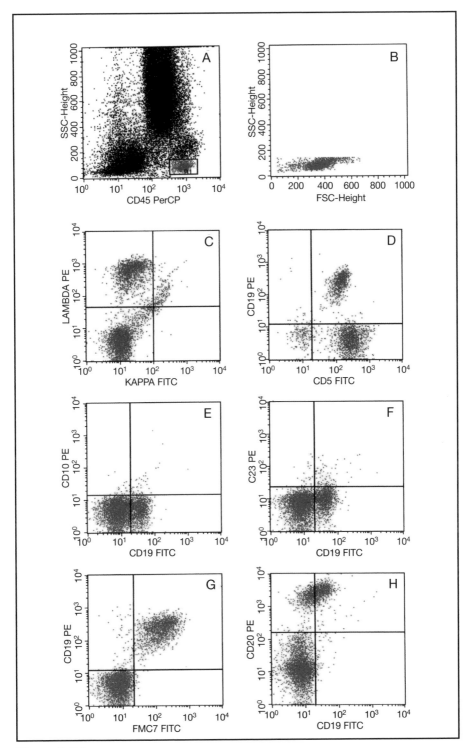

Figure 9-21

Case 9-7

History

A 57-year-old man presents with an enlarged axillary lymph node. Further physical and radiographic examination reveals other enlarged axillary and abdominal nodes. His CBC count and differential, serum biochemical profile, and protein electrophoresis are normal. A lymph node biopsy is obtained. A vaguely nodular proliferation of small and large lymphoid cells is seen, often without a distinct mantle zone. The nodules are closely opposed and extend into the tissue outside of the node capsule. No "zonation" of the nodular lymphoid cells is seen, nor are tingible body macrophages.

Given the clinical symptoms and morphologic features of the cells, an antibody panel directed primarily at B chronic lymphoid neoplasia is conducted (**Figure 9-22, A through H**, p 305). The cells with small and large lymphoid light scatter are analyzed (**Figure 9-22B**). There is a predominance of monoclonal B cells, with a composite antigen profile (> 20% B cells$^+$) of CD19$^+$, CD22$^+$ (bright), sIg$^+$ (kappa; bright), CD5$^-$, CD10$^+$ (dim), CD23$^+$ (half dim), and FMC7$^+$ (dim).

Interpretation

Realistically, this immunophenotyping did not have to be performed. The morphology is diagnostic of lymphoma in general and grade II FCL in particular. However, this is a particularly classic immunophenotypic profile. Specifically, the dim presence of CD10 has been found by various investigators to be present in 70% to 96% of cases. This difference may reflect case selection, antibody clone, cytometer sensitivity, and/or fluorochrome brightness. It should also be pointed out that correlation with cytomorphology is essential, because Burkitt's lymphoma and some B large cell lymphomas may also be dimly CD10$^+$. Lastly, a significant fraction of FCLs express FMC7 and CD23. Typically, this expression is dim and may be seen on only a minority of the cells (20% to 50%). CD23 is really useful only in the differential diagnosis of CD5$^+$ B-lymphoid neoplasms (B-CLL/SLL vs. MCL).

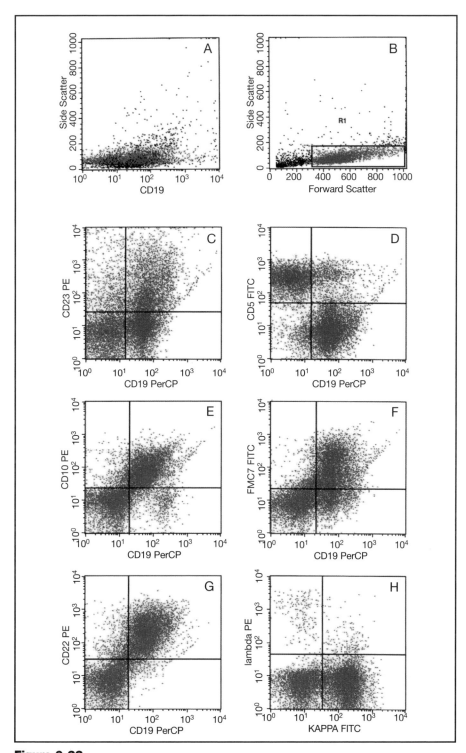

Figure 9-22

Case 9-8

History

A 57-year-old woman presents with an enlarged supraclavicular lymph node. The clinical and radiographic studies reveal a diffuse lymphadenopathy in the thoracic and abdominal spaces. An excisional biopsy of the supraclavicular node is performed. Because the biopsy is obtained on a Friday, it is elected to perform flow cytometric immunophenotyping before the routine histologic sections are available. However, the Wright-stained touch imprints reveal a mixed small- and large-cell lymphoproliferation. The histology seen on Monday reveals an effacement of the normal node architecture by a vaguely nodular small- and large-cell lymphoproliferation, very similar to what is seen in case 9-7.

Given the clinical symptoms and morphologic features of the cells, an antibody panel directed primarily at B chronic lymphoid neoplasia is performed (**Figure 9-23, A through H**, p 307). The bright CD45$^+$ cells with small (R2 region, green color) and large (R3 region, red color) lymphoid light scatter are analyzed (**Figure 9-23, A and B**). Both populations contain a predominance of monoclonal B cells. These have a composite antigen profile (> 20% B cells$^+$) of CD19$^+$, CD22$^+$ (bright), sIg$^+$ (lambda; dim to bright), CD5$^-$, CD10$^-$, CD23$^+$ (bright), and FMC7$^+$ (half dim).

Interpretation

This is an FCL. As in case 9-7, the morphology is diagnostic. The immunophenotyping is performed because of concerns about viability if the sample were held for approximately 3 days until Monday, when the routine histologic slides would be available. The light scatter is interesting in this case, as 2 lymphoid clusters (large and small) are seen. In the author's experience, this is unusual, as they typically merge, as seen in case 9-7. The immunophenotype is different from the norm in that there is no compelling expression of CD10 (**Figure 9-23G**), although there does appear to be a subtle shift, with a small minority of B cells being CD10$^+$ (< 20%). As mentioned in case 9-7, this profile is not rare (occurring in 4% to 30% of FCL cases) and should not be used to exclude the diagnosis.

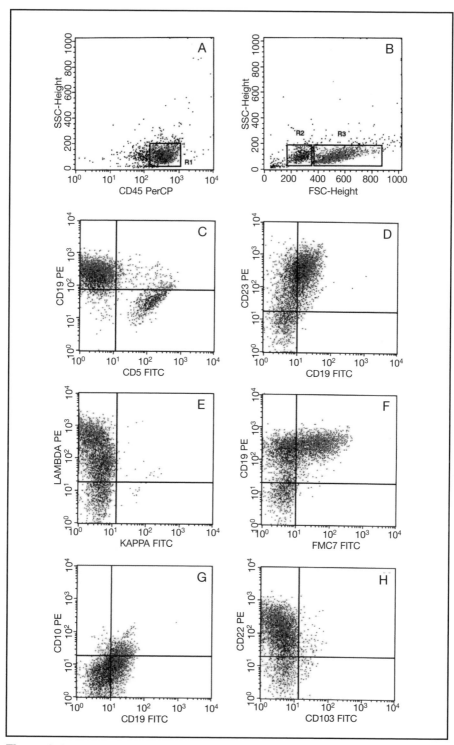

Figure 9-23

Case 9-9

History

The patient is a previously healthy 47-year-old woman who presents with left upper abdominal pain. Physical exam and radiographic scans reveal a marked splenomegaly. No lymphadenopathy is seen. The CBC count and differential reveal a moderate anemia and thrombocytopenia. Although the WBC count is normal, a minor fraction of the circulating lymphocytes are atypical. Serum protein electrophoresis reveals only an acute phase pattern. There is no monoclonal protein or suppression of polyclonal gammaglobulins. A bone marrow exam is performed and sample submitted for flow immunophenotyping of the lymphoid cells. Morphologically, there is a lymphoproliferation, composed of small and larger lymphoid cells. The latter have a moderate N/C ratio, mildly irregular nuclear contours, mature chromatin, and distinct nucleoli (although not the macronucleoli seen in B-PLL). Some lymphoid cells have irregular cytoplasmic projections.

Given the clinical symptoms and morphologic features of the cells, an antibody panel directed primarily at B chronic lymphoid neoplasia is performed (**Figure 9-24, A through H**, p 309). The bright CD45$^+$ cells with small to intermediate lymphoid light scatter (**Figure 9-24, A and B**) are analyzed (R1 plus R2 regions, fuchsia color). There is a predominant monoclonal B-cell proliferation, associated with a minor fraction of mature T cells (**Figure 9-24, C and G**). The B cells have a composite antigen profile (> 20% B cells$^+$) of CD19$^+$, CD20$^+$ (bright), CD22$^+$ (dim to bright), sIg$^+$ (dim to bright), CD5$^-$, CD10$^-$, CD23$^-$, CD103$^-$, and FMC7$^+$ (bright).

Interpretation

The combined immunomorphologic profile is of a mature B-cell leukemia/lymphoma. Given the absence of CD5, CD10, and CD103, along with the clinical history of isolated splenomegaly, normal WBC counts, and "veiled" or "hairy-like" lymphoid cells, the major differential diagnosis is a splenic marginal zone lymphoma (splenic lymphoma with veiled lymphocytes [SLVL]). One cannot consider an FCL, as a significant minority of cells lack CD5, CD10, and CD23. Although Waldenström macroglobulinemia may sometimes have this immunophenotype, it would not be a favored diagnosis, given the cytomorphology and absence of monoclonal proteinemia in this case. Base upon these results, a splenectomy is performed. It reveals a splenic marginal zone lymphoma.

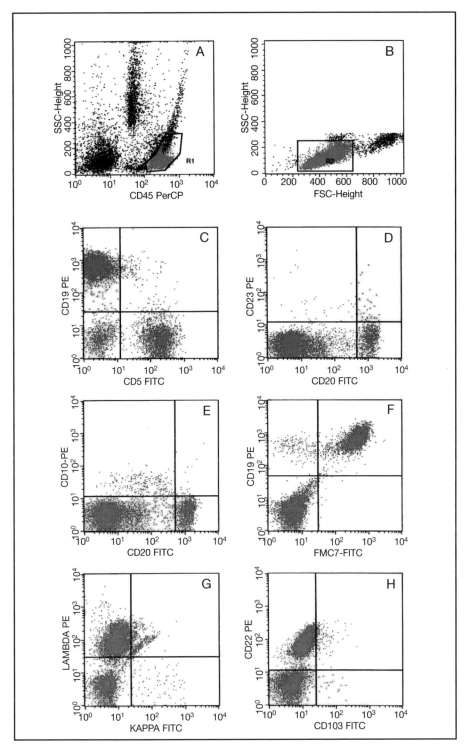

Figure 9-24

History

The patient is an 84-year-old woman who has had a mild lymphocytosis (13×10^9/L) for 5 months, with normal hemoglobin and platelet concentrations. The lymphocytosis was discovered upon a CBC count ordered for a routine health screen. No other clinical or physical exam data are provided. The Wright-stained peripheral smear reveals a mature lymphocytosis. The cells are intermediate in size, with a moderate-to-high N/C ratio and undifferentiated cytoplasm. The cellular borders are irregular, with "hairy" cytoplasmic extensions, varying from focal to more evenly distributed. The nuclei have essentially round contours. No nucleoli are seen.

Given the clinical symptoms and morphologic features of the cells, an antibody panel directed primarily at B chronic lymphoid neoplasia is conducted (**Figure 9-25, A through H**, p 311). The CD19$^+$ cells with small-to-intermediate lymphoid light scatter (**Figure 9-25 A and B**) are analyzed. These are virtually all a monoclonal B lymphoproliferation. They have a composite antigen profile (> 20% B cells$^+$) of CD19$^+$, CD20$^+$ (bright), CD22$^+$ (bright), sIg$^+$ (bright), CD5$^-$, CD10$^-$, CD11c$^+$ (bright), CD23$^-$, CD25$^-$, CD103$^-$, and FMC7$^+$ (bright).

Please note that the CD19 gating allows a very clear definition of the B-cell immunophenotype and essentially eliminates the effect of tube-to-tube variation in the fraction of B cells. The drawback is that the non-B cells are not able to serve as intrinsic (within tube) negative and positive controls. Fortunately, the panel is large enough that there is at least 1 test antigen for each fluorochrome that is nonreactive with the B cells and thus can serve as an intrinsic negative control. Should there be a concern about a lack of intrinsic positive controls (eg, for CD5, because this is not present on the B cells), then the operator can simply reanalyze the list mode file using just a lymphocyte light scatter gate, so that T lymphocytes are included.

Interpretation

The combined immunomorphologic profile is of a mature B-lymphoid leukemia/lymphoma. The major differential diagnoses would include marginal zone lymphoma and a variant HCL. The former is favored, given the lack of distinct nucleoli. An FCL cannot be totally excluded, although it is not favored based upon the cytomorphology. The morphology and/or lack of CD5 rule out B-CLL/SLL, MCL, and B-PLL, while the absence of CD25 and CD103 rule against HCL.

Unfortunately, no further follow-up is available on this patient. This is often the case in many practices. The challenges in this instance are (1) how "diag-

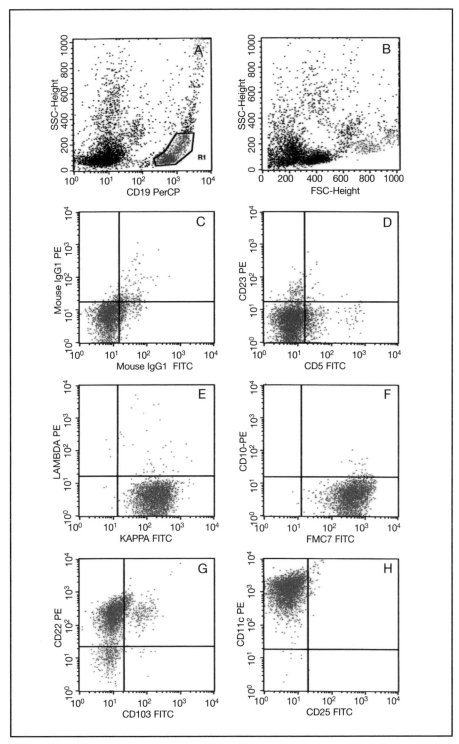

Figure 9-25

nostic" one should get and (2) what follow-up studies are suggested. In this case, the clearly monoclonal immunophenotype in the presence of a persistent absolute B-cell lymphocytosis is sufficient to conclude that there is a B-cell neoplasm. In such instances, the author prefers the terms "leukemia or lymphoma" to "lymphoproliferation" when the exact grade is not determined. Furthermore, the composite term "leukemia/lymphoma" is used here due to the incomplete data on the presence or absence of lymphadenopathy or organomegaly. What is recommended in this case is that if any lymphadenopathy or mucosal masses are detected, they should be biopsied. Cytogenetic exam of the blood may also be useful, particularly if a diagnostic translocation is detected (eg, t[14;18]).

Case 9-11

History

The patient is a 66-year-old man whose sample is submitted from an outside institution with a request to rule out leukemia. Other than data on WBC count, hemoglobin [Hgb], and platelet concentrations, no other clinical or laboratory information is immediately available. Review of the CBC count and Wright-stained peripheral smear reveal a leukoerythroblastic appearance associated with marked anemia and thrombocytopenia. The mature lymphoid cells are predominantly small round and large granular lymphocytes, admixed with a minor fraction of more atypical intermediate-sized cells. The latter have a moderate N/C ratio and deeply basophilic cytoplasm, with a hint of perinuclear clearing and mildly irregular cellular borders. The nuclei are essentially round with mature chromatin.

Given the clinical symptoms and morphologic features of the cells, an antibody panel directed primarily at B and T chronic lymphoid neoplasia is conducted; both large and small lymphoid light scatter gating and bright CD45$^+$ lymphoid gating are used. These reveal a mild NK lymphocytosis, admixed with mature heterogeneous T and polyclonal B cells (data not shown).

Just after the initial analysis, additional clinical information became available. The patient had presented with acute renal insufficiency associated with hypercalcemia. Given the newly enhanced impression of plasmacytoid cytomorphology of the atypical intermediate-sized cells, the gating for the existing flow data is altered to detect plasma cells (**Figure 9-26, A and B**, p 313). Because CD45 is in every tube, a 2-step approach is used. First, a region is drawn around the CD45$^-$ cells with low-to-intermediate side light scatter (**Figure 9-26A; R1**). Then, the forward and side light scatter of *only* the R1 cells is displayed and a second region drawn around the cells with larger lymphoid-to-monocytoid light scatter (**Figure 9-26B; R2**, red color). The initial panel now reveals a distinct

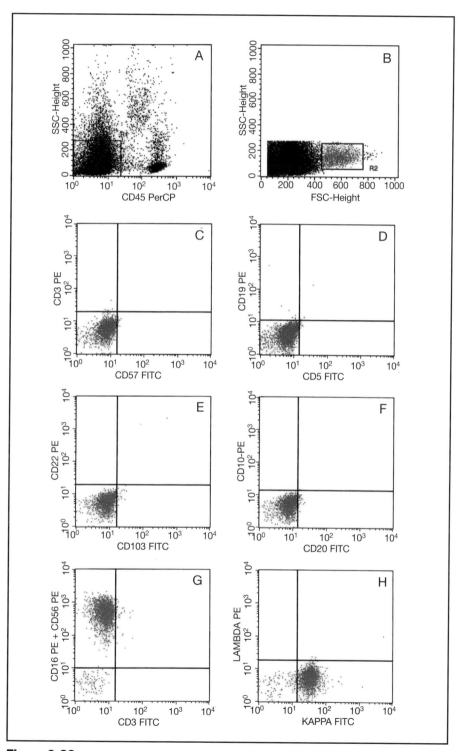

Figure 9-26

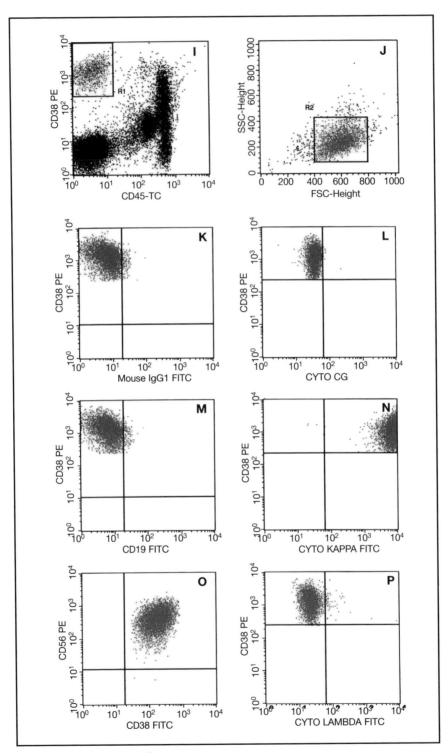

Figure 9-26 (continued)

population of cells that are CD16$^+$CD56$^+$ and sIg$^+$ (kappa; dim) and lack all other pan-B antigens (**Figure 9-26, C through H**, p 313, 314).

Based upon these results, a new panel is performed to examine the plasma cells (**Figure 9-26, I through P**). The CD45$^-$CD38$^{bright+}$ cells with plasmacytoid light scatter are analyzed (**Figure 9-26, I through J**). The membrane profile now clearly shows CD56 expression (**Figure 9-26O**) with clear, bright cytoplasmic kappa light chain monoclonality (**Figure 9-26N**).

Interpretation

There is a monoclonal CD56$^+$ plasma cell proliferation in the blood, representing a PCL. The expression of CD56 is not seen on normal/polyclonal plasma cells, and it augments the impression from the cytoplasmic light chain monoclonality that this is a malignant plasma-cell process. The large granular lymphocytosis seen in this case has been reported with myeloma and PCL by other investigators.

The apparent expression of dim sIg in this case has 2 possible explanations. First is that virtually all of the circulating immunoglobulin may be monoclonal. Hence, nonspecific absorption on the malignant cells would also be monoclonal in a kappa/lambda plot, not the linear dual expression seen with polyclonal immunoglobulins. The other possibility is that there is true sIg expression, simply reflecting the ability of an individual neoplasm to defy the standards set for classes of leukemias or lymphomas. Lastly, in the given clinical setting, this PCL is most likely secondary to a previously undiagnosed myeloma, now presenting with renal failure. Protein electrophoresis and immunofixation of the patient's serum and urine (if available) is recommended to the referring institution, along with a bone marrow biopsy.

Case 9-12

History

The patient is an 82-year-old woman whose only previous health issues revolved about the usual age-related problems of hypertension, hyperlipidemia, osteoarthritis, and esophageal reflux. Approximately 18 months prior, her CBC count and differential were completely normal. Now, at a routine visit to monitor her health problems, the CBC count reveals a marked lymphocytosis (lymphocytes: 81.71×10^9/L), with normal hemoglobin and platelet concentrations. She has no complaints of fatigue, weight loss, or night sweats. Physical exam does not reveal any lymphadenopathy, organomegaly, or skin lesions. A serum biochemical profile (including calcium) is normal with the exception of a mildly elevated lactate dehydrogenase (LDH).

The Wright-stained peripheral smear reveals a marked mature lymphocytosis. These are small cells with a high N/C ratio, undifferentiated cytoplasm, and sharp cellular borders. The nuclear contours are essentially round to mildly irregular and have mature, dense chromatin. Some cells have small indistinct nucleoli. Lastly, a very few smudge cells are seen.

Given the clinical history and morphology of the cells, a panel directed at B chronic lymphoid leukemia is performed. The bright CD45$^+$ cells with lymphoid light scatter are analyzed (**Figure 9-27, A and B**, p 317). The initial panel reveals that virtually all of the cells are of T lineage (**Figure 9-27, C and E**). The very few B cells have a polyclonal expression of immunoglobulin light chain (data not shown). Based upon established criteria, the technologist then performs a reflex panel of T and NK antigens (**Figure 9-27, D and F through H**). The T cells have a composite antigen profile (> 20% T cells+) of CD2$^+$, CD3$^+$, CD4$^+$, CD5$^+$, CD7$^+$ (uniformly bright), CD8$^-$ (not shown), CD11c$^-$ (not shown), CD16$^-$, CD25$^-$, CD56$^-$, and CD57$^-$.

Interpretation

The combined immunomorphologic profile in blood is virtually diagnostic of a T-cell malignancy in general and is fully consistent with the T-PLL/CLL grouping. The impression of neoplasia is based upon the marked absolute lymphocytosis and abnormal increase in CD4$^+$ and virtual absence of CD8$^+$ T cells. The abnormally uniform intensity of CD7 is a very soft indication of clonality, as CD7 expression usually ranges from absent to dim to bright on normal T cells.

Additional serologic studies reveal an absence of anti-HTLV-1 and -2 antibodies. This, along with the morphology, presence of CD7, and lack of CD25 expression, would rule out an ATCL. The lack of history of cutaneous T-cell

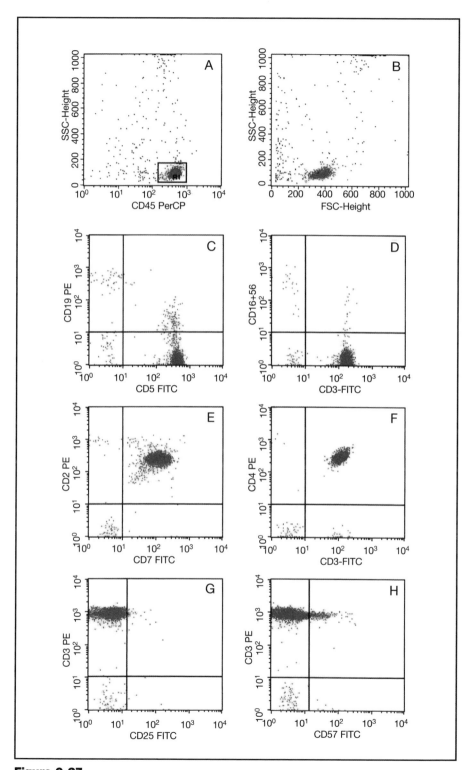

Figure 9-27

lymphoma and cytomorphology argue against either Sézary syndrome or a leukemia (SS/SL). Also, like ATCL, most SS/SL cases have significantly diminished CD7 expression. Radiographic studies fail to reveal any lymphadenopathy or organomegaly. The marrow reveals the same neoplastic T-cell infiltrate. This would argue against a peripheral T-cell lymphoma. Lastly, the cytomorphology and CD4⁺CD8⁻NK-antigen⁻ profile rule out a T- or NK-LGL.

Case 9-13

History

This is a 78-year-old Caucasian woman with a prior history of skin rash, diagnosed as a mycosis fungoides at an outside institution. She now has a diffuse scaling erythematous rash associated with a mild-to-moderate lymphocytosis (lymphocytes: 16×10^9/L), anemia (Hgb: 121 g/L), and normal platelet concentration. Enlarged supraclavicular and epitrochlear lymph nodes are observed. The Wright-stained peripheral smear reveals a mild lymphocytosis. These are small-to-intermediate sized cells with moderate-to-high N/C ratios, undifferentiated cytoplasm, and sharp cellular borders. Many nuclei have tight, deeply convoluted clefts, fully consistent with Sézary cells.

Given the clinical history, a panel directed at T-cell neoplasia is performed. The bright CD45⁺ cells with lymphoid light scatter (**Figure 9-28, A and B**, p 319) are virtually all atypical T cells. These have a composite antigen profile (> 20% T cells⁺) of CD2⁻, CD3⁺, CD4⁺, CD5⁺, CD7⁻, CD8⁻, CD16⁻ (not shown), CD25⁻, CD56⁻ (not shown), and CD57⁻ (**Figure 9-28, C through H**).

Interpretation

The presence of an absolute CD4⁺ T-cell lymphoproliferation in the blood with significant lack of expression of pan-T antigens (CD2, CD7) and the essential absence of any CD8 T cells is fully consistent with a diagnosis of T-cell leukemia/lymphoma. This, the cytomorphology, and the clinical history of cutaneous lymphoma along with the current presence of an extensive skin rash allow the diagnosis of Sézary syndrome or the leukemic phase of mycosis fungoides. The fact that the patient does not have any risk factors for HTLV infection, the absence of CD25 expression, and cytomorphology allow one to confidently exclude ATCL. Similarly, the cytomorphology and CD4⁺CD8⁻NK-antigen⁻ profile excludes T- and NK-LGLs.

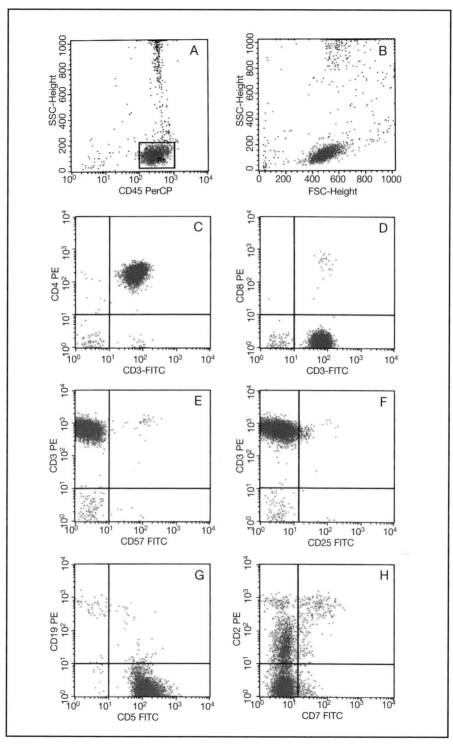

Figure 9-28

Case 9-14

History

The patient is a 75-year-old woman with a prior history of monoclonal gammopathy of undetermined significance (MGUS). She comes in for routine follow-up, which includes a CBC count, biochemical profile, and serum protein electrophoresis. Her MGUS persists, unchanged at 8 g/L, and without suppression of polyclonal gammaglobulins. A mild lymphocytosis is noted (lymphocytes: 5.1×10^9/L), associated with a mild, stable anemia (Hgb: 110 g/L) and normal platelet concentration. The neutrophil concentration is in the low normal range (2.6×10^9/L). A repeat CBC count 3 months later reveals that the lymphocytosis is unchanged. The referring hematologist orders a B-CLL immunophenotyping panel.

The bright CD45$^+$ cells with lymphoid light scatter predominate and are analyzed (**Figure 9-29, A and B**, p 321). These are virtually all CD5$^+$CD19$^-$ T cells (**Figure 9-29, H**). Based upon established criteria, the technologist then performs a reflex panel of T and NK antigens. The T cells are predominantly atypical CD8$^+$ lymphocytes, admixed with a minor fraction of CD4$^+$ cells. The former have a composite antigen profile (> 20% CD8$^+$ T cells) of CD2$^+$, CD3$^+$, CD4$^-$, CD5$^+$ (dim), CD7$^+$, CD8$^+$, CD16$^-$, CD25$^-$, CD56$^-$, and CD57$^+$.

Interpretation

Due to the reference nature of the sample, the morphology is examined by the flow interpreter only after immunophenotyping has been performed. The Wright-stained peripheral smear reveals a mild lymphocytosis. These are predominantly intermediate-sized lymphocytes with moderate N/C ratios, sharp cellular borders, and 2-5 distinct red granules in the cytoplasm. The nuclei are essentially round, with smooth mature chromatin and no nucleoli. This cytomorphology, in the setting of a persistent CD8$^+$NK-antigen$^+$ T lymphocytosis, is fully consistent with T-LGL. No loss of any the major pan-T cell antigens is seen, although the dimorphic CD5 expression is suggestive of a clonal process with residual normal T cells (in this case, probably the CD4$^+$ T lymphocytes).

While the expected neutropenia is not present, the neutrophil concentration is lower than would usually be expected. The major differential diagnoses would be a reactive T or NK lymphocytosis associated with neutropenia, rheumatoid arthritis (RA), and/or splenomegaly as part of Felty syndrome. If the history of RA is absent, there is neutropenia with no or minimal other cytopenias, and the clinical presentation is indolent, then T-LGL is the favored diagnosis. If this must be confirmed, PCR assay of the *TCRg* gene can be performed.

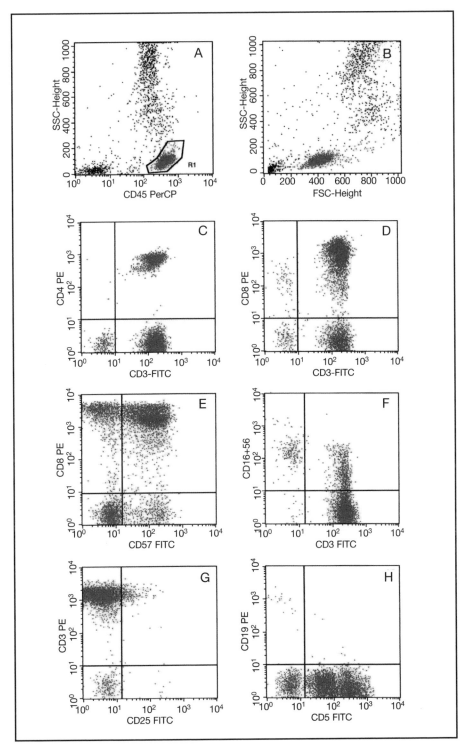

Figure 9-29

Case 9-15

History

The patient is a 79-year-old Caucasian man who over the past month has developed multiple skin nodules over his entire trunk and upper and lower extremities bilaterally. This is associated with mild cervical and inguinal lymphadenopathy. Organomegaly is not appreciated. The CBC count is remarkable only for mild thrombocytopenia and a few atypical lymphoid cells (see below). No other cytopenias are noted. A skin biopsy at an outside institution was read as consistent with nodular mycosis fungoides.

Due to the severity of his disease, a lymph node and repeat skin biopsies, along with a marrow exam, are performed. The lymph node biopsy reveals a diffuse lymphoproliferation characterized by small- and intermediate-sized cells. The larger lymphoid cells have moderate N/C ratios, sharp cellular borders, and undifferentiated cytoplasm. The nuclei are oval with an open but mature chromatin pattern. The small lymphocytes have typical small round lymph morphology. Similar large lymphoid cells are seen as clusters in the marrow. Circulating atypical lymphoid cells are also noted (9% of all leukocytes). These are intermediate-sized and have a few azurphilic granules in the cytoplasm.

The cell suspension from the lymph node is submitted for flow immunoanalysis. Based upon the clinical history, a panel directed primarily at T-cell lymphoma is performed (**Figure 9-30, A through M**, pp 323-324). Two major populations are seen (**Figure 9-30, A and B**): a bright CD45$^+$ cluster with small lymphoid light scatter (R2, green color) and a dimmer CD45$^+$ cluster with large lymphoid light scatter (R1, red color). Both populations are simultaneously displayed on each immunofluorescence dot plot.

The small lymphoid cells (R1, green color) are predominantly mature heterogeneous T and polyclonal B cells (**Figure 9-28, C through M**). The larger lymphoid cells (R2, red color) are an atypical T/NK population, with a composite antigen profile (> 20% R2 cells$^+$) of CD2$^-$, CD3$^-$, cytoplasmic CD3$^-$, CD4$^+$, CD5$^-$, CD7$^-$, CD8$^-$, CD16$^-$, CD25$^-$, CD56$^+$, CD57$^-$, and TdT$^-$. The simultaneous analysis of the small, presumably benign T and B cells is useful, because this population provides intrinsic positive controls, assuring that the multiple negative results are true-negative and not due to omission of antibodies and/or surface antigen degradation during cell isolation and transport.

Interpretation

The clinical history and immunomorphologic profile together consistent with a mature T/NK cell lymphoma. The phenotype is atypical in that the T/NK NHLs are either CD8$^+$CD4$^-$ or CD4$^-$CD8$^-$. These lymphomas usually have an

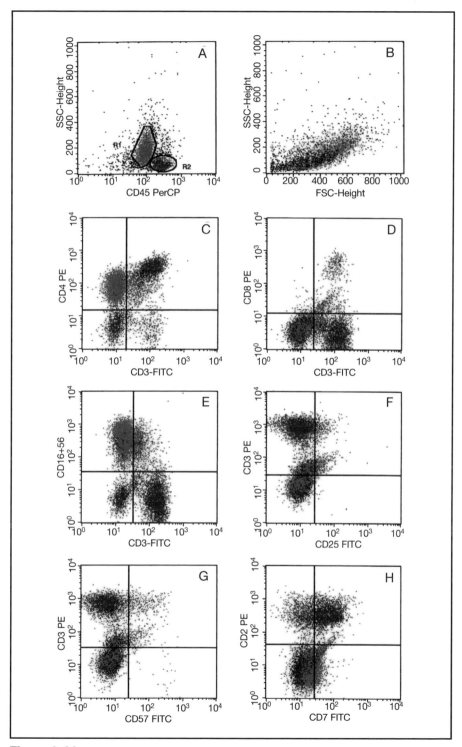

Figure 9-30

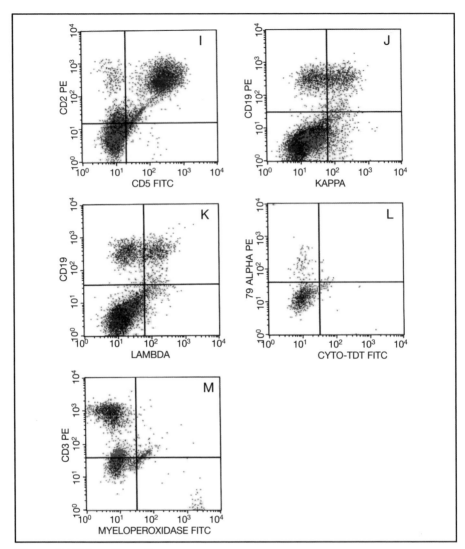

Figure 9-30 (continued)

aggressive clinical course and are associated with involvement of extranodal sites. As a corollary, newly developing mycosis fungoides would not be expected to disseminate so rapidly. Furthermore, virtually all MF cases are CD3+CD56− and express either CD2 or CD5. Review of the skin biopsy histology reveals a dense lymphoid infiltrate in the dermis, extensively extending into the subcutaneous tissue. However, there is a distinct lack of involvement of either the superficial dermis or epidermis, which would be very unusual in a case of advanced MF. Therefore, while the exact classification of this rare lymphoma is unclear, it is not, in the author's opinion, mycosis fungoides or Sézary syndrome.

Case 9-16

History

A 69-year-old woman who has a past history of rheumatoid arthritis (RA), presents with a 6-week history of bilateral inguinal lymphadenopathy. This is associated with clinical and radiographic evidence of axillary adenopathy. Furthermore, her CBC count reveals a mild anemia and marked neutropenia. An inguinal lymph node biopsy is performed, which reveals diffuse effacement of normal architecture by a mixed small, intermediate, and large cell lymphoproliferation. There are also scattered plasma cells and eosinophils. Intimately admixed with all of this is a high endothelial type vascular proliferation.

Given the clinical history and morphologic appearance of the cells, a panel directed at T-cell lymphoma is used to type the nodal lymphocytes. The cells with the light scatter small- to intermediate-sized lymphocytes are analyzed (**Figure 9-31A**). These are predominantly T cells (**Figure 9-31B**) admixed with a minor population of polyclonal B lymphocytes. The T cells are a roughly equal mixture of atypical $CD4^+$ cells and unremarkable $CD4^+$ and $CD8^+$ lymphocytes. Specifically, all T cells are $CD2^+$, $CD5^+$, and $CD7^+$. However, approximately 40% are $CD4^+CD3^-$cytoplasmic $CD3^+$ (**Figure 9-31, H through L**, pp 326-327). Thus, the composite (estimated) antigen profile of the atypical T cells is $CD2^+$, $CD3^-$, cytoplasmic $CD3^+$, $CD4^+$, $CD5^+$, $CD7^+$, $CD8^-$, $CD16^-$, $CD25^-$, $CD56^-$, and $CD57^-$.

Interpretation

This profile is quite complex, but is fully consistent with a mature T-cell lymphoma admixed with abundant reactive T and B cells. The absence of mem-

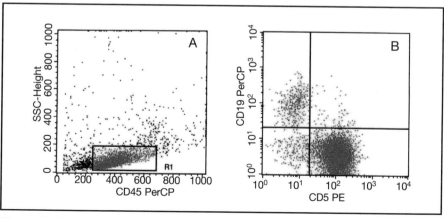

Figure 9-31

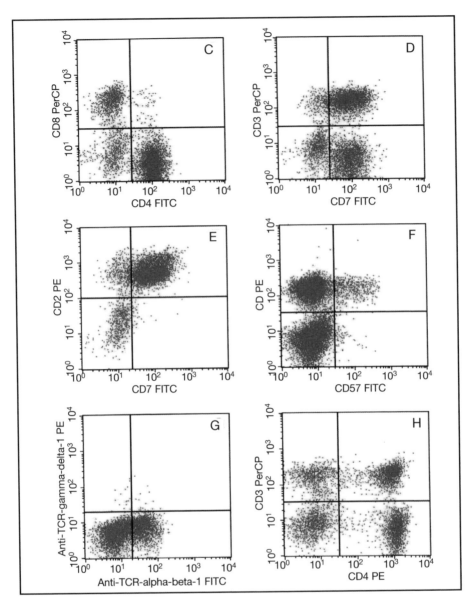

Figure 9-31 (continued)

brane CD3 on a significant proportion of cells is quite suggestive of a clonal pro-liferation. Southern blot analysis confirms this, revealing a clonal rearrangement of the *TCRb* gene.

The precise grading depends upon multiple features. The absence of NK and CD8 antigens combined with morphology in this case would tend to rule against a T/NK- or LGL-type neoplasm. The absence of CD25 and the mor-

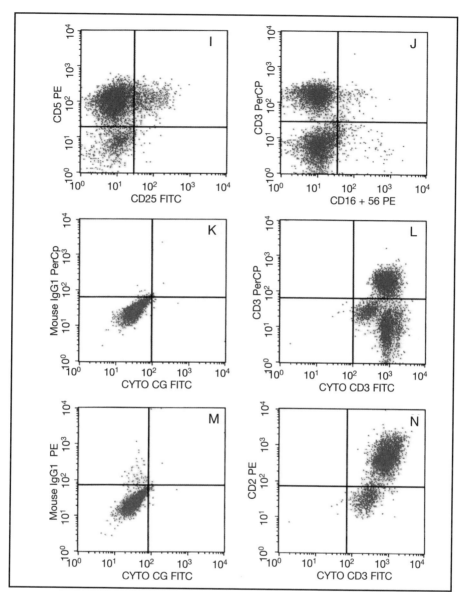

Figure 9-31 (continued)

phology would also stand against a diagnosis of adult T-cell lymphoma. The appearance is fully consistent with a diagnosis of angioimmunoblastic-like (AILD-like) T-cell lymphoma. In support of this, the serum protein electrophoresis reveals a marked polyclonal hypergammaglobulinemia of all major isotypes (IgG, IgA, and IgM). Therefore, the final diagnosis is AILD-like T-cell lymphoma.

References

1. Almasri NM, Zaer FS, Iturraspe JA, et al. Contribution of flow cytometry to the diagnosis of gastric lymphomas in endoscopic biopsy specimens. *Modern Pathol.* 1997;10:650–656.

2. Fletcher M, Baron G, Ashman M, et al. Use of whole blood methods in assessment of immune parameters in immunodeficiency states. *Diagn Clin Pathol.* 1987;5:69–81.

3. Kamat D, Laszewski M, Kemp J, et al. The diagnostic utility of immunophenotyping and immunogenotyping in the pathologic evaluation of lymphoid proliferations. *Modern Pathol.* 1990;3:105–112.

4. Carey JL, Linden MD, Maeda K, et al. Evaluation and reproducibility of criteria for leukemia and lymphoma immunophenotyping triage and interpretation by a quality assurance program. *Am J Clin Pathol.* 1993;100:338–339.

5. Harris NL, Jaffe ES, Stein H, et al. A revised European-American classification of lymphoid neoplasms: a proposal from the International Lymphoma Study Group. *Blood.* 1994;84:1361–1392.

6. Lai R, Weiss LM, Chang KL, et al. Frequency of CD43 expression in non-Hodgkin lymphoma: a survey of 742 cases and further characterization of rare CD43+ follicular lymphomas. *Am J Clin Pathol.* 1999;111:488–494.

7. Tworek JA, Singleton TP, Schnitzer B, et al. Flow cytometric and immunohistochemical analysis of small lymphocytic lymphoma, mantle cell lymphoma and plasmacytoid small lymphocytic lymphoma. *Am J Clin Pathol.* 1998;110:582–589.

8. Diaz De Leon E, Alkan S, Huang JC, et al. Usefulness of an immunohistochemical panel in paraffin-embedded tissues for the differentiation of B-cell non-Hodgkin's lymphomas of small lymphocytes. *Modern Pathol.* 1998;11:1046–1051.

9. Horny H-P, Campbell M, Steinke B, et al. Acute myeloid leukemia: immunohistologic findings in paraffin-embedded bone marrow biopsy specimens. *Hum Pathol.* 1990;21:648–655.

10. Pulford KA, Rigney EM, Micklem KJ, et al. KP1: a new monoclonal antibody that detects a monocyte/macrophage associated antigen in routinely processed tissue sections. *J Clin Pathol.* 1989;42:414–421.

11. Mason DY, Cordell J, Brown M, et al. Detection of T cells in paraffin wax embedded tissue using antibodies against a peptide sequence from the CD3 antigen. *J Clin Pathol.* 1989;42:1194–1200.

12. Mason DY, Comans-Bitter WM, Cordell JL, et al. Antibody L26 recognizes an intracellular epitope on the B-cell-associated CD20 antigen. *Am J Pathol.* 1990;136:1215–1222.

13. Warnke RA, Pulford KAF, Pallesen F, et al. Diagnosis of myelomonocytic and macrophage neoplasms in routinely processed tissue biopsies with monoclonal antibody KP1. *Am J Pathol.* 1990;135:1089–1095.

14. Linder J, Ye Y, Armitage J, Weisenburger D. Comprehensive immunohistochemical analysis of paraffin-embedded non-Hodgkin's lymphoma (NHL). *Modern Pathol.* 1988;1:29-34.

15. Salzman G, Crowell J, Martin J, et al. Cell classification by laser light scattering: identification and separation of unstained leukocytes. *Acta Cytologica.* 1973;19:374–377.

16. Nicholson JKA, McDougal JS, Hearn TL, et al. 1994 revised guidelines for the performance of CD4+ T-cell determinations in persons with human immunodeficiency virus (HIV) infections. *MMWR Morb Mortal Wkly Rep.* 1994;43(RR-3):1–21.

17. Shah V, Civin C, Loken M. Flow cytometric analysis of human marrow, IV: differential quantitative expression of T-200 common leukocyte antigen during normal hemopoiesis. *J Immunol.* 1988;140:1861–1867.

18. Loken M, Shah V, Dattilio D, et al. Flow cytometric analysis of human bone marrow, II: normal B lymphocyte development. *Blood.* 1987;70:1316–1324.

19. Borowitz M, Bach BA, Bauer KD, et al. Clinical applications of flow cytometry: immunophenotyping of leukemic cells; proposed guideline. In: Simson E, ed. *National Committee for Clinical Laboratory Standards.* Villanova, Pa: NCCLS; 1993:107.

20. Anderson K, Bates MP, Slaughenhoupf BL, et al. Expression of human B cell-associated antigens on leukemias and lymphomas: a model of human B cell differentiation. *Blood.* 1984;63:1424–1433.

21. Scheuermann RH, Racila E. CD19 antigen in leukemia and lymphoma diagnosis and immunotherapy. *Leukemia Lymphoma.* 1995;18:385–397.

22. Jackson N, Ling NR, Ball J, et al. An analysis of myeloma plasma cell phenotype using antibodies defined at the Third International Workshop on Human Leucocyte Differentiation Antigens. *Clin Exp Immunol.* 1988;72:351–356.

23. Witzig T, Kimlinger T, et al. Detection of peripheral blood myeloma cells by three-color flow cytometry. *Curr Top Microbiol Immunol.* 1995;194:3.

24. Almeida J, Orfao A, Mateo G, et al. Immunophenotypic and DNA content characteristics of plasma cells in multiple myeloma and monoclonal gammopathy of undetermined significance (review). *Pathologie Biologie.* 1999;47:119–127.

25. Sebestyen A, Berczi L, Mihalik R, et al. Syndecan-1 (CD138) expression in human non-Hodgkin lymphomas. *Br J Haematol.* 1999;104:412–419.

26. Loken M, Shah V, Dattilio K, et al. Flow cytometric analysis of human bone marrow, I: normal erythroid development. *Blood.* 1987;69:255–263.

27. Hata H, Xiao H, Petrucci M, et al. Interleukin-6 gene expression in multiple myeloma: a characteristic of immature tumor cells. *Blood.* 1993;81:3357-3364.

28. Chilosi M, Adami F, Lestani M, et al. CD138/syndecan-1: a useful immunohistochemical marker of normal and neoplastic plasma cells on routine trephine bone marrow biopsies. *Modern Pathol.* 1999;12:1101–1106.

29. Costes V, Magen V, Legouffe E, et al. The Mi15 monoclonal antibody (anti-syndecan-1) is a reliable marker for quantifying plasma cells in paraffin-embedded bone marrow biopsy specimens. *Hum Pathol.* 1999;30:1405–1411.

30. Anderson K, Boyd A, Fisher D, et al. Hairy cell leukemia: a tumor of pre-plasma cells. *Blood.* 1985;65:620–629.

31. Tefferi A, Li C-Y, Phyliky R. Immunotyping in chronic lymphocytosis: review of the natural history of the condition in 145 adult patients. *Mayo Clin Proc.* 1988;63:801–806.

32. Siebert JD, Mulvaney DA, Potter KL, et al. Relative frequencies and sites of presentation of lymphoid neoplasms in a community hospital according to the Revised European-American Classification. *Am J Clin Pathol.* 1999;111:379-386.

33. Jaffe ES, Krenacs L, Raffeld M. Classification of T-cell and NK-cell neoplasms based on the REAL classification. *Ann Oncol.* 1997;8(suppl 2):S17–S24.

34. Jennings CD, Foon KA. Recent advances in flow cytometry: application to the diagnosis of hematologic malignancy. *Blood.* 1997;90:2863–2892.

35. Algino KM, Thomason RW, King DE, et al. CD20 (pan-B cell antigen) expression on bone marrow-derived T cells. *Am J Clin Pathol.* 1996;106:78–81.

36. Hultin LE, Hausner MA, Hultin PM, et al. CD20 (pan-B cell) antigen is expressed at a low level on a subpopulation of human T lymphocytes. *Cytometry.* 1993;14:196–204.

37. Quintanilla-Martinez L, Preffer F, Rubin D, et al. CD20+ T-cell lymphoma: neoplastic transformation of a normal T-cell subset. *Am J Clin Pathol.* 1994;102:483–489.

38. Matutes E. Contribution of immunophenotype in the diagnosis and classification of hæmopoietic malignancies. *J Clin Pathol.* 1995;48:194–197.

39. Fukushima PI, Nguyen PKT, O'Grady P, et al. Flow cytometric analysis of k and l light chain expression in evaluation of specimens for B-cell neoplasia. *Cytometry.* 1996;26:243–252.

40. Stewart C. Multiparameter analysis of leukocytes by flow cytometry. In: Darzynkiewicz Z, Crissman H, eds. *Flow Cytometry.* San Diego, Calif: Academic Press; 1990:427–450.

41. Stewart C. Cell preparation for the identification of leukocytes. In: Darzynkiewicz Z, Crissman H, eds. *Flow Cytometry.* San Diego, Calif: Academic Press; 1990:411–426.

42. Medical devices; classification/reclassification; restricted devices; analyte specific reagents. *Federal Register.* 1997;62:62243–62260.

43. Bennett J, Catovsky D, Danial M-T, et al. Proposals for the classification of chronic (mature) B and T lymphoid leukemias. *J Clin Pathol.* 1989;42:567–584.

44. Dighiero G, Travade P, Chevret S, et al. B-cell chronic lymphocytic leukemia: present status and future directions (review). *Blood.* 1991;78:1901–1914.

45. Batata A, Shen B. Immunophenotyping of subtypes of B-chronic (mature) lymphoid leukemia: a study of 242 cases. *Cancer.* 1992;70:2436–2443.

46. Chan LC, Lam CK, Yeung TC, et al. The spectrum of chronic lymphoproliferative disorders in Hong Kong: a prospective study. *Leukemia.* 1997;11:1964–1972.

47. Pangalis GA, Angelopoulou MK, Vassilakopoulos TP, et al. B-chronic lymphocytic leukemia, small lymphocytic lymphoma and lymphoplasmacytic lymphoma, including Waldenström's macroglobulinemia: a clinical, morphologic and biologic spectrum of similar disorders. *Semin Hematol.* 1999;36:104–114.

48. Geisler C, Larsen J, Hansen N, et al. Prognostic importance of flow cytometric immunophenotyping of 540 consecutive patients with B-cell chronic lymphocytic leukemia. *Blood.* 1991;78:1795–1802.

49. Lens D, Dyer MJS, Garcia-Marco JM, et al. p53 abnormalities in CLL are associated with excess of prolymphocytes and poor prognosis. *Br J Haematol.* 1997;99:848–857.

50. Oscier DG, Matutes E, Copplestone A, et al. Atypical lymphocyte morphology: an adverse prognostic factor for disease progression in stage A CLL independent of trisomy 12. *Br J Haematol.* 1997;98:934–939.

51. Bullrich F, Negrini M, Croce CM. Molecular genetics of chronic lymphocytic leukemia. In: *Hematology 1999: The American Society of Hematology Education Program Book;* Schecter GP et al, eds. New Orleans, La: American Society of Hematology; 1999.

52. Banks PM, Chan J, Cleary ML, et al. Mantle cell lymphoma: a proposal for unification of morphologic, immunologic and molecular data. *Am J Surg Pathol.* 1992;16:637–640.

53. Robbins BA, Ellison DJ, Spinosa JC, et al. Diagnostic application of two-color flow cytometry in 161 cases of hairy cell leukemia. *Blood.* 1993;82:1277–1287.

54. Picker L, Weiss LM, Medeiros LJ, et al. Immunophenotypic criteria for the diagnosis of non-Hodgkin's lymphoma. *Am J Pathol.* 1987;128:181–201.

55. Tefferi A, Bartholmai BJ, Witzig TE, et al. Heterogeneity and clinical relevance of the intensity of CD20 and immunoglobulin light-chain expression in B-cell chronic lymphocytic leukemia. *Am J Clin Pathol.* 1996;106:457–461.

56. Miller M, Fishleder A, Tubbs R. The expression of CD22 (Leu14) and CD11c (LeuM5) in chronic lymphoproliferative disorders using two-color flow cytometric analysis. *Am J Clin Pathol.* 1991;96:100–108.

57. Moreau EJ, Matutes E, A'Hern RP, et al. Improvement of the chronic lymphocytic leukemia scoring system with the monoclonal antibody SN8 (CD79b). *Am J Clin Pathol.* 1997;108:378–382.

58. Ginaldi L, De Martinis M, Matutes E, et al. Levels of expression of CD19 and CD20 in chronic B cell leukaemias. *J Clin Pathol.* 1998;51:364–369.

59. Kurtin PJ, Hobday KS, Ziesmer S, et al. Demonstration of distinct antigenic profiles and small B-cell lymphomas by paraffin section immunohistochemistry. *Am J Clin Pathol.* 1999;112:319–329.

60. Zomas AP, Matutes E, Morilla R, et al. Expression of the immunoglobulin-associated protein B29 in B cell disorders with the monoclonal antibody SN8 (CD79b). *Leukemia.* 1996;10:1966–1970.

61. Bell PB, Rooney N, Bosanquet AG. CD79a detected by ZL7.4 separates chronic lymphocytic leukemia from mantle cell lymphoma in the leukemia phase. *Cytometry.* 1999;38:102–105.

62. Garcia Vela JA, Delgado I, Benito L, et al. CD79b expression in B cell chronic lymphocytic leukemia: its implication for minimal residual disease detection. *Leukemia.* 1999;13:1501–1505.

63. Thompson AA, Do HN, Saxon A, et al. Widespread B29 (CD79b) gene defects and loss of expression in chronic lymphocytic leukemia. *Leukemia Lymphoma.* 1998;32:561–569.

64. Alfarano A, Indraccolo S, Circosta P, et al. An alternatively spliced form of CD79b gene may account for altered B-cell receptor expression in B-chronic lymphocytic leukemia. *Blood.* 1999;93:2327–2335.

65. Catovsky D, Cherchi M, Brooks D, et al. Heterogeneity of B-cell leukemias demonstrated by the monoclonal antibody FMC7. *Blood.* 1981;58:406–408.

66. De la Hera A, Alvarez-Mon M, Sanchez-Madrid F, et al. Co-expression of Mac-1 and p150,95 on CD5$^+$ B cells: structural and functional characterization in a human chronic lymphocytic leukemia. *Eur J Immunol.* 1988;18:1131–1134.

67. Morabito F, Prasthofer E, Dunlap N, et al. Expression of myelomonocytic antigens on chronic lymphcytic leukemia B cells correlates with their ability to produce interleukin 1. *Blood.* 1987;70:1750–1757.

68. Chadburn A, Inghirami G, Knowles DM. Hairy cell leukemia-associated antigen LeuM5 (CD11c) is preferentially expressed by benign activated and neoplastic CD8 T cells. *Am J Pathol.* 1990;136:29–37.

69. Wormsley SB, Baird SM, Gadol N, et al. Characteristics of CD11c$^+$CD5$^+$ chronic B-cell leukemias and the identification of novel peripheral blood B-cell subsets with chronic lymphoid leukemia immunophenotypes. *Blood.* 1990;76:123–130.

70. Huh YO, Pugh WC, Kantarjian HM, et al. Detection of subgroups of chronic B-cell leukemias by FMC7 monoclonal antibody. *Am J Clin Pathol.* 1994;101:283–289.

71. Faguet G. Common chronic lymphatic leukemia antigen (cCLLa): distribution, fate and clinical applications. *Nouv Rev Fr Hematol.* 1988;30:305–310.

72. Mulligan SP, Dao LP, Francis SI, et al. B-cell chronic lymphocytic leukemia with CD8 expression: report of 10 cases and immunochemical analysis of the CD8 antigen. *Br J Haematol.* 1998;103:157–162.

73. Molica S, Levato D, Dattilo A, et al. Clinico-prognostic relevance of quantitative immunophenotyping in B-cell chronic lymphocytic leukemia with emphasis on the expression of CD20 antigen and surface immunoglobulins. *Eur J Haematol.* 1998;60:47–52.

74. Finn WG, Thangavelu M, Yelavarthi KK, et al. Karyotype correlates with peripheral blood morphology and immunophenotype in chronic lymphocytic leukemia. *Am J Clin Pathol.* 1996;105:458–467.

75. Damle RN, Wasil T, Fais F, et al. Ig V gene mutation status and CD38 expression as novel prognostic indicators in chronic lymphocytic leukemia. *Blood.* 1999;94:1840–1847.

76. Hamblin TJ, Davis Z, Gardiner A, et al. Unmutated Ig V$_h$ genes are associated with a more aggressive form of chronic lymphocytic leukemia. *Blood.* 1999;94:1848.

77. Ferry JA, Yang W-I, Zukerberg LR, et al. CD5+ extranodal marginal zone B-cell (MALT) lymphoma: a low grade neoplasm with a propensity for bone marrow involvement and relapse. *Am J Clin Pathol.* 1996;105:31–37.

78. Khalidi HS, Brynes RK, Browne P, et al. Intravascular large B-cell lymphoma: the CD5 antigen is expressed by a subset of cases. *Modern Pathol.* 1998;11:983–988.

79. Lin CW, O'Brien S, Faber J, et al. De novo CD5$^+$ Burkitt lymphoma, leukemia. *Am J Clin Pathol.* 1999;112:828–835.

80. Dorfman DM, Pinkus, GS. Distinction between small lymphocytic and mantle cell lymphoma by immunoreactivity for CD23. *Modern Pathol.* 1994;7:326–331.

81. Dunphy CH, Wheaton SE, Perkins SL. CD23 expression in transformed small lymphocytic lymphomas/chronic lymphocytic leukemias and blastic transformations of mantle cell lymphoma. *Modern Pathol.* 1997;10:818–822.

82. Kilo MN, Dorfman DM. The utility of flow cytometric analysis in the distinction of small lymphocytic leukemia from mantle cell lymphoma. *Am J Clin Pathol.* 1996;105:451–457.

83. Diaz de Leon E, Alkan S, Huang JC, et al. Usefulness of an immunohistochemical panel in paraffin-embedded tissues for the differentiation of B-cell non-Hodgkin's lymphomas of small lymphocytes. *Modern Pathol.* 1998;11:1046–1051.

84. Kidd PG, Calvelli T, Denny TN, et al. NIAID Division of AIDS Guidelines for Flow Cytometric Immunophenotyping. 1993, p. 1–25.

85. Shapiro JL, Miller ML, Pohlman B, et al. CD5⁻ B-cell lymphoproliferative disorders presenting in blood and bone marrow: a clinicopathologic study of 40 patients. *Am J Clin Pathol.* 1999;111:477–487.

86. Jaffe ES, Campo E, Raffeld M. Mantle cell lymphoma: biology and diagnosis. In: *Hematology 1999: The American Society of Hematology Education Program Book;* Schecter GP et al, eds. New Orleans, La: American Society of Hematology; 1999;319-328.

87. Weisenburger DD, Armitage JO. Mantle cell lymphoma – an entity comes of age. *Blood.* 1996;87:4483–4494.

88. Fisher RI. Mantle cell lymphoma: prognostic factors and treatment results. In: *Hematology 1999: The American Society of Hematology Education Program Book.* New Orleans, La: American Society of Hematology; 1999.

89. Coiffier B. Mantle cell lymphoma: new treatment possibilities. In: *Hematology 1999: The American Society of Hematology Education Program Book;* Schecter GP et al, eds. New Orleans, La: American Society of Hematology; 1999;329-334.

90. Soslow RA, Zukerberg LR, Harris NL, et al. BCL-1 (PRAD-1/Cyclin D-1) over-expression distinguishes the blastoid variant of mantle cell lymphoma from B-lineage lymphoblastic lymphoma. *Modern Pathol.* 1997;10:810–817.

91. Lardelli P, Bookman M, Sundeen J, et al. Lymphocytic lymphoma of intermediate differentiation: morphologic and immunophenotypic spectrum and clinical correlations. *Am J Surg Pathol.* 1990;14:752–763.

92. Kilo MN, Dorfman, DM. The utility of flow cytometric immunophenotypic analysis in the distinction of small lymphocytic lymphoma/chronic lymphocytic leukemia from mantle cell lymphoma. *Am J Clin Pathol.* 1996;105:451–457.

93. Pombo De Oliveira MS, Jaffe ES, Catovsky D. Leukaemic phase of mantle zone (intermediate) lymphoma: its characterization in 11 cases. *J Clin Pathol.* 1989;42:962–972.

94. Bain BJ, Catovsky D. The leukæmic phase of non-Hodgkin's lymphoma. *J Clin Pathol.* 1995;48:189–193.

95. Lai R, Arber DA, Chang KL, et al. Frequency of bcl-2 expression in non-Hodgkin's lymphoma: a study of 778 cases with comparison of marginal zone lymphoma and monocytoid B-cell hyperplasia. *Modern Pathol.* 1998;11:864–869.

96. Schnitzer B, Loesel L, Reed R. Lymphosarcoma cell leukemia: a clinicopathologic study. *Cancer.* 1970;26:1082–1096.

97. Mintzer D, Hauptman S. Lymphosarcoma cell leukemia and non-Hodgkin's lymphomas in leukemic phase. *Am J Med.* 1983;75:110–120.

98. Delia D, et al. Expression of the T1 (CD5, p67) surface antigen in B-CLL and B-NHL and its correlation with other B-cell differentiation markers. *Hematol Oncol.* 1986;4:237–248.

99. Sheibani K, Burke J, Swartz W, et al. Monocytoid B-cell lymphoma: clinico-pathologic study of 21 cases of a unique type of low-grade lymphoma. *Cancer.* 1988;62:1531–1538.

100. Catovsky D. Prolymphocytic leukemia. *Nouv Rev Fr Hematol.* 1982;24:343–347.

101. Galton D, Goldman J, Wiltshaw E, et al. Prolymphocytic leukaemia. *Br J Haematol.* 1975;27:2–23.

102. Melo J, Warde J, Chetty M, et al. The relationship between chronic lymphocytic leukemia and prolymphocytic leukemia, I: clinical and laboratory features of 300 patients and characterization of an intermediate group. *Br J Haematol.* 1986;63:377–387.

103. Berrebi A, Bassous-Buedj L, Vorst E, et al. Further characterization of prolympho-cytic leukemia cells as a tumor of activated B cells. *Am J Hematol.* 1990;34:181–185.

104. Enno A, Catovsky D, O'Brien M, et al. "Prolymphocytoid" transformation of chronic lymphocytic leukaemia. *Br J Haematol.* 1979;41:9–18.

105. Melo J, Catovsky D, Gregory W, et al. The relationship between chronic lym-phocytic leukemia and prolymphocytic leukemia, IV: analysis of survival and prognostic features. *Br J Haematol.* 1987;65:23–29.

106. Melo JV, Hegde U, Parreira A, et al. Splenic B cell lymphoma with circulating vil-lous lymphocytes: differential diagnosis of B cell leukemias with large spleens. *J Clin Pathol.* 1987;40:642–651.

107. Matutes E, Morilla R, Owusu-Ankomah K, et al. The immunophenotype of splenic lymphoma with villous lymphocytes and its relevance to the differential diagnosis with other B-cell disorders. *Blood.* 1994;83:1558–1562.

108. Golomb HM, Catovsky D, Golde DW. Hairy cell leukemia: a clinical review based on 71 cases. *Ann Intern Med.* 1978;89:677–683.

109. Chang KL, Stroup R, Weiss LM. Hairy cell leukemia: current status. *Am J Clin Pathol.* 1992;97:719–738.

110. Matutes E, Meeus P, McLennan K, et al. The significance of minimal residual dis-ease in hairy cell leukemia treated with deoxycoformycin: a long-term follow-up study. *Br J Haematol.* 1997;98:375–383.

111. Naeim F. Hairy cell leukemia: characteristics of the neoplastic cells. *Hum Pathol.* 1988;19:375–388.

112. Schwarting R, Stein H, Wang C-Y. The monoclonal antibodies S-HCL1 (Leu-14) and S-HCL 3 (Leu M5) allow the diagnosis of hairy cell leukemia. *Blood.* 1985;65:974–983.

113. Jansen J, Schuit H, Hermans J, et al. The prognostic significance of immunologic phenotype in hairy cell leukemia. *Blood.* 1984;63:1241–1244.

114. Sainati L, Matutes E, Mulligan S, et al. A variant form of hairy cell leukemia resist-ant to alpha-interferon: clinical and phenotypic characteristics of 17 patients. *Blood.* 1990;76:157–162.

115. Catovsky D, O'Brien M, Melo JV, et al. Hairy cell leukemia (HCL) variant: an intermediate disease between HCL and B prolymphocytic leukemia. *Semin Oncol.* 1984;11:362–369.

116. Troussard N, Valensi F, Duchayne E, et al. Splenic lymphoma with villous lymphocytes: clinical presentation, biology and prognostic factors in a series of 100 patients. *Br J Haematol.* 1996;93:731–739.

117. Kyle R. Multiple myeloma: review of 869 cases. *Mayo Clin Proc.* 1975;50:29–40.

118. Solomon A. Clinical implication of monoclonal light chains. *Semin Oncol.* 1986;13:341–349.

119. Kyle R, Garton J. The spectrum of IgM monoclonal gammopathy in 430 cases. *Mayo Clin Proc.* 1987;62:719–731.

120. Kyle R, Lust J. Monoclonal gammopathies of undetermined significance. *Semin Hematol.* 1989;26:176–200.

121. Barlogie B, Epstein J, Selvanayagam P, et al. Plasma cell myeloma— new biological insights and advances in therapy. *Blood.* 1989;73:865–879.

122. Kosmo M, Gale R. Plasma cell leukemia (review). *Semin Hematol.* 1987;24:202–208.

123. Parreira A, Robinson D, Melo J, et al. Primary plasma cell leukemia: immunological and ultrastructural studies in 6 cases. *Scand J Haematol.* 1985;35:570–578.

124. Toma V, Tetief F, Potgieter G, et al. Plasma cell leukemia. *Acta Haematol.* 1980;63:136–145.

125. Strickler JG, Audeh MW, Copenhaver CM, et al. Immunophenotypic differences between plasmacytoma/multiple myeloma and immunoblastic lymphoma. *Cancer.* 1988;61:1782–1786.

126. Garica-Sanz R, Orfao A, Gonzalez M, et al. Primary plasma cell leukemia: clinical immunophenotypic, DNA ploidy, and cytogenetic characteristics. *Blood.* 1999;93:1032–1037.

127. Alonso ML, Rubiol E, Mateu R, et al. cCD79a expression in a case of plasma cell leukemia. *Leukemia Res.* 1998;22:649–653.

128. Knapp W, Strobl H, Majdic O. Flow cytometric analysis of cell-surface and intracellular antigens in leukemia diagnosis. *Cytometry.* 1994;18:187–198.

129. Kanavaros P, Charlotte F, Martin N, et al. Expression of the immunoglobulin-associated MB-1 protein in non-Hodgkin's lymphomas. *Br J Haematol.* 1994;87(suppl 1):222.

130. Durie BGM, Grogan TM. CALLA-positive myeloma: an aggressive subtype with poor prognosis. *Blood.* 1985;66:229.

131. Grogan TM, Durie BGM, Spier CM, et al. Myelomonocytic antigen positive multiple myeloma. *Blood.* 1989;73:763.

132. Epstein J, Barlogie B, Katzmann J, et al. Phenotypic heterogeneity in aneuploid multiple myeloma indicates pre-B cell involvement. *Blood.* 1988;71:861.

133. Carbone A, Gaidano G, Gloghini A, et al. Differential expression of BCL-6, CD138/syndecan-1, and Epstein-Barr virus-encoded latent membrane protein-1 identifies distinct histogenetic subsets of acquired immunodeficiency syndrome-related non-Hodgkin's lymphomas. *Blood.* 1998;91:747–755.

134. Harada H, Kawano MM, Huang N, et al. Phenotypic difference of normal plasma cells from mature myeloma cells. *Blood.* 1993;81:2658–2663.

135. Caligaris-Cappio F, Bergui L, Tesio L, et al. Identification of malignant plasma cell precursors in the bone marrow of multiple myeloma. *J Clin Invest.* 1985:1243–1251.

136. Soneveld P, Durie BGM, Lokhorst HM, et al. Analysis of multidrug-resistance (MDR-1) glycoprotein and CD56 expression to separate monoclonal gammopathy from multiple myeloma. *Br J Haematol.* 1993;83:63–67.

137. Merlini G. Waldenström's macroglobulinemia – clinical manifestations and prognosis. In: *Hematology 1999: The American Society of Hematology Education Program Book;* Schechter GP et al, eds. New Orleans, La: American Society of Hematology; 1999:358-369.

138. Waldenstrom J. Incipient myelomatosis or "essential" hyperglobulinemia with fibrinogenopenia — a new syndrome? *Acta Med Scand.* 1944;117:216–247.

139. Fudenberg H, Virella G. Multiple myeloma and Waldenström's macroglobulinemia: unusual presentations. *Semin Hematol.* 1980;17:63–79.

140. Preud'Homme J-L, Seligmann M. Immunoglobulins on the surface of lymphoid cells in Waldenström's macroglobulinemia. *J Clin Invest.* 1972;51:701–705.

141. Chittal SM, Brousset P, Voigt J-J, et al. Large B-cell lymphoma rich in T-cells and simulating Hodgkin's disease. *Histopathology.* 1991;19:211–220.

142. Macon WR, Williams ME, Greer JP, et al. T-cell rich B-cell lymphomas: a clinicopathologic study of 19 cases. *Am J Surg Pathol.* 1992;16:351–363.

143. Hanson CA, Kurtin PJ, Hoyer JD, et al. Aberrant T-cell immunophenotype in viral infections: a limitation in the immunophenotypic diagnosis of T-cell lymphoproliferative disorders. *Modern Pathol.* 1998: 130A.

144. Hanson MN, Morrison VA, Peterson BA, et al. Posttransplant T-cell lymphoproliferative disorders: an aggressive late complication of solid organ transplantation. *Blood.* 1996;88:3626–3633.

145. Gentile TC, Hadlock KG, Uner AH, et al. Large granular lymphocyte leukaemia occurring after renal transplantation. *Br J Haematol.* 1998;101:507–512.

146. Sood R, Stewart CC, Aplan PD, et al. Neutropenia associated with T-cell large granular lymphocyte leukemia: long-term response to cyclosporine therapy despite persistence of abnormal cells. *Blood.* 1998;91:3372–3378.

147. McKenna RW, Arthur DC, Gajl-Peczalska KJ, et al. Granulated T cell lymphocytosis with neutropenia: malignant or benign chronic lymphoproliferative disorder? *Blood.* 1985;66:259–266.

148. Semenzato G, Pandolfi F, Chisesi T, et al. The lymphoproliferative disease of granular lymphocytes. *Cancer.* 1987;60:2971–2978.

149. Loughran T, Starkebaum G. Large granular lymphocyte leukemia: report of 38 cases and review of the literature. *Medicine.* 1987;66:397–405.

150. Gentile TC, Uner AH, Hutchison RE, et al. CD3+ CD56+ aggressive variant of large granular lymphocyte leukemia. *Blood.* 1994;84:2315–2321.

151. McKenna RW. Lymphoproliferative disorder of granular lymphocytes: more questions than answers. *Arch Pathol Lab Med.* 1992;116:235–237.

152. McDaniel HL, MacPherson BR, Tindle BH, et al. Lymphoproliferative disorder of granular lymphocytes: a heterogeneous disease. *Arch Pathol Lab Med.* 1992;116:242–248.

153. Lutzner M, Edelson R, Schein P, et al. Cutaneous T cell lymphomas: the Sézary syndrome, mycosis fungoides, and related disorders. *Ann Intern Med.* 1975;83:534–552.

154. Edelson R, Kirkpatrick C, Shevach E. Preferential cutaneous infiltration by neoplastic thymus-derived lymphocytes: morphologic and functional studies. *Ann Intern Med.* 1974;80:685.

155. Broder S, Edelson R, Lutzner M, et al. The Sézary syndrome: a malignant proliferation of helper T cells. *J Clin Invest.* 1976;58:1297–1306.

156. Berger C, Warburton D, Raafat J, et al. Cutaneous T-cell lymphoma: neoplasm of T cells with helper activity. *Blood.* 1979;53:642–651.

157. Weiss L, Wood G, Warnke R. Immunophenotypic differences between dermatopathic lymphadenopathy and lymph node involvement in mycosis fungoides. *Am J Pathol.* 1985;120:179–185.

158. van der Putte S, Toonstra J, van Wichen D, et al. Aberrant immunophenotypes in mycosis fungoides. *Arch Dermatol.* 1988;124:373–380.

159. Knowles D, Halper J. Human T cell malignancies: correlative clinical, histopathologic, immunologic and cytochemical analysis of 23 cases. *Am J Pathol.* 1982;106:187–203.

160. Carey J, Maeda K, Douglas M, et al. Immunophenotypic analysis of the leukemic phase of mycosis fungoides. *Lab Invest.* 1989;57:14A.

161. Matutes E, Brito-Babapulle V, Swansbury J, et al. Clinical and laboratory features of 78 cases of T-prolymphocytic leukemia. *Blood.* 1991;78:3269–3274.

162. Garand R, Goasguen J, Brizard A, et al. Indolent course as a relatively frequent presentation in T-prolymphocytic leukaemia. *Br J Haematol.* 1998;103:488–494.

163. Brunning RD. T-prolymphocytic leukemia (editorial). *Blood.* 1991;78:3111–3113.

164. Matutes E, Talavera J, O'Brien M, et al. The morphologic spectrum of T-prolymphocytic leukaemia. *Br J Haematol.* 1986;64:111–124.

165. Foa R, Pelicci P-G, Migone N, et al. Analysis of T-cell receptor beta chain (Tb) gene rearrangements demonstrates the monoclonal nature of T-cell chronic lymphoproliferative disorders. *Blood.* 1986;67:247–250.

166. Uchiyama T, Hori T, Tsudo M, et al. Interleukin-2 receptor (Tac antigen) expressed on adult T cell leukemia cells. *J Clin Invest.* 1985;76:446–453.

167. Takatsuki K, Uchiyama T, Ueshima Y, et al. Adult T cell leukemia: proposal as a new disease and cytogenetic, phenotypic and functional studies of leukemic cell. *GANN Monograph on Cancer Research.* 1982;28:13–22.

168. Waldmann T, Greene W, Sarin P, et al. Functional and phenotypic comparison of human T cell leukemia/lymphoma virus positive adult T cell leukemia with human T cell leukemia/lymphoma virus negative Sezary leukemia, and their distinction using Anti-Tac. *J Clin Invest.* 1984;73:1711–1718.

169. Witzig T, Phyliky R, Li C-Y, et al. T-Cell chronic lymphocytic leukemia with a helper/inducer membrane phenotype: a distinct clinicopathologic subtype with a poor prognosis. *Am J Hematol.* 1986;21:139–155.

170. Hoyer JD, Ross CW, Li C-Y, et al. True T-cell chronic lymphocytic leukemia: a morphologic and immunophenotypic study of 25 cases. *Blood.* 1995;86:1163–1169.

171. Lennert K, Kikuchi M, Sato E, et al. HTLV-positive and -negative T-cell lymphomas: morphological and immunohistochemical differences between European and HTLV-positive Japanese T-cell lymphomas. *Int J Cancer*. 1985;35:65–72.

172. Yamada Y. Phenotypic and functional analysis of leukemic cells from 16 patients with adult T-cell leukemia/lymphoma. *Blood*. 1988;61:192–199.

173. Morimoto C, Matsuyama T, Oshige C, et al. Functional and phenotypic studies of Japanese adult T cell leukemia cells. *J Clin Invest*. 1985;75:836–843.

174. Matsuoka M, Hattori T, Chosa T, et al. T3 surface molecules on adult T cell leukemia cells are modulated in vivo. *Blood*. 1986;67:1070–1076.

175. Nasu K, Said J, Vonderheid E, et al. Immunopathology of cutaneous T-cell lymphomas. *Am J Pathol*. 1985;119:436–447.

176. Schechter G, Sausville E, Fischmann B, et al. Evaluation of circulating malignant cells provides prognostic information in cutaneous T cell lymphoma. *Blood*. 1987;69:841.

177. Heulin C, Gonzalez M, Pedrinaci S, et al. Distribution of the CD45R antigen in the maturation of lymphoid and myeloid series: the CD45R negative phenotype is a constant finding in T CD4 positive lymphoproliferative disorders. *Br J Haematol*. 1988;69:173–179.

178. Worner I, Matutes E, Beverley P, et al. The distribution of CD45R, CD29 and CD45RO (UCHL1) antigens in mature CD4 positive T-cell leukaemias. *Br J Haematol*. 1990;74:439–444.

179. Bunn P. Diagnostic factors in intermediate and high-grade lymphomas: pathologic, immunologic and clinical (editorial). *J Clin Oncol*. 1988;6:1073–1075.

180. Shimoyama M, Ota K, Kikuchi M, et al. Major prognostic factors of adult patients with advanced T-cell lymphoma/leukemia. *J Clin Oncol*. 1988;6:1088–1097.

181. Clendenning W, Brecher G, Van Scott, E. Mycosis fungoides: relationship to malignant cutaneous reticulosis and the Sézary syndrome. *Arch Dermatol*. 1964;89:785.

182. Hui PK, Feller AC, Pileri S, et al. New aggressive variant of suppressor/cytotoxic T-CLL. *Am J Clin Pathol*. 1987;87:55–59.

183. Tajima K. Malignant lymphomas in Japan: epidemiological analysis of adult T-cell leukemia/lymphoma (ATL). *Cancer Metastasis Rev*. 1988;7:223–241.

184. Morimoto C, Matsuyama T, Oshige C, et al. Functional and phenotypic studies of Japanese adult T cell leukemia cells. *J Clin Invest*. 1985;75:836–843.

10

Flow Cytometric Analysis of Acute Leukemia

Catherine P. Leith
John Carey

Background

The modern diagnosis of acute leukemia requires a comprehensive approach, using morphology, immunophenotyping, cytology, cytogenetics, and/or nucleic acid-based diagnostic methods. Flow cytometric immunophenotyping is often critical for the correct diagnosis of acute leukemias. This necessity primarily reflects the undifferentiated morphology of these neoplasms and the therapeutic importance of defining acute myelogenous leukemia (AML) as opposed to acute lymphoblastic leukemia (ALL). The fundamental preanalytic and postanalytic issues dealing with specimen transport, processing, analysis, and reporting are covered in the chapter dealing with mature lymphoid leukemias and lymphomas (Chapter 9). Only a few issues specific to acute leukemias will be covered in this introductory section.

Triage

The 2 major issues in triage are as follows: (1) the decision as to whether to immunophenotype at all, and (2) the selection of the leukocyte antigen profile when immunophenotyping is required. A given laboratory's approach to these questions is closely related to the issues of the value of immunophenotyping for the diagnosis, prognosis, and follow-up of patients with acute leukemia. The correct diagnosis of AML or ALL is critically important in the work-up of a patient with newly diagnosed acute leukemia. Flow cytometric immunophenotyping is an extremely powerful and rapid method to achieve this and should always be used if there is any question about the lineage of the leukemia on the basis of morphologic and cytochemical studies alone. Immunophenotyping also defines T- and B-lineage ALL, which is very important in assigning patients to optimal treatment protocols. Additionally, immunophenotyping can identify the maturational stage of the leukemic blasts, which is quite useful in the treatment of B-lineage ALL. The utility of defining maturation of T-lineage ALLs or subtype of AMLs is a bit more controversial, with the exception of M0 and M7 AML (see below).

The prognostic utility of immunophenotyping, however, is limited once the nature of the disease, ALL versus AML, has been defined. In general, genomic lesions, defined by use of cytogenetic and nucleic acid testing, are more prognostic than antigen expression in AML and ALL. Characteristic immunophenotypic profiles have been associated with expression of important cytogenetic abnormalities. Specifically, in precursor B-cell ALL, some antigen profiles are strongly associated with certain molecular genetic lesions and might be used as a screen to define whether a particular molecular assay is needed.[1,2] Although the immunophenotype may give a clue to the underlying genetic abnormality, the sensitivity and specificity of the profile is not high enough to replace routine cytogenetic and/or molecular testing in patients with acute leukemia.[3]

Flow cytometric immunophenotyping can also often identify a characteristic immunophenotype of the leukemic blasts that may be used to monitor patients after therapy. This may be especially helpful in B-lineage ALL if there is difficulty in determining whether immature cells identified morphologically in posttreatment marrow represent regenerating normal elements (hematogones) or residual disease.[4-7] However, formal investigations evaluating the role of flow cytometry in the routine monitoring of minimal residual disease after therapy in acute leukemia are still ongoing. The results of these studies will help to determine how immunologic studies are used in routine posttreatment marrow surveillance.

Immunophenotyping: Method Selection

Immunophenotyping of acute leukemia is performed optimally by using flow cytometric immunofluorescence analysis. Leukemias, by definition, are already cell suspensions and therefore lend themselves readily to flow cytometric analysis. Flow cytometry allows objective evaluation of the sometimes dim immunofluorescence staining seen on leukemic blasts, rapid analysis of thousands of cells, and gating on specific populations of interest in patients with contaminating normal cells. These are all advantages over immunocytochemical staining of cytospin preparations. This is not to say that immunocytochemistry or immunohistochemistry cannot accurately distinguish ALL from AML. Indeed, immunohistochemistry of bone marrow biopsy specimens or immunocytochemistry of touch preparations may be essential in paucicellular marrows (eg, those with fibrosis in M7 AML).[8] However, the much larger repertoire of antibodies available for flow cytometry compared with immunohistochemical evaluation of fixed tissue, as well as the speed and ease of flow cytometric analysis of leukemic specimens, make this the method of choice in the great majority of cases.

Flow Gating Strategies: Acute Leukemia Blasts

The identification of acute leukemia cells using light scatter characteristics is usually straightforward because the majority of cases are composed predominantly of blasts. Occasionally, the presence of many benign cells in the specimen can lead to a failure to identify blasts using light scattering properties alone. In particular, ALL blasts usually have a continuously variable forward light scatter, ranging from that of small lymphocytes to large blasts. If light scatter gating alone is used, small benign lymphocytes will be included in the gate and may give rise to confusion about the lineage of the blasts.

Borowitz et al[9] have shown that in 80% of patients with ALL and AML, the blasts show characteristically dim CD45 expression compared with mature lymphocytes (which show brighter-positive CD45) and erythroid cells, platelets, and their precursors (which show nondetectable CD45) (**Figure 10-1**). The intensity of CD45 on the blasts is similar to that of mature neutrophils, with the former being differentiated from the latter by having significantly lower side light

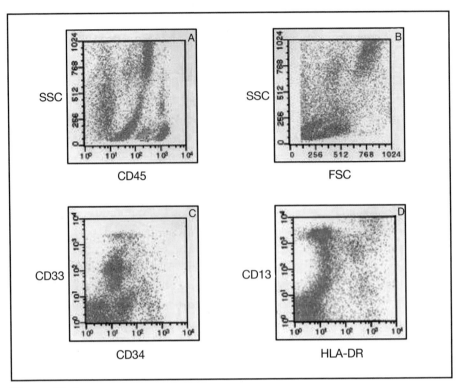

Figure 10-1

Utility of CD45 gating in identification of leukemic blasts.

This is an example of a patient with suspected AML where the aspirate was very hemodilute, and contained only a small percentage of blasts. In such cases in particular, CD45 gating is helpful in distinguishing leukemic blasts from other cells in the sample. **A.** CD45 versus side scatter (SSC): The blasts are identified as having low side scatter, and dim CD45 staining (red population). **B.** Forward scatter (FSC) versus side scatter: The light scattering properties of the blasts identified in A are shown. These have low SSC with a range of FSC, overlapping with other cells in the low SSC region. Gating on light scatter properties alone would thus not identify this single population. **C.** Phenotype of the identified blasts. The blasts identified by CD45 and SSC gating in A are clearly identified as having CD34 but no CD33 expression. **D.** The blasts identified by CD45/SSC gating also express CD13 and HLA-DR.

scatter. Therefore, in cases in which the light scatter identification of the blasts is questionable, CD45 gating can be quite helpful. This alone, or in combination with standard light scatter gating, will usually allow a sensitive and specific blast gate. Indeed, when working with complex samples (eg, bone marrow), CD45 gating is the optimum gating technique.

The major drawbacks to the CD45 gate are (1) sensitivity, (2) cost, and (3) limitation of the number of unique markers in each tube. In approximately 20% of acute leukemias, typically B-cell precursor ALL, the neoplastic cells are CD45⁻ and show low side scatter, and therefore they cocluster with erythroid cells. However, the phenotype of the blasts in such cases should be clearly identifiable as B-cell precursors, and thus in practice this circumstance should not cause confusion.[9] As flow cytometric analysis moves increasingly to 3- or 4-color analysis and as the repertoire of directly conjugated antibodies in different colors increases, the limitations of the number of unique markers in each tube will no longer be a problem.

A final issue is the utility of a surveillance tube, a unique combination of antigens that will define most major differentiation clusters of hematolymphoid cells, whether benign or neoplastic. CD45/GPA/CD14 and CD45/CD33/CD71, combined with light scatter, are excellent surveillance tubes for bone marrow examination in all cases of acute leukemia. Indeed, one or the other can be applied to all bone marrow samples submitted for flow cytometric evaluation, and both allow for a rapid assessment of the relative proportions of different elements in the marrow, as well as an assessment of their maturity.

Flow Immunophenotyping: Panels and Analysis

The panel of antibodies chosen will depend on the role immunophenotyping is going to play in the diagnosis, prognosis, or monitoring of minimal residual disease (MRD). For diagnosis, 2 main factors need to be considered in antibody selection: (1) the heterogeneity of expression of lineage-associated markers between different leukemias of the same lineage and (2) the necessity of distinguishing malignant blasts from residual normal hematolymphoid cells in the specimen.

Acute leukemias, even of the same lineage and French-American-British (FAB) subtype, may express different lineage-associated antigens on their surface. Additionally, acute leukemic blasts quite frequently express antigens associated with different lineages. For example, the expression of the T cell-associated antigens CD2, CD4, CD5, and CD7 has been well described on AML blasts. Therefore the panel, at a minimum, must contain sufficient markers of each lineage to discriminate accurately, for example, between AML expressing T-cell antigens and T-lineage ALL.[3,10] In addition, the panel and gating strategy must allow distinction of leukemic blasts from residual normal marrow or peripheral blood white cells. If MRD monitoring is going to be considered in the future, the diagnostic panel needs to be sufficiently extensive to identify a unique leukemia phenotype that may be used for subsequent analysis.

The approach used in each laboratory will depend on which is the most efficient means of workflow through the laboratory and the immunophenotypic detail required in each case. In some cases a screening panel to assign lineage may be performed first, followed by a more detailed analysis with further lineage-associated markers, whereas in other laboratories it may be more efficient to perform a larger initial panel, with follow-up studies only performed in unusual cases. In general, lineage assignment can be based on both surface and intracellular antigen-staining patterns. Again, each laboratory needs to define the method that best suits its caseload and case mix.

Membrane (Cell Surface) Analysis

Membrane antigen analysis typically includes monoclonal antibodies to at least 2 different antigens for each of the major cell lines in the clinical differential (myeloid vs T vs B) (**Table 10-1**). No consensus has been reached about which antigens should be included and the particular combinations to use. Most panels do include the antibodies to the following leukocyte antigens to define the these lineages:

- **B:** CD19 and CD22
- **T:** CD7 with either CD5 and/or CD2
- **Myeloid / Monocytic:** CD13, CD14 and CD33
- **Megakaryocytic:** CD61 and/or CD41

Finally, membrane panels usually include a CD19/CD10 combination and anti-CD34. Other antibodies to membrane antigens may be included on the primary or follow-up panels in order to refine the diagnostic certainty.

CD4, CD56, and CD117 expression have been used to support the diagnosis of AML, given the relative lack of specificity of CD13 and CD33 for AML.[11-15] Furthermore, the coexpression of CD56 and CD34 on AML can be used as a marker for evaluation of MRD.[12,16]

Table 10-1

Acute Leukemias: Useful Antigens for Flow Cytometry Panels

Antigens	ALL vs AML	ALL Subtype	AML Type M0*	AML Type M7*	AML Type M4/5*	AML Type M3*	AML Type M6*
CD10/19	Yes†	Yes	Yes				
CD20 or 22	±‡	±					
CD7/5 (2)	Yes	Yes					
CD34 and 56	±	±	±	±	±	±	±
CD13, CD14, CD33	Yes		Yes	Yes	Yes	Yes	Yes
CD61 (41)	Yes			Yes			
CD45/GPA	Yes		Yes	±	Yes	±	Yes
kappa/lambda		Yes					
Cyt. CD22 or CD79 alpha	±	±	Yes				
Cyt. CD3	±	±	Yes				
Cyt. MPO	±		Yes				
Cyt. mu		±					
Other†	CD1, CD2, CD3, CD117, TdT	TdT, CD9	CD117	CD41, CD42, factor VIII (IHC)**	CD11b, CD11c, CD24	HLA Dr, CD9	CD71

Items in parentheses are alternative or additional markers.
*M0, M3, M4, M5, M6, M7 = FAB subclasses of AML.[16,17]
†Yes = always included in panel.
‡± or other = optional inclusion in panel.
¶cyt. = cytoplasmic and membrane.
**IHC = immunohistochemistry.

Surface immunoglobulin light chain (sIg) expression is prognostically important in B-lineage ALL, although the relative rarity of non-L3 B-lineage ALL means many years or decades may pass before a morphologically unsuspected B-lineage ALL will be detected by routine inclusion of sIg on the primary acute leukemia panel.[17-19] In addition, inclusion of surface light chains will detect cases of blastic mantle cell lymphoma presenting in leukemia phase, which can closely resemble ALL.[20]

The inclusion of CD1 and/or CD4/CD8 (coexpression of both or CD8 only) may aid in the definition of T-lineage ALL when only one pan-T antigen is otherwise expressed and/or there is coexpression of myeloid-associated antigens.[17,21]

Lastly, the inclusion of an erythroid-associated antigen, such as glycophorin A (GPA) or CD71, may be helpful in rare cases of M6 AML, particularly the M6b variant (see below).[22-24] GPA is more specific for erythroid lineage than CD71, although diagnostic cases of M1, M4/4, and M7 AML have been reported to be GPA+.[25] Also, the inclusion of either of these with CD45 serves as an excellent surveillance/gating combination (see above).

Cytoplasmic/Intracellular Flow Analysis

There are several antigens that are expressed predominantly within the cell that have excellent sensitivity and specificity for lymphoblastic or myelomonocytic differentiation. These cytoplasmic antigens may be used as follow-up markers, particularly when membrane analysis is inconclusive, or as markers in a concise primary panel. Because standard flow immunofluorescence techniques for cytoplasmic antigen analysis also measure residual surface membrane expression, antigens that could have membrane and/or cytoplasmic expression, such as CD22 or CD3, must be assessed by both membrane and cytoplasmic analysis (**Figure 10-2**).

The expression of certain antigens has been shown to be very sensitive and specific for T- (cytoplasmic [c]CD3) and B-lineage (cCD22 and cCD79 alpha)ALLs and lymphoblastic lymphomas .[3,26,27] The presence of myeloperoxidase (MPO) antigen is quite specific for AML.[28,29] This includes most patients with AML with myelomonocytic or monocytic differentiation (M4/5), as well as the M1-3 types of AML. The apparent discrepancy between MPO antigen and function in M4/5 disease has been confirmed using cytochemical staining. However, not all cases of AML, including FAB M0 AML, will be cMPO+, while MPO immunoreactivity has been reported in some ALLs. Furthermore, if a nonfixative lysing reagent is used, artificial-positive MPO immunoreactivity can be seen if residual benign myeloid cells comprise greater than 20% of all nucleated cells.[26] This is due to release of MPO from these cells, with electrostatic binding of the MPO by the DNA in the nuclei of any cell, including the neoplastic cells.

Nuclear terminal deoxynucleotidyl transferase (TdT) is a sensitive marker of lymphoblastic differentiation, which can be readily detected by means of flow cytometry.[30-33] Although bright TdT antigen expression has a good predictive

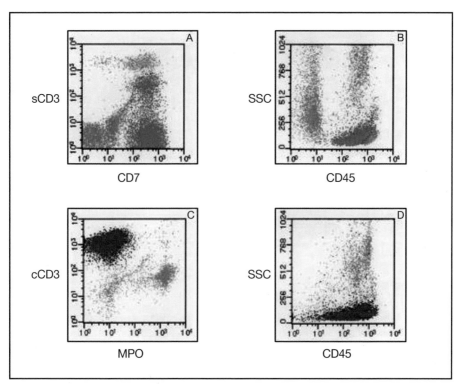

Figure 10-2

Use of surface and cytoplasmic staining in the lineage assignment of leukemic blasts. This was a pediatric patient whose marrow was effaced by acute leukemia. Staining of the blasts for both surface and cytoplasmic CD3 was performed. **A.** Staining of the blasts for surface CD3 and CD7 reveals a predominant population of cells, which express CD7 but have dim or negative CD3 expression (turquoise population). A much smaller population of cells with both CD7 and bright CD3 expression are also identified (red population). **B.** Back-gating on these populations shows that the CD3 negative/dim cells have low SSC and low CD45 expression, characteristic of blasts, while the surface CD3 bright cells have bright CD45/low SSC characteristic of mature lymphocytes (red population). **C.** The marrow was stained for cytoplasmic CD3 and for myeloperoxidase. A predominant population of cCD3-positive cells was identified. **D.** These cCD3-psotive cells have the dim CD45 and low SSC staining characteristic of blasts. Thus the leukemic blasts in this case show cytoplasmic but not surface CD3 expression, typical of an immature T-lymphoblastic leukemia.

value for ALL, dim staining can be seen in patients with both ALL and AML, with up to 40% of the latter being reported as TdT[+].[3,34-36] Furthermore, high background staining in AML may make interpretation quite difficult. The inclusion of surface markers such as CD19 with TdT staining can help better define TdT expression on the cells of interest.

Acute Leukemias: Antigen Phenotyping for Diagnosis

The diagnosis of AML according to the standard FAB criteria can be made on morphologic and cytochemical studies, and immunophenotyping is required only for the diagnosis of AML M0 and M7 and minimally differentiated AML M6.[37-40] In contrast, ALL always requires immunophenotyping for its correct diagnosis and its distinction from M0 or, less commonly, M6 or M7 AML. Immunophenotyping can accurately distinguish T- and B-lineage ALL and AML and can also identify occasional cases of true biphenotypic leukemia or undifferentiated leukemia.

ALL Typing

The primary question to be answered is usually one of the lineage of the acute leukemia. Occasionally, the maturation is also in question. Profiles indicating immaturity of acute leukemia are as follows:

- the absence of sIg, particularly combined with bright CD10 expression in B-lineage ALL;
- the strong presence of CD7 and absence of membrane CD3, the expression of CD1, and/or the coexpresssion of CD4 and CD8 in T-lineage ALL; and
- the presence of membrane CD34 and/or intracellular (nuclear) TdT.

B-lineage ALL

Patients with B-cell precursor ALL characteristically express membrane CD19 and cytoplasmic CD22 and CD79 alpha (**Figure 10-3**).[3,41-44] CD19 expression is characteristically bright, which is in contrast to the dim expression that may be seen in AML with the t(8;21) translocation. Surface, as well as cytoplasmic, CD22 can also frequently be detected if the more sensitive phycoerythrin-labeled reagents are used for its detection. CD20, an antigen expressed later in B-cell differentiation than CD19, is only expressed in a subset of cases, while surface light chains are by definition absent. The presence of these pan-B antigens in the absence of CD7, CD13, CD14, and CD33 is virtually diagnostic of B-lineage ALL.

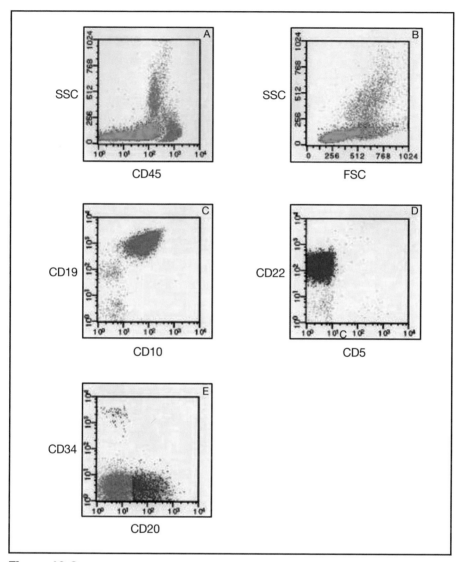

Figure 10-3

Pediatric patient with B-cell precursor ALL with a phenotype suggestive of a t (1;19) translocation. **A.** The leukemic blasts are identified by CD45/SSC gating in each case. The blasts have dim to absent CD45 expression, and low SSC. **B.** Light scattering properties of these gated blasts show low SSC with a range of FSC properties. **C.** The gated leukemic blasts show bright CD19 expression, as well as expression of CD10. **D.** CD22 is expressed while CD5 is absent. Use of a PE-conjugated CD22 often allows identification of CD22 expression in B-precursor ALL without the necessity of performing cytoplasmic CD22 staining. **E.** The blasts are CD34 negative, and show a subpopulation that is CD20-positive (green) and another subset that is CD20-negative (gray). The combination of lack of CD34 expression, together with lack of CD20 expression in at least some of the blasts is suggestive of B-precursor ALL harboring a t(1;19). The presence of this fusion was demonstrated in this patient by RT-PCR methods.

Additional markers frequently expressed in B-precursor ALL are CD10 and CD34. CD10 is characteristically expressed in ALL and not AML; therefore its expression in conjunction with pan-B antigens is useful supporting evidence for an ALL diagnosis in cases in which the leukemic blasts coexpress myeloid-associated antigens. Detection of CD34 expression by the leukemic blasts confirms their immaturity and may be useful later in monitoring MRD after therapy.

Analysis of surface light chain expression can also be useful in the evaluation of patients with acute leukemia because this will identify occasional cases of L3 ALL/Burkitt's lymphoma unrecognized by morphologic examination. Additionally, mantle cell lymphoma rarely may present as an acute leukemic process without any history or clinical manifestations of lymphoma. Identification of monoclonal surface immunoglobulin in these cases is crucial and should prompt the pathologist to examine CD5 expression on the leukemic cells; these mantle cell leukemias, like their lymphomatous counterparts, characteristically coexpress CD5.[20]

Thirty to fifty percent of patients with B-precursor ALL show coexpression of a single myeloid-associated antigen, such as CD13 and CD33, whereas 2 or more myeloid antigens are expressed in approximately 8% of cases.[42,44-47] Cytoplasmic MPO has also been described in B-lineage ALL, but it is usually very weak in comparison with the level of expression in AML.[48] The reliable identification of B lineage in these cases depends upon interpretation of the entire profile. Typically, such cases involve only one or occasionally 2 dimly expressed myeloid antigens, whereas there are usually 2 or more brightly expressed B or lymphoid lineage antigens (eg, CD10, CD19, CD22, or cCD79 alpha). These features, combined with the absence of significant cytoplasmic granulation or Auer rods, allow a confident diagnosis of B-lineage ALL with myeloid antigen expression.

Genotypic Markers in B-lineage ALL

Genotype is prognostically very important in B-lineage ALL. Specific antigenic profiles have been associated with specific genotypes in ALL, and in some cases these antigenic profiles are sufficiently sensitive and specific for a particular genotype that they have been advocated as a screening tool for selective cytogenetic/molecular testing for specific genotypic abnormalities. One of the first associations recognized was that of the pre-B (cytoplasmic mu positive) phenotype with the t(1;19) translocation. It is now recognized that the t(1;19) translocation, rather than the pre-B phenotype, confers poor prognosis, and therefore cytogenetic/molecular analyses for this translocation have superseded cytoplasmic mu detection to correctly identify patients who may require more aggressive therapy.[49,50]

Patients with the t(1;19) translocation have a characteristic immunophenotypic profile. The blasts of these patients homogeneously express CD19, CD10, and CD9. CD34 is completely absent, and CD20 is absent or expressed only by a subset of the blasts, with a significant fraction of the blasts being CD20⁻.[2] This CD19⁺/CD10⁺/CD9⁺/CD34⁻/CD20-partial-negative phenotype is sufficiently distinctive that its recognition should prompt further testing, such as molecular studies, particularly if cytogenetic studies fail to identify a t(1;19) translocation. Specific monoclonal antibodies to the E2A/pbx1 chimeric protein derived from the t(1;19) translocation may also be useful.[51,52]

A predictive phenotype for the t(12;21) TEL-AML1 fusion in patients with precursor B-lineage ALL has also been described. In these patients the leukemic blasts lack or show only partial expression of CD9 or CD20. This phenotype has a sensitivity of 88% and a specificity of 71% for the t(12;21) translocation.[1] Pediatric patients with a t(12;21) translocation also show an increased frequency of CD13 and/or CD33.[46]

Although myeloid antigen expression has not been found to be prognostically useful in pediatric B-lineage ALL, its expression may predict an *MLL* gene rearrangement.[45,46] About 80% of patients with an *MLL* gene rearrangement express the myeloid antigens CD65, CD15, or CD33, whereas they generally lack CD13 or CD14.[46,53,54] The t(4;11) translocation that occurs particularly in infants has in addition been associated with a lack of CD10 and low or absent CD24 expression.[53,55] Among pediatric patients with ALL, no phenotype pathognomonic of the t(9;22) translocation has been identified. However, among adult patients, the CD19⁺CD10⁺CD34⁺ phenotype is associated with the t(9;22) translocation, although this phenotype is by no means exclusive to this group.[47]

Prognostic Markers in B-lineage ALL

Historically, the CD10⁺ phenotype was regarded as a good prognostic indicator in B-lineage ALL, and expression of myeloid-associated antigens was viewed as a marker of poor prognosis. However, after one accounts for clinical factors, such as age, white blood cell count, and sex, CD10 expression is no longer independently prognostic.[42] Similarly, although initial studies suggested some difference in clinical response in B-lineage ALL with myeloid antigen expression, recent studies on large groups of patients have found no differences in clinical outcome in these myeloid antigen-positive cases.[42,46,56] Therefore, it is important to recognize myeloid antigen positive ALL to correctly distinguish it from AML with lymphoid antigen coexpression, but not for prognosis.

Recently, interest has focused on the correlation between the level of expression of different antigens by leukemic blasts and clinical outcome. By using fluorescent microparticles for standardization, patients with B-lineage ALL whose blasts express bright CD20 or CD45 have been found to have a poorer response than those patients whose blasts have lower levels of these antigens. However, accurate assessment of fluorescent intensity requires the use of fluorescent microparticles, and therefore, to date, it is not routinely used in clinical flow cytometry laboratories.[57]

T-lineage ALL

T-lineage ALL comprises about 15% of pediatric ALL cases.[58] Although historically T-lineage ALL had a poor response to therapy, this disease has shown a remarkable improvement in clinical outcome with the advent of risk-adjusted multiagent chemotherapy. The antigens expressed by T lineage ALL depend on the degree of maturation of the T lymphoblasts. The most primitive T lymphoblasts (prothymocyte stage) express CD7 and usually CD2, whereas blasts at the immature thymocyte stage also typically express CD5 and CD1, coexpress CD4 and CD8, and express cytoplasmic, but not surface, CD3 (see **Figure 10-4**). Lymphoblasts at the mature T-cell stage express surface CD3 in addition to CD2, CD5, and CD7. However, phenotypic aberrations can be seen, so that the phenotype of cells at a particular stage of development may not always be accurately recapitulated by the leukemic blasts. In addition to expression of varying numbers of T cell–associated antigens, the blasts of patients with T-lineage ALL typically do not express HLA-DR.

Problems with lineage assignment of a T-lineage ALL can arise because the T cell–associated antigens CD7, CD2, CD4, and CD5 can all also be expressed by AML blasts. In addition, expression of myeloid antigens, such as CD13 and CD33, is quite frequently observed in T-lineage ALL; about 10% to 20% of patients express a single myeloid antigen, with a small percentage (6%) expressing 2 or more myeloid antigens.[42,44,46,56] Myeloid antigen expression may be more frequent among patients with very immature (prothymocyte) T-lineage ALL. Cytoplasmic CD3 staining can be particularly useful in problematic cases expressing both myeloid and T-cell antigens because cCD3 is a sensitive and highly specific marker for T-cell, rather than myeloid, lineage.[3,26,27] Other markers that can be helpful in distinguishing myeloid antigen-positive T-lineage ALL from T-lymphoid antigen–positive AML include HLA-DR (frequently negative in T-lineage ALL, particularly in pediatric patients, but positive in AML), bright

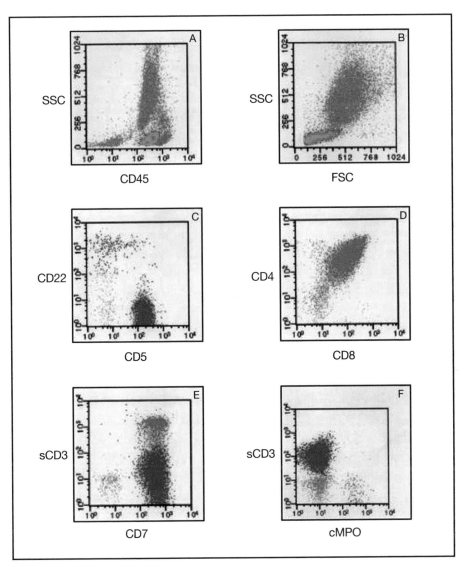

Figure 10-4

50-year-old adult male who presented with fatigue, and was found to have pancytopenia with circulating blasts. There was no adenopathy or mediastinal mass. **A.** CD45 staining identifies a population of blasts with dim CD45 expression and low SSC characteristics (red population). **B.** This population is also quite readily identified by FSC/SSC but would overlap with normal mature lymphocytes. **C.** With the CD45 gate applied, the leukemic blasts are analyzed for expression of CD22 and CD5. The blasts express CD5 but not CD22. **D.** The blasts co-stain with CD4 and CD8. This is characteristic of an immature T-cell at the immature thymocyte stage of differentiation. **E.** As expected for immature T-cells at this stage of differentiation, the blasts express CD7 but show almost no surface CD3 expression (green population). **F.** The blasts show cytoplasmic CD3 expression, confirming their immature T-cell lineage. In this case, the blasts were also negative for HLA-DR and for CD13 and CD33.

TdT, and CD10 (expressed in 30% of patients with T-lineage ALL).[59] The level of expression of particular antigens may also be useful: both CD7 and CD4 expression is brighter in T-lineage ALL than in AML.

Genotypic Markers in T-lineage ALL

Unlike in B-lineage ALL, no specific immunophenotypic markers indicative of genotype have been described in T-lineage ALL.

Prognostic Markers in T-lineage ALL

Various studies have attempted to correlate the degree of T-lymphoblast differentiation in ALL with clinical response. Although historical studies found no differences in clinical outcome with maturational stage, a more recent study analyzing clinical response in patients treated with contemporary Childhood Cancer Group (CCG) protocols suggests a lower event-free survival rate for patients with very immature T-cell (prothymocyte T-cell; CD7$^+$/CD2$^-$/CD5$^-$) ALL.[21,60] However, because in some patients the blasts also expressed myeloid antigens, it is unclear whether all of these patients would still be classified as having T-lineage ALL rather than AML. More recently, this issue has been refined by the identification of a *selection-related* phenotype corresponding to the phenotype of T-cell precursors undergoing thymic cortical selection. This phenotype, defined as either expression of CD1 or coexpression of CD4 and CD8 by the leukemic blasts, has been associated with an improved clinical response in pediatric patients.[61]

Expression of CD2 by leukemic blasts has also been associated with an improved clinical response in pediatric patients. Among adult patients with T-lineage ALL, expression of 6 or more T cell-associated antigens has been associated with an improved survival versus patients with 3 or fewer antigens expressed.[47,62] As in B-lineage ALL, it has been controversial whether expression of myeloid antigens confers poor prognosis in T-cell ALL. Most recent studies suggest that with current therapies, coexpression of myeloid antigens is probably not clinically significant.[56,58]

Changes in ALL Phenotype at Relapse

Patients with ALL frequently show some differences in phenotype between diagnosis and relapse, with such changes being reported in 50% to 75% of cases. These changes in phenotype almost universally are changes in stage of differentiation of the leukemic blasts rather than alterations in cell lineage and appear to be more frequent in patients with T-lineage ALL.[63,64] Phenotypic changes may include loss or gain of antigens, including loss or gain of myeloid-associated antigens, such as CD13 and CD33. Phenotypic changes in leukemic blasts can be problematic if coexpression of particular markers is being used for MRD detection (see below).

In only a very small percentage of cases (5% in one study) does the phenotype change sufficiently to alter lineage assignment, including switches from ALL (B-lineage) to AML.[64] Because such lineage switches can rarely occur, it is probably worthwhile to perform at least limited studies in relapsed disease, particularly if the clinical presentation is unusual, to confirm that the lineage of the disease has remained the same.

AML

Currently, the key role of immunophenotyping in AML lies in its use in correctly discriminating AML from ALL or other entities. Immunophenotyping is therefore essential in the correct assignment of lineage to AML cases without differentiation (AML FAB M0) or with megakaryocytic differentiation (AML M7), because these leukemias cannot be identified by means of traditional cytochemical staining techniques alone. The role of immunophenotyping in the subclassification of other AML subtypes has been much more limited. There is not a good correlation between immunophenotyping and traditional FAB morphologic classification of AML, with the exception of a few subtypes with specific underlying cytogenetic abnormalities, such as acute promyelocytic leukemia (APL) with the t(15;17) translocation, and even these correlations are not sufficiently sensitive and specific to take the place of cytogenetic testing (see below). In addition, it is controversial whether expression of specific antigens can help to identify patients with good or poor clinical prognosis.

AML Diagnosis and Classification

The blasts in patients with AML can be heterogeneous in their expression of both myeloid- and lymphoid-associated antigens (**Figure 10-5**). The myeloid antigens most frequently expressed are CD33 and/or CD13 (> 90% of cases), and these should be studied in all cases.[65] However, some patients show aberrant loss of one of these myeloid antigens, and therefore, as for ALL typing, the

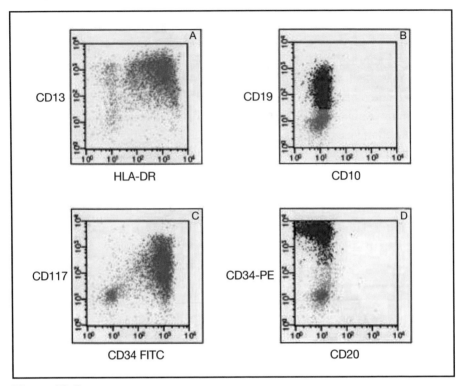

Figure 10-5
Phenotype of AML with t(8;21). Patient who presented with leucocytosis, and with 25% marrow blasts, with evidence of maturation. The leukemia was classified as AML M2. A t(8;21) was subsequently revealed by cytogenetics. The blasts in this case have been identified using CD45/SSC gating, and only this population is identified in the histograms. **A.** CD13 versus HLA-DR. The leukemic blasts express both HLA-DR and CD13 as is characteristic of AML. **B.** CD19 versus CD10. The blasts show expression of CD19 without CD10 co-staining. Note that the CD19 expression is much weaker than that seen in B-precursor ALL (Figure 10-3 C). **C.** CD117 versus CD34-FITC. The blasts show staining with both CD117 and with CD34. Staining with this CD34-FITC-labeled reagent is very bright. **D.** CD34-PE versus CD20. The PE-labeled CD34 reagent show even brighter staining. This very bright staining with CD34, combined with dim CD19 expression is quite characteristic of AML with a t(8;21). The use of PE-labeled CD34 will identify CD34 expression much more sensitively than a FITC-labeled reagent.

phenotypic panel must include several myeloid markers to ensure that such patients with aberrant antigen loss are not misidentified as having ALL.[66] CD117 is another excellent and very specific marker for AML. It is expressed in 65% to 90% of patients with AML and, in contrast to CD13 and CD33, CD117 is expressed very infrequently in ALL, being expressed only occasionally in T-lineage ALL.[11,13,15] Other myeloid antigens frequently expressed in patients with AML include CD15 (60%) and CD4 (67%). CD4 expression is characteristically dim, similar to the level of expression on monocytes. When expressed in this dim fashion, it is now well recognized as a myeloid marker and should not cause confusion with T-lineage ALL. In fact, dim CD4 expression is a quite useful myeloid-specific marker in AML diagnosis.[14,65,67]

Several other myeloid markers may be useful in diagnosis or to more accurately assess the maturation pathway in AML. Both CD14 and CD24 are characteristically expressed in AML with monocytic differentiation, of which CD24 appears more sensitive in predicting monocytic lineage.[68] CD64 is expressed on cells committed to the granulocyte-monocytic lineages and appears more specific for these lineages than CD13 and CD33, which are also expressed on non-committed progenitor cells.[69]

The pattern of myeloid antigens expressed in AML is quite frequently asynchronous, so that antigens normally expressed at different stages in myeloid cell development are coexpressed by the leukemic blasts. CD34 and CD15 coexpression can be identified in up to 20% of cases and has been particularly associated with AML with the t(8;21) translocation.[65,66,70] In addition, expression of CD16 by nongranular monomyeloid cells, rather than its usual expression by granulated cells undergoing neutrophil maturation, can be identified in about 15% of cases.[66] In addition to the asynchronous expression of myeloid antigens, some patients with AML may show unusually bright expression of some markers. For example, CD34 expression in the leukemic blasts is much brighter than that seen in normal bone marrow progenitors in AML with the t(8;21) translocation.[66,71]

In the same way that patients with ALL frequently coexpress myeloid antigens, patients with AML quite frequently express lymphoid-associated antigens. The T cell-related antigens CD7, CD5, and CD2 (in decreasing order of frequency of expression) are expressed in about 20% to 40% of cases, whereas the B-lineage antigens CD19 and CD20 occur in about 10% to 25% of cases. CD19 expression is more frequent among patients with childhood AML (35%) than those with adult AML (10%).[71] CD10 is also rarely expressed. Usually, there is only one lymphoid antigen expressed, and it typically has dim intensity. In contrast, there are usually 2 or more AML antigens with bright intensity. This, along with the morphology (granulation, Auer rods) and/or cytochemistry, can clearly distinguish lymphoid antigen-positive AML from ALL. In difficult cases (eg, one bright lymphoid and myeloid antigen with undifferentiated morphology and cytochemistry), the demonstration of cytoplasmic MPO expression along with the absence of B (cCD79 alpha/cCD22) and T antigens (cCD3) is definitive.

Correlation of Immunophenotype with Morphologic Classification

Overall, there are not very close correlations between FAB subtype and immunophenotype, and therefore, although some phenotypes are more characteristically associated with certain morphologic subtypes, the phenotype alone is not diagnostic of a particular FAB subtype. Exceptions to this are the M0 and M7 subtypes, which must be immunophenotyped for identification, and, to a lesser extent, the M6 subtype of AML.

AML M0

Minimally differentiated or M0 AML presents really not so much an issue of subtyping AML as it does of making the proper diagnosis of AML versus ALL.[37,39] According to the FAB, M0 AML lacks morphologic and cytochemical features of myeloid, monocytic or erythroid differentiation. Therefore, diagnosis requires the presence of one or more myeloid-associated antigens (eg, CD13, CD14, CD33, or cMPO) and the absence of T or B lymphoid-associated antigens (eg, CD19, CD22, cCD3, or cCD79 alpha). The latter should not include TdT and others (eg, CD2 and CD7) that have significant lineage infidelity.

M7 AML

The acute megakaryocytic leukemias (M7 AML) are part of the spectrum of neoplastic disorders of megakaryocytes, which include essential thrombocythemia and chronic idiopathic myelofibrosis.[72] M7 AML comprises about 5% to 10% of all *de novo* AMLs. Although there is some controversy regarding the prognosis for patients with M7 AML, it generally appears to be similar to that of AML in general.[73]

The diagnosis of M7 AML requires morphologic, cytochemical, and immunophenotypic evidence. Because of the frequency of nonproductive marrow taps, immunohistochemical methods may need to be used. The M1 through M6 AMLs should first be excluded by means of traditional FAB criteria. Next, a clear demonstration of one or more megakaryocyte-associated antigens on or in the neoplastic blasts is required.[38] Typically, these include membrane CD41 or CD61 or cytoplasmic expression of CD61 or factor VIII antigen.[74-76] The latter 2 antigens can be examined by means of immunohistochemistry, even in fixed material. The expression of CD42, although specific, lacks sensitivity.[75,76] A majority of megakaryoblastic leukemia cases are CD13+, CD33+, and/or CD34+. However, monocytic (CD11b and CD14) and myeloid antigens (CD15) are only rarely expressed. Nuclear TdT and B (CD19 and CD20) and T (CD2, CD5, and CD7) antigens are almost always absent.

Caution should be exercised when interpreting flow cytometric expression of platelet antigens on blasts. Nonspecific binding of platelets to blasts may result in typically low-intensity staining of some or all blasts for CD41, CD42, and CD61.[77] Manual immunofluorescence examination of the blasts for true linear membrane staining (vs focal globular staining with platelet binding) or immunohistochemical demonstration of cytoplasmic CD61 or factor VIII staining in the blasts in the marrow biopsy specimen or aspirate smear should be performed to confirm blast membrane staining for platelet antigens. Lastly, M7 AMLs may express erythroid-associated antigens (glycophorin A), whereas M6 AMLs can express platelet antigens (CD41 and CD42), probably reflecting the close relation of normal erythroid and megakaryocytic differentiation.[22,74] Insistence on first excluding M6 AML on the basis of FAB morphologic criteria should clarify such cases.

AML with Erythroid Differentiation (AML M6)

The acute erythroblastic leukemias are uncommon, comprising no more than 4% of all AMLs. The FAB system currently classifies these leukemias entirely by morphologic and cytochemical criteria, although it is now recognized that some AML M6 types (AML M6b) show minimal differentiation and must be identified by immunophenotypic means.[22,39] The FAB system will be modified so that pure erythroblastic leukemias will be classified as M6b, with the original classification being M6a.[24] Typically, M6 AML is variably positive for CD13, CD33, and/or CD34 and negative for CD15. Erythroid antigens, such as GPA and cytoplasmic hemoglobin, are found in a majority of cases, although any one antigen has a significant lack of sensitivity. Megakaryocyte-associated antigens (CD41 and CD61) may occasionally be seen in M6 AML, perhaps reflecting the close lineage association between normal erythropoiesis and megkaryocytopoiesis.[22,74,78]

Other Correlations of Immunophenotype with Morphology

The correlation between immunophenotype and FAB in other AML subsets is quite poor, although there are some general associations between expression of particular markers and pattern of differentiation. CD117, for example, is expressed more frequently in AML blasts with myeloid differentiation (FAB M0, M1, M2, and M3) and is very infrequently expressed in blasts with monocytic or megakaryocytic differentiation (M5 [particularly M5b AML] and M7).[11,13,15] In contrast, CD4, CD14, and CD15 are more often seen in monocytic leukemias, with CD15 expression in particular associated with M5b, AML whereas CD34 expression is infrequent in both monocytic leukemias and in M3 AML. CD2 and CD19 are seen with increased frequency in M3 and in AML M4eo. In the latter, almost all cases express CD2 and/or CD19. [79-81]

Correlations of Immunophenotype with Genotype in AML

In general, with the exception of APL, neither morphology nor phenotype is strongly predictive of genotype in AML. The best known and clearest association is that of APL with the t(15;17) translocation. Not only does this type of AML have a distinct morphology, but it also has a characteristic immunophenotype. The characteristic phenotype is CD13[+]CD33[+], without CD34, HLA-DR, or CD14. Lack of HLA-DR expression is a clue to a patient having APL but is not in itself diagnostic. In addition, the blasts in microgranular APL may express CD2.[78,80,82,83]

Other genotypes associated with somewhat distinctive phenotypes include AML with the t(8;21) translocation in which the leukemic blasts characteristically show strong CD34 expression, with weak expression of CD19 and/or expression of CD56 (see **Figure 10-5**, p 356). These blasts lack CD14 or CD4 expression.[71,78,84]

In AML M4eo associated with the inv[16] cytogenetic lesion, the blasts express either CD34 and/or CD13 with CD14/CD4. In addition, the blasts generally express CD2 or CD19.[78,80] However, expression of any single antigen is not predictive of genotype; CD19 expression is also seen in AML lacking the t[8;21] translocation, as is CD2 in cases lacking a t[15;17] translocation.[81,85]

Translocations involving 11q23 are recurring abnormalities seen in both AML and ALL, and in both cases the *MLL* gene is involved. AML blasts which harbor 11q23 lesions almost always show myelomonocytic differentiation. The leukemic blasts characteristically express CD15, CD64, and dim CD4, as well as CD13 and CD33. CD34 is expressed in a minority of cases. However, this phenotype is also frequently seen in M4/M5 cases without 11q23 abnormalities and therefore is not specific for this entity.[78,86,87]

Specific Immunophenotypic Subtypes of AML

CD56 expression is well-recognized in AML and has been associated with monocytic differentiation and background dysplasia.[88] Additionally, rare CD56[+]acute leukemias show distinctive features. In some cases these patients present with primarily extramedullary disease and only subsequently develop marrow involvement. The course is characteristically aggressive. The blasts express CD7, CD33, CD34, and often HLA-DR, with or without cytoplasmic

CD3, as well as CD56.[31,89] Other patients present with disease that morphologically resembles the microgranular variant of APL, although there is no underlying t[15;17] translocation. In these patients the blasts express CD56 and myeloid markers and lack expression of HLA-DR.[90]

Correlation of Immunophenotype with Prognosis

There are conflicting results regarding the prognostic importance of immunophenotype in AML. These differing results may in part be due to different antibodies used, definition of antigen expression, patient treatment groups, and treatment type. Historically, CD34 has been associated with worse outcome in adult AML, but this may be through its high association with other markers of poor prognosis, such as expression of *p*-glycoprotein.[91,92] Other markers that have been implicated as portending poor prognosis include CD7, CD2, and CD11c, although no consistent association has been found between their expression and response to therapy.[35,78,80,93-95]

Acute Mixed Lineage, Biphenotypic, and Undifferentiated Leukemias

Modern immunophenotyping has made the diagnosis of acute undifferentiated leukemia very rare. However, because of the lack of specificity of many of the antigens, a significant minority of patients with ALL with myeloid antigen coexpression (myeloid antigen-positive ALL) and AML with lymphoid antigen coexpression (lymphoid antigen-positive AML) are seen. Although there is some degree of controversy, most cases of lymphoid antigen-positive AML and myeloid antigen-positive ALL behave like pure AMLs and ALLs, respectively, when corrected for age and cytogenetic findings. This includes responses to therapies tailored for ALL or AML. The approach to the differential diagnosis of these patients has been discussed above. To briefly reiterate, the laboratory worker should include consideration of patient age, morphology, and/or cytochemistry, along with the relative predominance of either myeloid or lymphoid antigens and their intensities; for example, a patient with multiple bright lymphoid antigens with one dim myeloid antigen probably has ALL.

With these excluded, there are rare cases of acute mixed lineage leukemia that do not have a predominant AML or ALL differentiation, as well as rare cases of true biphenotypic leukemia, where some of the blasts phenotype as myeloblasts and others as lymphoblasts.

The diagnosis of acute mixed lineage leukemia requires the following:

- morphology of M0, L1, or L2 (no Auer rods);
- negative cytochemistries (specific and nonspecific esterases and Sudan black); and
- essentially equivalent expression in numbers and intensities of myeloid and lymphoid antigens, as assessed by both membrane and cytoplasmic antigen analysis.

The diagnosis of biphenotypic acute leukemia requires identification of 2 blast populations, one expressing myeloid markers and the other expressing lymphoid markers (**Figure 10-6**).

The diagnosis of acute undifferentiated leukemia requires the following:

- morphology of M0, L1, or L2 (no Auer rods);
- lack of expression of standard cytochemistries; and
- lack of reactivity with an extended antigen profile of well-defined T, B, megakaryocytic, myelomonocytic, and erythroid antigens, including cytoplasmic antigens (see **Table 10-1**, p 345).

The blasts may express antigens that have very low specificity for lineage, such as TdT, HLA-DR, CD7, and CD34.

The definition of these entities will be to a certain degree arbitrary, and there may be multiple possible ways to define them. The key point for the laboratory worker is to pick a method and stick with it.

Multidrug Resistance

One of the primary causes of failure of chemotherapy of leukemias and lymphomas is the development of drug resistance by the tumor cells. Mechanisms of drug resistance can be considered broadly as follows.

- Decreased delivery of drug to target
- Dimished vascular supply to tumor
- Efflux of drug from the cell (p-glycoprotein and related efflux pumps)
- Increased drug catabolism by the cell
- Increased resistance of target to drug
    Mutated target proteins
    Increased resistance to chemotherapy-mediated apoptosis

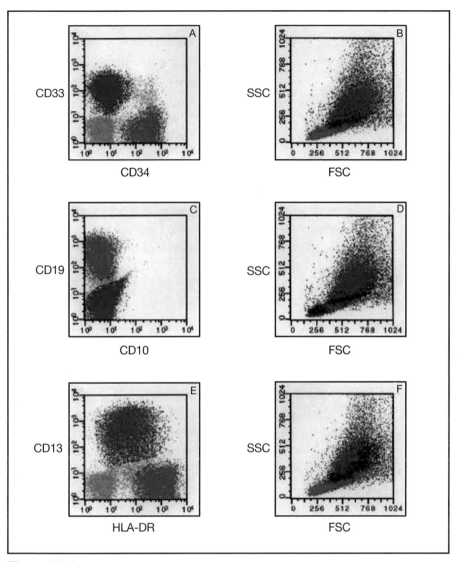

Figure 10-6

Biphenotypic Acute Leukemia. In this unusual case, the marrow was essentially 100% replaced by leukemic blasts with distinct morphology. There was a population of small blasts with scant cytoplasm and quite indistinct nucleoli that resembled lymphoblasts, and a second population of larger blasts with more abundant cytoplasm, some with a few cytoplasmic granules. Staining of this case showed 2 quite distinct blast phenotypes. The phenotype is shown in the left panel in each case. Backgating on the distinct phenotypic populations identified allows identification of the light scattering properties of each blast subset (corresponding right panel). **A & B.** CD33 versus CD34. A distinct population of CD34-positive/CD33-negative blasts is identified (green population) which is seen to have low SSC on backgating. A second population of CD33-positive/CD34-negative cells is present (blue population). These are larger with more granularity when examined by light scattering properties (B). **C & D:** CD19 versus CD10: The smaller blasts (green) express CD19 but not CD10. The larger blasts (blue) are negative for both markers. **E & F:** CD13 versus HLA-DR. The smaller blasts (green) are HLA-DR-positive and CD13 negative. In contrast the larger blasts (blue) are positive for both markers.

One of the most widely studied mechanisms of drug resistance is that mediated by the multidrug resistance protein (MDR1 or P-glycoprotein). The *MDR1* gene encodes an energy-dependent efflux pump, which can pump numerous chemically unrelated substances, including daunomycin, which is key in AML therapy, from the cell. [96] P-glycoprotein expression has been associated with increased resistance to therapy and poor clinical outcome in many studies of patients with AML.[92,97-99] One of the reasons there is particular interest in P-glycoprotein-mediated resistance is that drugs such as cyclosporine A or its nonimmunosuppressive analogue PSC 833 can block P-glycoprotein–mediated drug efflux in vitro and thus may be useful adjuncts in overcoming drug resistance in vivo. In fact, the first large, phase III, randomized trial examining the effect of cyclosporine A on outcome in AML found that addition of cyclosporine A improved clinical response and overall survival among patients with high-risk AML.[100]

However, 2 factors currently limit the utility of measuring MDR1 expression in the clinical laboratory. First, MDR1 measurement is technically difficult because of its low level of expression on leukemic blasts, as well as its expression on other cells, such as suppressor T cells and natural killer cells. The consensus recommendation is to use 2 methods of analysis (eg, protein expression and functional drug efflux) to analyze MDR1 on clinical samples.[101] However, even with multiple methods, it is difficult to attain interlaboratory standardization of results. Thus, the current inherent difficulty in comparing results from one laboratory to another precludes the routine measurement of MDR1 in clinical laboratories. Second, drug resistance in AML is highly complex, involving efflux-mediated resistance conferred by a variety of transmembrane transporters and also other mechanisms, such as resistance to apoptosis.[102-107] This complexity is highlighted in the recent trial with cyclosporine A as an adjunct to AML therapy in which incorporation of cyclosporine A benefited not only patients with MDR1$^+$ AML but also those with MDR1$^-$ disease. Until both technical and biologic issues are better understood, routine measurement of drug resistance is not warranted in a clinical flow cytometry laboratory.

Minimal Residual Disease (MRD)

Cytoreductive chemotherapy allows the majority of leukemias to be put into clinical complete remission after one course of induction chemotherapy.

However, essentially all of these patients will subsequently relapse and die of their disease unless further systemic therapy is given. This is because residual disease is still present after successful induction chemotherapy, although the tumor burden has fallen below that detected by morphologic examination of the marrow (< 5% marrow blasts). Historically, following induction therapy, patients are treated with consolidation with or without intensification therapy for a certain number of cycles before they are considered cured of their disease. However, using standard morphologic approaches, it is not possible to determine whether the patient's tumor burden is falling, stable, or slowly rising during this time. As a result, therapies tailored to the tumor response to therapy have not been possible. The goal of MRD testing is to assess more accurately the tumor burden in the patient and thus better determine the type of therapy needed by each individual patient in the future. Therefore, one issue with analysis of MRD by flow cytometry or other methods is the need to establish the clinical significance of differences in MRD with large multicenter trials. A second issue and a corollary of the first is that the methods used to detect MRD need to be standardized. Several issues need to be studied, including the extent and combination of the various monoclonal antibodies, cytometry calibration, and the gating protocols needed for cell identification. Unless these are dealt with adequately, it will be difficult to define the value of flow cytometry-based MRD detection and reproducibly define MRD routinely in the clinical flow laboratory.

Three major techniques for MRD testing have been advocated:

- immunophenotyping
- detection of cells with karyotypic abnormalities by cytogenetics or fluorescence in situ hybridization (FISH) techniques and
- detection of genetic abnormalities with polymerase chain reaction (PCR).

The sensitivity of detection of abnormal karyotypes in malignant cells by classical cytogenetics or FISH techniques tends to be quite low (approximately 1% to 5%) unless marrow is manipulated to enrich for leukemic cells. PCR-based molecular methods are very sensitive and may be particularly useful if serial MRD measurements are made to assess whether the tumor burden is going up, is stabilized, or is going down. Several reviews discuss PCR-based MRD assays.[108-110] MRD detection with both flow cytometry- and PCR-based methodologies may be useful in ALL monitoring because the 2 technologies are to some extent complimentary, with flow cytometry being informative in some cases that lack a genotypic marker to follow and vice versa.[111]

Multiparameter flow cytometry-based MRD detection relies on the identification of cells with phenotypes not normally seen or that are present only at much lower levels in bone marrow, blood, or other tissue sites (eg, cerebrospinal fluid). Several investigators have shown that ALL and AML frequently show atypical antigen profiles, and these atypical phenotypes (leukemia-associated phenotypes) can be exploited to detect small numbers of leukemic cells (from 1 in 10^2 to 1 in 10^4 cells) in otherwise morphologically normal marrow.[109,112] Initial results of flow-based MRD testing have clearly shown that detection of leukemic cells in patients whose marrow is in morphologic remission is associated with an increased risk of subsequent relapse in both AML and ALL.[6,12,28,65,113-115]

In AML, specific leukemia-associated phenotypes have been exploited for MRD detection. These include expression of nonmyeloid antigens (eg, the T-cell associated antigens CD2 or CD7), asynchronous expression of myeloid antigens (eg, CD56 with CD34), overexpression of myeloid antigens, and absence of expression of myeloid antigens.[109,113,115-117] These all require that a specific neoplastic phenotype be identified at diagnosis for an individual leukemia, as well as a knowledge of the frequency of unusual phenotypes among normal bone marrow progenitor cells. $CD7^+$ myeloid cells, for example, can make up a small fraction of normal marrow constituents and should not be confused with neoplastic $CD7^+$ AML blasts.

In ALL, specific leukemia-associated phenotypes have also been used to identify residual disease.[115,118] Among patients with T-lineage ALL, detection of immature T lymphoblasts at even very low percentages in the marrow has been associated with MRD because such immature T cells are not a normal marrow constituent. In patients with B-precursor ALL, the situation is slightly more complex, because normal bone marrow contains a small percentage of nonmalignant B-cell precursor cells (often called hematogones [HGs]), which can be confused not only morphologically but also immunophenotypically with B-lineage ALL blasts.

HGs are $CD19^+/CD10^+$ B-cell precursors (surface Ig-negative) with a subset expressing TdT and CD20 and CD34.[119] The normal HG population can expand, particularly in marrow in pediatric patients recovering from chemotherapy, as well as in some viral and reactive states.[7] Therefore, MRD detection in B-lineage ALL must be able to differentiate normal HGs from leukemic blasts. This can be achieved because of the presence of qualitative differences in the staining pattern between leukemic blasts and normal HGs that can be detected with multiparameter flow cytometry (**Figure 10-7**).[120] Normal HG differentiation is highly reproducible and shows different stages of differentiation with characteristic staining patterns (eg, from bright $CD10^+/CD20^-$ to dimmer $CD10^+$/dim $CD20^+$ to bright $CD20^+/CD10^-$, with the latter often having a minor fraction of polyclonal sIg expression).[4] In contrast, leukemic blasts show

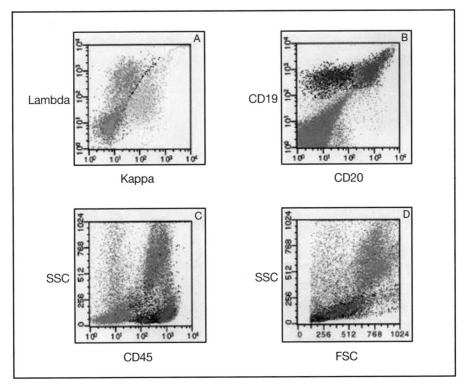

Figure 10-7

Identification of hematogones in the bone marrow. Hematogones (normal B-cell precursors) are present in all marrows in small numbers. The percent of hematogones may be increased quite dramatically, particularly in pediatric ALL patients after chemotherapy. These large numbers of hematogones can cause confusion with leukemic blasts, but phenotyping can aid in their distinction. **A.** Bone marrow stained with CD19, kappa and lambda. A CD19 gate has been applied, so only CD19-positive cells are shown. As well as kappa+ (orange) and lambda+ (purple) cells, some of the CD19+ cells identified lack surface immunoglobulin (red population). These cells either represent normal hematogones, or leukemic blasts. **B, C, D.** The same marrow stained with CD19, CD20 and CD45. **B.** Staining with CD19 and CD20 shows that the CD19+ cells have a range of CD20 expression from negative (blue population) to positive (green population). This range of expression of CD20 is characteristic of hematogones. **C.** The same CD19+/CD20-positive and negative populations can be readily identified with CD45 staining. The CD20+ cells (green) show bright CD45 expression characteristic of mature lymphoid cells, while the CD19-negative population shows dim CD45 expression (blue). **D.** Distinct light scattering properties of the B-cell populations identifed. The CD19+/CD20+ B-cells show low SSC and intermediate FSC characteristic of mature lymphoid cells. In contrast the CD19+/CD20- cells show very low FSC. This low FSC is characteristic of hematogones, and is different from the higher FSC seen with leukemic blasts.

qualitative differences in staining, such as higher levels of expression of CD19 and CD10 and lower expression of TdT compared with normal HGs. In addition, leukemic blasts tend to show uniform expression of antigens, in contrast to variable expression among HGs.[121,122] Such phenotypic differences can be exploited to detect MRD and reliably distinguish it from normal HG after therapy for B-precursor ALL.[4,6,121,123,124]

Flow DNA Analysis

Unlike in non-Hodgkin's lymphomas, DNA analysis appears to have a better-defined role in the prognostication of ALLs.[125] However, in AMLs and, increasingly, in ALLs, cytogenetic and molecular analysis allows a better discrimination of DNA lesions. The latter can detect translocations and/or small quantitative changes that are prognostically adverse in ALL (t[9;22], t[8;14], t[4;11], t[1;19]) and favorable (t[8;21], t[15;17], inv[16]) or less favorable (+8, t[9;22], –5q, –7q, and other random translocations) in AML.[126-128] These would not be detected with flow cytometric DNA analysis because of the lack of a sufficient quantitative change in total DNA (> 4 chromosomes). In addition, the cytogenetic approach allows quantitation of DNA through a chromosome count.

Cytogenetic analysis does have some technical drawbacks compared with flow cytometric DNA analysis. It is slower, analyzes only a handful of cells, is labor intensive, and is more costly on a case-by-case basis. In addition, cytogenetic analysis may be unsuccessful if the cells of interest do not grow. Quantitation of DNA by flow cytometric or karyotypic analysis has indicated some promise of prognostically useful information in ALL. Look et al[129] evaluated 205 standard-risk childhood ALLs (white blood cell count < 10^6/microliter; non-T non-B phenotype; no mediastinal or central nervous system involvement). Patients with hyperdiploidy (DI ≥ 1.16 or ≥ 53 average chromosomes) had a significantly better prognosis than those with DIs in the diploid or peridiploid region (1.01-1.15). An S-phase fraction (SPF) of 6.8% or less predicted a significantly better induction of remission and continuous complete remission. However, only a DNA Index (DI) of 1.16 or greater remained significant for continuous complete remission after multivariate analysis.

A later study by this group was based on karyotypic analysis of 722 childhood ALLs of all types.[130] These investigators found that hyperdiploidy (> 50 chromosomes) was associated with a significantly greater length of continuous complete remission than diploidy, pseudodiploidy, or hyperdiploidy of 50 or fewer chromosomes. However, after multivariate analysis, only the leukocyte count and presence or absence of a chromosomal translocation were found to be independent prognostic features. Unlike the patient group in the earlier study, this patient group was treated with several different protocols.

The pediatric oncology group evaluated karyotype with the outcome of 685 early pre-B (CD10$^+$/cyt. mu$^-$) and pre-B (cyt. mu$^+$) childhood ALLs.[131] These patients were treated with a uniform chemotherapeutic protocol. Karyotypic hyperdiploidy (either > 46 or > 50 chromosomes) was not a significant predictor of continuous complete remission in either type of ALL. Pseudodiploidy was independently correlated with a shorter continuous complete remission in early pre-B, but not pre-B, ALL. In adults karyotypic hyperdiploidy (> 50 chromosomes) has been correlated with greater continuous complete remission and survival.[126]

In ALL or AML, the proliferative fraction has not been demonstrated to be a reliable independent predictor of continuous complete remission. Similarly, the flow DNA ploidy status of AML appears to have no current value. The flow cytometric DNA and/or karyotypic ploidy status does appear to have some predictive value of the duration of continuous complete remission. However, in ALL not all studies agree as to the range of ALLs in which ploidy is an independent prognostic feature. Lastly, only karyotypic analysis is able to define the small prognostically significant DNA lesions, which are not detectable by current flow cytometric DNA analysis. Future studies, with uniform protocols and including large numbers of patients, will be necessary to truly define the use of flow cytometric DNA analysis in acute leukemias.

References

1. Borowitz M, Rubnitz J, Nash M, et al. Surface antigen phenotype can predict TEL-AML1 rearrangement in childhood B-precursor ALL: a Pediatric Oncology Group study. *Leukemia*. 1998;12:1764–1770.

2. Borowitz M, Hunger S, Carroll A, et al. Predictability of the t(1;19)(q23;p13) from surface antigen phenotype: implications for screening cases of childhood acute lymphoblastic leukemia for molecular analysis. A Pediatric Oncology Group Study. *Blood*. 1993;82:1086–1091.

3. Rothe G, Schmitz G. Consensus protocol for the flow cytometric immunophenotyping of hematopoietic malignancies. *Leukemia*. 1996;10:877–895.

4. Weir EG, Cowan K, Le Beau P, Borowitz MJ. A limited antibody panel can distinguish B-precursor acute lymphoblastic leukemia from normal B precursors with four color flow cytometry: implications for residual disease detection. *Leukemia.* 1999;13:558–567.

5. Dworzak MN, Fritsch G, Froschl G, et al. Four-color flow cytometric investigation of terminal deoxynucleotidyl transferase-positive lymphoid precursors in pediatric bone marrow: CD79a expression precedes CD19 in early B-cell ontogeny. *Blood.* 1998;92:3203–3209.

6. Farahat N, Morilla A, Owusu-Ankomah K, et al. Detection of minimal residual disease in B-lineage acute lymphoblastic leukaemia by quantitative flow cytometry. *Br J Haematol.* 1998;101:158–164.

7. Rimsza LM, Larson RS, Foucar K, et al. Florid hematogone proliferations can be distinguished from B-lineage ALL by immunophenotypic and architectural features. *Am J Clin Pathol.* 2000;114:66-75.

8. Pileri SA, Ascani S, Milani M, et al. Acute leukaemia immunophenotyping in bone-marrow routine sections. *Br J Haematol.* 1999;105:394–401.

9. Borowitz M, Guenther K, Shults K, et al. Immunophenotyping of acute leukemia by flow cytometric analysis: use of CD45 and right-angle light scatter to gate on leukemic blasts in three-color analysis. *Am J Clin Pathol.* 1993;100:534–540.

10. Stewart CC, Behm FG, Carey JL, et al. U.S.-Canadian consensus recommendations on the immunophenotypic analysis of hematologic neoplasia by flow cytometry: selection of antibody combinations. *Cytometry.* 1997;30:231–235.

11. Bene M, Bernier M, Casasnovas R, et al. The reliability and specificity of c-kit for the diagnosis of acute myeloid leukemias and undifferentiated leukemias. *Blood.* 1998;92:596–599.

12. Campana D. Monitoring minimal residual disease in acute leukemia: expectations, possibilities and initial clinical results. *Int J Clin Lab Res.* 1994;24:132–138.

13. Cascavilla N, Musto P, D'Arena G, et al. CD117 (c-kit) is a restricted antigen of acute myeloid leukemia and characterizes early differentiative levels of M5 FAB subtype. *Haematologica.* 1998;83:392–397.

14. Larson R, McCurley T. CD4 predicts nonlymphocytic lineage in acute leukemia: insights from analysis of 125 cases using two-color flow cytometry. *Am J Clin Pathol.* 1995;104:204–211.

15. Nomdedeu J, Mateu R, Altes A, et al. Enhanced myeloid specificity of CD 117 compared with CD13 and CD33. *Leuk Res.* 1999;23:341–347.

16. Coustan-Smith E, Behm FG, Hurwitz CA, et al. N-CAM (CD56) expression by CD34+ malignant myeloblasts has implications for minimal residual disease detection in acute myeloid leukemia. *Leukemia.* 1993;7:853–858.

17. Pui CH, Behm FG, Crist WM. Clinical and biologic relevance of immunologic marker studies in childhood acute lymphoblastic leukemia. *Blood.* 1993;82:343–362.

18. Michiels JJ, Adriaansen HJ, Hagemeijer A, et al. TdT positive B-cell acute lymphoblastic leukaemia (B-ALL) without Burkitt characteristics. *Br J Haematol.* 1988;68:423–426.

19. Finley J, Borcherding W. Acute B-lymphocytic leukemia with L1 morphology: a report of two pediatric cases. *Leukemia.* 1987;2:60–62.

20. Viswanatha DS, Foucar K, Berry B, et al. Blastic mantle cell leukemia: an unusual variant of blastic mantle cell lymphoma. *Mod Pathol.* 2000;13:825–833.

21. Uckun F, Gaynon P, Sensel M, et al. Clinical features and treatment outcome of childhood T-lineage acute lymphoblastic leukemia according to the apparent maturational stage of T-lineage leukemic blasts: a Children's Cancer Group Study. *J Clin Oncol.* 1997;15:2214–2221.

22. Linari S, Vannucchi AM, Ciolli S, et al. Coexpression of erythroid and megakaryocytic genes in acute erythroblastic (FAB M6) and megakaryoblastic (FAB M7) leukaemias. *Br J Haematol.* 1998;102:1335–1337.

23. Mazzella FM, Kowal-Vern A, Shrit MA, et al. Acute erythroleukemia: evaluation of 48 cases with reference to classification, cell proliferation, cytogenetics, and prognosis. *Am J Clin Pathol.* 1998;110:590–598.

24. Goldberg SL, Noel P, Klumpp TR, et al. The erythroid leukemias: a comparative study of erythroleukemia (FAB M6) and Di Guglielmo disease. *Am J Clin Oncol.* 1998;21:42–47.

25. Sieff C, Bicknell D, Caine G, et al. Antigen expression on normal and leukaemic erythroid precursors. *Hamatologie und Bluttransfusion.* 1983;28:397–402.

26. Drach D, Drach J, Glassl H, et al. Flow cytometric detection of cytoplasmic antigens in acute leukemias: implications for lineage assignment. *Leuk Res.* 1993;17:455–461.

27. Janossy G, Coustan-Smith E, Campana D. The reliability of cytoplasmic CD3 and CD22 antigen expression in the immunodiagnosis of acute leukemia: a study of 500 cases. *Leukemia.* 1989;3:170–181.

28. Drach J, Drach D, Glassl H, et al. Flow cytometric determination of atypical antigen expression in acute leukemia for the study of minimal residual disease. *Cytometry.* 1992;13:893–901.

29. Urbano-Ispizua A, Matutes E, Villamor N, et al. The value of detecting surface and cytoplasmic antigens in acute myeloid leukaemia. *Br J Haematol.* 1992;81:178–183.

30. Groeneveld, TE, Marvelde JG, van den Beemd MWM, et al. Flow cytometric detection of intracellular antigens for immunophenotyping of normal and malignant leukocytes. *Leukemia.* 1996;10:1383–1389.

31. Suzuki R, Yamamoto K, Seto M, et al. CD7+ and CD56+ myeloid/natural killer cell precursor acute leukemia: a distinct hematolymphoid disease entity. *Blood.* 1997;90:2417–2428.

32. Syrjala MT, Tiirikainen M, Jansson SE, et al. Flow cytometric analysis of terminal deoxynucleotidyl transferase. *Am J Clin Pathol.* 1993;99:298–303.

33. Huard TK. Clinically useful nontraditional applications of flow cytometry. In: Keren, DF, et al, eds. *Flow Cytometry and Clinical Diagnosis.* Chicago, IL: American Society of Clinical Pathologists Press; 1994;390–424.

34. Benedetto P, Mertelsmann R, Szatrowski TH, et al. Prognostic significance of terminal deoxynucleotidyl transferase activity in acute nonlymphoblastic leukemia. *J Clin Oncol.* 1986;4:489–495.

35. Legrand O, Perrot JY, Simonin G, et al. Adult biphenotypic acute leukaemia: an entity with poor prognosis which is related to unfavourable cytogenetics and P-glycoprotein over-expression. *Br J Haematol.* 1998;100:147–155.

36. Parreira A, Pombo de Oliveira MS, Matutes E, et al. Terminal deoxynucleotidyl transferase positive acute myeloid leukaemia: an association with immature myeloblastic leukaemia. *Br J Haematol.* 1988;69:219–224.

37. Bennett JM, Catovsky D, Daniel MT, et al. Proposal for the recognition of minimally differentiated acute myeloid leukaemia (AML-MO). *Br J Haematol.* 1991;78:325–329.

38. Bennett JM, Catovsky D, Daniel MT, et al. Criteria for the diagnosis of acute leukemia of megakaryocyte lineage (M7). A report of the French-American-British Cooperative Group. *Ann Intern Med.* 1985;103:460–462.

39. Bennett JM, Catovsky D, Daniel MT, et al. Proposed revised criteria for the classification of acute myeloid leukemia. A report of the French-American-British Cooperative Group. *Ann Intern Med.* 1985;103:620–625.

40. Garand R, Duchayne E, Blanchard D, et al. Minimally differentiated erythroleukaemia (AML M6 'variant'): a rare subset of AML distinct from AML M6. Groupe Francais d'Hematologie Cellulaire. *Br J Haematol.* 1995;90:868–875.

41. Bene MC, Castoldi G, Knapp W, et al. Proposals for the immunological classification of acute leukemias. *Leukemia.* 1995;9:1783–1786.

42. Hann IM, Richards SM, Eden OB, et al. Analysis of the immunophenotype of children treated on the Medical Research Council United Kingdom ALL Trial X1 (MRCUK ALL X1) . *Leukemia.* 1998;12:1249–1255.

43. Knapp W, Strobl H, Majdic O. Flow cytometric analysis of cell-surface and intracellular antigens in leukemia diagnosis. *Cytometry.* 1994;18:187–198.

44. Khalidi H, Chang K, Medeiros J, et al. Acute lymphoblastic leukemia survey of immunophenotype, French-American-British classification, frequency of myeloid antigen expression, and karyotypic abnormalities in 210 pediatric and adult cases. *Am J Clin Pathol.* 1999;111:467–476.

45. Lauria F, Raspadori D, Martinelli G, et al. Increased expression of myeloid antigen markers in adult acute lymphoblastic leukaemia patients: diagnostic and prognostic implications. *Br J Haematol.* 1994;87:286–292.

46. Pui C, Rubnitz J, Hancock M, et al. Reappraisal of the clinical and biologic significance of myeloid-associated antigen expression in childhood acute lymphoblastic leukemia. *J Clin Oncol.* 1998;16:3768–3773.

47. Czuczman M, Dodge R, Stewart C, et al. Value of immunophenotype in intensively treated adult acute lymphoblastic leukemia: Cancer and Leukemia Group B Study 8364. *Blood.* 1999;93:3931–3939.

48. Nakase K, Sartor M, Bradstock K. Detection of myeloperoxidase by flow cytometry in acute leukemia. *Cytometry.* 1998;34:198–202.

49. Hunger SP. Chromosomal translocations involving the *E2A* gene in acute lymphoblastic leukemia: clinical features and molecular pathogenesis. *Blood.* 1996;87:1211–1224.

50. Pui CH, Raimondi SC, Hancock ML, et al. Immunologic, cytogenetic, and clinical characterization of childhood acute lymphoblastic leukemia with the t(1;19)(q23;p13) or its derivative. *J Clin Oncol.* 1994;12:2601–2606.

51. Sang B-C, Shi L, Dias P, et al. Monoclonal antibodies specific to the acute lymphoblastic leukemia t(1;19)-associated E2A/pbx1 chimeric protein: characterization and diagnostic utility. *Blood.* 1997;89:2909–2914.

52. Berendes P, Hoogeveen A, van Dijk M, et al. Specific immunologic recognition of the *tumor-specific* E2A-PBX1 fusion-point antigen in t(1;19)-positive pre-B cells. *Leukemia.* 1995;9:1321–1327.

53. Ludwig WD, Rieder H, Bartram CR, et al. Immunophenotypic and genotypic features, clinical characteristics, and treatment outcome of adult pro-B acute lymphoblastic leukemia: results of the German multicenter trials GMALL 03/87 and 04/89. *Blood.* 1998;92:1898–1909.

54. Behm FG, Raimondi SC, Frestedt JL, et al. Rearrangement of the MLL gene confers a poor prognosis in childhood acute lymphoblastic leukemia, regardless of presenting age. *Blood.* 1996;87:2870–2877.

55. Chen CS, Sorensen PH, Domer PH, et al. Molecular rearrangements on chromosome 11q23 predominate in infant acute lymphoblastic leukemia and are associated with specific biologic variables and poor outcome. *Blood.* 1993;81:2386–2393.

56. Uckun F, Sather H, Gaynon P, et al. Clinical features and treatment outcome of children with myeloid antigen positive acute lymphoblastic leukemia: a report from the Children's Cancer Group. *Blood.* 1997;90:28–35.

57. Borowitz M, Shuster J, Carroll A, et al. Prognostic significance of fluorescence intensity of surface marker expression in childhood B-precursor acute lymphoblastic leukemia. A Pediatric Oncology Group Study. *Blood.* 1997;89:3960–3966.

58. Uckun F, Sensel M, Sun L, et al. Biology and treatment of childhood T-lineage acute lymphoblastic leukemia. *Blood.* 1998;91:735–746.

59. Dowell BL, Borowitz MJ, Boyett JM, et al. Immunologic and clinicopathologic features of common acute lymphoblastic leukemia antigen-positive childhood T-cell leukemia. A Pediatric Oncology. *Cancer.* 1987;59:2020–2026.

60. Crist WM, Shuster JJ, Falletta J, et al. Clinical features and outcome in childhood T-cell leukemia-lymphoma according to stage of thymocyte differentiation: a Pediatric Oncology Group. *Blood.* 1988;72:1891–1897.

61. Niehues T, Kapaun P, Harms D, et al. A classification based on T cell selection-related phenotypes identifies a subgroup of childhood T-ALL with favorable outcome in the COALL studies. *Leukemia.* 1999;13:614–617.

62. Uckun F, Steinherz P, Sather H, et al. CD2 antigen expression on leukemic cells as a predictor of event-free survival after chemotherapy for T-lineage acute lymphoblastic leukemia: a Children's Cancer Group Study. *Blood.* 1996;88:4288–4295.

63. Guglielmi C, Cordone I, Boecklin F, et al. Immunophenotype of adult and childhood acute lymphoblastic leukemia: changes at first relapse and clinico-prognostic implications. *Leukemia.* 1997;11:1501–1507.

64. van Wering E, Beishuizen A, Roeffen E, et al. Immunophenotypic changes between diagnosis and relapse in childhood acute lymphoblastic leukemia. *Leukemia.* 1995;9:1523-1533.

65. Reading CL, Estey EH, Huh YO, et al. Expression of unusual immunophenotype combinations in acute myelogenous leukemia. *Blood.* 1993;81:3083–3090.

66. Terstappen L, Safford M, Konemann S, et al. Flow cytometric characterization of acute myeloid leukemia. Part II. Phenotypic heterogeneity at diagnosis. *Leukemia.* 1991;5:757–767.

67. Vinante F, Pizzolo G, Rigo A, et al. The CD4 molecule belongs to the phenotypic repertoire of most cases of acute myeloid leukemia. *Leukemia.* 1992;6:1257–1262.

68. Raife T, Lager D, Kemp J, et al. Expression of CD24 (BA-1) predicts monocytic lineage in acute myeloid leukemia. *Am J Clin Pathol* 1994;101:296–299.

69. Olweus J, Lund-Johansen F, Terstappen L. CD64/FcyRI is a granulo-monocytic lineage marker on CD34+ hematopoietic progenitor cells. *Blood.* 1995;85:2402–2413.

70. Andrieu V, Radford-Weiss I, Troussard X, et al. Molecular detection of t(8;21)/AML1-ETO in AML M1/M2: correlation with cytogenetics, morphology and immunophenotype. *Br J Haematol* 1996;92:855–865.

71. Porwit-MacDonald A, Janossy G, Ivory K, et al. Leukemia-associated changes identified by quantitative flow cytometry. IV. CD34 overexpression in acute myelogenous leukemia M2 with t(8;21). *Blood.* 1996;87:1162–1169.

72. Harris NL, Jaffe ES, Diebold J, et al. World Health Organization classification of neoplastic diseases of the hematopoietic and lymphoid tissues: report of the Clinical Advisory. *J Clin Oncol* 1999;17:3835–3849.

73. Ruiz-Arguelles GJ, Lobato-Mendizabal E, San Miguel JF, et al. Long-term treatment results for acute megakaryoblastic leukaemia patients: a multicentre study. *Br J Haematol* 1992;82:671–675.

74. Helleberg C, Knudsen H, Hansen PB, et al. CD34+ megakaryoblastic leukaemic cells are CD38-, but CD61+ and glycophorin A+: improved criteria for diagnosis of AML-M7? *Leukemia.* 1997;11:830–834.

75. Breton-Gorius J, Villeval JL, Kieffer N, et al. Limits of phenotypic markers for the diagnosis of megakaryoblastic leukemia. *Blood Cells.* 1989;15:259–277.

76. Cuneo A, Mecucci C, Kerim S, et al. Multipotent stem cell involvement in megakaryoblastic leukemia: cytologic and cytogenetic evidence in 15 patients. *Blood.* 1989;74:1781–1790.

77. Betz SA, Foucar K, Head DR, et al. False-positive flow cytometric platelet glycoprotein IIb/IIIa expression in myeloid leukemias secondary to platelet adherence to blasts. *Blood.* 1992;79:2399–2403.

78. Creutzig U, Harbott J, Sperling C, et al. Clinical significance of surface antigen expression in children with acute myeloid leukemia: results of study AML-BFM-87. *Blood.* 1995;86:3097–3108.

79. Smith F, Lampkin B, Versteeg C, et al. Expression of lymphoid-associated cell surface antigens by childhood acute myeloid leukemia cells lacks prognostic significance. *Blood.* 1992;79:2415–2422.

80. Ball E, Davis R, Griffin J, et al. Prognostic value of lymphocyte surface markers in acute myeloid leukemia. *Blood.* 1991;77:2242–2250.

81. Khalidi H, Medeiros J, Chang K, et al. The immunophenotype of adult acute myeloid leukemia. High frequency of lymphoid antigen expression and comparison of immunophenotype, French-American-British classification, and karyotypic abnormalities. *Am J Clin Pathol.* 1998;109:211-220.

82. Biondi A, Luciano A, Bassan R, et al. CD2 expression in acute promyelocytic leukemia is associated with microgranular morphology (FAB M3v) but not with any PML gene breakpoint. *Leukemia.* 1995;9:1461–1466.

83. Tallman MS. Differentiating therapy in acute myeloid leukemia. *Leukemia.* 1996;10:1262–1268.

84. Hurwitz CA, Raimondi SC, Head D, et al. Distinctive immunophenotypic features of t(8;21)(q22;q22) acute myeloblastic leukemia in children. *Blood.* 1992;80:3182–3188.

85. Brandt J, Tisone J, Bohman J, et al. Abberant expression of CD19 as a marker of monocytic lineage in acute myelogenous leukemia. *Am J Clin Pathol.* 1997;107:283–291.

86. Baer MR, Stewart CC, Lawrence D, et al. Acute myeloid leukemia with 11q23 translocations: myelomonocytic immunophenotype by multiparameter flow cytometry. *Leukemia.* 1998;12:317–325.

87. Sorensen PH, Chen CS, Smith FO, et al. Molecular rearrangements of the MLL gene are present in most cases of infant acute myeloid leukemia and are strongly correlated with monocytic or myelomonocytic phenotypes. *J Clin Invest.* 1994;93:429–437.

88. Mann KP, DeCastro CM, Liu J, et al. Neural cell adhesion molecule (CD56)-positive acute myelogenous leukemia and myelodysplastic and myeloproliferative syndromes. *Am J Clin Pathol.* 1997;107:653–660.

89. Dunphy CH, Gregowicz AJ, Rodriguez G Jr. Natural killer cell acute leukemia with myeloid antigen expression. A previously undescribed form of acute leukemia. *Am J Clin Pathol.* 1995;104:212–215.

90. Scott AA, Head DR, Kopecky KJ, et al. HLA-DR-, CD33+, CD56+, CD16- myeloid/natural killer cell acute leukemia: a previously unrecognized form of acute leukemia potentially misdiagnosed as French-American-British acute myeloid leukemia-M3. *Blood.* 1994;84:244–255.

91. Geller R, Zahurak M, Hurwitz C, et al. Prognostic importance of immunophenotyping in adults with acute myelocytic leukaemia: the significance of the stem-cell glycoprotein CD34 (My10). *Br J Haematol.* 1990;76:340–347.

92. Leith CP, Kopecky KJ, Godwin JE, et al. Acute myeloid leukemia in the elderly: assessment of multidrug resistance (MDR1) and cytogenetics distinguishes biologic subgroups with remarkably distinct responses to standard chemotherapy. A Southwest Oncology Group study. *Blood.* 1997;89:3323–3329.

93. Kornblau S, Thall P, Huh Y, et al. Analysis of CD7 expression in acute myelogenous leukemia: martingale residual plots combined with 'optimal' cutpoint analysis reveals absence of prognostic significance. *Leukemia.* 1995;9:1735–1741.

94. Bradstock K, Matthews J, Benson E, et al. Prognostic value of immunophenotyping in acute myeloid leukemia. *Blood.* 1994;84:1220–1225.

95. Paietta E, Anderson J, Yunis J, et al. Acute myeloid leukaemia expressing the leucocyte integrin CD11b—a new leukaemic syndrome with poor prognosis: result of an ECOG database analysis. *Br J Haematol.* 1998;100:265–272.

96. Chin KV, Pastan I, Gottesman MM. Function and regulation of the human multidrug resistance gene. *Adv Cancer Res.* 1993;60:157–180.

97. Leith CP, Kopecky KJ, Chen IM, et al. Frequency and clinical significance of expression of the multidrug resistance proteins, MDR1/p-glycoprotein, MRP1 and LRP in acute myeloid leukemia. A Southwest Oncology Group study. *Blood.* 1999;94:1086–1099.

98. Campos L, Guyotat D, Archimbaud E, et al. Clinical significance of multidrug resistance P-glycoprotein expression on acute nonlymphoblastic leukemia cells at diagnosis. *Blood.* 1992;79:473-476.

99. Legrand O, Simonin G, Perrot J, et al. Pgp and MRP activities using calcein-AM are prognostic factors in adult acute myeloid leukemia patients. *Blood.* 1998;91:4480–4488.

100. List AF, Kopecky KJ, Willman CL, et al. Benefit of cyclosporine (CsA) modulation of anthracycline resistance in high-risk AML: a Southwest Oncology Group (SWOG) study [abstract]. *Blood.* 1999;92:312a.

101. Beck WT, Grogan TM, Willman CL, et al. Methods to detect P-glycoprotein-associated multidrug resistance in patient tumors: consensus recommendations. *Cancer Res.* 1996;56:3010–3020.

102. Allikmets R, Schriml LM, Hutchinson A, et al. A human placenta-specific ATP-binding cassette gene (ABCP) on chromosome 4q22 that is involved in multidrug resistance. *Cancer Res.* 1998;58:5337–5339.

103. Filipits M, Pohl G, Stranzl T, et al. Expression of the lung resistance protein predicts poor outcome in de novo acute myeloid leukemia. *Blood.* 1998;91:1508–1513.

104. Filipits M, Stranzl T, Pohl G, et al. Drug resistance factors in acute myeloid leukemia: a comparative analysis. *Leukemia.* 2000;14:68–76.

105. Johnstone RW, Cretney E, Smyth MJ. P-glycoprotein protects leukemia cells against caspase-dependent, but not caspase-independent, cell death. *Blood.* 1999;93:1075-1085.

106. Kuss BJ, O'Neill GM, Eyre H, et al. ARA, a novel ABC transporter, is located at 16p13.1, is deleted in inv(16) leukemias, and is shown to be expressed in primitive hematopoietic precursors. *Genomics* 1998;51:455-458.

107. List AF. Non-P-glycoprotein drug export mechanisms of multidrug resistance. *Semin Hematol.* 1997;34:20–24.

108. Foroni L, Harrison CJ, Hoffbrand AV, et al. Investigation of minimal residual disease in childhood and adult acute lymphoblastic leukaemia by molecular analysis. *Br J Haematol.* 1999;105:7–24.

109. Yin JA, Tobal K. Detection of minimal residual disease in acute myeloid leukaemia: methodologies, clinical and biological significance. *Br J Haematol.* 1999;106:578–590.

110. Campana D, Pui CH. Detection of minimal residual disease in acute leukemia: methodologic advances and clinical significance. *Blood.* 1995;85:1416–1434.

111. Neale GA, Coustan-Smith E, Pan Q, et al. Tandem application of flow cytometry and polymerase chain reaction for comprehensive detection of minimal residual disease in childhood acute lymphoblastic leukemia. *Leukemia.* 1999;13:1221–1226.

112. Terstappen LW, Safford M, Unterhalt M, et al. Flow cytometric characterization of acute myeloid leukemia: IV. Comparison to the differentiation pathway of normal hematopoietic progenitor cells. *Leukemia.* 1992;6:993–1000.

113. San Miguel JF, Martinez A, Macedo A, et al. Immunophenotyping investigation of minimal residual disease is a useful approach for predicting relapse in acute myeloid leukemia patients. *Blood.* 1997;90:2465–2470.

114. Sievers EL, Lange BJ, Buckley JD, et al. Prediction of relapse of pediatric acute myeloid leukemia by use of multidimensional flow cytometry. *J Natl Cancer Inst.* 1996;88:1483–1488.

115. Coustan-Smith E, Behm FG, Sanchez J, et al. Immunological detection of minimal residual disease in children with acute lymphoblastic leukaemia. *Lancet.* 1998;351:550-554.

116. Macedo A, Orfao A, Gonzalez M, et al. Immunological detection of blast cell subpopulations in acute myeloblastic leukemia at diagnosis: implications for minimal residual disease studies. *Leukemia.* 1995;9:993–998.

117. Macedo A, Orfao A, Martinez A, et al. Immunophenotype of c-kit cells in normal human bone marrow: implications for the detection of minimal residual disease in AML. *Br J Haematol.* 1995;89:338–341.

118. Ciudad J, San Miguel JF, Lopez-Berges MC, et al. Prognostic value of immunophenotypic detection of minimal residual disease in acute lymphoblastic leukemia. *J Clin Oncol.* 1998;16:3774–3781.

119. Dworzak MN, Fritsch G, Fleischer C, et al. Multiparameter phenotype mapping of normal and post-chemotherapy B lymphopoiesis in pediatric bone marrow. *Leukemia.* 1997;11:1266–1273.

120. Dworzak MN, Fritsch G, Fleischer C, et al. Comparative phenotype mapping of normal vs. malignant pediatric B-lymphopoiesis unveils leukemia-associated aberrations. *Exp Hematol.* 1998;26:305–313.

121. Farahat N, Lens D, Zomas A, et al. Quantitative flow cytometry can distinguish between normal and leukaemic B-cell precursors. *Br J Haematol.* 1995;91:640–646.

122. Rego EM, Tone LG, Garcia AB, et al. CD10 and CD19 fluorescence intensity of B-cell precursors in normal and leukemic bone marrow. Clinical characterization of CD10(+strong) and CD10(+weak) common acute lymphoblastic leukemia. *Leuk Res.* 1999;23:441–450.

123. Griesinger F, Piro-Noack M, Kaib N, et al. Leukaemia-associated immunophenotypes (LAIP) are observed in 90% of adult and childhood acute lymphoblastic leukaemia: detection in remission marrow predicts outcome. *Br J Haematol.* 1999;105:241–255.

124. Wells DA, Sale GE, Shulman HM, et al. Multidimensional flow cytometry of marrow can differentiate leukemic from normal lymphoblasts and myeloblasts after chemotherapy and bone marrow transplantation. *Am J Clin Pathol* 1998;110:84–94.

125. Pui C-H, Behm F, Crist W. Clinical and biologic relevance of immunologic marker studies in childhood acute lymphoblastic leukemia. *Blood.* 1993;82:343–362.

126. Hoelzer D, Gale P. Acute lymphoblastic leukemia in adults: recent progress, future directions. *Semin Hematol.* 1987;24:27–39.

127. Keating MJ, Smith TL, Kantarjian H, et al. Cytogenetic pattern in acute myelogenous leukemia: a major reproducible determinant of outcome. *Leukemia.* 1988;2:403–412.

128. Schiffer CA, Lee EJ, Takafumi T, et al. Prognostic impact of cytogenetic abnormalities in patients with de novo acute nonlymphocytic leukemia. *Blood.* 1989;73:263-270.

129. Look AT, Roberson PK, Williams DL, et al. Prognostic importance of blast cell DNA content in childhood acute lymphoblastic leukemia. *Blood.* 1985;65:1079-1086.

130. Pui CH, Williams DL, Roberson PK, et al. Correlation of karyotype and immunophenotype in childhood acute lymphoblastic leukemia. *J Clin Oncol.* 1988;6:56-61.

131. Crist W, Boyett J, Jackson J, et al. Prognostic importance of the pre-B cell immunophenotype and other presenting features of B-lineage childhood acute lymphoblastic leukemia: a Pediatric Oncology Group Study. *Blood.* 1989;74:1252-1259.

11

Flow Cytometry for Primary Immunodeficiency Diseases

Richard Schiff
Sherrie E. Schiff

Introduction

Patients with immunodeficiency diseases may present with recurrent or persistent infections, especially with opportunistic organisms, or with a bewildering variety of autoimmune and inflammatory conditions. Many of these diseases can be effectively treated, but a successful outcome requires early recognition and treatment before permanent tissue damage or severe, untreatable infections occur. The final classification of the particular immunodeficiency disease usually requires referral to a specialist in such disorders, but the physician in primary care must recognize the signs and symptoms of immune dysregulation and identify the patient who needs further evaluation.

The first human immunodeficiency disease was reported in 1952 by Colonel Ogden Bruton, who recognized that a child with recurrent infections lacked the gamma globulin fraction in his serum. Since then, a variety of congenital immunodeficiency diseases have been described, and in the last 15 years, the genetic causes of many have been elucidated. Evaluation of these experiments of nature has provided invaluable information about the normal function of the immune system.

Genetically determined immunodeficiency diseases are rare. It has been estimated that hypogammaglobulinemia occurs with a frequency of 1 in 50, 000 and
severe combined immunodeficiency (SCID) with a frequency of 1 in 500, 000
live births. The most common immune deficiency, selective immunoglobulin A
(IgA) deficiency, has a reported frequency of 1 in 300 to 1 in 3000, depending on
the population studied. The incidence of many of these diseases may be much
higher, as many of the children die of infections before immune deficiency is suspected. Early recognition is vital, for many of these diseases can be treated by
replacement immunoglobulin or cytokines, or they may be cured by bone marrow transplantation. In the near future, gene therapy will provide a cure for many
immune system defects.

Diagnosis of immunodeficiency diseases is based on clinical features and on
characterization of the immunologic defect. The use of flow cytometry has vastly
improved our ability to evaluate the cells of the immune system. In the last 20
years, many of the cell surface proteins and glycoproteins have been identified
with monoclonal antibodies. Flow cytometry using these antibodies has been
invaluable in enumerating neutrophils, monocytes, natural killer (NK) cells, and
subsets of lymphocytes. Some of the proteins are present only on activated cells.
Therefore, expression of these proteins is a marker for cell activation and proliferation, enabling flow cytometry to be used to measure cell function. If cell
membranes are made permeable, monoclonal antibodies and various chemical
dyes can bind to proteins within the cell, allowing the use of flow cytometry to
measure functions as diverse as calcium fluxes, cytokine production, and cell
death. This chapter will review the congenital, or primary, immunodeficiency
diseases and indicate how flow cytometry can be used to help make a diagnosis
and determine the appropriate therapy.

Clinical Features of Primary Immunodeficiency Diseases

The most recent classification of the primary immunodeficiency diseases
was proposed by a committee of the World Health Organization in 1997.[1] The
classification (**Table 11-1**), based on the clinical and immunologic evaluation of
patients and current knowledge of the genetic defects, undoubtedly will change
as the genetic abnormality for each disease is identified. Our concept of the
organization of the lymphocyte-mediated immune system was developed from
studies in animals. The loss of delayed hypersensitivity reactions and other

TABLE 11-1

Disorders of Humoral and Cellular Immunity

Disorder	Functional Deficiency	Cellular or Genetic Defect	Gene Defect/ Linkage
Predominantly Antibody Defects			
X-linked agamma-globulinemia	Absent antibody. No B cells. Recurrent infections.	Absent B lympho-cytes	Bruton tyrosine kinase deficiency (Btk), Xq22
X-linked agamma-globulinemia with hyper-IgM	Antibody deficiency. Low IgA and IgG.	Inability of T cells to provide switch signal to B cells	CD40 ligand defect, Xq26
Common variable immunodeficiency	Hypogammaglobu-linemia. Poor anti-body formation. Recurrent infections. Autoimmunity	Unknown; variable defects in B cells, T helper cells, or excessive T suppressor cells	Unknown
IgG subclass deficiency	May be associated with antibody defi-ciency. May have recurrent infections	Unknown: may be a defect in antigen processing, switch T cells, or switch region in heavy chain	Unknown
Poor response to polysaccharide antigens	Specific antibody deficiency. Recurrent infections.	Unknown, possibly defect in antigen processing	Unknown
Selective IgA deficiency	IgA antibody defi-ciency, allergy, autoimmunity	Possible switch defect. Possible abnormal switch T cells	Unknown, possibly 6p21.3
Transient hypogam-maglobulinemia of infancy	Prolonged physio-logic IgG trough; usually no antibody deficiency	Unknown; slow mat-uration of B and T lymphocytes. Persis-tent CD5+ B cells.	Unknown
X-linked lymphoprolif-erative syndrome Thymic hypoplasia	Abnormal response to Epstein-Barr virus, immune deficiency, malignancy	Inability of T cells to control EBV-activated B cells	Xq24-26

so-called cellular immune functions following the removal of the thymus in mice led to the identification of the thymus-derived or T lymphocyte. Similarly, studies in chickens indicated that removal of the bursa of Fabricius led to a selec-tive defect in antibody formation due to the loss of bursal or B lymphocytes. Although this concept has been immensely useful, there are few examples of a pure defect in human disease. The pattern of human disease does differ, however, depending on whether the primary defect affects the T cells, B cells,

TABLE 11-1 (continued)

Disorder	Functional Deficiency	Cellular or Genetic Defect	Gene Defect/ Linkage
Primary Defect in Cellular Immunity-Combined Immunodeficiency			
(DiGeorge anomaly)	Variable T and (secondary) B cell defects. Opportunistic infections in the most severe cases.	Developmental field defect involving all brachial arches. Variable development of the thymus	Deletion on chromosome 22q11 (80%)
Severe combined immune deficiency	Opportunistic infections. Failure to thrive. Death by age 2		
X-linked	Severe B and T cell defects	Absent T and NK cells, elevated B cells	Defect in gamma-chain of the common cytokine receptor, Xq13
JAK-3 deficiency	Severe T and B cell defects	Absent T and NK cells, elevated B cells. Signal transduction defect.	19q13.1
IL7 receptor deficiency	Severe B and T cell defects	Absent T with normal B and NK	
ZAP-70 deficiency	Severe T and variable B cell defects	CD8 lymphopenia	2q12
Adenosine deaminase deficiency	Severe B and T cell defects	Deletions or base substitutions in ADA gene	20q13-ter
Defective expression of HLA antigens	Severe B and T cell defects	Absent expression of class I antigens	TAP1 and TAP2 defects
		Absent expression of class I antigens	MCH2TA, RFX5, RFXAP
Deficiency of T cell receptors	Variable B and T cell defects	Defective expression of CD3 epsilon	11
Cellular immunodeficiency with immunoglobulins (Nezelof syndrome)	Severe T cell, variable B cell defects; autoimmune disease	Unknown; variable	Unknown
PNP deficiency	Severe T cell, variable B cell defects; autoimmune disease	Defect in gene for purine nucleoside phosphorylase	PNP gene defect, 14q13.1

phagocytic cells, or complement system. Many of the biochemical abnormalities that cause significant defects in lymphocyte function also affect other cells that

TABLE 11-1 (continued)

Disorder	Functional Deficiency	Cellular or Genetic Defect	Gene Defect/ Linkage
Other Well-defined Immune Deficiencies			
Omenn syndrome	Variable T cell and antibody defects; "GVH-like" syndrome	Recombinase activat- ing gene defect, RAG1 and RAG2	11p13
Wiskott-Aldrich syndrome	Variable T cell defect; poor antibody response to antigens, thrombocytopenia; malignancy	Defect in CD43 expression. Defi- ciency of the WASP protein involved in actin polymerization Gene identified on X-chromosome but not yet characterized.	WASP, Xp11.22- 11.23
Chronic mucocuta- neous candidiasis	Chronic Candida infections. Some with antibody deficiency.	Variable response to Candida. Possible defect in processing of mannan.	Unknown
Hyper-IgE syndrome	Excessive IgE; poor specific antibody responses	Unknown; possible defect in T cell regulation or possible over-expression of IL-4	Unknown
Ataxia-telangiectasia	Variable T and B cell defect; malignancy	Unknown; defect in DNA repair involving many cells	11q22.3
Cartilage-hair hypoplasia	Moderate-to-severe T and B cell defect	Unknown; defect in G1 cycle of many cells, including lymphocytes	Unknown

are not involved in host defense. Therefore, other abnormalities, such as cerebellar ataxia in ataxia telangiectasia, or thrombocytopenia and eczema in Wiskott-Aldrich syndrome, may provide the clue to the immunologic defect. In addition to the well-characterized immunodeficiency syndromes, immune defects may be found in a variety of neurologic and metabolic diseases, chromosomal abnormalities, and in skeletal dysplasias (**Table 11-2**).[1,2] In the majority of these diseases, the relationship between the biochemical abnormality and the immune defect is not known. In some cases, the impairment in immunity may be of clinical significance, so early recognition and diagnosis is of great importance.

TABLE 11-2

Immune Deficiencies Associated with Other Disorders

Disorder	Functional Deficiency	Cellular or Genetic Defect	Gene Defect/ Linkage
Down syndrome	Mental retardation, cardiac defects, recurrent infections	Variable antibody defects, Low IgM, abnormal DH reactions	Trisomy 21
Turner syndrome	Short stature, transient lymphoedema, recurrent infections,	Decreased IgG and IgM	XO
Bloom syndrome	Low birth weight, retarded growth, sensitivity to light, frequent infections	Decreased IgM. Decreased T cell function. Possible defect in maturation of B cell.	11q23
Fanconi's anemia	Bone marrow failure, increased leukemia, café au lait spots	Decreased IgA, decreased T and NK function	
Acrodermatitis enteropathica	Eczema, diarrhea, malabsorption, recurrent infections	Decreased T numbers and function. Impaired chemotaxis	Unknown
Anhidrotic ectodermal dysplasia	Hypohidrosis, faulty dentition	Low zinc levelsVariable antibody and DH abnormalities	
Transcobalamine 2 deficiency	Diarrhea, failure to thrive, megaloblastic anemia	Defective lymphocyte proliferation, decreased antibody formation. Defective B12 transport protein	
Glycogen storage disease, type 2	Neutropenia, recurrent infections	Neutrophil dysfunction	alpha-1,4-glucosidase deficiency

Infections in Patients with Immunodeficiency Diseases

For the most part, the pattern of susceptibility to infections in patients with immunodeficiency diseases has a specific cause that depends on the nature of the immune deficiency; however, important exceptions exist. Patients with antibody deficiency most commonly suffer from purulent bacterial infections, including pneumonia, meningitis, arthritis, sinusitis, otitis, conjunctivitis, and gastroenteritis. These infections are most frequently caused by encapsulated organisms such as *Haemophilus influenzae* and *Streptococcus pneumoniae,* but other organisms, including *Staphylococcus aureus, Meningococcus, Pseudomonas, Campylobacter, Ureaplasma,* and *Mycoplasma,* are commonly isolated. Most viral infections are adequately controlled by T lymphocytes and NK cells, but several viruses can result in devastating consequences. Poliomyelitis, often secondary to live virus vaccine, results in several cases of paralytic disease each year. Viral hepatitis, particularly hepatitis C, is particularly severe in patients with agammaglobulinemia. Another important exception is chronic meningoencephalitis caused by enteroviruses of the echovirus and coxsackievirus species, which occurs primarily in patients with X-linked agammaglobulinemia but has also occurred in a few patients with other forms of agammaglobulinemia. Some protozoal infections, notably *Giardia lamblia,* cause significant difficulty for patients with humoral immunodeficiency, and *Pneumocystis carinii* infections occasionally occur despite apparently normal T-cell function.

Patients with T-cell immunodeficiency are susceptible to a variety of opportunistic organisms. Growth failure and early death occur more frequently in these patients than in patients with humoral immunodeficiency. Oral and cutaneous candidiasis is common, and disseminated infections with *Candida* species, *Cryptococcus, Histoplasma,* and *Nocardia* occur frequently. Protozoal infections, particularly with *P. carinii,* are a frequent cause of death unless recognized and rapidly treated. *Toxoplasma* can cause chronic infections leading to blindness, and *Cryptosporidium* is a common cause of chronic diarrhea. T-cell immunity is particularly important for defense against a variety of viral infections, especially the herpesviruses: cytomegalovirus (CMV), herpes simplex virus, and varicella zoster virus. The respiratory viruses—adenovirus, parainfluenza virus, and respiratory syncytial virus—often cause fulminant pneumonia and may disseminate throughout the body. Infections with both pathogenic and nonpathogenic bacteria are a significant problem, probably because nearly all patients have associated deficiency in antibody formation. However, atypical organisms such as *Mycobacterium tuberculosis, Mycobacterium intracellulare,* and *Listeria monocytogenes* cause infections primarily in patients with cellular immunodeficiencies.

Defects in the phagocytic system and complement result in increased susceptibility to bacterial and fungal infections. Decreased numbers of phagocytes or a reduction in their ability to ingest organisms results in sepsis or disseminated infections with a variety of gram-negative and gram-positive bacteria and fungi such as *Candida albicans* and *Aspergillus.* Defective killing, as in chronic granulomatous disease, can also result in granulomatous lesions or abscesses. Absence of the early complement components results in susceptibility to gram-positive bacteria, whereas the lack of the late components leads to a high incidence of *Neisseria* infections. Defects in the early components of the complement cascade are also associated with autoimmune disease caused by failure to clear immune complexes.

Immunodeficiency Diseases with Primary Defect in Humoral Immunity

Defects in this category include a primary defect in the ability to make immunoglobulins or specific antibodies, but some of the following diseases are also characterized by T-cell defects. The genetic defect has been identified for X-linked agammaglobulinemia and X-linked hyperimmunoglobulinemia-M (hyper-IgM) syndrome, but for the majority of antibody deficiencies, the biochemical defect is unknown.

X-linked Agammaglobulinemia

Boys afflicted with X-linked agammaglobulinemia (XAG) usually present after the sixth month of life, after the transplacentally derived IgG has been catabolized.[3] They acquire pyogenic infections with high-grade bacteria such as pneumococci, *Haemophilus,* and streptococci. Unusual organisms may be seen as well, such as *Ureaplasma urealyticum,* which causes an erosive septic arthritis. Infections of the sinopulmonary tract predominate, including sinusitis, pharyngitis, otitis, bronchitis, and pneumonia, but others, such as furunculosis, arthritis, and meningitis, also frequently occur. Growth failure is not a common problem unless chronic diarrhea is present, often because of infection with *G. lamblia.* These patients handle most viral infections as well as normal hosts, but a few viruses can lead to devastating illness. Poliovirus, either wild-type or live vaccine strain, can cause paralytic disease; nearly all cases of vaccine-related paralytic poliomyelitis occur in patients with immunodeficiency. Children excrete the virus in stool for weeks to months after immunization, which increases the opportunity for the virus to mutate to a more neurotropic form. The hepatitis viruses can also cause severe, even fatal, chronic active hepatitis. Enteroviruses of the echovirus and coxsackievirus species can cause chronic meningoencephalitis.[4] This central nervous system (CNS) disease is chronic and often leads to progressive neurologic deterioration despite high doses of intravenous gamma globulin. Some patients have improved when gamma globulin has been infused directly into the cerebral ventricles,[5] but the disease can never be totally cured. Patients may also develop a dermatomyositis-like illness and progress to sclerodermatous changes with atrophic skin and joint contractures. The disease is almost exclusively confined to patients with XAG, although a few females lacking B lymphocytes and others with forms of common variable immune deficiency have also contracted this illness.

Patients with XAG have a nearly complete absence of immunoglobulins of all isotypes, although small amounts of IgM may be present. Isohemagglutinins are absent, and there is no response to immunizations with a variety of antigens, including tetanus and diphtheria, *H. influenzae, S. pneumoniae,* poliomyelitis, measles, or bacteriophage φ/χ-174. A few exceptional families have been described whose members have immunoglobulins and even some specific antibody early in life, but progress to typical XAG within a few years.[6] One family was described with genetically proven XAG in 3 affected males, the oldest of whom was 51 years old at diagnosis.[7] The mechanism of this "late-onset" illness is not known, but these observations provide a cautionary note when evaluating young infants; longitudinal follow-up is crucial for all infants suspected of having immunodeficiency.

In diagnosing XAG, the most characteristic immunologic finding is the nearly complete absence of B lymphocytes as detected by surface immunoglobulins or surface receptors CD21 (Epstein-Barr virus [EBV] receptor), CD19, or CD20. No germinal centers can be identified upon histologic examination of lymph nodes or tonsils, which accounts for the absence of these structures on physical examination. T-cell percentages are increased as a result of the loss of B cells; T-cell activity is usually normal and thymic architecture is intact. The disease is caused by an absence of an enzyme, Bruton tyrosine kinase (BTK), that is necessary for the progression of pre-B cells to mature B cells.[3,8,9] Patients have been identified with milder forms of the disease; there is a suggestion that patients with less severe manifestations have defects in the SH2 or kinase domains of the gene.[10] Identification of the gene defect is very important for genetic counseling. Because this is an X-linked disease, there is a high probability that the boy's mother is a carrier for the defect and therefore is at risk of having another boy with the same disease. Daughters of a carrier may also be carriers and at risk of having affected children. There is a high rate of spontaneous mutation, however, so it is important to evaluate the mother as well as the child to give accurate counseling.

The diagnosis of immune deficiency is based on the absence of immunoglobulins. Flow cytometry is used to indicate the absence of B lymphocytes and distinguish X-linked agammaglobulinemia from common variable immune deficiency. All of the markers found on mature B cells—CD19, CD20, and CD21—are absent. In addition, patients lack cells with surface IgM and IgD. The definitive diagnosis is now made by identifying the defect in the *BTK* gene in both the patient and his mother. Genetic testing is necessary to distinguish X-linked agammaglobulinemia from a rarer autosomal defect that is also characterized by absence of mature B lymphocytes. Several girls as well as boys have been identified who have a defect in the mu heavy-chain locus itself[11]; these patients also have a complete absence of B lymphocytes and very low levels of immunoglobulins and are at risk of developing echovirus meningoencephalitis.

X-linked Immunodeficiency with Hyper-IgM

Patients with X-linked immunodeficiency with hyper-IgM (HIM) have a clinical presentation similar to those with X-linked agammaglobulinemia. They present within the first few months of life with pyogenic infections, including pneumonia, otitis, sinusitis, and pharyngitis.[12] However, other infections may dominate. Clinically significant diarrhea occurs in up to 40% of patients[13] and they may need total parenteral nutrition to prevent failure to thrive. Chronic watery diarrhea has been associated with *Cryptosporidium* infections[14] that may lead to fatal sclerosing cholangitis. *P. carinii* pneumonia has also been reported in a significant number of patients.[13,15] In addition to *Pneumocystis*, patients with HIM have increased susceptibility to a variety of opportunistic infections, such as candidiasis, disseminated cryptococcosis, histoplasmosis, and cryptococcal meningitis, diseases that are usually associated with defects in cellular immunity.[12] This suggests that the defect might be in the T cell rather than the B cell, despite initial clinical observations.

IgG and IgA concentrations in serum are usually extremely low, and antibody responses are absent. IgM concentrations can be normal to markedly elevated, usually with a polyclonal pattern. T-lymphocyte numbers are normal by flow cytometry, and T-cell function is normal by standard assays of proliferation. B-cell numbers may be normal or slightly reduced. When stimulated with polyclonal activators such as EBV, B cells of affected patients synthesize only IgM, which is similar to the immature B cell of the neonate. This finding suggested that the defect is intrinsic to the B cell despite the clinical problems that pointed to a defect in T-cell function.

The solution to this discrepancy was found when an abnormality was identified in the ligand for CD40 (gp39), found on T cells, that interacts with CD40 on B cells.[16,17] If B cells from those patients are stimulated with anti-CD40, they produce immunoglobulins normally. Interaction of CD40 ligand (CD40-L) on T cells with CD40 delivers an anti-apoptotic signal to immature B cells. In the presence of stimulants such as phorbol esters, anti-CD20 monoclonal antibodies, or anti-IgM, binding of CD40 by anti-CD40 or CD40-L sends a progression signal to immature B cells. Engagement of CD40, in the presence of IL-4, causes B-cell proliferation, upregulates the costimulatory molecule B7, induces CD23 expression, and ultimately induces immunoglobulin class switching.[12]

CD40 is present on cells other than B cells, including thymic epithelium, follicular dendritic cells, monocytes, and macrophages, which may explain the diverse clinical manifestations that go far beyond the B-cell defect.

Distinguishing XAG from HIM may be difficult, particularly in the young child, because the IgM concentrations may initially be normal or even low. However, unlike patients with XAG, patients with hyper-IgM often have lymphoid hypertrophy. Autoimmune hematologic diseases, including hemolytic anemia, thrombocytopenia, and cyclic or persistent neutropenia, are frequent. Not every patient has had an abnormal CD40-L, and the presence of females with the hyper-IgM phenotype indicates that there is more than one genetic cause.

Flow cytometry is used to enumerate B and T lymphocytes, but it has limited utility in the diagnosis of HIM. B- and T-cell numbers are normal in the majority of patients with HIM. Recently it has been possible to use flow cytometry to demonstrate the lack of CD40-L on T lymphocytes.[18] CD40-L is present on the surface of activated $CD4^+$ T lymphocytes. Using a whole blood technique, O'Gorman and colleagues were able to demonstrate that the majority of phorbol-activated T cells expressed the CD40-L, whereas it was found on fewer than 5% of cells from patients with HIM. The presence of CD40-L by monoclonal antibody does not exclude the presence of HIM, however, because point mutations may allow expression but interfere with function. Definitive diagnosis requires molecular analysis.

Common Variable Immune Deficiency

Common variable immune deficiency (CVID) represents a variety of immune defects that undoubtedly have different genetic origins.[19] The onset can be early in infancy, like that of XAG, or the disease may present later in life. In a few patients the evolution of the immunodeficiency has been documented, often first with a decrease in the ability to form specific antibodies and later a decline in immunoglobulin concentrations. The spectrum and severity of infections is similar to that of patients with XAG except that echovirus meningoencephalitis is uncommon. On physical examination lymphoid tissue is present and may be increased, with lymphadenopathy, enlarged tonsils, nodular lymphoid hyperplasia of the intestine, and splenomegaly. Some patients have an interstitial pneumonitis due to B-cell hyperplasia. This nonmalignant condition resolves once gamma globulin therapy is initiated.[20,21]

CVID is more complex than XAG, with a high incidence of autoimmune disorders that may dominate the clinical picture. Nearly every organ system can be involved. Hematologic disorders include hemolytic anemia, thrombocytopenia, and neutropenia. Alopecia areata and vitiligo are relatively common, and the incidence of other skin diseases such as warts is increased. Autoimmune endocrine disorders and collagen vascular disease, such as rheumatoid arthritis, sicca syndrome, and systemic lupus erythematosus, are seen with increased frequency. Gastrointestinal disorders are common, including a sprue-like syndrome, with or without lymphoid hyperplasia, atrophic gastritis, achlorhydria, and pernicious anemia. Bowel infections with unusual organisms such as *Giardia, Helicobacter pylori,* and *H. jejuni* are frequent and resistant to therapy. Malignancy is also common, with non-Hodgkin's lymphoma, gastric carcinoma, and a variety of carcinomas of the skin and genital tract predominating. In a series of 248 adult and pediatric patients observed for 1 to 25 years by Cunningham-Rundles and Bodian, 27% developed chronic lung disease, 22% autoimmune disease, 16% cancer, 11% hepatitis, and 4% malabsorption.[19]

The mechanism of the immune defect in CVID is unknown. Although the severity varies, all patients have a marked reduction in serum immunoglobulin concentrations and poor responses to specific antigens. The number of B lymphocytes present in the peripheral blood usually is normal. B cells taken from patients with CVID fail to synthesize normal amounts of immunoglobulins when stimulated with the polyclonal activator pokeweed mitogen.[22] Because pokeweed mitogen-induced immunoglobulin production is dependent on T-cell help, this system could not distinguish whether the defect was in the B or T lymphocyte. Coculture of B cells from patients with T cells from normal donors failed to restore immunoglobulin production, indicating that the B lymphocytes were abnormal.[23] Using conventional assays, T-cell activity, including T-cell help, appears normal in most patients with CVID. However, on more careful evaluation, T cells from patients with CVID produce less IL-2 and gamma interferon than T cells from normal donors,[24] indicating that there may be a common defect that affects both B and T lymphocytes. A subset of patients had an inverted CD4/CD8 ratio caused by an increase in CD8[hi] T cells. These patients were characterized by a higher incidence of splenomegaly and depressed in vivo responses to recall antigens.[22] On further analysis, the CD8[hi] T cells displayed increased expression of CD57, associated with cytotoxic and suppressor cell activity, and HLA-DR, a marker of activation.[25] Functional analysis of these T cells demonstrated that the CD4 cells produced IL-2 normally and the CD8[hi] cells produced increased amounts of gamma interferon and were potent suppressors of immunoglobulin production in vitro. However, the B cells from these patients were also abnormal, indicating that increased suppressor activity is not the cause of impaired immunoglobulin production.

Another possible clue to the etiology of CVID, as well as IgA deficiency, is the observation that many patients with both diseases have in common a high incidence of CFA gene deletions and *C2* rare gene alleles.[26] Twenty-one families were investigated. In 5 families more than one member was affected, and all affected individuals demonstrated both CVID and IgA deficiency. Two major histocompatibility complex (MHC) haplotypes were shared by 24 of 31 affected individuals, suggesting that a susceptibility gene for both diseases may exist between the *C4B* and *C2* genes. These observations suggest that CVID and IgA deficiency may be opposite ends of a clinical spectrum with a common genetic defect.

Selective IgA Deficiency

Isolated deficiency of IgA is the most common of the primary immunodeficiency diseases; its incidence has been reported to be as high as 1 in 333 blood donors. Most investigators do not consider a patient deficient unless the serum concentration of IgA is less than 0.1 or 0.15 g/L. Many patients with IgA deficiency are clinically normal, but there are higher incidences of infectious allergic, collagen-vascular, and gastrointestinal (GI) disorders in patients with reduced IgA concentrations.[27,28] There is also an increased incidence of malignancy, particularly of the GI tract. The increased incidence of respiratory genitourinary tract infection is to be expected because IgA is an immunoglobulin found primarily in external secretions. Bacterial infections predominate, with a spectrum of organisms that is similar to that of other humoral immunodeficiency diseases. Antibodies to food antigens, especially cow milk and ruminant serum proteins, are common and may be related to the high incidence of malabsorption and a sprue-like condition in these patients.[29] Autoantibodies are also frequent and often result in clinically relevant autoimmune disease. Antibodies to DNA and rheumatoid factor are present in many patients, even those without clinical manifestations of disease.[30,31] Antibodies may also be formed to IgA, presumably by exposure to maternal serum during pregnancy, and can be associated with anaphylactic reactions when patients are given blood products.[32] Such reactions can be avoided by using blood products from IgA-deficient donors or by washing packed red blood cells. Patients with selective IgA deficiency should not be infused with intravenous gamma globulin unless they have an associated antibody deficiency. The use of gamma globulin products that have very low concentrations of IgA, such as Gammagard® (Baxter Healthcare Corp., Glendale, CA), can reduce the risk of serious allergic reactions.

IgA deficiency may also be secondary to treatment with some medications, such as phenytoin, gold, or penicillamine.[27,33] The decrease in IgA usually resolves when the drug is withdrawn, but occasionally the deficiency is permanent. IgA levels have been noted to fluctuate, and patients have improved spontaneously.[34] IgA deficiency is more common in families with other immune deficiencies, especially common variable immune deficiency.[26,35] It has been linked to certain HLA types, particularly HLA-A28, A1, and B8,[36] and with certain haplotypes of the MHC class III genes that code for complement components, as was discussed in the section on CVID.[26] IgA deficiency is also linked to IgG subclass deficiency, both clinically[37] and by its association with C4 null alleles.[35]

T-cell numbers and subsets and B-cell numbers are normal.[38] IgA is expressed on the surface of B lymphocytes, but the cells cannot be induced to synthesize IgA. IgA is near the end of the immunoglobulin heavy-chain gene region, so that errors in switching are likely to be more common. Recent studies indicate that T cells are involved in immunoglobulin isotype switching,[39] suggesting that the primary defect may be in the regulatory T cell rather than the B cell. The concurrence of other forms of immune dysregulation such as autoimmune disease lends support to this hypothesis. Occasional reports of excessive T-cell suppressor activity also point to a T-cell defect[40]; however, most evidence points to a primary defect in the B lymphocyte.

Evaluation of patients with selective IgA deficiency begins with the measurement of serum immunoglobulins. Levels below 0.05 g/L are of clinical relevance. The significance of levels that are slightly more than 2 standard deviations below normal is unknown, but these may indicate a defect in regulation. Such patients are not considered to be at risk of anaphylactic reactions to IgA. Measurement of IgA levels may be complicated by the presence of antiruminant antibodies that can cause immune complexes with the anti-IgA antibody used to measure the immunoglobulin levels. When antiruminant antibodies are suspected, it is necessary to use rabbit anti-IgA to clarify the situation and accurately determine the IgA concentrations. Determination of IgA subclasses is poorly standardized and of no clinical utility.[1] Levels of IgA in secretions usually reflect the serum concentrations. Rare patients have been identified who lack the secretory component necessary to move the IgA from the lamina propria into the lumen of the GI or respiratory tracts.[41] In general, the determination of secretory IgA or secretory component is not of benefit and is so poorly standardized that it should not be part of the routine evaluation. Measurement of IgG subclasses may be of some utility, because there is a higher incidence of antibody deficiency in patients who have both IgA and IgG subclass deficiency.[37] However, antibody deficiency may exist even if the IgG subclasses are normal,[42] again emphasizing that determination of antibody formation is more important than measurement of IgG subclasses. Therefore, measurement of the ability to make a specific antibody is important to prove that a patient has isolated IgA deficiency and does not have CVID. Measurement of lymphocyte subsets is of limited utility and should be reserved for those patients in whom a more serious immune defect is suspected.

IgG Subclass Deficiency

Selective deficiency of IgG subclasses in patients with normal total IgG concentrations was first described in 1968. Within a few years, there were numerous reports of an association of frequent infections, primarily of the sinopulmonary tract, with a deficiency of one or more IgG subclasses.[43-45] Nearly every combination of subclass deficiency has been described, but some appear to be more relevant than others. Deficiency of IgG2 with or without concurrent IgA deficiency seems to have greatest association with recurrent infections.[37,46-48] IgG2 and IgG4 subclass deficiency has been associated with chronic mucocutaneous candidiasis and bronchiectasis.[49] Beck and Heiner described several patients with complete absence of IgG4 who developed recurrent sinusitis and pneumonia that often progressed to bronchiectasis.[50] Others concluded that IgA deficiency or low IgG2 subclass levels are more likely to be associated with infections than is IgG4 deficiency.[51] Deficiency of IgG1 was associated with pyogenic infections of the lung, and deficiency of IgG3 with recurrent respiratory infections and viral infections of the urinary tract.[44] Other disorders have been associated with a variety of subclass deficiencies. Autoimmune cytopenias are associated with IgG2 deficiency,[52] juvenile diabetes is associated with IgG2,3 deficiency,[53] idiopathic thrombocytopenic purpura and systemic lupus with decreased IgG2 and absent IgG4,[53] childhood epilepsy with IgG2 deficiency,[54] and deficiency of IgG1,2,3 is associated with mothers who give birth to infants who have group B streptococcal sepsis.[53] Despite these clinical associations, it is still not clear if the absent subclass is of clinical significance or if subclass deficiency is merely an indicator of immune dysregulation. Completely healthy individuals have been identified with absent IgG1,2,4 due to gene deletions. This suggests that it is not the lack of a subclass *per se* that is relevant to the increased incidence of infection. Responses to certain antigens are made preferentially in a particular subclass. For example, in adults, responses to polysaccharide antigens such as *H. influenzae* are preferentially of the IgG2 subclass; however, children or IgG2-deficient patients make perfectly functional antipolysaccharide antibody of the IgG1 subclass.[55,56] There are biologic differences between the subclasses, but no subclass has a biologic activity that is so unique that other subclasses cannot assume its function. As stated, there is a higher incidence of poor antibody responses, particularly to polysaccharide antigens, in patients with subclass deficiencies. However, when groups of patients were studied, the increased incidence of infection was related to poor antibody responses regardless of IgG subclass concentrations.[57]

Evaluation of patients with IgG subclass deficiency obviously includes measurement of immunoglobulins and IgG subclasses, but determination of the ability to make antibodies to specific antigens is crucial to determining which patients might require therapy with intravenous gamma globulin.[58] Measurement of IgG subclasses alone does not accurately predict the ability to respond to specific antigens and adds little to the evaluation of patients.[59] Determination of IgG subclasses is not precise; normal ranges of subclasses have been published for children[60,61] and adults.[61,62] Most commercial laboratories rely on published normal ranges that do not necessarily apply to the technique they use to determine the subclass values and do not consider variations among ethnic groups. Lymphocyte subsets and T-cell function are normal and their determination is not relevant to the evaluation of these patients.

Antibody Deficiency with Normal Immunoglobulin Concentrations

Some patients have normal serum immunoglobulin concentrations but poor specific antibody titers to a variety of antigens, including tetanus and diphtheria, blood group substances, and pneumococcal polysaccharides. Primary responses to bacteriophage φ/χ-174 are also far below normal. In some patients, abnormalities of IgG subclasses are present, but the critical abnormality is the inability to respond to antigen challenge. Despite the normal immunoglobulin concentrations, these patients should be treated with intravenous gamma globulin if they cannot produce functional antibodies.[58,63]

A great deal of attention has been paid to the ability to respond to polysaccharide antigens. As discussed in the preceding section, there is an association between IgG2 subclass deficiency and poor responses to polysaccharides.[37,46-48] All infants fail to respond to polysaccharides, and a normal response is not achieved until at least 3 years of age.[64] A number of children between the ages of 2 and 5 years have been identified who have poor responses to polysaccharide antigens such as unconjugated H. influenzae vaccine.[57] Most of these children eventually develop a normal antibody response, so this may represent a delay in maturation rather than a true immunodeficiency. These patients are different from the children with transient hypogammaglobulinemia of infancy (THI) in that these children have normal immunoglobulin concentrations but fail to respond appropriately to antigens, whereas those with THI have low immunoglobulins but normal antibody responses. Patients who fail to respond to polysaccharides may suffer from recurrent and severe infections, and, if they fail to improve with antibiotics and reduced exposure in day care, may benefit from therapy with intravenous gamma globulin.

Transient Hypogammaglobulinemia of Infancy

If compared to normal adults, all children are immunodeficient at birth and require several years for immunoglobulins and antibody responses to become "normal." A small number of children with recurrent infections have been identified who have depressed immunoglobulin concentrations that eventually normalize. This disorder, transient hypogammaglobulinemia of infancy (THI), appears to be relatively rare. Only 11 patients were reported by Tiller and Buckley [65] over a 13-year period, and 5 patients were described by Dressler and his colleagues in 8000 sera tested over an 11-year period.[66] By definition, all of these patients recover, usually by age 2 to 4 years. These patients can be distinguished from those with more serious immunodeficiencies in that their ability to form specific antibodies to immunization is intact despite their low immunoglobulin levels. Unfortunately, it is not possible to make a definitive diagnosis without a prolonged period of reevaluation.

A subset of patients with low immunoglobulins has been described who do not show complete recovery. Some develop selective IgA deficiency. Others have depressed responses to antigens, especially the carbohydrate antigens from *H. influenzae* and *S. pneumoniae*.[67,68] In one study, many had symptoms of either atopic disease or food allergy, and 3 of 15 had gastrointestinal symptoms without evidence of atopic disease.[68] Immune dysregulation is suggested by alterations in cytokine production[69] and helper T cell activity.[70] It is likely that these patients represent one end of the spectrum of immunologic maturation, and although most eventually recover, they are at increased risk of infection as long as antibody production is abnormal. The decision to treat such patients should be based on the incidence of infection and severity of the antibody deficiency, not immunoglobulin concentrations alone.

Immunodeficiency with Thymoma

Immunodeficiency associated with thymoma, known as Good syndrome, is a disease predominantly of adults in the fourth decade or older in association with benign thymoma of the spindle-cell variety.[1,2] Patients may develop eosinophilia or eosinopenia, hemolytic or agenerative anemia, agranulocytosis, thrombocytopenia, or pancytopenia. Recurrent infections occur and are associated with pan-hypogammaglobulinemia and poor antibody responses. The percentage of B cells is low or even absent. T-cell numbers and function appear to be normal, although excessive suppressor activity has been reported in some patients. There was one reported case in an 8-year-old boy who died of disseminate varicella.[71]

Immunodeficiency Diseases with Primary Defect in Cellular Immunity

Isolated defects in T cell function are rare because T cells are required for normal B cell function. Thymic hypoplasia and the DiGeorge anomaly primarily involve T cell number and function, although if the defect is severe enough, B cell function is also involved. In all other diseases B cell function is impaired either because a single gene defect affects both B and T cells, such as in X-linked severe combined immune deficiency, or because T cell help for B cells is impaired. The genetic cause has been identified for several of these diseases, but many are understood only in terms of the cellular defect.

Thymic Hypoplasia (DiGeorge Anomaly)

DiGeorge anomaly (DGA) was initially described as the combination of congenital heart defects, hypocalcemia, and T-cell immunodeficiency.[72,73] It is now known to encompass a much broader constellation of defects that can be associated with any or all of the derivatives of the brachial arches. In 80% to 90% of the children with this defect, it is possible to demonstrate a 22q11 deletion. Whether the remaining patients have a different genetic disorder or the deletion is too small to be detected is presently unknown. A few patients, particularly infants of diabetic mothers, have been shown to have a deletion in 10p13. A similar syndrome has been described after in utero exposure to teratogenic agents such as ethanol or isotretinoin. Over the years, this syndrome DGA has also been termed velo-cardio-facial syndrome, conotruncal face syndrome, CHARGE anomalad, and CATCH22 syndrome. Currently, the name 22q11 deletion syndrome is in vogue.[73] The most common cardiac defects are truncus arteriosus, interrupted aortic arch type B, and tetralogy of Fallot. Hypoparathyroidism may lead to severe hypocalcemia in infancy, but parathyroid function often improves with the passage of time. There is a high incidence of palatal dysfunction and swallowing defects, leading to difficulty with speech and feeding. As more children with DGA survive the cardiac defects, it has become apparent that there is an increased incidence of neuropsychiatric defects, including developmental delay, mental retardation, and behavior disorders. The immunologic abnormality is due to the failure of the thymus to develop from the fourth brachial pouch and results in a variable decrease in the number of T lymphocytes. The T cells that are present function normally, but if the T-cell numbers are sufficiently low, the child is at risk from opportunistic infections such as *P. carinii* pneumonia or *C. albicans*.

The immunologic defect in DGA is variable and is not confined to cellular immune function.[74] In a review of 18 patients, only 4 had a severe, permanent T-cell defect, even though no thymus could be identified at surgery in 11 of 14 patients; the histology of the thymus in the other 3 was normal. Several patients had reduced T-cell numbers or function, which improved over the first few months of life. Immunoglobulin levels were often normal, but no specific antibody was formed after appropriate immunization in the 4 children with severe T-cell dysfunction. The overall experience with DGA suggests that many of the children will improve over time and that only a small subset have sufficient abnormality of T-cell function to put them at risk of serious infections. However, those patients with no T lymphocytes are at very high risk of life-threatening infections and their treatment should be handled as a medical emergency.

Patients with conotruncal cardiac defects and hypocalcemia should be evaluated for possible immunologic defects and other stigmata of DiGeorge anomaly. Blood counts may reveal significant lymphopenia, although a T-cell defect could be masked by a high number of B cells. Evaluation for the 22q11 deletion by fluorescence in situ hybridization (FISH) is very helpful in making the diagnosis, but it is still crucial to evaluate T-cell numbers and function to determine if the T-cell defect is of clinical significance. Most cases of DiGeorge anomaly can be distinguished from SCID by the clinical presentation and the normal function of the residual T lymphocytes. However, the distinction may be difficult in children with complete absence of T lymphocytes. Children with severe

T-cell defects are at risk of developing graft-versus-host disease (GvHD) if given nonirradiated blood, so it is important to consider the diagnosis before the child has surgery to correct the cardiac defect.

The variability in the expression of the immunologic defect and the tendency for improvement over time has made evaluation of therapy difficult. During the past two decades patients were treated with thymic implants, thymic epithelium, or thymic hormones such as thymosin. Although some of them demonstrated improvement in immunologic function, it was not possible to prove that it was due to the therapy. Patients with severe immunologic defects do require reconstitution, but the best form of therapy is still a controversial issue. Markert and colleagues recently transplanted lymphocyte-free cultured thymic epithelium into several patients with complete T-cell defects and were able to demonstrate that the patients' pre-T cells migrated to the donor epithelium and underwent normal maturation.[75] The immune system of one patient was reconstituted with a bone marrow transplant from an HLA-identical sibling.[76] T-depleted unmatched transplants are not effective because the defect is not due to a lack of stem cells, but from an inability of the stem cells to mature into T lymphocytes.

Severe Combined Immunodeficiency Disease

Severe combined immunodeficiency (SCID) actually represents a large number of heterogeneous syndromes characterized by severe deficiency of both B- and T-cell function. T lymphocytes are severely reduced in nearly all patients, but B-cell and NK-cell numbers are variable. B-cell function is probably normal in all but patients with X-linked SCID, as indicated by the ability of patients' B cells to cooperate with normal donor T cells in posttransplant bone marrow chimeras; however, B-cell function is reduced prior to transplant because of the lack of T-cell help.[77] These are the most severe of the immunologic disorders; onset is early in life, and nearly all patients die of opportunistic infection or malignancy before their first birthday unless they are kept in isolation and their immune system is reconstituted with normal bone marrow.

Patients with SCID usually present within the first few months of life with mucocutaneous candidiasis, recurrent sepsis, pneumonia, otitis, and diarrhea. Early growth is normal, but once infections start the infants exhibit extreme wasting. Opportunistic infections arise, especially *P. carinii* pneumonia, *C. albicans,* and overwhelming infections with vaccinia, varicella, measles, and bacille Calmette-Guérin (BCG), occur and provide the strongest clue to the diagnosis. These infants are susceptible to GvHD if given histoincompatible immunocompetent lymphocytes, and they may die of overwhelming GvHD if transfused with nonirradiated blood products.

Nearly all patients are severely lymphopenic, but only if one uses age-related normal values rather than the lymphocyte count of $1.0 \times 10^9/L$ that is considered to be the lower limit of normal for adults.[78] Some patients have normal lymphocyte counts, however, and that may delay diagnosis if a high index of suspicion is not maintained. In most cases, the lymphocytes are either B cells or NK cells; T-cell numbers are usually low. An exception is the infant in whom maternal T cells have crossed the placenta and engrafted. Responses to mitogens and antigens in vitro are uniformly very low or absent and are the most reliable means of making the diagnosis of SCID. Serum immunoglobulin levels are severely depressed and there is no response to specific antigens.

In addition to the lymphopenia, patients exhibit cutaneous anergy and the inability to reject skin grafts. On examination, lymphoid tissue is absent, and no thymus is detectable by x-ray examination; at surgery or autopsy a very tiny thymus may be found, usually in the neck, that histologically lacks corticomedullary distinction and Hassall's corpuscles.

The etiologies of several forms of SCID are known at the molecular level: X-linked SCID, which is due to a defect in the common gamma chain; JAK-3 deficiency; ZAP-70 deficiency; IL-7 receptor deficiency; and adenosine deaminase deficiency. Other diseases characterized by severe defects in B- and T-cell function include defective expression of histocompatibility antigens (bare lymphocyte syndrome), defective expression of the T-cell receptor, purine nucleoside phosphorylase deficiency, Omenn syndrome, and Nezelof syndrome. A few patients have been described who have a block at the level of production of IL-2; some of these patients improve with injections of recombinant IL-2, although there is never complete restoration of function. Regardless of the phenotype, bone marrow transplantation is the ,most effective means of therapy.[79,80] Success in treating these patients depends on making an early diagnosis and transplanting before serious infections occur.

X-linked SCID

The majority of patients with SCID are male. Their lymphocyte subpopulations are characterized by flow cytometry by the absence of T and NK cells but normal numbers of B cells ($T^-NK^-B^+$). T-cell and NK-cell functions are absent, and B-cell function is severely reduced.[81] The defect has been mapped to the short arm of the X chromosome and is caused by mutations in the gamma chain of the IL-2 receptor.[82] However, lack of the IL-2 receptor in mice does not cause severe combined immune deficiency. It is now known that the gamma chain is shared by a family of cytokine receptors. Defective signaling through receptors for IL-4, IL-7, IL-9, IL-13, and IL-15 results in abnormal functions of B and NK cells. X-linked SCID, like the other genetic forms of this disease, can be cured by bone marrow transplantation, though B-cell function may remain low despite good T-cell function and excellent clinical response.

JAK-3 Defect

Another subgroup of patients with SCID is characterized by the virtual absence of T lymphocytes and NK cells but normal numbers of B lymphocytes, a profile similar to that of X-linked SCID. However, these patients have normal gamma chain and autosomal inheritance. Clinically, these patients are indistinguishable from those with X-linked disease. They suffer opportunistic infections and most die if they are not transplanted with bone marrow from a normal donor. This form of SCID is now known to be caused by a defect in a protein kinase, JAK3, that binds to the common gamma chain.[83] Thus, although the gamma chain is present, it cannot send a signal downstream to activate the cell. JAK3 maps to 19p12 and is part of a family of kinases that are involved in T-cell activation. This gene defect should be suspected in female T⁻NK⁻B⁺ SCID patients or in males with a normal gamma chain.

ZAP-70 Deficiency

ZAP-70 deficiency is an autosomal recessive form of SCID characterized by an absence of CD8⁺ T cells and normal-to-elevated numbers of CD4⁺ cells. The CD4⁺ cells are unresponsive to stimulation through the T-cell receptor.[84] Patients present within the first 2 years of life with recurrent infections and failure to thrive. Unlike patients with most other forms of SCID, patients with ZAP-70 deficiency have lymphoid tissue; their thymuses have normal histologic architecture. However, with immunophenotyping the thymus is abnormal, with normal numbers of CD4⁺CD8⁺ thymocytes and CD4⁺ T cells, but no CD8⁺ cells. B-cell numbers are normal, but patients have severe hypogammaglobulinemia and no antibody responses to specific antigens. Most of these patients are treated with bone marrow transplantation.

ZAP-70 is a protein tyrosine kinase (PTK) that is associated with the T-cell receptor. A non-Src kinase, it is found in association with the kinases Lck, Syk, and Fyn and has structural homology to Syk. These kinases bind to the activated T-cell receptor and therefore are critical for signal transduction. The paradox of normal numbers of double-positive thymocytes, absence of CD8⁺ cells, and nonfunctional CD4$^+$ cells may be explained by the role of Syk. Levels of Syk are very high in thymocytes, where it substitutes for ZAP-70. ZAP-70 is crucial for selection of CD8$^+$ T cells, but Syk is adequate for selection of CD4$^+$ cells. In the periphery, the level of Syk falls, and, in the absence of ZAP-70, signal transduction does not take place. Hence, the T cells cannot respond to activation through the T-cell receptor, though they do proliferate normally if the receptor is bypassed by activation through phorbol and ionomycin.

Deficiency of ZAP-70 should be suspected in a child with no CD8$^+$ T cells but normal or even elevated numbers of CD3$^+$CD4$^+$ T cells, normal numbers of B cells, and normal numbers of NK cells. NK function is normal, and in all but one of the patients reported, B-cell function was absent. The T cells fail to proliferate or make cytokines when stimulated with phytohemagglutinin (PHA), anti-CD3, or other mitogens that bind to the T-cell receptor, but proliferate and make IL-2 if exposed to phorbol and ionomycin, which directly stimulate phospholipase C.

IL-7 Receptor Deficiency

A few patients with SCID have no T cells but a normal number of B and NK cells. Thus, they differ from patients with the X-linked and JAK-3 genetic forms, in which the common cytokine pathway is defective. These patients were found to have mutations in the IL-7 receptor.[85] The IL-7 pathway is now known to be crucial to the development of T cells, but not B or NK cells. IL-4 signaling is important for function but not development of B lymphocytes, whereas IL-15 appears to be most relevant for production of NK cells. As in the other forms of SCID, characterization of the lymphocyte phenotype by flow cytometry not only is crucial for the diagnosis of SCID, but also provides important clues to the underlying genetic defect.

Adenosine Deaminase Deficiency

Approximately 15% of patients with SCID have been found to lack this enzyme in the purine salvage pathway.[86] Adenosine deaminase (ADA) deficiency leads to a buildup of high levels of 2'-adenosine, which leads to expansion of intracellular pools of deoxyadenosine triphosphate (dATP) and S-adenosylhomocysteine. dATP is toxic to many cells, but T cells are particularly sensitive. Patients are severely lymphopenic, with essentially no B, T, or NK cells. Immunoglobulin levels are very low. ADA-deficient patients usually present early in life, but a few have been reported in whom serious infections did not begin for several years. Even in this disease, in which the genetic defect has been identified, there is heterogeneity. Patients with major deletions in the *ADA* gene have a more severe form than those with a point mutation, which may be "leaky" and allow some active enzyme to be produced. This is an autosomal recessive condition, and parents have half the normal level of enzyme in their cells, which permits carrier detection. Only a small percentage of enzyme is necessary to prevent the buildup of toxic metabolites and prevent immunodeficiency.

The majority of ADA-deficient patients are similar to other patients with SCID. Some patients differ, however, in that they have skeletal abnormalities, which include a rib cage abnormality similar to rachitic rosary and chondro-osseous dysplasia of long bones throughout the body. Unlike in patients treated with the ADA inhibitor deoxycoformycin, other tissues of the body are relatively healthy in ADA-deficient patients; only the T cells are severely affected.

The treatment of choice for this form of SCID is also bone marrow transplant, although there is a higher incidence of graft failure in ADA-deficient patients than in patients with other forms of SCID unless some form of cytoreduction is done before the transplant. Patients can also be treated with enzyme replacement. Initially, infusions of normal red blood cells were used, but the levels of ADA that were achieved were not adequate to reduce the adenosine to acceptable levels, and patients suffered from iron overload from the many transfusions. Patients are now treated with bovine ADA linked to polyethylene glycol (PEG-ADA), which prolongs its half-life.[87] Patients treated with PEG-ADA achieve good levels of ADA, and the adenosine levels fall to normal. There is clinical and immunologic improvement, although the level of reconstitution is not as good as that achieved with bone marrow transplant. PEG-ADA is a valuable form of therapy for these children, but should be reserved for those in whom bone marrow transplant is contraindicated or has failed.

Defective Expression of Major Histocompatibility Antigens

The lack of class I (bare lymphocyte syndrome [BLS] type I) , class II (BLS type II), or class I plus class II (BLS type III) major histocompatibility antigens prevents cooperation between cells of the immune system and results in a syndrome similar to other forms of SCID. Patients present with *P. carinii* pneumonia; oral candidiasis; recurrent bacterial pneumonia and septicemia; increased susceptibility to viral infections, especially the herpesviruses and enteroviruses; and chronic diarrhea and malabsorption. For the most severely affected, survival is unlikely unless the patient can be successfully treated with bone marrow.

Defects in class I expression—HLA class I molecules present antigens to cytotoxic CD8$^+$ T cells. The lack of detectable class I molecules has been termed bare lymphocyte syndrome (BLS). Patients with BLS may be healthy for the first year or two of life. Chronic lung disease may develop in late childhood.[88,89] A few patients with BLS have developed nasal polyposis; 1 patient presented with vasculitis.[90] Only 9 patients have been reported, so it is difficult to know the full spectrum of the defect.

Class I molecules are composed of a polymorphic heavy chain encoded by the *HLA-A, HLA-B,* and *HLA-C* genes, associated with beta-2-microglobulin. The molecules are synthesized and assembled in the endoplasmic reticulum, where they are associated with the chaperone molecules calnexin and calreticulin. The complexes are loaded with peptides derived from the degradation of antigens that were taken into the cytoplasm. The peptides are transported from the cytosol into the endoplasmic reticulum by a peptide transporter protein composed of 2 subunits, TAP1 and TAP2. The interaction of the peptides with the TAP proteins is controlled by a newly discovered protein, tapasin. The cases of BLS studied to date have been caused by 2 defects. In 2 patients[91] the HLA class I genes were constitutively expressed poorly. In 5 other patients the class I antigens were unstable, and in at least 2 of the patients the defect was a stop codon in the *TAP2* gene.[92] Expression of class I antigens can be determined by flow cytometry using a pan-anti-HLA class I monoclonal antibody. The magnitude of the expression can be deduced from the intensity of the signal; patients with BLS express only 10% as much class I antigen as do healthy individuals.[91]

Defects in class II expression—The class II antigens present exogenous peptides to CD4$^+$ T cells and thus are crucial for the activation of T-cell immunity. The lack of class II antigens is sometimes termed bare lymphocyte syndrome type II, or BLS type II. Approximately 70 patients have been described worldwide, primarily from Northern Africa, the Middle East, and Mediterranean countries.[93,94] Patients with BLS type II develop sepsis and chronic infections of the gastrointestinal, pulmonary, upper respiratory, and urinary tracts.[93] Infections begin within the first few months of life and continue unabated until death. Few children have lived beyond 5 years of age. Infections result from a variety of bacteria, fungi, and viruses. *Pseudomonas* and *Salmonella* are the most common bacteria and cytomegalovirus the most common virus seen in these patients. Chronic diarrhea with villous atrophy is a frequent problem. Several patients have had cholangitis. Recurrent bronchopulmonary infections with both viruses and bacteria occur in all patients. Many patients develop meningitis caused by viruses, including poliovirus, despite immunization. Others develop meningitis caused by enterovirus, herpes simplex, and adenovirus.

The immunologic defects result from the lack of class II antigen and defective cell interaction.[93,95,96] There is a significant reduction in the number of CD4[+] cells, although the total number of B and T lymphocytes is normal. T cells proliferate normally to mitogens but not to antigens, and delayed hypersensitivity skin tests are negative. The majority of patients are pan-hypogammaglobulinemic, and antibody responses are absent or severely reduced. As would be expected, the most characteristic finding is a complete absence of class II or DR antigens on the cell surface.

HLA class II expression is under very complex regulation. Transcription is controlled by an upstream promoter region consisting of 4 cis-acting DNA elements, the S, X, X2, and Y boxes. The protein complexes RFX, X2BP, and NF-Y bind to the X, X2, and Y boxes, respectively. The majority of patients have a defect in the RFX protein or in its binding to the X box.[97] The molecular defect is not known for the majority of these patients. In a few patients there is a defect in an RFX-associated protein that is important for binding of RFX (RFXAP gene).[98] In others, there was a lack of the MHCII transactivator, CIITA.[99] In yet another group of patients, the defect was found to reside in the 75-kd subunit of RFX (RFX5).[100] These mutations have been instrumental in the elucidation of the regulation of transcription of the MHC class II genes, but the diversity of defects will make correction by gene therapy very challenging.

BLS type II can be corrected with bone marrow transplantation, but it is very important to make the diagnosis early, before severe infections supervene. The disease should be suspected in patients with low CD4 counts and can be confirmed by demonstrating lack of MHCII expression on lymphocytes. Other findings, such as a lack of specific antigen responses, help confirm the diagnosis. Bone marrow transplant is the only effective therapy for this disorder. Eleven of 16 patients who did not undergo transplant died of infections, and no patient has survived beyond 14 years without transplant.[101] The overall outcome for patients who have been transplanted is poor, with only 8 of 21 patients surviving with a normal immune system.[101,102] However, the outcome is best for children transplanted before 2 years of age and for those with an HLA-identical sibling.[102]

Deficiency of T-Cell Receptors

Several patients with a clinical syndrome of SCID have been found to have decreased expression of the T-cell receptor-CD3 complex (TCR-CD3).[103,104] The first patient developed severe diarrhea with a biopsy consistent with celiac disease and subsequently had recurrent infections with a variety of gram-negative organisms. He died at 32 months of age from bronchopneumonia. Another child had recurrent infections with *H. influenzae*. In one family, 3 children died of viral infections before the diagnosis was made in a younger sibling. Interestingly, an older sibling in one family had no CD3$^+$ cells but was clinically very healthy.

In these patients, numbers of CD4$^+$ and CD8$^+$ lymphocytes are normal, but all of the cells are CD3$^-$.[105] Lymphocytes from most of these patients fail to proliferate in response to mitogens, but respond to TCR-independent signals such as anti-CD2, phorbol esters, or IL-2. Some patients are able to respond to specific antigens such as tetanus. The TCR-CD3 complex consists of at least 7 chains. Two chains form the clonotypic heterodimer, which determines antigen specificity. The other chains comprise the CD3 complex, which is important for signal transduction. In one family the biochemical defect was found to be localized to expression of the CD3 epsilon chain, and in 2 others the CD3 gamma chain was defective. Expression of CD3 varies depending on which chain is abnormal and which monoclonal antibodies are used for analysis. It is important to evaluate not only the number of cells positive for CD3, but also the intensity of expression of the CD3 molecule on the cell surface.

Cellular Immunodeficiency with Immunoglobulins (Nezelof Syndrome)

Severe but incomplete T-cell dysfunction results in a clinical syndrome characterized by failure to thrive, chronic mucocutaneous candidiasis, diarrhea, and susceptibility to viral infections, especially the herpesviruses varicella and herpes simplex. These patients develop chronic progressive pulmonary infections, gram-negative sepsis, and urinary tract infections. Autoimmune disorders, especially hemolytic anemia and thrombocytopenia, are common, and there is an increased incidence of lymphoreticular malignancies. Most patients are profoundly lymphopenic, with proportional reductions in CD4 and CD8 T cells. T-cell responses in vivo and in vitro to mitogens and antigens is markedly reduced but is not absent, as in classic SCID. Serum immunoglobulins are normal or elevated, but specific antibody formation is absent. This variant of SCID can be treated with bone marrow transplantation, but it is always necessary to use myeloablative therapy to eliminate the residual T-cell function so that the transplant will not be rejected.

This syndrome is distinguished from other forms of SCID by the presence of immunoglobulins and lymphoid tissue. The histologic structure of the thymus and lymph nodes is abnormal, with poor corticomedullary distinction and reduced or absent Hassall's corpuscles in the thymus and poor follicle formation in peripheral lymphoid organs. Some patients present with lymphadenopathy and hepatosplenomegaly. This description is obviously suggestive of acquired immunodeficiency syndrome (AIDS), but this is a genetic disorder distinguished by several features. Total T cells are reduced, but there usually is a normal CD4/CD8 ratio. While T-cell function is usually relatively normal early in human immunodeficiency virus (HIV) infection, it is low at all times in the genetic disorder. The architecture of the thymus is different, but this is not usually known antemortem. Because antibody formation may be poor, lack of antibody to HIV-1 is an unreliable indicator in the patient, but can be evaluated in the mother because vertical transmission is the most likely mode of infection. Tests for HIV antigen, such as polymerase chain reaction (PCR), are most useful for distinguishing between congenital and acquired immune deficiency. The pathogenesis of this disorder is not known, and it is most likely that what is now termed Nezelof syndrome will ultimately be found to have multiple genetic causes.

Purine Nucleoside Phosphorylase Deficiency

A small number of patients with severe cellular immunodeficiency with immunoglobulins lack an important purine salvage pathway enzyme called purine nucleoside phosphorylase (PNP).[106,107] In addition to severe susceptibility to infections, these patients have a very high incidence of lymphoreticular malignancies, and more than 50% have neurologic complications. The neurologic problems, which include ataxia, spastic diplegia, mental retardation, and retarded motor development, are not secondary to infections. Autoimmune diseases are also common, and include thrombocytopenia, hemolytic anemia, neutropenia, and vasculitis in the central nervous system.

On physical examination, lymphoid tissue is sparse. Thymic architecture is usually abnormal, though Hassall's corpuscles are present. Immunologically, T-cell numbers are severely reduced, but NK- and B-cell numbers are normal or increased. T-cell function is markedly reduced, and B-cell function, though variable, is usually poor and declines with age. NK-cell function is normal. This disorder differs from ADA deficiency in that B and NK cells are present and immunoglobulin levels are usually normal. Uric acid is low or absent, and there are no associated skeletal abnormalities. The outcome for patients with PNP deficiency has been very poor. Twenty-nine of the 34 patients reported by Markert had died at the time of the report.[106] Enzyme replacement therapy has not been as successful in this disease as it has been in ADA deficiency. Bone marrow transplantation is still the treatment of choice, but the success rate is very low due to failure of engraftment and the occurrence of overwhelming infections. Transplantation has not halted the progression of the neurologic complications. If transplantation is to be beneficial, patients should be transplanted when young and before complications ensue.

Recombination Defects: Omenn Syndrome

In 1965 Gilbert Omenn reported 12 patients in 6 sibling relationships who had developed a fatal illness characterized by a generalized erythematous scaling skin eruption, hepatosplenomegaly, generalized lymphadenopathy, eosinophilia, and fever.[108] Death was usually secondary to overwhelming infection with *S. aureus, C. albicans, P. carinii* pneumonia, and a variety of other organisms. Subsequent immunologic studies revealed B lymphopenia with reduced serum concentrations of IgG, IgA, and IgM; increased levels of IgE; and a marked depression of T-cell activation not restored by the addition of exogenous IL-2.[109] IL-2 and interferon gamma production were depressed. Lymphocyte counts were normal or elevated in many patients, with normal percentages of T cells and variable CD4/CD8 ratios. When patients were compared with normal family members, they had reduced numbers of $CD3^+$ and $CD4^+$ T cells, with an increase in $CD8^+$ T cells.[110] Biopsy of lymph nodes showed effacement of the normal architecture with a proliferation of histiocytes that were positive for the surface antigens S100, T6, and Ia, which are characteristic of Langerhans or interdigitating reticulum cells.

The pathologic findings are similar to those of acute GvHD, and some studies have suggested that this is the etiology of Omenn syndrome.[111] Indeed, these patients clinically resemble patients with severe combined immunodeficiency and maternal engraftment. However, the familial association with an autosomal recessive mode of inheritance and the inability to detect maternal cells in the majority of patients who have been studied support this as a distinct disease entity. It is reminiscent of patients with Letterer-Siwe syndrome and SCID.[112] DNA haplotype analysis of the T cells showed a variable number of tandem repeats, indicating that the cells were derived from the patients.[113] A given T-cell subset, TCR alpha-beta$^+$, $CD4^+CD8^+$, or TCR gamma-delta$^+$, was predominant in each patient, and there was oligoclonality of the T-cell receptor gene usage.[113]

It is now believed that Omenn syndrome is caused by defects in recombination of the T-cell receptor. Immunoglobulin molecules and T-cell receptors are similar in that they are composed of disparate sections of DNA that are brought together and joined using enzymes known as recombinases and ligases. This allows greater genetic diversity by bringing together one of many variable regions with one of several constant regions. If recombination does not take place, the B cell or T cell fails to develop. The genes responsible for the recombination are the recombinase activating genes 1 and 2 (*RAG1* and *RAG2*). Complete *RAG1* and *RAG2* deficiency results in a T⁻B⁻NK⁺ SCID.[114] However, partial deficiency leads to Omenn syndrome. This was first suspected when a child who had a sibling with T⁻B⁻ SCID was diagnosed with Omenn syndrome.[113]

The defects in recombination lead to dysregulation of both B- and T-lymphocyte development. Lymph nodes are enlarged due to activated T cells that are $CD3^+CD45RO^+DR^+$ and that often coexpress CD30, CD95, and/or CD25.[115,116] The cells have a T_H2 phenotype and produce IL-4 and IL-5. T cells from patients with Omenn syndrome have reduced proliferative responses to mitogens and increased susceptibility to cell death,[117] particularly through CD95 signaling. They have also been noted to have an increased incidence of $CD4^-CD8^-$ T cells[118] and expansion of a limited number of T-cell receptor families, as detected by flow cytometry.[119]

Reticular Dysgenesis

This extremely rare disorder is the most severe form of SCID. Patients have severe lymphopenia and depressed B- and T-cell function, but also lack granulocytes. Red cells and platelets are usually normal. Some patients have had small numbers of granulocytes or T cells, arguing against a stem cell defect. Seven of the 8 patients reported to date have died of overwhelming infections within the first 3 months of life; only one patient who was treated with a bone marrow transplant has survived.[120,121]

Combined Immunodeficiency Diseases

X-linked Lymphoproliferative Disease

X-linked lymphoproliferative disease (XLP) is characterized by selective inability to respond to infection with Epstein-Barr virus (EBV), which results in severe or fatal infectious mononucleosis and acquired immunodeficiency.[122] The disease was originally reported by Purtilo in 1975 in the male children of 3 families of the Duncan kindred.[123,124] Since then, more than 80 kindred with more than 272 affected males have been reported to the international registry. The XLP gene locus has been mapped to Xq25, but to date the gene has not been cloned.

The most common presentation, which occurs in approximately 78% of patients, is fatal mononucleosis with hepatic necrosis and bone marrow aplasia. If they survive the initial infection, many patients have severe defects in humoral immunity; 30% develop lymphomas.[125] Prior to exposure to EBV, the majority of patients are immunologically intact, with normal proliferative responses to mitogens and normal NK-cell activity.[122] After exposure, patients have a marked impairment in the ability to make specific antibodies to EBV nuclear antigen

(EBNA), whereas anticapsid antibody levels are normal or elevated. T-cell immunity is impaired, with inverted CD4/CD8 ratios[126] and decreased proliferative responses to mitogens.[123] In one study, however, some patients demonstrated decreased cytotoxic responses to EBV-infected cells[127] in an outgrowth inhibition assay. NK-cell activity was increased during, but significantly depressed after, EBV infection in many of the patients studied.[123,128,129] In the healthy individual, cytotoxic and suppressor cells generated during acute viral infection inhibit immunoglobulin production and limit the course of the infection. In XLP, the CD8$^+$ cells develop into aberrant self-destructive killer cells that cause tissue and organ destruction and irreparably damage the immune system.

There is no effective therapy for XLP. Acyclovir and ganciclovir have not been particularly effective, probably because EBV is no longer in the replication phase. Patients who survive the initial infection and do not develop lymphomas are likely to develop agammaglobulinemia and recurrent infections. These symptoms improve markedly after the patients begin treatment with intravenous gamma globulin. There have been reports of a beneficial response to alpha-interferon,[129] but overall the results have not been encouraging. Prophylactic administration of gamma globulin with high titers of antibody to EBV is being used in patients found to have an abnormal XLP gene in an attempt to prevent the initial infection, but again, the results have been disappointing.[125,129] Trials have been proposed using cytotoxic agents to eliminate the activated CD8 cytotoxic cells, but no data are yet available. Most recently, bone marrow transplant has been used to correct the defect and prevent the onset of the lymphoproliferative syndrome.[130-132] The transplant must be done early in life because most of the boys transplanted after 15 years of age died within 90 days of complications from the transplant.[125,133]

Wiskott-Aldrich Syndrome

The combination of eczema, thrombocytopenia, and recurrent pyogenic infections is an X-linked disorder first reported in the United States in 1957.[134] In 1994, a multinational survey of 154 patients reported the disease's clinical and immunologic characteristics.[135] The gene for Wiskott-Aldrich syndrome (WAS) and a closely related but milder disease, X-linked thrombocytopenia, has been mapped to Xp11.22; the defective gene encoding the WAS protein (WASP), has now been identified.[136]

Clinically, boys who have WAS present with bloody diarrhea and petechiae early in infancy.[135] Platelet numbers are reduced and individual platelets are small. Platelets from patients with WAS have abnormal survival times, whereas normal platelets infused into patients with WAS have normal survival times.

Eczema also develops early in life and may be related to a specific allergy, although often no allergen can be identified. The most striking abnormality is the high incidence of bacterial infections, especially otitis, sinusitis, pneumonia, and meningitis, often caused by encapsulated organisms such as *S. pneumoniae* and *H. influenzae.* There is often increased susceptibility to viruses such as varicella and *P. carinii;* however, mucocutaneous candidiasis and other opportunistic infections are uncommon. There is an extremely high incidence of malignancy—nearly 15% in the immunodeficiency registry.[137] The majority of the tumors have been lymphomas, including those in the CNS that were initially thought to be brain tumors but were actually lymphomas metastatic from the abdomen.

The most consistent immunologic abnormality in these patients is an impaired humoral response to polysaccharide antigens, with diminished or absent isohemagglutinins, low concentrations of natural antibodies to *Escherichia coli,* and poor antibody response following immunization with carbohydrate antigens such as *H. influenzae* and pneumococcal polysaccharide.[138,139] The response to other antigens, including polio, diphtheria, and tetanus, is also reduced, but not as severely as that to carbohydrate antigens. The response to bacteriophage φ/χ-171 is abnormal, with impaired immunoglobulin isotype switching from IgM to IgG.[140] Serum concentrations of IgG are usually normal, IgM is slightly low, and IgA and IgE often elevated. All immunoglobulins are catabolized at a markedly increased rate; IgG at 3 times and IgA and IgM at twice the usual rate.[141] Thus, the synthetic rates are increased in proportion to maintain the serum concentrations. The concentrations of IgG2 have been found to be normal, despite the poor response to polysaccharide antigens and the apparent linkage of IgG2 to responses to those antigens.[142]

Patients with WAS frequently have cutaneous anergy in delayed hypersensitivity skin testing.[139,143] Proliferative responses to the usual mitogens and antigens, as well as allogeneic cells, are moderately decreased.[135,140] Cells from these patients do not proliferate in response to periodate, which oxidizes carbohydrate residues on glycoproteins.[144] In addition, the response to immobilized anti-CD3 is abnormal,[145] again indicating that there is a subtle defect in T-cell function. The numbers and proportions of T lymphocytes in peripheral blood are modestly decreased, with normal CD4/CD8 ratios.[135] However, the proportion of NK cells and non-MHC-restricted gamma/delta-bearing cytotoxic T cells is increased.[146] These T cells are unique in that they do not express CD5. The numbers of B lymphocytes, as indicated by CD20, are normal, although a high proportion of these are negative for CD21, the complement and EBV receptor, a pattern seen on immature B cells.[147] The number of CD23+ B cells is increased. B-cell lines derived from patients with WAS respond normally to IL-4, IL-6, and low-molecular-weight B-cell growth factor,[148] but do not produce immunoglobulin normally when stimulated with pokeweed mitogen (PWM) or *Staphylococcus aureus* Cowan I (SAC).[149]

Lymphocytes and platelets from patients with WAS have been reported to lack a 115-kd surface sialoglycoprotein known as gpLI15 or sialophorin and now designated CD43.[150] The gene for sialophorin is located in the p11.2 band of chromosome 16. Because WAS is an X-linked disease, the reduced expression of sialophorin cannot be the primary defect. With the identification of the *WASP* gene, it is now known that the gene codes for a protein that interacts with the actin in the cell cytoskeleton.[151,152]

WAS has a very high mortality rate due to bleeding in infants, infection in older children, and malignancy in children and young adults. Many patients develop other complications, such as vasculitis, and the immunosuppressive agents used to treat the vasculitis increase the risk of infection and malignancy. Treatment has been mainly supportive, with bone marrow transplantation reserved for those with an HLA-identical sibling. Survival rates for WAS patients treated with marrow transplanted from parents or unrelated donors are very poor (usually less than 10%). However, with improvements in techniques for transplantation and the fact that younger patients respond better to transplantation, all WAS patients should be considered for transplant in the first five years of life.

Chronic Mucocutaneous Candidiasis

Chronic mucocutaneous candidiasis (CMC) is a group of syndromes that are characterized by persistent infections of the skin, nails, and mucous membranes with *Candida* species and occasionally other fungal organisms.[153] Although many other defects of cellular immunity are associated with an increased susceptibility to fungal infection, only in CMC do patients develop disfiguring hyperkeratotic lesions. Despite the extensive superficial infection, disseminated infection leading to pneumonia, sepsis, or parenchymal organs is unusual. Six subgroups were identified by Kirkpatrick based on associated abnormalities and the pattern of the candidiasis: (1) chronic oral candidiasis; (2) mucocutaneous candidiasis with endocrinopathy; (3) localized mucocutaneous candidiasis; (4) chronic diffuse candidiasis; (5) chronic candidiasis associated with thymoma; and (6) chronic candidiasis and keratitis. Endocrine abnormalities are common, especially in the second group, and include hypoparathyroidism, hypothyroidism, hypoadrenalism, gonadal dysfunction, and polyendocrinopathy syndromes. Autoimmune disease is also a common feature, and may involve the endocrine organs, with antibodies to thyroid, adrenal, and islet cells. Anti-parietal cell antibody can lead to pernicious anemia, and autoimmune disease in the skin can result in alopecia totalis, vitiligo, and chronic keratitis. Gastrointestinal disorders also occur, with chronic malabsorption that may be related to gluten sensitivity, chronic active hepatitis, and dental enamel dysplasia.[154] Despite the initial impression that infection in CMC patients is confined to *Candida* species, the majority of patients suffer from multiple infections, including pyogenic infections of the skin, sinopulmonary tract, and urinary tract.[154,155] Recurrent pneumonia with bronchiectasis has been a significant cause of morbidity and mortality.[154,156] Isolated cases of bacterial sepsis and meningitis have been reported. A few patients have had severe infections with varicella, herpes simplex, measles, and respiratory syncytial virus, suggesting a defect in cell-mediated immunity. Superficial but persistent infections with dermatophytes are relatively common. Although disseminated infections with fungi are uncommon, at least 5 children are known to have had life-threatening disseminated infections with *Histoplasma capsulatum*.[157]

The underlying immunologic defect is yet uncharacterized. The majority of patients are anergic to *Candida* in vivo,[154] but some demonstrate positive responses, especially if tested while the disease is under good control. Similar results are observed when their lymphocytes are stimulated with *Candida* antigen in vitro. Although some patients are completely anergic, the majority can respond to other recall antigens such as tetanus or streptokinase. Responses to mitogens are normal in the majority of patients.[154] Serum immunoglobulins and antibody responses are normal in most patients, but isolated defects, including IgG subclass deficiency, have been reported.[156] B-and T-cell numbers and subsets have also been within normal limits, but transient abnormalities have been observed in patients tested during the acute phase of their illness. Durandy and colleagues[158] found that in vitro production of antibody to mannan isolated from the cell wall of *C. albicans* was absent during the active phase of the disease. T lymphocytes from patients with CMC were not able to proliferate in response to mannan or provide helper activity for B-cell antibody activity. This was associated with the presence of mannan-specific suppressor T cells. They hypothesized that defective processing of mannan by monocytes could lead to the accumulation of mannan and the induction of suppressor T lymphocytes. The serum of patients in the active phase of the disease contained a factor that could inhibit the response of normal cells to *Candida* antigens.[159] The factor was a polysaccharide from the cell wall of *Candida* and disappeared with successful antifungal therapy. More recently, evaluation of cytokine profiles in patients with CMC indicates that although they can recognize and respond to *Candida*, it is a T_H2 rather than a T_H1 response.[160,161] CMC patients have impaired cytokine production when stimulated with *Candida* antigens, resulting in low or absent IL-2, increased IL-6, and variable amounts of interferon gamma.[160] Evaluation of T-cell subsets indicates that CMC patients have increased percentages of $CD4^+CD45RA^+$ cells and a significant decrease in the number of $CD4^+CD29^+$ cells.[161] T cells from the patients produced more IL-4 and less IL-2R, again suggesting a T_H2 predominance.

Hyperimmunoglobulinemia E Syndrome

Patients with hyperimmunoglobulinemia E (hyper-IgE) syndrome suffer from recurrent severe staphylococcal abscesses of the skin and lung and an eczematous skin rash.[162-164] They have extremely high serum concentrations of IgE, usually several thousand units per milliliter. The hallmark of the disease is severe, recurrent infections in the skin, lungs, liver, and other sites that lead to abscesses and pneumatoceles. Most infections are caused by *S. aureus,* but a variety of other bacteria and fungi, especially *C. albicans* and *Aspergillus,* have been isolated. Some patients develop skin infections with *Candida* that are similar to those of patients with chronic mucocutaneous candidiasis. Both males and females are affected, as are members of successive generations, suggesting an autosomal dominant form of inheritance with incomplete penetrance.

The underlying immunologic defect has not been identified. Disorders of phagocytosis and chemotaxis have been reported.[165,166] Serum immunoglobulin concentrations are usually normal, except for the elevated IgE; specific antibody responses to a wide variety of protein and carbohydrate antigens are variable but often impaired.[167] Some patients fail to switch from IgM to IgG when immunized with bacteriophage ϕ/χ-174, and others show a rapid decline in antibody titers.[167] Most patients have normal numbers of circulating B and T lymphocytes and subsets, and responses to mitogens are usually normal.[162,168] When T cells from patients with hyper-IgE are stimulated with PHA, they produce less interferon gamma and TNF-alpha than normal controls.[169] Production of IL-4 is enhanced and interferon gamma reduced, and levels of soluble CD23 (IgE receptor) are elevated in the patients compared with healthy controls.[170] Mononuclear cells from patients produce IgE in vitro but do not increase production when stimulated with IL-4, suggesting that they are already maximally stimulated.[171] IgE antibodies to staphylococci are elevated in patients with hyper-IgE,[172] leading to speculation that the antibody initiates an inflammatory response. However, the importance of these immunologic abnormalities and elevated IgE and their relationship to the high incidence of abscess and pneumatocele formation is still unclear.

Ataxia Telangiectasia

Ataxia telangiectasia (AT) is a complex multisystem disease in which the immune system is variably involved.[173,174] The predominant abnormality is progressive cerebellar ataxia, which is manifest about the time the child starts to walk and, in severe cases, progresses until he or she is confined to a wheelchair, usually by 10 or 12 years of age. Oculomotor abnormalities are prominent and may precede truncal ataxia. Oculocutaneous telangiectasias develop between the ages of 3 and 6 years and help distinguish this form from other forms of ataxia. Immunologic abnormalities manifest as recurrent sinopulmonary infections; chronic pneumonia and bronchiectasis are a frequent cause of death. Although these are the cardinal manifestations of the disease, all organ systems are involved. The skin and hair show progeric changes, with graying of the hair and loss of elastic tissue. The skin may become atrophic, and even begin to resemble skin affected by mild scleroderma. Nearly all patients develop seborrheic dermatitis and common warts. One of the most dramatic and devastating aspects of AT is the remarkable incidence of malignancy. Nearly 15% of patients develop malignancy, often of the lymphoreticular system; T-cell malignancies are especially common.[175,176] Cutaneous, hepatic, and renal tumors are also common, especially in patients over 15 years of age. Radiomimetic chemotherapy drugs and irradiation lead to severe, ultimately fatal reactions and are therefore contraindicated in these patients. The common pathogenic link appears to be defective DNA repair, leading to a high frequency of mutations.[177,178]

Sinopulmonary infections are very common. There is not a high incidence of infections with opportunistic organisms and the response to most viral infections is normal, although one patient died from disseminated varicella. The immunologic abnormalities are highly variable.[179] The most frequent humoral abnormality is absent IgA, found in 50% to 80% of AT patients. IgE levels are also often low, and IgM levels, while normal, may be monomeric. IgG concentrations are usually normal, but subclass deficiency, especially of IgG2, is common.[180] Specific antibody titers may be reduced but are seldom absent. T-cell immunity is mildly decreased in vivo, as evidenced by cutaneous anergy and prolonged allograft survival. Percentages of T cells in the peripheral blood are only mildly reduced, although there may be a selective decrease in CD4 lymphocytes.[181] There is an increase in the number of T cells expressing gamma/delta receptors compared with alpha/beta receptors.[93] Proliferative responses to mitogens and antigens in vitro are also significantly reduced, but never absent.[182,183] Production of interferon gamma and IL-2 are also reduced. Thymic histology is abnormal, with poor corticomedullary distinction and absence of Hassall's corpuscles. Serum alpha-fetoprotein levels are markedly elevated, aiding in the diagnosis.[174]

Cartilage-Hair Hypoplasia

Immune deficiency has been associated with short-limbed dwarfism, especially those patients with cartilage-hair hypoplasia (CHH).[184,185] The biochemical defect is not known, but at least with regard to the immune response, there is a defect in early gene activation.[186,187] Patients have short and pudgy hands, hyperextensible joints of the hands and feet, sparse light hair, and redundant skin. Some have megacolon or other gastrointestinal disorders. Radiologically, the bones show sclerotic or cystic changes in the metaphysis and flaring of the costochondral junctions. Patients may develop severe, often fatal infections with varicella, vaccinia, and poliovirus, and opportunistic infections such as oral candidiasis can occur.[184,188] There appears to be a defect in cellular proliferation that affects all cells of the body, including those of the immune system.[187]

The immunologic defect is highly variable, ranging from nearly normal to a clinical picture resembling that of SCID.[185] Some patients have only defective humoral immunity, which nonetheless may be severe enough to require replacement with gamma globulin. A subset of patients has severe T-cell defects with decreased T-cell numbers.[185,187,188] Proliferative responses to mitogens are impaired due to an arrest in the G0 phase of the cell cycle.[189] NK-cell activity is normal or increased,[184] which has been speculated to account for the lack of an increased incidence of malignancy in this disorder. However, some researchers have reported that up to 10% of patients with CHH may develop malignancies, which is nearly as high as in WAS and ataxia telangiectasia.[190] Early attempts to correct the immune defect with thymosin were not successful.[191] Bone marrow transplant has been effective in correcting the T-cell abnormality, though the achondroplasia was unaffected.[79,192]

Disorders of Complement

Complement deficiency is one of the rarest of the immunologic disorders. The complement system comprises more than 25 plasma and membrane-bound glycoproteins, and defects have been described for most of these components.[193,194] In general, absence of one of the early components of the classic complement pathway results in autoimmune disease such as systemic lupus erythematosus (SLE) or increased susceptibility to infection with gram-positive bacteria, whereas defects in the later components of the classic pathway or in the alternative pathway result in an increased incidence of *Neisseria* infections. A defect in one of the inhibitory proteins can result in secondary defects in one of the other components due to uncontrolled utilization.

Defects Resulting in Autoimmune Disease

The most common manifestation of C1q deficiency is SLE, often with renal involvement. Absence of C1r, C1s, C4, or C2 may also result in a SLE-like syndrome. Patients with C2 deficiency, which is the most common complement deficiency, also have an increased incidence of rheumatoid arthritis. Absence of C3 is extremely rare, with only 16 patients reported, 5 of whom had glomerulonephritis or an SLE-like syndrome. The reason these defects lead to autoimmune disease is unknown, but it is thought to be due to an inability to clear immune complexes via C1q or C3 receptors on phagocytic cells. Absence of C1 inhibitor results in uncontrolled activation of C1, C2, and C4, and results in hereditary angioedema, characterized by recurrent episodes of nonpruritic, nonurticarial swelling of the face, extremities, upper airways, and abdominal viscera. Patients may present with upper airway obstruction, occasionally leading to death. Episodes involving abdominal viscera may result in symptoms suggestive of an acute abdomen and have led to needless surgery when the true cause of the pain was overlooked.

Defects Resulting in Recurrent Infections

A defect in one of the early components of the classic pathway—C1, C4, C2, or C3—may result in an increased incidence of pyogenic infections with the gram-positive bacteria *Streptococcus* and *Staphylococcus*. This suggests that phagocytosis and intracellular killing are critical for host defense against these organisms. Patients with the most common defect, C2 deficiency, may present with sepsis, pneumonia, meningitis, or pyogenic arthritis with *S. pneumoniae*. Several of these patients have been unable to make specific antibodies to the pneumococcal polysaccharide antigens when immunized with the pneumococcal vaccine. This suggests that development of immune complexes with complement is critical for the antigen processing that leads to antibody formation against these antigens.

Defects in C3, the alternative pathway components, or any of the terminal components of the classic pathway result in an increased incidence of *Neisseria* infections, including meningitis, sepsis, and pyogenic arthritis. Infections with other organisms, such as brucellosis and toxoplasmosis, have also been reported. Defects in the C3 regulatory factors, factor I and factor H, result in decreased levels of C3 and a similar clinical presentation. Because the terminal complement components are necessary for the development of the membrane attack complex, susceptibility to *Neisseria* suggests that extracellular lysis by complement is important for defense against these organisms. However, some patients with deficiency of complement are healthy, and the rarity of these defects makes it difficult to understand the mechanisms that lead to increased susceptibility.

Deficiency in Cell-Surface Complement Receptors

Membrane receptors for activated complement components mediate many of the biologic activities of the system, such as chemotaxis, phagocytosis, and leukocyte activation. CR1 is a receptor for C3b and serves as an adhesion receptor to enhance phagocytosis by macrophages. However, the bulk of CR1 is on erythrocytes, where its primary purpose appears to be transporting and clearing immune complexes from the circulation. CR3 and CR4 are receptors for iC3b and belong to the integrin family of adhesion molecules. Defects in these proteins are associated with lack of the CD18 molecule, known as leukocyte function antigen 1 (LFA-1) deficiency, and lead to the disease leukocyte adhesion defect (LAD), discussed in the chapter on phagocytic disorders. Because isolated defects of CR3 and CR4 have not been described, the relative importance of defective complement binding compared with intracellular adhesion is not known.

Defects in Cell-Surface Complement Components

Several complement components are found on the surfaces of cells and serve to regulate complements and protect cells from the consequences of complement activation. Some, such as decay accelerating factor, C8bp, and CD59, serve to limit complement damage to homologous cells. Defects in these proteins lead to paroxysmal nocturnal hemoglobinuria, a clonal bone marrow disorder characterized by chronic intravascular hemolysis and thrombosis. The underlying defect is an abnormality in the synthesis of the glycolipid anchors, which attach proteins to the cell membrane. These molecules are found on leukocytes and platelets as well as on red blood cells, which may explain the thrombocytopenia, leukopenia, and thrombosis seen in this disease.

Immunodeficiency Associated with Other Disorders

Chromosomal Abnormalities

Immunologic defects have been identified in association with a variety of chromosomal disorders,[2] but none has been well characterized. Patients with Down syndrome have an increased incidence of respiratory infections, hepatitis, and leukemia.[195] IgG subclass deficiencies, impaired antibody responses, deficient T-cell function (especially decreased interferon production), and abnormal phagocytic function have all been reported in Down syndrome, but no consistent abnormality has been identified. Patients with Bloom syndrome, xeroderma pigmentosum, and Fanconi's anemia all have chromosomal repair abnormalities and increased incidences of malignancies that are reminiscent of the malignancies seen in ataxia telangiectasia. They also have increased incidences of sinopulmonary infections. Patients with Bloom syndrome may have decreased concentrations of one or more immunoglobulin isotypes and impaired antibody responses.[196] Some have decreased in vitro cellular immune responses. Similar abnormalities have been observed in Fanconi's anemia, but few patients have been studied in detail.

Nutritional Disorders

Severe protein-calorie malnutrition can result in profound B- and T-cell defects, but this problem is beyond the scope of this chapter. Of the inherited nutritional defects, an inability to absorb zinc is an autosomal recessive disease that leads to a clinical syndrome known as acrodermatitis enteropathica. The disease is characterized by eczema, especially around the mouth and rectum, chronic diarrhea and malabsorption, and recurrent sinopulmonary infections.[197] Patients may have hypogammaglobulinemia, but it may be secondary to enteric losses.[198] There also may be an associated T-lymphocyte defect with decreased response to PHA and impaired delayed hypersensitivity skin test reactions.[197] Therapy with parenteral zinc or high doses of oral zinc results in clearing of the diarrhea, skin rash, and immunologic defect.

Metabolic Diseases

Several hereditary metabolic disorders have associated immunologic defects.[2] Few patients have been studied, and the relationships of the metabolic defects to the immune dysfunctions are not clear. Biotin-dependent carboxylase deficiency results in convulsions, ataxia, alopecia, and keratoconjunctivitis. Patients may have *Candida* dermatitis, isolated IgA deficiency, and a reduced number of T cells in the peripheral blood. Biotin corrects both the biochemical and clinical abnormalities.[199] Patients with type I hereditary orotic aciduria have growth failure, recurrent diarrhea, megaloblastic anemia, and an increased incidence of infections, including meningitis and severe varicella. They are lymphopenic, with decreased numbers of T cells and impaired T-cell function.[200,201] Transcobalamin II deficiency leads to severe megaloblastic anemia, failure to thrive, diarrhea, vomiting, and lethargy. Hypogammaglobulinemia is frequently present,[202] with IgG levels in the serum between 0 and 2.26 g/L. IgA and IgM also may be decreased.[203]

Immunobiology of the Neonate

Immaturity is the most common cause of immune "deficiency," at least if adult levels of immune function are used as the measuring standard. Neonates are both immunologically immature and naïve. Development of the immune system begins in the first trimester of gestation, and immune cell numbers rise rapidly in the last months of pregnancy. However, although the cells of neonates are capable of carrying out all the functions of the cells of adults, the magnitude and rapidity of the neonatal immune response is much reduced. Some of the mechanisms responsible for this impaired function are understood, and others are being investigated, aided by information that we learn from studying patients with congenital immunodeficiency diseases.

Development of the Neutrophil and Macrophage System

Phagocytosis is the most primitive host defense mechanism, but mammalian neutrophils and monocytes have evolved complex functions that go far beyond phagocytosis. In addition to producing an array of enzymes that are capable of killing bacteria and viruses, these cells generate oxygen free radicals that can kill even highly resistant bacteria; produce cytokines that activate lymphocytes, endothelial cells, and stromal cells such as fibroblasts; and process and present antigen to B and T lymphocytes. In order to function appropriately, the neutrophils and macrophages must be able to respond to a chemotactic stimulus, adhere to endothelial cells or intracellular matrix, deform to fit between the endothelial cells, bind to the target, and ingest and kill the organism. The phagocytic cells of the neonate are defective to some degree in all of these functions.[204]

The first step in the inflammatory response is adhesion of neutrophils to endothelium at the site of inflammation. Adhesion is mediated largely by a family of cell surface glycoproteins, the integrins, that include the iC3b receptor (Mac-1, CR3, or CD11b/18), LFA-1 (CD11a/18), and p150,95. These receptors interact with intracellular adhesion molecules (ICAMs) that have been upregulated on the endothelial cells by IL-1 and TNF-alpha. After adhering to a substrate, the phagocyte must be able to recognize and migrate along a concentration gradient of an attractant substance. Stimulation of the cell upregulates receptors, causes ruffling of the membrane, and increases random movement. Receptors for the chemoattractant are concentrated along the leading edge of the cell; after interaction with the ligand, the receptor-ligand complex is moved to the uropod or trailing foot of the cell. There it is ingested and broken down. New receptor is synthesized and fused with the cell membrane to allow further recognition of the gradient. The cell moves by attaching the leading edge to the substrate using adhesion molecules and then contracting the cytoskeleton, which consists of microfilaments of actin and myosin. The cells must be deformable to fit between endothelial cells and through the extracellular matrix. Once the cell reaches the site of infection, it must attach to the organism or infected cell. Attachment requires that the organism be opsonized with substances such as IgG, complement, or fibronectin; therefore, the cell must express specific receptors such as FcgammaIII, CR3, CR4, or the fibronectin receptor. The cell engulfs the attached organism by extending pseudopods to surround the particle and forming a phagocytic vesicle that subsequently fuses with the primary granules to form phagolysosomes. Organisms are killed using a variety of methods involving both oxidative and nonoxidative mechanisms. The former require generation of oxygen free radicals through the hexose monophosphate shunt and NADPH oxidase. These are converted to hydrogen peroxide, then

•OH, and subsequently to hypochlorous acid (OCl⁻) by myeloperoxidase.

•OH, and subsequently to hypochlorous acid (OCl^-) by myeloperoxidase. Organisms are also killed by numerous enzymes contained within the granules, such as lysozyme, cathepsin, defensins, and bactericidal/permeability-inducing protein. Neutrophils and mononuclear phagocytes share most of these functions; in addition, mononuclear phagocytic cells process and present antigen to T lymphocytes. There is evidence that neutrophils and monocytes from preterm neonates, and to a lesser extent term infants, are defective in most of these functions.

Ontogeny of Neutrophils and Monocytes

Precursors of neutrophils can first be detected in the yolk sac within the first weeks after implantation, and mature neutrophils are detected in the peripheral blood by 12 to 14 weeks' gestation.[205] The number of cells rises rapidly during the ensuing 12 weeks.[206] Premature infants of birth weight < 1000 g have neutrophil counts of approximately 8×10^9/L at birth, whereas small-for-gestational-age infants have neutrophil counts of only 2×10^9/L, which may fall even further during the first few days of life.[207] Term infants have much higher counts, averaging 24×10^9/L at 4 hours after birth in one study,[208] though others[209,210] found absolute neutrophil counts to be closer to 8×10^9/L at birth, rising over the first 3 days and then declining to approximately 4×10^9/L. Despite these values, which are greater than those for adults, neonates are prone to develop neutropenia when septic.[205,211] Neonates have very small storage pools of immature neutrophils in the marrow; only approximately twice the number in the peripheral circulation, compared with adults, who have 14 times the peripheral number.[212] Once the storage pool is depleted by an infection, infants are at risk for developing overwhelming sepsis that is often fatal.

The development of monocytes and tissue macrophages has not been studied as extensively as that of neutrophils. Mean monocyte counts at birth range from 6 to 9×10^9/L.[209,213]

Neutrophil Function

Adhesion—Early studies indicated that adherence by neonatal neutrophils was significantly diminished compared with neutrophils from children and adults,[214,215] but these studies measured adherence to glass beads or nylon wool, which do not require specific receptor interactions. Studies using human umbilical vein endothelial cells (HUVECs) indicated that baseline adherence by neonatal cells that is dependent on LFA-1 is normal, but baseline adherence through CD11b/18 is impaired.[216] Chemotactic stimulation greatly increased adhesion of adult but not neonatal neutrophils, perhaps due to both a deficiency in the expression of CR3[217] and the lack of upregulation when the cells are stimulated.[218] On the other hand, granulocyte-monocyte stimulating factor (GM-CSF) primes the neonatal neutrophils so that stimulation with the peptide formyl-methionyl-leucyl-phenylalanine (f-MLP) upregulates CR3 expression and improves adhesion.[219] Hence, although the neonatal cells are deficient compared with those of adults, under some circumstances they can be induced to normal activity.

Locomotion and chemotaxis—As discussed in the previous section, migration across the endothelial membrane is abnormal in neonates, at least in part, because of defective expression of adhesion molecules.[216] However, the cells are defective in several other ways. Diapedesis requires energy utilization, a contractile system that involves actin and myosin, and regulation of membrane fluidity[220] by proteins such as gelsolin.[221] Neutrophils from neonates show abnormal actin polymerization[222] and decreased deformability when measured by elastometry.[223] These abnormalities undoubtedly contribute to the observed impaired random migration[224] and abnormal response to a chemotactic stimulus that may persist until a child is 6 years old.[225-227]

The degree to which the response of neonatal cells to a chemotactic stimulus is abnormal may depend on the assay used.[224-228] Using a Boyden chamber, migration of neutrophils from preterm infants was equivalent to that of term infants, about 20% of adult values.[229] Chemotaxis improved when the infants developed superficial bacterial infections, but was absent when they were septic. Migration through a 3-micrometer pore filter indicated a greater degree of abnormality than when 8-micrometer pores were used,[228] suggesting that the cells recognized the chemoattractant and began movement, but that fluidity of the cell was abnormal. The degree of abnormality was greater if zymosan was used as the stimulant rather than *E. coli* chemotactic factor.[225] Binding of the chemotactic stimulant f-MLP was the same in adult and neonatal cells, suggesting that the cells were capable of recognizing the chemoattractant.[230] However, fewer receptors are placed on the membrane from the intracellular granules and signal transduction through the f-MLP receptor is reduced in neonatal cells compared with cells from adults.[231] In addition, cells from neonates do not upregulate CR3 receptors normally[232] and fail to generate additional levels of actin upon stimulation.[233] In summary, the abnormalities in diapedesis, random migration, and directed migration are due to defective upregulation of adhesion and chemoattractant molecules, impaired membrane fluidity, and decreased actin polymerization.

Phagocytosis—Attachment to particulate antigens uses receptors for complement C3b and iC3b and the Fc portion of the IgG molecule. Neonatal neutrophils express significantly lower levels of the IgG receptor FcγRIII, though the levels of FcγRI and FcγRII are normal or elevated.[234] However, there may not be a close correlation between the levels of these receptors and phagocytosis. In one study, phagocytic rates and number of *E. coli* bacteria ingested were slightly lower in neonates compared with adult neutrophils, but were significantly impaired in premature infants.[235] Although the researchers confirmed the decreased receptor numbers, they could not find a correlation between the number of receptors and the degree of impairment. Most studies have shown that phagocytosis by neutrophils from term infants of a variety of organisms is equivalent to that of older children and adults.[236-239] When neonatal cells are stimulated by infection or artificial stimulants such as f-MLP, phagocytosis is stimulated.[238,240] Most studies have demonstrated that even preterm infants' neutrophils have normal phagocytic activity,[236,241] though they may be more easily overcome when the number of infectious organisms is high.[231]

Killing—The ability of neutrophils to kill microorganisms can be determined directly in bactericidal or fungicidal assays or indirectly by measuring the ability to generate an oxidative burst using nitro blue tetrazolium (NBT) dye reduction, chemiluminescence, or measurement of free radicals. Studies measuring NBT dye reduction in resting leukocytes indicated that leukocytes from term and premature infants reduced dye normally, although the percentage of positive cells decreased significantly in septic infants.[242] All the cells increased appropriately when they were stimulated. Chemiluminescence of zymosan-stimulated neutrophils from term infants was significantly reduced compared with that of their mothers or normal controls.[243] Neutrophils from premature infants were abnormal for up to 2 months after birth; the degree of abnormality correlated with a higher frequency of serious infections.[244] Neutrophils from neonates generated higher-than-normal $\bullet O_2^-$ radicals but much less $\bullet OH$ than adults.[245] The cause of the defective conversion is unknown but would result in poor production of OCl^-. Generation of superoxide anion was greatly enhanced in neonatal neutrophils after preincubation in recombinant human granulocyte colony stimulating factor (G-CSF),[246] although bactericidal activity was not increased. Other studies have found that chemiluminescence by neonatal neutrophils was equivalent to that of adults when they were stimulated with f-MLP, but that they did not increase appropriately when primed with lipopolysaccharide (LPS) or TNF-alpha.[247] Binding affinity for LPS and TNF-alpha was the same for adult and neonatal cells, but the number of binding sites for f-MLP was decreased in neonatal neutrophils. However, although the number of binding sites for LPS (designated CD14) was similar between the adult and neonatal cells, the neonatal cells did not upregulate the number of CD14 receptors on the surface after stimulation with LPS.[248]

Intracellular killing of microorganisms by healthy term neonates is considered to be normal.[249] Even premature infants showed normal killing if they were healthy.[250] However, stressed infants showed a marked impairment of killing of *E. coli* and *Staphylococcus*.[214] When high bacteria-neutrophil ratios were used, the ability to kill *E. coli* was significantly impaired,[243] indicating that neonatal cells have little reserve. The ability of neutrophils from neonates to kill microorganisms such as group B streptococci was also reduced compared with adults.[251] On the other hand, killing of *C. albicans* was normal in healthy term infants.[252] Therefore, killing of microorganisms by the neutrophils of healthy infants is equivalent to that of adults as long as the neonates are healthy and the assay system is not stressed by adding a high multiplicity of organisms. The significance of these in vitro findings is not entirely known, but it does suggest that neonates can be more easily overwhelmed by bacterial infection, and that once sick they become even more deficient in their ability to resist the infection.

Macrophage Function

Mononuclear phagocytes have functions similar to those of polymorphonuclear leukocytes. In addition, they are important sources of cytokines and are crucial as antigen-presenting cells. The function of the mononuclear phagocyte system has been reviewed in detail by Yoder and his colleagues.[253]

Chemotaxis, phagocytosis, and killing—Studies of monocytes from both preterm and term neonates demonstrate both normal and impaired chemotaxis, phagocytosis, and killing, similar to the findings for neutrophils. In one study, all of these functions were entirely normal.[254] Random movement was normal[226] but chemotaxis in a gradient was significantly decreased and did not achieve adult levels for up to 6 years.[227,255] The expression of CD14, the receptor for LPS, was normal in monocytes from term neonates, but the density of the adhesion molecules CD11a, CD11b, and CD11c was less than that of adult monocytes.[256] Since the adhesion molecules are important to phagocytosis, the lower density could contribute to impaired ability to ingest particles. Phagocytosis by term neonates has been reported to be both normal[257] and impaired.[258,259] Ingestion of polystyrene particles was delayed in neonatal monocytes, though eventually it was equivalent to those from adults.[258] Phagocytosis of *Streptococcus agalactiae* was significantly lower in cord blood monocytes,[259] but ingestion of a wide variety of particles and microorganisms, including latex particles, opsonized sheep erythrocytes, *S. aureus*, *Toxoplasma gondii*, and herpes simplex virus II, was equivalent in cord blood and adult monocytes.[257] Cord blood monocytes were capable of killing *C. albicans* to an equivalent degree as adult monocytes, but did not demonstrate augmentation when stimulated with interferon gamma .[260] Similarly, cord blood monocytes can kill a variety of bacteria.[257] Others found less efficient killing of *S. aureus* and type III group B streptococci by cord blood monocytes[259]; the lack of correlation between these findings may be due to differences in assay conditions.

Antigen presentation—Mononuclear macrophages play a critical role in presenting antigen to T cells. Antigen is processed within the macrophage and presented to CD4 cells in the context of class II (HLA-DR) antigens or to CD8 cells in the context of class I (HLA-A and HLA-B) antigens. Interaction of the T cell and the macrophage induces the macrophage to elaborate IL-1, which subsequently stimulates the T cell to proliferate and produce IL-2. HLA-DR expression is deficient in cord blood monocytes, but is increased to normal levels when the cells are stimulated with lymphokines such as IFN-alpha.[261] Cord blood monocytes cocultured with maternal or paternal T cells were fully capable of presenting tetanus toxoid[262,263] or *E. coli*[264] to induce the T cells to proliferate. However, when the monocytes were "pulsed" with antigen the response was significantly decreased when cord blood monocytes were used compared with those from adults. The significance of this difference in technique is not clear, but it may suggest a difference in the kinetics of antigen presentation by cord blood monocytes.

Monokine production—Monocytes are important sources of inflammatory cytokines including IL-1beta, TNF-alpha, IL-6, and IL-8, as well as leukotrienes. IL-1 activity has been reported to be both normal[265] and diminished.[266] In the first study, monocytes from 27 infants of gestational age 31 to 41 weeks produced normal amounts of IL-1 when stimulated with LPS; unstimulated levels were elevated in infants with perinatal stress or infections.[265] In the second study, both IL-1 and TNF-alpha were significantly reduced in term and preterm infants compared with adult controls.[266] Both studies measured IL-1 using an IL-1-dependent mouse T-cell line; TNF-alpha was measured by enzyme-linked immunosorbent assay (ELISA). There is no ready explanation for the discrepancy but several other studies showed similar dichotomy,[266] which may be due to selection of the infant populations to be studied. IL-6 is a monocyte-derived cytokine that is produced in response to IL-1 stimulation and is involved in B- and T-cell maturation and cycling of hematopoietic progenitor cells. Purified monocytes from term neonates produced only 50% and premature infants only 25% as much IL-6 as adult controls.[267] Other studies did not find a significant difference when using whole blood rather than purified monocytes.[268] It is possible that other cells in the mixture bound or degraded the IL-6 in the adult cell suspensions. Levels of both IL-8 and messenger RNA (mRNA) were decreased in purified monocytes from preterm and term infants.[269,270] In one study the cells were stimulated with IL-1alpha, TNF-alpha, and LPS,[269] whereas in the other study the cells were stimulated with group B streptococci.[270] The monocytes also produced less leukotriene B_4 in response to stimulation with streptococci.[270] Both IL-8 and leukotriene B_4 are potent chemoattractants, and the decreased levels may contribute to the poor response of neonates to infection.

Development of the Complement System

The complement system consists of a complex series of proteins that serve 2 major functions, to directly lyse cells and microorganisms and to act as potent opsonins.[271] C3 is crucial to the complement cascade. Fragments of C3-C3b, iC3b, and C3d-attach to target cells and bind to specific receptors on phagocytic cells, thereby greatly enhancing phagocytosis. Another C3 fragment, C3a, serves as a mediator of inflammation, stimulating chemotaxis and increasing vascular permeability. After C3 is activated, it can initiate the rest of the cascade, C5 to C9, which ultimately leads to lysis of red cells and some microorganisms. C3 can be activated through one of two pathways. The so-called classical pathway is initiated by antibody-antigen complexes that fix the complement components C1, C4, and C2, which form an enzyme that cleaves a thioester on the inactive C3 molecule to form active C3. This pathway is dependent on the presence of specific antibody, especially IgM, so it is less active in the neonate who lacks IgM and has limited amounts of specific IgG. However, some gram-positive and gram-negative bacteria, mycoplasma, and RNA viruses are capable of directly activating C1q and bypassing the need for antibody in the classical pathway. The other pathway to activate C3 is known as the alternative pathway and is independent of antibody. Factor B binds to small amounts of cleaved C3 that are spontaneously generated in the plasma. Normally this C3-factor B complex is degraded, but if the interaction takes place on an appropriate cell surface, the complex is protected and, in concert with other proteins such as factor D and properdin, acts as a potent enzyme to cleave additional C3 and initiate the remainder of the complement cascade. Most mammalian cells have complement regulatory proteins on their surfaces to prevent activation of the alternative pathway. However, if the interaction takes place on a bacterial or fungal cell surface, C3 is activated and the remainder of the complement system is directed against the organism.

Because the complement system is a cascade involving many different proteins, a severe deficiency of one protein or a relative deficiency of many proteins can result in decreased function of the entire system. Complement is present early in fetal development. Most of the complement components have been detected in cultures of fetal tissues: C5 from lung and liver at 8 to 9 weeks of gestation; C4, C2, and C3 from liver at 8 to 14 weeks; C1q from spleen at 14 weeks; and C1 from small intestine and colon at 19 weeks.[271] None of the complement components cross the placenta, as shown by studies of allotypic markers on the proteins, so the levels in the infant reflect synthesis.[271,272] The concentrations of the various components increase throughout gestation and reach approximately 50% to 90% of adult values by term, though preterm infants have significantly lower levels of all components, especially those of the alternative pathway.[231,271] Concentrations of the later components, especially C6, C8, and C9, are more affected in both term and preterm infants, ranging from 10% to 47% of adult values.[271] In one study, measurements of complement obtained using the functional assay CH_{50} ranged from 50% to 81% of adult values, depending on whether the infants were compared to normal adults or the higher values found in their postpartum mothers.[271] Levels of activation products, C3a-desArg from the classical pathway and C3bBbP from the alternative, were similar in term infants and adults and increased transiently in infected newborns,[273] suggesting that the lower levels were due to low synthesis rather than consumption. This study also showed that the infants were capable of activating complement in response to infection, but only the early steps in the cascade were evaluated. The serum of newborns had decreased opsonic activity[274] and production of chemotactic factors.[275] The decreased generation of chemoattractant was not due to lack of specific antibody since addition of antigen-antibody complexes did not overcome the defect.[275] Adding specific antibody did not normalize generation of C5a, but normal levels of the chemoattractant could be achieved by adding C3.[276] Thus, the levels of the complement components are sufficiently low to impair function, especially in premature infants and, together with decreased levels of specific antibodies and impaired levels of other opsonins, are a significant cause of increased infection in young children.

Development of Humoral Immunity

The humoral immune system consists of the B lymphocytes and their secreted products, the immunoglobulins. B cells begin development very early in fetal development, but in humans the humoral system is very immature at birth, and full maturation does not occur until around the time of puberty. Our understanding of B-cell development has been greatly enhanced by molecular biology techniques that have elucidated the complex gene rearrangements that are unique among the genes of the immunoglobulin supergene family. The primary purpose of B cells is to produce immunoglobulins that are specific antibodies. B cells also present antigen to T cells and produce a joining or J chain polypeptide that helps hold the dimeric IgA and pentameric IgM together.

B-cell development occurs in 2 stages.[231] In the initial stages, precursor cells rearrange the heavy-chain mu genes and express cytoplasmic mu chains and are termed pre-B cells. Next, the light chain rearranges and the cell can express IgM on the surface (sIgM). At this point the cell is an immature B cell. Up to this point the maturation process is antigen-independent and can occur in the total absence of T cells. Indeed, exposure of these immature B cells to antigens, in the absence of T-cell help, leads to clonal deletion. This is a mechanism for eliminating cells that are capable of reacting to self-antigens. Isotype switching occurs and the immature B cell can express IgA and IgG on the surface, though the number of cells is low and these immunoglobulins are coexpressed with IgM and often IgD. This isotype switching is also T-independent, though later T-cell help is required for isotype switching of mature B cells to IgG- or IgA-producing plasma cells. After the mature B cell has formed, further exposure to antigen results in clonal expansion of cells whose surface immunoglobulin binds to that antigen and development of plasma cells producing specific antibody.

Ontogeny of B Cells

B-cell precursors originate in yolk sac and initially develop in the fetal liver.[277-282] The first recognizable cell is a large cycling lymphoid cell with cytoplasmic mu heavy chains but no light chains. These cells appear in the human fetal liver at about 8 weeks' gestation. By 12 weeks' gestation these cells can be identified in fetal bone marrow. The large pre-B cells give rise to small, resting pre-B cells that express HLA-DR and about this time begin to express the receptor for EBV, CD21.[277] The pre-B cell rearranges either a kappa or lambda light chain and is able to express sIgM;[278,279] it is then an immature B cell. A small proportion of sIgM⁻ cells have cytoplasmic light chains; these cells represent an intermediate stage in transition between a pre-B and B lymphocyte. Immature sIgM⁺ B cells are the predominant type from the 9th to the 12th week of gestation. Pre-B cells are numerous in fetal liver but are far outnumbered by B cells in spleen, blood, and lymph nodes. By the second half of gestation the major site of pre-B-cell production shifts from the liver to the bone marrow.[280] By the thirteenth week of gestation the majority of cells express both IgM and IgD, and a few sIgA and sIgG cells begin to appear at about this time.[277] The frequency of B cells expressing the various isotypes achieves adult proportions by the 15th week, but nearly all coexpress sIgM, which is an immature phenotype. The shift toward cells expressing a single isotype does not occur until after birth. For example, IgA-bearing cells that do not coexpress sIgM appear at 3 to 5 months of age.[277] The number of IgA-secreting cells is reduced at birth, especially in premature infants, although the number is significantly increased if the neonate is infected.[283]

B-cell development can be further characterized using monoclonal antibodies. The pre-B cells and immature B cells in fetal liver express IgM, CD19, CD20, and CD24, but are negative for CD21 and CD22.[281,282] However, CD21, which is the receptor for C3b and EBV, develops at about this time because EBV infection of these cells leads to proliferation.[277] These early pre-B and some immature B cells are positive for the surface enzyme TdT (terminal deoxynucleotidyl transferase) and for CD10, or CALLA (common acute lymphoblastic leukemia antigen).[282] These surface antigens largely disappear early in B-cell development, though some CD10[+] cells can be found in peripheral blood B lymphocytes. HLA-DR also is present at the pre-B-cell stage.[284] Greater numbers of HLA-DR cells than HLA-DP or HLA-DQ cells are present at 12 weeks' gestation. Expression of HLA-DQ occurs about the same time as expression of sIgD and is coincident with the development of follicles.[284] Both lymph node cells at 17 weeks' and spleen at 16-21 weeks' gestation are positive for all of these antigens but are negative for CD5, an antigen that is shared by T cells. After 17 weeks the B cells in lymph nodes are positive for CD5.[281] In the fetal spleen, up to 40%-60% of the B cells are CD5[+]. CD5[+] B cells are increased following bone marrow transplantation, HIV infection, and some autoimmune diseases.[285] The percentage and absolute number of CD5[+] B cells are markedly elevated in the blood of term or premature infants.[283] A late marker of B-cell maturation is the enzyme ecto-5'-nucleotidase (ecto-5'-NT).[286] Activity of ecto-5'-NT is decreased in a variety of B-cell disorders such as X-linked agammaglobulinemia and common variable CVID and is low on neonatal B cells, but reaches normal adult levels by the time infants are 6 months of age.[286] Isotype switching is dependent on CD40-L on the T cell interacting with CD40 on B cells. Although CD40 is present on the surface of neonatal B cells, they are unable to switch to IgG or IgA by stimulation with CD40 agonists such as anti-CD40 or soluble CD40-L in the presence of IL-4 or IL-10.[287]

The development of B cells can be evaluated by their ability to synthesize immunoglobulin in response to a variety of stimuli. Some stimuli, such as PWM, require T-cell help and thus are difficult to use in neonates, whose T cells are also immature. Others, such as *Nocardia* water-soluble mitogen (NWSM) and *Staphylococcus aureus* Cowan I (SAC), are relatively independent of T cells, and infection with EBV is completely T-independent. Transformation of both sIgM[+] and sIgM[-] cells from neonatal blood resulted in secretion of IgM, whereas stimulation of only sIgM[+] adult cells resulted in IgM production.[288] B cells from the peripheral blood of adults produced predominantly IgM, whereas production of other isotypes depended on the tissue source of the B cells; splenocytes produced IgG but B cells from the appendix produced IgA. Cord blood B lymphocytes developed into cells with cytoplasmic IgM but not IgA or IgG, though IgG-secreting cells were detected in the cultures by a reverse hemolytic plaque assay.[289] NWSM stimulated cord and newborn peripheral blood to produce small numbers of IgM-producing B cells but only rare IgA- or IgG-producing cells.[290] The number of IgM-producing cells reached adult levels by 1 month of age, whereas the number of IgG-producing cells was not normal until 5 to 8 years of age and IgA-producing cells by 9 to 12 years. Purified B cells from adults produced immunoglobulins poorly but were significantly augmented when either adult or neonatal T cells were added. Similar results were obtained using cord blood B cells, though only IgM-secreting cells were produced and the magnitude was much lower than when using adult B cells. The addition of T cells from adults did not increase the number of cells synthesizing IgG or IgA.[290] Stimulation of unfractionated cord cells with PWM yielded similar results, though none of the isotypes were normal by 3 years of age.[290] The total number of immunoglobulin-producing cells was about 50% of adult values at 3 years of age and was equivalent to that of adults by 5 years. It was found that cord blood T lymphocytes were suppressive and that their removal resulted in greater numbers of IgM-producing B cells.[290] The suppressive effect was absent when infants were tested between 1 and 2 years of age. The addition of hydrocortisone decreased the suppressive activity and enhanced immunoglobulin in a majority of neonates tested.[291,292] Depletion of monocytes did not have an effect.[292] Substituting adult T cells for cord blood T cells increased the production of Ig plaque-forming cells, particularly of the IgG and IgA classes.[293,294]

SAC stimulates a subset of B cells that rosette with mouse erythrocytes to proliferate, but these cells do not proceed to immunoglobulin production.[295] SAC does not stimulate the nonrosetting B cells in the presence or absence of T cells. The addition of PWM in the presence of T cells resulted in immunoglobulin synthesis by the rosette-negative B cells only.[295] The combination of PWM and SAC enhanced the production of immunoglobulin by unfractionated cord cells compared with PWM alone.[296] Addition of IL-1 could substitute for SAC, and various elements of T-cell-conditioned medium, now known to be IL-2, IL-4, and IL-6, could replace PWM. In a more recent study, B cells from fetal liver, spleen, and bone marrow could be induced to produce IgM, IgG, and IgE, but not IgA, in response to IL-4 and either anti-CD40 or cloned CD4[+] T cells.[297] The majority of the responding cells had the phenotype CD19⁺CD10⁺CD5⁺. Addition of IL-6 did not have an effect. Pre-B cells that were sIgM⁻ could not be induced to produce immunoglobulin. Thus, poor immunoglobulin production in the neonate is due in part to immaturity of the B cells, which produce mainly IgM, but suppressor activity by neonatal T cells and T-cell immaturity also are significant factors.

Immunoglobulin Production

Normally, the fetus produces very little immunoglobulin prior to birth. The fetus is capable of producing antibody in response to infection, but nearly all is of the IgM isotype. Maternal antibody is specifically transferred across the placenta beginning at the end of the first trimester, though the majority of IgG enters the fetus in the last 12 weeks. Immunoglobulin production begins at the time of birth, probably as a result of antigen stimulation, regardless of whether the child is term or premature.[298] However, premature infants do not receive as much IgG from their mothers. Therefore, premature infants begin life with low IgG levels and remain hypogammaglobulinemic for more than 6 months.[299] IgM production is only slightly delayed compared with that of normal full-term children, whereas IgA production is severely impaired.[299] In the term infant, the levels of IgG approach those of adults by 5 or 6 years of age, IgM by 2 or 3 years, and IgA by 10 to 12 years.[300] The secretory IgA system develops slowly after birth.[301] There are no IgA plasma cells in the lamina propria at birth, but within a short time IgA⁺ cells appear and IgA can be detected by immunofluorescence.[302] There was more IgM than IgA antibody in intestinal secretions after peroral immunization with *E. coli*.[303] IgA was detectable in the tears of infants as young as 10 to 20 days of age[304] and in saliva by the second week.[305] The concentration of sIgA increased slowly, reaching adult levels by 6 to 8 years of age.[306]

Specific Antibody Formation

The fetus is able to synthesize IgM antibodies in response to infection by the 20th week of gestation.[307,308] Immunization of the mother with tetanus toxoid has induced IgM antitetanus antibody in the fetus,[309] presumably on the basis of antigen that has crossed the placenta. However, the presence of secretory IgA and IgM antibodies to *E. coli* and poliovirus in neonates suggests that the infant was responding to anti-idiotype antibodies from the mother, since it was unlikely that the mother was exposed to polio antigen and therefore could not have transmitted it to the fetus.[310] This interesting observation has not been confirmed in other systems, but does raise questions about interpretation of antibody responses in neonates.

Neonates are capable of responding to protein antigens such as tetanus toxoid or conjugated *H. influenzae* vaccine within a few weeks of birth.[311-313] However, there is little response to the T-independent polysaccharide antigens until the child is at least 24 months of age[314-316]; younger children are capable of producing transient IgG1 antibodies but are unable to develop immunologic memory. Premature infants produced antibodies to ingested protein antigens, such as bovine serum albumin,[298] and premature infants also produced antibodies to routine immunizations, though the levels were lower than in term infants.[317] In the premature infants, IgG antibodies to tetanus and diphtheria fell from birth to 4 months of age and then rose significantly by 9 months, 2 months after the third diphtheria-pertussis-tetanus (DPT) immunization. However, the levels were lower than in term infants. Levels of IgG antibody to staphylococci were comparable to those of term babies. IgM opsonic activity in response to natural exposure to *E. coli* was low in both term and preterm infants at birth and rose comparably by 9 months of chronologic age. Thus, the preterm infants matured in relation to postnatal chronologic age rather than gestational age.[317]

Development of the Cellular Immune System

The cellular immune system comprises the thymus-derived or T lymphocytes. T cells are responsible for protection against viral, fungal, and parasitic organisms and neoplastic cells, and in addition play a crucial role in the regulation of B cells. Development of the thymus and T cells begins early in fetal life, and the early T cells have many of the functions of mature cells; however, at the time of birth human T cells are functionally immature, with impaired capacity to produce cytokines, poor ability to provide help for B cells, and excessive suppressor activity.[318-320]

Ontogeny of T Cells

T cells arise from lymphoid precursors that develop within the thymus. The primitive thymic rudiment forms at about 4 weeks' gestation from the ectoderm of the third brachial cleft and the endoderm of the third brachial pouch.[321] The right and left rudiments enlarge and fuse by the eighth week, and at about that time the first precursors from the fetal liver and bone marrow begin to colonize the epithelial rudiment. Mesodermal cells invade the rudimentary thymus in the 10th week, effecting lobulation and inducing proliferation of the epithelial cells. Corticomedullary distinction is present by 14 weeks and the first Hassall's bodies by 16 weeks. The epithelial cells in the 7-week thymic rudiment express class II determinants and by 8.5 weeks both class I and class II. If the hematopoietic precursors are not normal and cannot interact with the other thymic elements, as occurs in babies with SCID, development is arrested and the thymus remains epithelial and primitive. Thus, mutual interactions between all of the elements—epithelial, mesenchymal, and hematopoietic—are required for normal thymic development.

The first cells that can be considered pre-T cells are present in the 7-week thymus and are CD7[+] but negative for the classical T-cell antigens CD3, CD4, and CD8. By 8.5 weeks a subset is positive for the sheep red blood cell receptor CD2. These cells are at thymocyte stage I.[321] Development proceeds rapidly and by 10 weeks thymocytes are positive for CD5, CD3, CD25, and both CD4 and CD8, and a subset are positive for the transferrin receptor CD71. The IL-2 receptor, CD25 or Tac, is present on both B and T cells, though in higher density on the T cell. The majority of Tac[+] cells in the thymus are present in the medulla.[322] Few cells are positive in the fetal liver or spleen at 18-20 weeks' gestation. Rearrangements of TCR alpha/beta occur at about the same time as expression of the CD3 molecule, but some of the CD3[+] cells express TCR gamma/delta; the percentage of gamma/delta[+] cells peaks at about 15 weeks' gestation and then decreases toward adult levels by birth. However, these cells are found in higher proportion in the mucosal lymphoid areas. At 10 weeks, 47% of the CD3[+] cells express TCR beta and 25% are positive for TCR alpha/beta.[320] CD1, another marker of T cells, also appears shortly after CD3, at about 12 weeks' gestation. As the thymocytes mature, the density of CD3 on the surface increases to that seen in peripheral blood T cells.[320] Occasional CD3[+] cells are present in the blood from the end of the 12th week, their proportion rising from 20%-30% at 14 weeks to 50% by 22 weeks. These cells are positive for either CD4 or CD8, but not both. Nearly all of the T cells are positive for the CD45RA phenotype characteristic of naive T cells. The appearance of T cells in the blood is paralleled by the presence of T cells in the spleen and liver.

Lymphoid cells obtained from fetal thymus as early as 10 to 12 weeks' or from peripheral blood at 14 weeks' gestation are capable of responding to mitogens such as PHA or concanavalin A (Con A), or to allogeneic cells.[323-325] Responses to Con A develop more slowly, as is seen in some animal models.[326] Because proliferation of T cells is dependent on production of IL-2, it is clear that fetal cells are capable of synthesizing that cytokine. By the time of birth the cord blood T cells can respond to mitogen stimulation as well as those of adults, though some investigators have reported reduced responses in premature infants, perhaps due to excessive suppressor activity.[326] The T cells from 15-22 weeks are capable of developing specific cell-mediated cytotoxicity following stimulation with alloantigens, though much more poorly than those from term infants or adults.[327] Despite the ability of these cells to proliferate, as is discussed in the following sections, these T cells are both naïve and immature.

Postnatal Development of T-Cell Function

Maturation of the T-cell repertoire

Maturation of the T cells–Neonatal T cells express CD3, CD4, and CD8 in proportions that approximate those of adult T cells, yet the cells are phenotypically and functionally immature. In early studies it was shown that cord blood T cells had a lower percentage of the helper-inducer phenotype, 2H4$^-$4B4$^+$, whereas the percentage of the suppressor-inducer phenotype 2H4$^+$4B4$^-$ was slightly higher than in adult T cells.[328] More recently it has been shown that the majority of the cord blood T cells are CD45RA$^+$CD45RO$^-$, which is characteristic of virgin or naive T cells.[329] Many of these cells displayed a low level of fluorescence when stained with an anti-CD45 antibody; this CD45RO^{dim+} population is not seen in older children or adults. The amount of CD45RO could be upregulated by stimulation with PHA or allogeneic cells. The percentage of CD3$^+$ cells with CD45RO increases logarithmically during the first several years of life, from < 10% at birth to 40% at 10 years of age to > 60% in adulthood. Infants who became atopic in the first years of life tended to have lower levels of the mature CD45RO$^+$ T cells,[330] perhaps leading to poorer T-cell regulation.

There is a higher proportion of gamma-delta T cells in the neonate than in the adult or older child.[318,331] Neonatal gamma-delta T cells are phenotypically and functionally different from gamma-delta T cells in the adult.[331] They are weakly cytotoxic to K-562, an NK-sensitive line, and display poor lectin-mediated cytolysis and redirected cytolysis. They express lower levels of CD2, LFA-1, and CD45RO than adult cells and are therefore more similar to the small population of CD4$^+$ gamma-delta T cells in the adult. The neonatal T cells express a diverse V_γ and V_δ gene segments rather than the predominant $V_\gamma 2V_\delta 2$ commonly seen in adult gamma-delta T cells. A large proportion of these neonatal cells respond to mycobacterial heat shock proteins, and their numbers can be increased by immunization, especially with pertussis.[318]

T cells from newborns are deficient in their ability to provide B-cell help. It is now known that interaction of CD40-L on T cells with CD40 on B cells is critical for immunoglobulin isotype switching and normal production of antibody. Expression of CD40-L was lower in newborn lymphocytes than in adult cells after stimulation with phorbol ester and ionomycin.[332,333] The activated cord T cells also had lower levels of mRNA for CD40-L. Neonatal B cells were able to synthesize IgE when they were provided with IL-4 and their CD40 receptors were engaged by anti-CD40, indicating that the defect is primarily in the T cell.[332] Neonatal cells could not express CD40-L although they expressed other activation markers such as CD69.[287] CD40-L was expressed on 19- to 28-week fetuses and could be expressed on newborns' T-lymphocyte cell lines generated with PHA and IL-2. CD40-L mRNA transcripts and intracytoplasmic protein expression were reduced, indicating a possible transcriptional down-regulation of CD40-L expression.[287]

Neonatal T cells have reduced expression of the IL-2Rγ chain, which is correlated with decreased IL-2-dependent T-cell activation.[334,335] This is in contrast to fetal cells and those from preterm infants who had high expression of CD25 along with an immature phenotype, CD1$^+$CD38$^+$CD71$^+$, which is more characteristic of mature thymic cells.[336] The immaturity of the cord blood T cells is further shown by the upregulation of CD38 on neonatal but not adult T cells,[337] a higher proportion of double-positive CD4$^+$CD8$^+$CD3$^+$ cells,[338] and binding to peanut agglutinin characteristic of mature thymocytes.[339] Cord blood lymphocytes also have reduced expression of receptors for IL-2, IL-4, IL-6, IL-7, TNF-alpha, and IFN-gamma.[340] None of the receptors was absent, but the reduced expression might be responsible for the decreased responsiveness to those cytokines.

Normal values for T lymphocytes in infancy and childhood

Infants have a marked lymphocytosis at birth. One study reported that the mean (SD) lymphocyte count for healthy newborn infants was 4.185×10^9/L (2.017 to 7.261×10^9/L).[213] By 5 days the number had increased to 5.616×10^9/L (2.856 to 9.125×10^9/L). The normal numbers of lymphocytes, T cells, B cells, and NK cells are summarized in **Table 11-3**.[341] The relative percentage of T cells is decreased in neonates compared with adults, but the absolute number is increased due to the lymphocytosis, and the number remains higher than adult values until nearly 7 years of age. The same is true of B cells and NK cells, although the latter fall within the adult range within 1 year of birth.[341] CD4 and CD8 counts were determined from a large group of infants from 0 to 4 years of age by the European Collaborative Study.[342] Though focused on providing normal values for evaluating children for HIV infection, the resulting graphs are nonetheless useful in evaluating children with suspected primary immunodeficiency diseases. In this study, CD4 counts peaked at around 6 months of age, with a median of 2.0×10^9/L. CD8 counts peaked much later, at around 1 year of age. More extensive evaluation of lymphocyte subsets was done, comparing cord blood values to those obtained from infants at 5 days of age.[343] For the majority of children the CD3$^+$, CD4$^+$, and CD5$^+$ counts and percentages were higher in the sample obtained at 5 days than in their cord blood. B-cell numbers and

Table 11-3
Absolute Numbers of Lymphocyte Subsets from Birth to Adulthood*

Lymphocyte Subset	< 1 year of age		1 to 3 years of age		3 to 5 years of age		5 to 13 years of age	
CD3	5026	± 2996	2971	± 2188	2641	± 1739	1890	± 872
CD4	3817	± 2570	2094	± 1527	1798	± 1372	1104	± 616
CD8	1614	± 1131	1019	± 990	1003	± 779	865	± 530
CD20	1149	1278	591	811	362	476	233	242
CD57	852	± 1517	531	± 704	717	± 408	599	± 649
HLA-DR	2337	± 2266	1625	± 1363	1189	± 784	910	± 556

*Mean ± 2 SD.
Abbreviations: CD3 = pan T cells; CD4 = helper/inducer T cells; CD8 = suppressor/cytotoxic T cells, subset of NK cells; CD21= B cells; CD57 = subset of NK cells and subset of activated T cytotoxic cells.
Adapted from Yanase, et al.[346]

percentages decreased, as did the number and percentage of NK cells determined by anti-CD16+CD56+. Another study of 53 newborns reported the normal values of T-cell, B-cell, and NK-cell percentages and absolute numbers, as well as the values for CD71, CD25, TCR alpha/beta, and CD11a.[344] The values in this study were comparable to those obtained in the previous studies. Cytotoxic T cells and NK cells were studied in 12 neonates using 2-color flow cytometric analysis.[345] Both the percentages and absolute numbers of CD57+ lymphocytes and non-MHC-restricted cytotoxic T cells (CD3+CD56+) were reduced. The phenotype of the NK cells was different from that of adults' cells, with higher levels of CD11b+ and lower levels of CD57+ among the CD16+ lymphocytes. The percentages and absolute numbers of CD4+, CD8+, CD3+, CD16+, CD19+, CD20+, and HLA-DR+ cells were reported in 72 Japanese infants and children from 2 months to 13 years of age.[346]

Proliferation

Cord blood T cells from term infants proliferate in response to mitogens such as PHA or allogeneic cells as well as, or better than, adult T cells.[347-350] The responses decrease into the normal adult range late in infancy.[349,350] A subpopulation of activated T cells in cord blood that are HLA-DR+ and CD25+ and coexpress both CD4 and CD8 undergo strong IL-2-induced proliferation and may be a mechanism to provide strong responses to an otherwise compromised immune system.[351] Although the responses to classical mitogens are normal, the responses to other stimuli, such as anti-CD2[352] or anti-CD3,[349,353,354] are markedly reduced. The response to anti-CD2 can be augmented by the addition of calcium ionophore[352] or IL-1[355] into the culture, indicating that the poor response is due to defective upregulation of IL-2 production. In contrast to the response to mitogens by T cells from term infants, in most studies T cells from premature neonates have reduced responses.[356,357] In one study, 50% of infants < 1000 g had impaired responses to PHA and Con A, whereas infants from 1251 to 1500 g had normal responses.[358] In another study of very low birth weight infants (700 to 1300 g), nearly all had significantly reduced responses to PHA that did not rise into the normal range until 8 weeks after birth.[356] However, in another study by Herrod and his coworkers of 16 healthy premature infants < 1350 g, nearly all had responses equivalent to those of healthy term infants.[359] The difference between this study and the others may be the health of the infants and the fact that they all received enteral nutritional support. Neonatal cells are much more sensitive to the effects of dexamethasone than are adult cells, but the inhibition can be reversed by adding IL-2.[360] Therefore, although responses to routine mitogens or allogeneic cells suggest that neonates are normal, there are several lines of evidence, such as the poor response to anti-CD3 or anti-CD2 and the sensitivity to corticosteroids, that indicate that the cells are functionally immature.

Helper and suppressor activity

One of the more interesting aspects of the neonatal immune response is the strong suppressor activity, even within the so-called helper or CD4$^+$ subset of T cells. The first indication of the suppressor function of neonatal cells was the observation by Olding and Oldstone that lymphocytes from neonates strongly decreased proliferation of their mothers' cells.[361] Suppressor activity was present in fetal liver as early as the 8th week of gestation and in fetal blood by the 14th week, and persisted until the infant was about 1 year of age.[362] Supernatants of cord blood T cells were capable of suppressing immunoglobulin production by adult B cells in a PWM-driven system.[363] Initially the primary suppressor activity was identified to be within the CD8$^+$ population[364]; resting T cells were not suppressive and had to be activated by PWM or allogeneic cells before they could exert their activity.[365] These observations are in contrast to those of a large number of studies that conclusively demonstrated that nearly all of the suppressor activity resided in the CD4$^+$CD8$^-$ population of T cells.[366-370] Cord blood mononuclear cells depleted of CD8$^+$ cells still showed strong suppression of immunoglobulin production by adult B cells, whereas depletion of CD4$^+$ T cells abrogated suppression in a PWM-driven system.[366,368] Cord mononuclear cells activated with PWM or allogeneic cells were also capable of suppressing mitogen-induced proliferation of adult cells,[367] but Con A, which stimulates predominantly CD8$^+$ cells, did not induce suppressor activity in cord blood.[369] The suppressor activity was eliminated by irradiation or hydrocortisone.[368,371]

The neonatal cells are relatively resistant to their own suppressive activity.[372] Cord blood CD4$^+$ cells exert their suppressive activity directly, not by inducing adult CD8$^+$ suppressor cells.[367] Maternal mononuclear cells depleted of CD4 or CD8 T cells were highly sensitive to suppression by prostaglandin E$_2$ (PGE$_2$), whereas similar cord blood populations were resistant.[367,373,374] The mechanism of the PGE$_2$-induced suppression is not known, but it was shown that PGE$_2$ could suppress proliferation by calcium ionophore or various mitogens, but not phorbol ester.[375] This differential sensitivity to PGE$_2$ could provide a mechanism for fetal and neonatal cells to suppress graft-versus-host activity of maternal lymphocytes without inhibiting their own T-cell-mediated functions.

In contrast to the strong suppressor activity exerted by cord blood CD4$^+$ cells, they have poor ability to provide help for either neonatal or adult B cells.[366,371,376] This inability to provide help is independent of the suppressor activity and may be due, at least in part, to deficiencies in cytokine production,[376] as is discussed in the next section.

Cytokine Production

The majority of studies of cord blood and young infants indicate that production of the cytokines is defective (both the T$_H$1 cytokines such as IFN-gamma and IL-2 and the T$_H$2 cytokines involved in helper activity for B cells). Early studies indicated that the production of immune or IFN-gamma was defective,[319,377-380] whereas production of classical or alpha interferon (IFN-alpha) was normal.[377] The defect in IFN-gamma production may be due to immaturity of the macrophages rather than an intrinsic T-cell defect.[381] Production of IFN-gamma remains abnormal for several months[379] and perhaps years[380] after birth. Production of IFN-gamma in response to natural infection with herpes simplex virus was significantly impaired in neonates and postpartum women for up to 6 weeks.[382] In contrast to these studies, Stephens and coworkers found IFN-gamma production to be normal in 30 term infants from birth to 9 months of age.[383] Wu and colleagues found that the CD45RA or naive T cells in cord blood could be induced to produce IFN-gamma when cultured in the presence of IL-12.[384] Production was enhanced in the presence of IL-1 or macrophages, IL-2, and TNF-alpha. In the presence of IL-12 the T cells become activated and express CD25, CD71, and HLA-DR. The IL-12 enhances the production of IL-2 and IFN-gamma, but not IL-4, and thus favors maturation into the T$_H$1 phenotype.[384]

Cord blood cells stimulated with PHA or phorbol myristate acetate produced less IL-2 and IL-6, and provided less growth and differentiating activity for B cells than T cells from adults.[385] Decreased IL-2 production can lead to failure to expand antigen-specific precursor cell populations and hence poor responses to antigens.[386] Augmentation of IL-2 production by addition of IL-1 markedly improved the otherwise poor response of neonatal cells to anti-CD2,[355] again indicating that diminished IL-2 production is central to the hyporesponsiveness of neonatal cells. IL-4 production also was reduced, which may, at least in part, be responsible for the poor ability to provide help for B cells.[319,380] Other cytokines, such as macrophage-inhibiting factor (MIF) and lymphocyte-inhibiting factor (LIF), also were decreased, though these factors remain poorly characterized and the early studies have not been confirmed.[387]

Natural Killer Cells and Cytotoxicity

Natural killer cells are defined as a population of cells that are capable of spontaneous cytotoxicity against a variety of target cells. NK cells resemble large granular lymphocytes, but their exact origin is unknown. They express the CD2 antigen, which is present on the majority of T lymphocytes, but also express CD16, the FcγRIII on granulocytes. Currently they are defined as CD3epsilon⁻, CD16⁺, and/or CD56⁺ lymphocytes that mediate MHC-unrestricted cytotoxicity. NK cells do not rearrange the T-cell antigen receptor genes and thus differ from cytotoxic T cells. NK cells are active against tumor cells and virally infected cells, regardless of whether they express HLA antigens, and thus may play an important role in immune surveillance. NK activity develops early in fetal life. Activity was detected in the liver as early as 9 weeks' gestation,[388] though functional NK cells could not be detected in the fetal blood until approximately 27 weeks' gestation.[389] Cord blood from 3 of 4 premature infants of gestational age 28 to 33 weeks demonstrated activity comparable to that of term infants.[388] The fetal NK cells and a subset of cord blood NK cells differed from adult NK cells in that they expressed substantial amounts of CD3 delta and CD3 epsilon proteins in the cytoplasm.[390] The fetal cells also differed from the adult in their response to IL-2 and IFN-gamma[389]; the activity of adult cells is boosted by both cytokines, whereas the NK cells obtained from early fetuses responded to IL-2 but not the interferon.

The proportion of CD16⁺ cells in cord blood or the blood of infants is diminished compared with adult values, but the absolute numbers are not significantly different.[345] The NK cells from the newborn are phenotypically different, with much higher levels of CD11b and lower levels of CD57. The NK activity of normal term infants was diminished in several studies.[391-394] Some studies have demonstrated a bimodal distribution, with 12 of 20 cord blood samples exhibiting normal NK activity and the remaining 8 virtually no

NK function in one study,[391] and a similar proportion in a more recent study.[395] Other studies have shown that the overall NK activity of the neonate is significantly reduced; for example, 16% specific activity compared with 36% in adults in one study[392] or 27% compared to 39% in adults.[393] NK activity remains lower than adult levels for at least 4 years.[396] If the cord blood cells are incubated overnight in IFN-alpha, NK activity increases significantly and approximates that of the adult.[392,393] Similarly, incubation in IL-2 increases killing by cord blood NK cells to the normal range.[397] These observations suggest that the NK cells are present but fail to mature because of lack of T-cell-derived cytokines. It is likely that in premature and even in term infants 2 populations of NK cells exist.[395] Normal activity was associated with cells that were CD16$^+$CD56$^+$. The cord blood cells were responsive to IL-2, but not to IFN-gamma, unlike adult cells, which respond to both. Although no study has shown a direct correlation between the reduced NK activity and clinical disease, it may be responsible for the increased incidence of malignancy and overwhelming viral infections in the neonatal period.

The other cytotoxic mechanisms have been less well studied in the neonate. Lectin-dependent T-lymphocyte cytotoxicity was significantly reduced in cord and neonatal blood, whereas lectin-dependent cytotoxicity by non-T cells was normal or even enhanced.[394] Similarly, antibody-dependent cellular cytotoxicity was markedly reduced in infants,[398,399] improving over the first weeks of life. Others found that NK activity was low in neonates but that antibody-mediated cytotoxicity and NK-like activity generated in mixed lymphocyte cultures were equivalent to those of adults, and that lymphokine-activated killer (LAK) cell activity was high in the neonate.[400] While these defects may explain the increased susceptibility to viral infections that is observed in neonates, the biologic relevance of these assays is far from clear.

Clinical and Laboratory Evaluation of the Patient with Suspected Immunodeficiency Disease

History and Physical Examination

Immune deficiency diseases can present at any age, though the majority of the severe congenital diseases become manifest within the first few years of life.

Severe defects in cellular immunity or neutrophils may present within hours to days of birth. In general, primary humoral immunodeficiencies do not present in the perinatal period since the maternal antibodies transferred across the placenta help to protect the newborn infant from infection for the first 3-6 months of life. CVID can present in infancy or the onset may be delayed for years. Some diseases, such as chronic granulomatous disease, hyper-IgE syndrome, and ataxia telangiectasia, often do not present for several years. In many cases, the onset may be an autoimmune disease or unusual response to a typical infection. The clinician must have a high index of suspicion to make the diagnosis of immune deficiency before serious infections and permanent tissue damage occur.

Specific points in the history, physical examination, and laboratory evaluation can be helpful in determining whether a patient has an immune defect (**Table 11-4**). All children are at risk of developing infections, but the frequency, severity, and infectious agent can give important clues when deciding who should undergo an immunologic evaluation. Infections with opportunistic agents such as *P. carinii* or *C. albicans* should always lead to an evaluation of the immune system. Recurrent or persistent infections or infections that are unusually severe also should be an indication for initiating an evaluation. A history of chronic diarrhea, rash, or failure to thrive is of special concern. As was discussed in the previous sections, many of the immune deficiency diseases are associated with specific abnormalities. Therefore, hypocalcemia, congenital heart disease, and abnormal facial features would suggest DiGeorge anomaly. Similarly, an eczematous rash, petechiae or bleeding, and sinopulmonary infections in a boy would be consistent with Wiskott-Aldrich syndrome. Babies with SCID can present with thrush, diarrhea, and failure to thrive, but may also have an erythematous morbilliform rash due to GvHD from transplacentally acquired maternal T lymphocytes. The constellation of omphalitis or delayed separation of the umbilical cord and a marked leukocytosis is very suggestive of leukocyte adhesion defect, or LAD. Recurrent sepsis suggests a defect in phagocytosis or complement. It is important to realize that children can initially present with a very benign history, and thus a very high index of suspicion and a willingness to evaluate children with unusual features is critical if the diagnosis is to be made early, before serious complications can develop.

A careful family history of immunodeficiency should be obtained, with special emphasis on a history of recurrent infections or early childhood deaths. It is especially important to ask about infections among male members of the family since many of the primary immunodeficiency diseases are inherited in an X-linked fashion. However, many of the X-linked defects arise from spontaneous mutations in the patient so that the family history is negative. Risk factors for AIDS also must be explored and in most cases followed by specific testing of the

Table 11-4
Evaluation of Host Defense in Patients with Suspected Immune Deficiency

General	
Detailed history	*Chest X-ray*
Physical examination	Sinus X-ray or CT scan
Family history	Tests for allergy

Humoral Immunity	
Screening Tests	*Advanced Tests*
White blood count and differential	B cell phenotyping
Quantitative immunoglobulins	Antibodies to vaccine antigens
Isoagglutinins (anti-A and anti-B)	(eg, tetanus, diphtheria, H. influenzae)
CH50 or CH100	Specific complement components
	Response to bacteriophage φ/χ-174
	In vitro immunoglobulin synthesis

Cellular Immunity	
Screening Tests	*Advanced Tests*
White blood count and differential	Lymphocyte phenotyping
Delayed hypersensitivity skin tests	Proliferation to mitogens, antigens,
	allogeneic cells
	In vitro immunoglobulin synthesis
	Cytokine production
	Cellular cytotoxicity (eg, NK assay)

Phagocytic System	
Screening Tests	*Advanced Tests*
White blood count and differential	Oxidative burst assay
NBT	Quantitative NBT
	Cell surface receptors by flow cytometry
	Chemotaxis
	Phagocytosis
	Bactericidal assay
	Cellular adhesion

infant and the mother. The physical exam should focus on the general health and nutrition of the patient and include an evaluation of lymphoid tissue, as either absence or hypertrophy of these tissues may indicate an immune defect.

If a primary immunodeficiency disease is suspected in an infant, several precautions should be taken until the diagnosis is clarified. These include the avoidance of live virus vaccines to minimize the risk of infection and the exclusive use of irradiated blood products to preclude transfusion-acquired GvHD.

Strict isolation is seldom indicated unless SCID is suspected, but removal from daycare might be wise. Common respiratory viruses such as respiratory syncytial virus, parainfluenza, and adenovirus can be deadly in children with T-cell disorders. Therefore, relative isolation is warranted until a specific diagnosis can be made.

Laboratory Evaluation

General Laboratory Testing

Properly conducted and interpreted laboratory studies are an important part of the immunologic evaluation. The presence of a thymic shadow can be evaluated by a chest roentgenogram. A complete blood cell count with differential is a crucial and cost-effective screening test. An absolute lymphocyte count can be an important clue as to the presence of SCID, DiGeorge anomaly, or other T-cell disorders. A leukocytosis might suggest either a severe infection or LAD. Similarly, quantitative measurement of immunoglobulins is an inexpensive screening test for B-cell and combined immune disorders. It is important to remember that in the first few months of life the IgG is likely maternal in origin. However, a low IgA or IgM level can be suggestive. The values must be compared with the age-adjusted normal reference ranges.[300] Measurement of IgG subclasses offers little, especially if the total IgG is low, and has no place as a screening test. Most children can be evaluated for their ability to make specific antibody to vaccine antigens. The tests are readily available through commercial laboratories, but it is necessary to be sure that the same laboratory is used consistently. It also is important to understood that the "normal" values that are listed in the reports are those considered to be protective, not necessarily the levels achieved by the normal child. Hence, a level that is barely protective might be very abnormal. The CH_{50} is an adequate screen for congenital defects in the complement system, as all children with a complete absence of one component will have an abnormal CH_{50} or CH_{100}. Delayed hypersensitivity skin tests, using recall antigens such as tetanus, diphtheria, or measles, or common antigens such as *Candida,* are a useful screen in infants over one year of age. Even then, as many as 20% of subjects will respond poorly, especially if only 1 or 2 antigens are used.[401] A positive test is reassuring, however. Children under a year of age cannot be reliably tested by intradermal skin tests, though Kniker and colleagues claimed that infants could be evaluated using the Multitest-® CMI device (Mérieux Institute, Inc., France), which employs 7 recall antigens.[402]

Evaluation of Cellular Immunity

More specific diagnoses can be made through functional studies of the immune system, including lymphocyte subset enumeration by flow cytometry, T-cell proliferative responses to mitogens or specific antigens, and more exotic tests such as in vitro immunoglobulin synthesis or cytokine production. Monoclonal antibodies and flow cytometry are used to evaluate T- and B-cell subsets, but also to identify unusual or immature populations. For example, patients with selective deficiency in the ability to respond to polysaccharide antigens were found to have a predominance of B cells positive for CD5, which normally is seen only in young infants.[403] In another use of flow cytometry, platelets from children with Wiskott-Aldrich syndrome were shown to have defective expression of CD62p and CD63, which may relate to the reduced ability to modulate platelet glycoprotein IIb/IIIa complex expression.[404] Hyper-IgM syndrome may be diagnosed by determining expression of CD40-L on the surface of T cells by flow cytometry.[18] However, some patients express nonfunctional protein, so although absence of expression is diagnostic, patients with CD40-L must be evaluated by molecular biology techniques.

Flow cytometry can be used not only to evaluate subsets of lymphocytes, but also to determine cell activation, cytotoxicity, and cytokine expression. T-cell function is most commonly measured by determining the ability of the cells to proliferate when stimulated with nonspecific mitogens such as PHA, Con A, or PWM, specific antigens such as tetanus toxoid or *Candida albicans,* or allogeneic cells. These agents bind to the T-cell receptor and activate the cells to undergo mitosis. Typically, proliferation is determined by measuring the incorporation of tritiated thymidine into the DNA. This has proven reliable, but does require the use of a radioactive isotope and cannot be used to evaluate the response of specific subsets. DNA synthesis can be quantitated by staining cells with ethidium bromide and measuring with a flow cytometer.[405] This obviates the need for radioisotopes, but requires a computer program to calculate the DNA content and cannot be done on intact cells. Mitogen and antigen-specific responses also can be determined by labeling the cell membrane with a fluorescent dye, PKH26, and following the label as it is distributed to the daughter cells.[406] This technique is especially useful for analysis of cell cycles and can be combined with monoclonal antibodies to label individual subsets. Immediately after lymphocytes are activated there are changes in calcium fluxes followed by protein synthesis, expression of new receptors on the cell surface, RNA synthesis, and finally DNA synthesis. Thus, determination of the early events allows measurement of function more rapidly than does determination of DNA synthesis. CD69 is expressed within 2 hours of activation and thus provides a rapid indicator of cell proliferation.[407-409] Measurement of CD69 can be combined with determination of other activation markers such as CD25 and CD71, as well as adhesion molecules such as L-selectin.[410] New applications of flow cytometry have made it possible to evaluate intracytoplasmic events, such as the detection of intracellular phosphorylated STAT-1.[411] Monoclonal antibodies were developed that can distinguish between phosphorylated and native STAT-1 protein, allowing rapid detection of cell activation and correlation with specific cell subsets. Cytokine production and cytokine receptor expression also can be measured by flow cytometry.[412,413] Up to 6 cytokines can be evaluated simultaneously and cell receptor expression measured concurrently.[412] The use of flow cytometry is not only more rapid and more sensitive than measuring cytokine levels in the culture supernatant by ELISA, but production by specific subsets can be measured. For example, patients with CVID were found to have excessive production of IFN-gamma in the CD8$^+$CD28$^+$ cytotoxic subset of T lymphocytes, which may impair the ability of the CD4$^+$ cells to provide help for the B cells.[413]

Cellular cytotoxicity, both by NK cells and cytotoxic lymphocytes, is typically determined by measuring the release of radiolabeled chromium from the target cells. This method has been reliable, but cumbersome. Because ^{51}Cr does not have a very long half-life, it is necessary to order new material frequently. The background release of the label is a problem during incubations–which last several days. Several methods have been developed to use flow cytometry in the evaluation of cellular cytotoxicity. Intact cells do not allow entry of propidium iodide, so its incorporation into the nucleus is a measure of damage to the target cell. Targets are labeled with a stable dye such as PKH26, and uptake of propidium into the nucleus is measured by flow cytometry.[414] For long incubations, where many of the effector cells also will die, both cell populations can be labeled with contrasting dyes.[415] A new method utilizes annexin V, which binds to phosphatidylserine, an early marker of apoptosis.[416] These apoptotic events occur rapidly after mixing the target and effector cells, and by labeling the effector cells with monoclonal antibodies, killing can be evaluated at the cellular level.

Although these methods have been validated in healthy subjects, it has not been proven that they are valid in all patients with immunodeficiency diseases. For example, if the defect occurs late in the activation pathway, it may be possible for the cell to express CD69 yet not enter into mitosis. These flow cytometric techniques can be very useful in evaluating patients with immunodeficiency diseases, but it is important to correlate them with conventional techniques in each disorder.

References

1. Anonymous. Primary immunodeficiency diseases: report of a WHO scientific group. *Clin Exp Immunol.* 1997;109(suppl 1):1–28.

2. Ming JE, Stiehm ER, Graham JM. Immunodeficiency as a component of recognizable syndromes. *Am J Med Genetics.* 1996;66:378–398.

3. Smith CIE, Bäckesjö C-M, Berglöf A, et al. X-linked agammaglobulinemia: lack of mature B lineage cells caused by mutations in the Btk kinase. *Springer Semin Immunopathol.* 1998;19:369–381.

4. McKinney RE, Katz SL, Wilfert CM. Chronic enteroviral meningoencephalitis in agammaglobulinemic patients. *Rev Infect Dis.* 1987;9:334–356.

5. Dwyer JM, Erlendsson K. Intraventricular gamma-globulin for the management of enterovirus encephalitis. *Pediatr Infect Dis J.* 1988;7:S30–33.

6. Leickly FE, Buckley RH. Variability in B cell maturation and differentiation in X-linked agammaglobulinemia. *Clin Exp Immunol.* 1986;65:90–99.

7. Kornfeld SJ, Haire RN, Strong SJ, et al. Extreme variation in X-linked agammaglobulinemia phenotype in a three-generation family. *J Allergy Clin Immunol.* 1997;100:702–706.

8. Vetrie D, Vorechovsky I, Sideras P, et al. The gene involved in X-linked agammaglobulinaemia is a member of the src family of protein-tyrosine kinases. *Nature.* 1993;361:226–233.

9. Tsukada N, Saffran DC, Rawlings DJ. Deficient expression of a B cell cytoplasmic tyrosine kinase in human X-linked agammaglobulinemia. *Cell.* 1993;72:279–290.

10. Vihinen M, Brooimans RA, Kwan S-P. BTKbase: XLA mutation registry. *Immunol Today.* 1996;17:502–506.

11. Yel L, Minegishi Y, Coustan SE, et al. Mutations in the mu heavy-chain gene in patients with agammaglobulinemia [see comments]. *N Engl J Med.* 1996;335:1486–1493.

12. Ramesh N, Seki M, Notarangelo LD, Geha RS. The hyper-IgM (HIM) syndrome. *Springer Semin Immunopathol.* 1998;19:383–399.

13. Notarangelo LD, Duse M, Ugazio AG. Immunodeficiency with hyper-IgM (HIM). *Immunodefic Rev.* 1992;3:101–125.

14. Stiehm ER, Chin TW, Haas A, et al. Infectious complications of the primary immunodeficiencies. *Clin Immunol Immunopathol.* 1986;40:69–86.

15. Banatvala N, Davies J, Kanariou M, et al. Hypogammaglobulinemia associated with normal or increased IgM (hyper IgM syndrome): a case review. *Arch Dis Child.* 1994;71:150–154.

16. Allen RC, Armitage RJ, Conley ME, et al. CD40 ligand gene defects responsible for X-linked hyper-IgM syndrome. *Science.* 1993;259:990–998.

17. Aruffo A, Farrington M, Hollenbaugh D, et al. The CD40 ligand, gp39, is defective in activated T cells from patients with X-linked hyper-IgM syndrome. *Cell.* 1993;72:291–300.

18. O'Gorman MRG, Zass D, Paniagua M, et al. Development of a whole blood flow cytometry procedure for the diagnosis of X-linked hyper IgM syndrome (XHIM) in patients and carriers. *Clin Immunol Immunopathol.* 1997;85:172–181.

19. Cunningham-Rundles C, Bodian C. Common variable immunodeficiency: clinical and immunological features of 248 patients. *Clin Immunol.* 1999;92:34–48.

20. Church JA, Isaacs H, Saxon A. Lymphoid interstitial pneumonitis and hypogammaglobulinemia in children. *Am Rev Respir Dis.* 1981;124:491–496.

21. Levinson AL, Hopewell PC, Stites DP. Coexistent lymphoid interstitial pneumonia, pernicious anemia, and agammaglobulinemia. *Arch Intern Med.* 1976;1976:213–216.

22. Strober W, Eisenstein E, Jaffe JS, et al. New insights into common variable immunodeficiency. *Ann Intern Med.* 1993;118:720–730.

23. de la Concha EG, Oldham G, Webster ADB, et al. Quantitative measurement of T- and B-cell function in "variable" primary hypogammaglobulinemia: evidence for a consistent B cell defect. *Clin Exp Immunol.* 1977;27:208–215.

24. Sneller MC, Strober W. Abnormalities of lymphokine gene expression in patients with common variable immunodeficiency. *J Immunol.* 1990;144:3762–3769.

25. Wright JJ, Wagner DK, Blaese RM, et al. Characterization of common variable immunodeficiency: identification of patients with distinctive immunophenotypic and clinical features. *Blood.* 1990;76:2046–2051.

26. Volanakis JE, Zhu Z-B, Schaffer FM, et al. Major histocompatibility complex class III genes and susceptibility to immunoglobulin A deficiency and common variable immunodeficiency. *J Clin Invest.* 1992;89:1914–1922.

27. Burks AW, Steele RW. Selective IgA deficiency. *Ann Allergy.* 1986;57:3–8.

28. Hanson LÅ, Björkander J, Carlsson B, et al. The heterogeneity of IgA deficiency. *J Clin Immunol.* 1988;8:159–162.

29. Cunningham-Rundles C, Brandeis WE, Pudifin DJ. Autoimmunity in selective IgA deficiency: relationship to anti-bovine protein antibodies, circulating immune complexes and clinical disease. *Clin Exp Immunol.* 1981;45:299–305.

30. Ammann AJ, Hong R. Selective IgA deficiency: presentation of 30 cases and a review of the literature. *Medicine (Baltimore).* 1971;60:223–236.

31. Ammann AJ, Wara DW, Pillarisetty RJ. The prevalence of autoantibodies in T-cell, B-cell, and phagocytic immunodeficiency disorders. *Clin Immunol Immunopathol.* 1979;14:456–466.

32. Burks AW, Sampson HA, Buckley RH. Anaphylactic reactions after gamma globulin administration in patients with hypogammaglobulinemia. *N Engl J Med.* 1986;314:560–564.

33. Seager J, Jamison DL, Wilson J. IgA deficiency, epilepsy and phenytoin treatment. *Lancet.* 1975;2:632–634.

34. Plebani A, Monafo V, Ugazio A, et al. Clinical heterogeneity and reversibility of selective immunoglobulin A deficiency in 80 children. *Lancet.* 1986;1:829–831.

35. Cunningham-Rundles C, Fotino M, Rosina O, et al. Selective IgA deficiency, IgG subclass deficiency, and the major histocompatibility complex. *Clin Immunol Immunopathol.* 1991;61(2, part 2):S61–S69.

36. Ambrus M, Hernadi E, Baker CJ. Prevalence of HLA-A1 and HLA-B8 antigens in selective IgA deficiency. *Clin Immunol Immunopathol.* 1977;7:311–314.

37. Oxelius VA, Laurell AB, Lindquist B. IgG subclasses in selective IgA deficiency. *N Engl J Med.* 1981;304:1476–1477.

38. Tedder TF, Crain MJ, Kubagawa H. Evaluation of lymphocyte differentiation in primary and secondary immunodeficiency diseases. *J Immunol.* 1985;135:1786–1791.

39. Schwartz SA. Heavy chain-specific suppression of immunoglobulin synthesis and secretion by lymphocytes from patients with selective IgA deficiency. *J Immunol.* 1980;24:2034–2036.

40. Atwater JS, Tomasi TBJ. Suppressor cells and IgA deficiency. *Clin Immunol Immunopathol.* 1978;9:379–384.

41. Strober W, Krakauer R, Klaeveman HL, et al. Secretory component deficiency: a disorder of the IgA immune system. *N Engl J Med.* 1976;294:351–356.

42. Lane PJL, MacLennan ICM. Impaired IgG2 anti-pneumococcal antibody responses in patients with recurrent infection and normal IgG2 levels but no IgA. *Clin Exp Immunol.* 1986;65:427–433.

43. Jefferis R, Kumararatne DS. Selective IgG subclass deficiency: quantification and clinical relevance. *Clin Exp Immunol.* 1990;81:357–367.

44. Oxelius V-A, Hanson LÅ, Björkander J, et al. IgG3 deficiency: common in obstructive lung disease. *Monogr Allergy.* 1986;20:106–115.

45. Preud'Homme JL, Hanson LA. IgG subclass deficiency. *Immunodefic Rev.* 1990;2:129–149.

46. Bass JL, Nuss R, Mehta KA, et al. Recurrent meningococcemia associated with IgG2-subclass deficiency. *N Engl J Med.* 1983;309:430.

47. Umetsu DT, Ambrosino DM, Quinti I, et al. Recurrent sinopulmonary infection and impaired antibody response to bacterial capsular polysaccharide antigen in children with selective IgG-subclass deficiency. *N Engl J Med.* 1985;313:1247–1251.

48. Freijd A, Oxelius V-A, Rynnel-Dagöö B. A prospective study demonstrating an association between plasma IgG2 concentrations and susceptibility to otitis media in children. *Scand J Infect Dis.* 1985;17:115–120.

49. Bragger C, Seger RA, Aeppli R, et al. IgG2/IgG4 subclass deficiency in a patient with chronic mucocutaneous candidiasis and bronchiectases. *Eur J Pediatr.* 1989;149:168–169.

50. Beck CS, Heiner DC. Selective immunoglobulin G4 deficiency and recurrent infections of the respiratory tract. *Am Rev Respir Dis.* 1981;124:94–96.

51. Bartmann P, Kleihauer E. Undetectable IgG4 in immunoprecipitation: association with repeated infections in children? *Eur J Pediatr.* 1988;148:211–214.

52. Bussel J, Morell A, Skvaril F. IgG2 deficiency in autoimmune cytopenias. *Monogr Allergy.* 1986;20:116–118.

53. Oxelius V-A: Immunoglobulin G (IgG) subclasses and human disease. *Am J Med.* 1984;76:7–18.

54. Duse M, Tiberti S, Plebani A, et al. IgG2 deficiency and intractable epilepsy of childhood. *Monogr Allergy.* 1986;20:128–134.

55. Hammarström L, Smith CIE. IgG subclasses in bacterial infections. *Monogr Allergy.* 1986;19:122–133.

56. Hammarström L, Lefranc G, Lefranc MP, et al. Aberrant pattern of anti-carbohydrate antibodies in immunoglobulin class or subclass-deficient donors. *Monogr Allergy.* 1986;20:50–56.

57. Ambrosino DM, Umetsu DT, Siber GR, et al. Selective defect in the antibody response to *Haemophilus influenzae* type b in children with recurrent infections and normal IgG subclass levels. *J Allergy Clin Immunol.* 1988;81:1175–1179.

58. Herrod HG. Management of the patient with IgG subclass deficiency and/or selective antibody deficiency. *Ann Allergy.* 1993;70:3–8.

59. Gross S, Blaiss MS, Herrod HG. Role of immunoglobulin subclasses and specific antibody determinations in the evaluation of recurrent infection in children. *J Pediatr.* 1992;121:516–522.

60. Oxelius V-A. IgG subclass levels in infancy and childhood. *Acta Paediatr Scand.* 1979;68:23–27.

61. Van der Giessen M, Rossouw E, Algra-van Veen T, et al. Quantification of IgG subclasses in sera of normal adults and healthy children between 4 and 12 years of age. *Clin Exp Immunol.* 1975;21:501–509.

62. French M. Serum IgG subclasses in normal adults. *Monogr Allergy.* 1986;19:100–107.

63. Silk HJ, Ambrosino D, Geha RS. Effect of intravenous gammaglobulin therapy in IgG2 deficient and IgG2 sufficient children with recurrent infections and poor response to immunization with *Hemophilus influenzae* type b capsular polysaccharide antigen. *Ann Allergy.* 1990;64:21–25.

64. Sell SH, Wright PF, Vaughn WK, Thompson J, Schiffman G. Clinical studies of pneumococcal vaccines in infants, I: reactogenicity and immunogenicity of two polyvalent polysaccharide vaccines. *Rev Infect Dis.* 1981;3:S97–S107.

65. Tiller TL, Buckley RH. Transient hypogammaglobulinemia of infancy: review of the literature, clinical and immunologic features of 11 new cases, and long-term follow-up. *J Pediatr.* 1978;92:347–353.

66. Dressler F, Peter HH, Müller W, et al. Transient hypogammaglobulinemia of infancy. *Acta Paediatr Scand.* 1989;78:767–774.

67. McGeady SJ. Transient hypogammaglobulinemia of infancy: need to reconsider name and definition. *J Pediatr.* 1987;110:47–50.

68. Walker AM, Kemp AS, Hill DJ, et al. Features of transient hypogammaglobulinemia in infants screened for immunologic abnormalities. *Arch Dis Child.* 1994;70:183–186.

69. Kowalczyk D, Mytar B, Zembala M. Cytokine production in transient hypogammaglobulinemia and isolated IgA deficiency. *J Allergy Clin Immunol.* 1997;100:556–562.

70. Siegel RL, Issekutz T, Schwaber J, et al. Deficiency of T helper cells in transient hypogammaglobulinemia of infancy. *N Engl J Med.* 1981;305:1307–1313.

71. Watts RG, Kelly DR. Fatal varicella infection in a child associated with thymoma and immunodeficiency (Good's syndrome). *Med Pediatr Oncol.* 1990;18:246–251.

72. Hong R. The DiGeorge anomaly. *Immunodefic Rev.* 1991;3:1–14.

73. Thomas JA, Graham JM. Chromosome 22q11 deletion syndrome: an update and review for the primary pediatrician. *Clin Pediatr.* May 1997:253–266.

74. Bastian J, Law S, Vogler LB, et al. Prediction of persistent immunodeficiency in the DiGeorge anomaly. *J Pediatr.* 1989;115:391–396.

75. Markert ML, Boeck A, Hale LP, et al. Transplantation of thymus tissue in complete DiGeorge syndrome. *N Engl J Med.* 1999;341:1180–1189.

76. Goldsobel AB, Haas A, Stiehm ER. Bone marrow transplantation in DiGeorge syndrome. *J Pediatr.* 1987;111:40–44.

77. Buckley RH, Gard S, Schiff RI, et al. T cells and T cell subsets in a large population of patients with primary immunodeficiency. In: Wedgwood R, Rosen FS, eds. *Primary Immunodeficiencies.* New York, NY: Alan R Liss; 1983:187–191.

78. Gossage DL, Buckley RH. Prevalence of lymphocytopenia in severe combined immunodeficiency. *N Engl J Med.* 1990;323:1422–1423.

79. Buckley R, Schiff SE, Schiff RI, et al. Hematopoietic stem-cell transplantation for the treatment of severe combined immunodeficiency. *N Engl J Med.* 1999;340:508–516.

80. Fischer A, Haddad E, Jabado N, et al. Stem cell transplantation for immunodeficiency. *Springer Semin Immunopathol.* 1998;19:479–492.

81. Buckley RH, Schiff RI, Schiff SE, et al. Human severe combined immunodeficiency: genetic, phenotypic, and functional diversity in one hundred eight infants. *J Pediatr.* 1997;130:378–387.

82. Takeshita T, Asao H, Ohtani K. Cloning of the γ chain of the human IL-2 receptor. *Science.* 1992;257:379–382.

83. Candotti F, O'Shea JJ, Villa A. Severe combined immune deficiencies due to defects of the common γ chain-JAK3 signalling pathway. *Springer Semin Immunopathol.* 1998;19:401–415.

84. Mazer B, Harbeck RJ, Franklin R, et al. Phenotypic features of selective T cell deficiency characterized by absence of CD8+ T lymphocytes and undetectable mRNA for ZAP-70 kinase. *Clin Immunol Immunopathol.* 1997;84:129–138.

85. Puel A, Ziegler SF, Buckley RH, et al. Defective IL7R expression in T(-)B(+)NK(+) severe combined immunodeficiency. *Nat Genet.* 1998;20:394-397.

86. Hirschhorn R. Adenosine deaminase deficiency. *Immunodefic Rev.* 1990;2:175–198.

87. Hershfield MS, Buckley RH, Greenberg ML, et al. Treatment of adenosine deaminase deficiency with polyethylene glycol-modified adenosine deaminase (PEG-ADA). *N Engl J Med.* 1987;316:589–596.

88. Touraine JL, Betuel H, Souillet G, et al. Combined immunodeficiency disease associated with absence of cell surface HLA-A and -B antigens. *J Pediatr.* 1978;93:47–51.

89. Plebani A, Monafo V, Cattaneo R, et al. Defective expression of HLA class I and CD1a molecules in a boy with Marfan-like phenotype and deep skin ulcers. *J Am Acad Dermatol.* 1996;35:814–818.

90. Teisserenc H, Schmitt W, Blake N, et al. A case of primary immunodeficiency due to a defect of the major histocompatibility gene complex class I processing and presentation pathway. *Immunol Lett.* 1997;57:183–187.

91. Payne R, Brodsky FM, Peterlin BM, et al. "Bare lymphocytes" without immunodeficiency. *Hum Immunol.* 1983;6:219–227.

92. de la Salle H, Hanau D, Fricker D, et al. Homozygous human TAP peptide transporter mutation in HLA class I deficiency. *Science.* 1994;265:237–241.

93. Carbonari M, Cherchi M, Paganelli R, et al. Relative increase of T cells expressing the gamma/delta rather than the alpha/beta receptor in ataxia telangiectasia. *N Engl J Med.* 1990;322:73–76.

94. Lisowska-Grospierre B, Durandy A, Virelizier J-L, et al. Combined immunodeficiency with defective expression of HLA: modulations of an abnormal HLA synthesis and functional studies. *Birth Defects.* 1983;19:87–92.

95. Touraine J-L, Marseglia GL, Betuel H, et al. The bare lymphocyte syndrome. *Bone Marrow Transplant.* 1992;9(suppl 1):54–56.

96. Klein C, Lisowska-Grospierre B, LeDeist F, et al. Major histocompatibility complex class II deficiency: clinical manifestations, immunologic features, and outcome. *J Pediatr.* 1993;123:921–928.

97. Reith W, Steimle V, Mach B. Molecular defects in the bare lymphocyte syndrome and regulation of MHC class II genes. *Immunol Today.* 1995;16:539–546.

98. Lisowska-Grospierre B, Fondaneche MC, Rols MP, et al. Two complementation groups account for most cases of inherited MHC class II deficiency. *Hum Mol Genetics.* 1994;3:953–958.

99. Steimle V, Otten LA, Zufferey M, et al. Complementation cloning of an MHC class II transactivator mutated in hereditary MHC class II deficiency (or bare lymphocyte syndrome). *Cell.* 1993;75:135–146.

100. Steimle V, Durand B, Barras E, et al. A novel DNA binding regulatory factor is mutated in primary MHC class II deficiency (bare lymphocyte syndrome). *Genes Dev.* 1995;9:1021–1032.

101. Reith W, Steimle V, Lisowska-Grospierre B, et al. Molecular basis of major histocompatibility complex class II deficiency. In: Ochs HD, Smith CIE, Puck JM, eds. *Primary Immunodeficiency Diseases: A Molecular and Genetic Approach.* New York, NY: Oxford University Press; 1999:167–180.

102. Klein C, Cavazzana-Calvo M, LeDeist F, et al. Bone marrow transplantation in major histocompatibility complex class II deficiency: a single-center study of 19 patients. *Blood.* 1995;85:580–587.

103. Fischer A. Primary T-cell immunodeficiencies. *Curr Opin Immunol.* 1993;5:569–578.

104. van Tol MTL, Berkel AI, Vossen JM, et al. CD3γ chain deficiency leads to a cellular immunodeficiency with mild clinical presentation. *The Immunologist.* 1997;1:41.

105. Regueiro JR, Lopez-Botet M, De Landazuri MO, et al. An in vivo functional immune system lacking polyclonal T cell surface expression of the CD3/Ti(WT31) complex. *Scand J Immunol.* 1987;26:699–707.

106. Markert ML. Purine nucleoside phosphorylase deficiency. *Immunodefic Rev.* 1991;3:45–81.

107. Giblett ER, Ammann AJ, Wara DW, et al. Nucleoside phosphorylase deficiency in a child with severely defective T cell immunity and normal B cell immunity. *Lancet.* 1975;1:1010–1013.

108. Omenn GS. Familial reticuloendotheliosis with eosinophilia. *N Engl J Med.* 1965;273:427–432.

109. Businco L, Di Frazio A, Ziruolo MG, et al. Clinical and immunologic findings in four infants with Omenn's syndrome: a form of severe combined immunodeficiency with phenotypically normal T cells, elevated IgE, and eosinophilia. *Clin Immunol Immunopathol.* 1987;44:123–133.

110. Karol RA, Eng J, Cooper JB, et al. Imbalances in subsets of T lymphocytes in an inbred pedigree with Omenn's syndrome. *Clin Immunol Immunopathol.* 1983;27:412–427.

111. Jouan H, Le Deist F, Nezelof C. Omenn's syndrome—pathologic arguments in favor of a graft versus host pathogenesis: a report of nine cases. *Hum Pathol.* 1987;18:1101–1108.

112. Cederbaum SD, Niwayama G, Stiehm ER, et al. Combined immunodeficiency presenting as the Letterer-Siwe syndrome. *J Pediatr.* 1974;85:466–471.

113. de Saint-Basile G, Le Deist F, de Vallartay J-P, et al. Restricted heterogeneity of T lymphocytes in combined immunodeficiency with hypereosinophilia (Omenn's syndrome). *J Clin Invest.* 1991;87:1352–1359.

114. Schwartz K, Gaus GH, Ludwig L, et al. RAG mutations in human B cell-negative SCID. *Science.* 1996;274:97–99.

115. Chilosi M, Pizzolo G, Facchetti F, et al. The pathology of Omenn's syndrome. *Am J Surg Pathol.* 1996;20:773–774.

116. Chilosi M, Facchetti F, Notarangelo LD, et al. CD30 expression and abnormal soluble CD30 serum accumulation in Omenn's syndrome: evidence for a T helper 2-mediated condition. *Eur J Immunol.* 1966;26:329–334.

117. Brugnoni D, Airò P, Facchetti F, et al. In vitro cell death of activated lymphocytes in Omenn's syndrome. *Eur J Immunol.* 1997;27:2765–2773.

118. Wirt DP, Brooks EG, Vaidya S, et al. Novel T-lymphocyte population in combined immunodeficiency with features of graft-versus-host disease. *N Engl J Med.* 1989;321:370–374.

119. Markert ML, Finkel BD, McLaughlin TM, et al. Mutations in the purine nucleoside phosphorylase deficiency. *Hum Mutat.* 1997;9:118–121.

120. Ownby DR, Pizzo S, Blackmon L, et al. Severe combined immunodeficiency with leukopenia (reticular dysgenesis) in siblings: immunologic and histopathologic findings. *J Pediatr.* 1976;89:382–387.

121. Ammann AJ, Hong R. Disorders of the T cell system. In: Stiehm ER, Fulginiti VA, eds. *Immunologic Disorders in Infants and Children.* Philadelphia, Pa: WB Saunders; 1980:286–348.

122. Sullivan JL, Woda BA. X-linked lymphoproliferative syndrome. *Immunodefic Rev.* 1989;1:325–347.

123. Purtilo DT, Cassel CK, Yang JP, Harper R. X-linked recessive progressive combined variable immunodeficiency (Duncan's disease). *Lancet.* 1975;1:935–940.

124. Purtilo DT. Epstein-Barr virus-induced diseases in the X-linked lymphoproliferative syndrome and related disorders. *Biomed Pharmacother.* 1985;39:52.

125. Seemayer TA, Gross TG, Egeler RM, et al. X-linked lymphoproliferative disease: twenty-five years after the discovery. *Pediatr Res.* 1995;38:471–477.

126. Lindsten T, Seeley JK, Ballow M, et al. Immune deficiency in the X-linked lymphoproliferative syndrome, II: immunoregulatory T cell defects. *J Immunol.* 1982;129:2536–2540.

127. Harada S, Sakamoto K, Seeley JK, et al. Immune deficiency in the X-linked lymphoproliferative syndrome. I: Epstein-Barr virus specific defects. *J Immunol.* 1982;129:2532.

128. Argov S, Johnson DR, Collins M, et al. Defective natural killing activity but retention of lymphocyte-mediated antibody-dependent cellular cytotoxicity in patients with the X-linked lymphoproliferative syndrome. *Cell Immunol.* 1986;100:1–9.

129. Okano M, Pirruccello SJ, Grierson HL, et al. Immunovirological studies of fatal infectious mononucleosis in a patient with X-linked lymphoproliferative syndrome treated with intravenous immunoglobulin and interferon-alpha. *Clin Immunol Immunopathol.* 1990;54:410–418.

130. Williams LL, Rooney CM, Conley ME, et al. Correction of Duncan's syndrome by allogeneic bone marrow transplantation. *Lancet.* 1993;342:587–588.

131. Pracher E, Grümayer-Panzer ER, Zoubek A, et al. Bone marrow transplantation in a boy with X-linked lymphoproliferative syndrome and acute severe infectious mononucleosis. *Bone Marrow Transplant.* 1994;13:655–658.

132. Vowels MR, Lam-Po-Tang R, Berdoukas V, et al. Correction of X-linked lymphoproliferative disease by transplantation of cord-blood stem cells. *N Engl J Med.* 1993;329:1623–1625.

133. Gross TG, Filipovich AH, Conley ME, et al. Cure of X-linked lymphoproliferative disease (XLP) with allogeneic hematopoietic stem cell transplantation (HSCT)—report from the XLP registry. *Bone Marrow Transplant.* 1996;17:741–744.

134. Huntley CC, Dees SC. Eczema associated with thrombocytopenic purpura and purulent otitis media. *Pediatrics.* 1957;19:351–361.

135. Sullivan KE, Mullen CA, Blaese RM, et al. A multiinstitutional survey of the Wiskott Aldrich syndrome. *J Pediatr.* 1994;125:876–885.

136. Derry JMJ, Ochs HD, Francke U. Isolation of a novel gene mutated in Wiskott-Aldrich syndrome. *Cell.* 1994;78:635–644.

137. Kersey JH, Shapiro RS, Filipovich AH. Relationship of immunodeficiency to lymphoid malignancy. *Pediatr Infect Dis J.* 1988;7:510–512.

138. Blaese RM, Strober W, Waldmann TA. Immunodeficiency in the Wiskott-Aldrich syndrome. *Birth Defects.* 1975;XI:250–254.

139. Cooper MD, Chase HP, Lowman JT, et al. Wiskott-Aldrich syndrome: an immunologic deficiency disease involving the afferent limb of immunity. *Am J Med.* 1968;44:499–513.

140. Ochs HD, Slichter SJ, Harker LA, et al. The Wiskott-Aldrich syndrome: studies of lymphocytes, granulocytes, and platelets. *Blood.* 1980;55:243–252.

141. Waldmann TA, Strober W. Metabolism of immunoglobulins. *Prog Allergy.* 1969;13:1–110.

142. Nahm MH, Blaese RM, Crain MJ, et al. Patients with Wiskott-Aldrich syndrome have normal IgG2 levels. *J Immunol.* 1986;137:3484–3487.

143. Spitler LE, Levin AS, Stites DP, et al. The Wiskott-Aldrich syndrome: immunologic studies in nine patients and selected family members. *Cell Immunol.* 1975;19:201–218.

144. Siminovitch KA, Greer WL, Novogrodsky A, et al. A diagnostic assay for the Wiskott-Aldrich syndrome and its variant forms. *J Investig Med.* 1995;43:159–169.

145. Molina IJ, Sancho J, Terhorst C, et al. T cells of patients with the Wiskott-Aldrich syndrome have a restricted defect in proliferative responses. *J Immunol.* 1993;151:4383–4390.

146. Morio T, Takase K, Okawa H, et al. The increase of non-MHC-restricted cytotoxic cells (g/d-TCR-bearing T cells or NK cells) and the abnormal differentiation of B cells in Wiskott-Aldrich syndrome. *Clin Immunol Immunopathol.* 1989;52:279–290.

147. Simon HU, Mills GB, Hasimoto S, et al. Evidence for defective transmembrane signaling in B cells from patients with Wiskott-Aldrich syndrome. *J Clin Invest.* 1992;90:1396–1405.

148. Lau YL, Shields JG, Levinsky RJ, et al. Epstein-Barr virus transformed lymphoblastoid cell lines derived from patients with X-linked agammaglobulinaemia and Wiskott-Aldrich syndrome: responses to B cell growth and differentiation factors. *Clin Exp Immunol.* 1989;75:190–195.

149. Lau YL, Jones BM, Low LCK, et al. Defective B-cell regulatory T-cell function in Wiskott-Aldrich syndrome. *Eur J Pediatr.* 1992;151:680–683.

150. Remold-O'Donnell E, Rosen RS. Sialophorin (CD43) and the Wiskott-Aldrich syndrome. *Immunol Rev.* 1990;2:151–174.

151. Yonemura S, Nagafuchi A, Sato N, et al. Concentration of an integral membrane protein, CD43 (leukosialin, sialophorin), in the cleavage furrow through the interaction of its cytoplasmic domain with actin-based cytoskeletons. *J Cell Biol.* 1993;120:437–449.

152. Thrasher AJ, Jones GE, Kinnon C, et al. Is Wiskott-Aldrich syndrome a cell trafficking disorder? *Immunol Today.* 1998;19:537–539.

153. Kirkpatrick CH. Chronic mucocutaneous candidiasis: immunologic and antibiotic therapy. *Ann N Y Acad Sci.* 1988;S44:471–480.

154. Herrod HG. Chronic mucocutaneous candidiasis in childhood and complications of non-Candida infection: a report of the Pediatric Immunodeficiency Collaborative Study Group. *J Pediatr.* 1990;116:377–382.

155. Chipps BE, Saulsbury FT, Hsu SH, et al. Non-candidial infections in children with chronic mucocutaneous candidiasis. *Johns Hopkins Med J.* 1979;144:175–179.

156. Bentur L, Nisbet-Brown E, Levison H, et al. Lung disease associated with IgG subclass deficiency in chronic mucocutaneous candidiasis. *J Pediatr.* 1991;118:82–86.

157. Flynn PM, Barrett FF, Herrod HG. Disseminated histoplasmosis in two patients with chronic mucocutaneous candidiasis. *Pediatr Infect Dis J.* 1987;6:691–693.

158. Durandy A, Fischer A, Le Deist F, et al. Mannan-specific and mannan-induced T-cell suppressive activity in patients with chronic mucocutaneous candidiasis. *J Clin Immunol.* 1987;7:400–409.

159. Fischer A, Ballet JJ, Griscelli C. Specific inhibition of in vitro *Candida*-induced lymphocyte proliferation by polysaccharidic antigens present in the serum of patients with chronic mucocutaneous candidiasis. *J Clin Invest.* 1978;62:1005–1013.

160. Lilic D, Cant AJ, Abinun M, et al. Chronic mucocutaneous candidiasis, I: altered antigen-stimulated IL-2, IL-4, IL-6 and interferon gamma (IFN-gamma) production. *Clin Exp Immunol.* 1996;105:205–212.

161. Kobrynski LJ, Tanimune L, Kilpatrick L, et al. Production of T-helper cell subsets and cytokines by lymphocytes from patients with chronic mucocutaneous candidiasis. *Clin Diagn Lab Immunol.* 1996;3:740–745.

162. Buckley RH, Sampson HA. The hyperimmunoglobulinemia E syndrome. In: Franklin EC, ed. *Clinical Immunology Update.* New York, NY: Elsevier North-Holland Inc; 1981:147–167.

163. Buckley RH, Wray BB, Belmaker EZ. Extreme hyperimmunoglobulinemia E and undue susceptibility to infection. *Pediatrics.* 1972;49:59–70.

164. Grimbacher B, Holland SM, Gallin JI, et al. Hyper IgE syndrome with recurrent infections—an autosomal dominant multisystem disorder. *N Engl J Med.* 1999;340:692–702.

165. Clark RA, Root RK, Kimball HR, et al. Defective neutrophil chemotaxis and cellular immunity in a child with recurrent infections. *Ann Intern Med.* 1973;78:515–519.

166. Constantopoulos A, Karpouzas J, Xypolita A, et al. Defective neutrophil chemotaxis and hyperimmunoglobulinemia E in a child with recurrent infections. *Helv Paediatr Acta.* 1978;33:81–84.

167. Sheerin KA, Buckley RH. Antibody responses to protein, polysaccharide, and ØX-174 antigens in the hyperimmunoglobulinemia E (hyper IgE) syndrome. *J Allergy Clin Immunol.* 1991;87:803–811.

168. Leung DYM, Geha RS. Clinical and immunologic aspects of the hyperimmunoglobulin E syndrome. *Hematol/Oncol Clin North Am.* 1988;2:81.

169. Del Prete G, Tiri A, Maggi E, et al. Defective in vitro production of gamma interferon and tumor necrosis factor alpha by circulating T cells from patients with the hyper immunoglobulin E syndrome. *J Clin Invest.* 1989;84:1830–1835.

170. Rousset F, Robert J, Andary M, et al. Shifts in interleukin-4 and interferon-g production by T cells of patients with elevated serum IgE levels and the modulatory effects of these lymphokines on spontaneous IgE synthesis. *J Allergy Clin Immunol.* 1991;87:58–69.

171. Claassen JL, Levine AD, Schiff SE, et al. Mononuclear cells from patients with the hyper IgE syndrome produce little IgE when stimulated with recombinant interleukin 4 in vitro. *J Allergy Clin Immunol.* 1991;88:713–721.

172. Berger M, Kirkpatrick CH, Goldsmith PK, et al. IgE antibodies to *Staphylococcus aureus* and *Candida albicans* in patients with the syndrome of hyperimmunoglobulin E and recurrent infections. *J Immunol.* 1980;125:2437–2443.

173. Swift M. Genetic aspects of ataxia telangiectasia. *Immunodefic Rev.* 1990;2:67–81.

174. Boder E. Ataxia-telangiectasia: an overview. In: Gatti R, Swift M, eds. *Ataxia-Telangiectasia: Genetics, Neuropathology, and Immunology of a Degenerative Disease of Childhood.* New York, NY: Alan R Liss; 1985;19:1–63.

175. Swift M, Morrell D, Massey RB, et al. Incidence of cancer in 161 families affected by ataxia telangiectasia. *N Engl J Med.* 1991;325:18831–1836.

176. Filipovich AH, Mathur A, Kamat D, et al. Lymphoproliferative disorders and other tumors complicating immunodeficiencies. *Immunodef.* 1994;5:91–112.

177. Utsumi H, Sasaki MS. Deficient repair of potentially lethal damage in actively growing ataxia telangiectasia cells. *Radiat Res.* 1984;97:407–413.

178. Lavin MF, Khanna KK, Beamish H, et al. Defect in radiation signal transduction in ataxia-telangiectasia. *Int J Radiat Biol.* 1994;66:S151–S156.

179. Roifman CM, Gelfand EW. Heterogeneity of the immunological deficiency in ataxia-telangiectasia: absence of a clinical-pathological correlation. In: Gatti R, Swift M, eds. *Ataxia-Telangiectasia: Genetics, Neuropathology, and Immunology of a Degenerative Disease of Childhood.* New York, NY: Alan R Liss; 1985;19:273–285.

180. Oxelius V-A, Berkel AI, Hanson LÅ. IgG2 deficiency in ataxia-telangiectasia. *N Engl J Med.* 1982;306:515–517.

181. Fiorilli M, Businco L, Pandolfi F, et al. Heterogeneity of immunological abnormalities in ataxia-telangiectasia. *J Clin Immunol.* 1983;3:135–141.

182. Gatti RA, Bick M, Tam CF, et al. ataxia-telangiectasia: a multiparameter analysis of eight families. *Clin Immunol Immunopathol.* 1982;23:501–516.

183. Levis WR, Dattner AM, Shaw JS. Selective defects in T cell function in ataxia-telangiectasia. *Clin Exp Immunol.* 1978;37:44–49.

184. Polmar SH, Pierce GF. Cartilage hair hypoplasia: immunological aspects and their clinical implications. *Clin Immunol Immunopathol.* 1986;40:87–93.

185. Mäkitie O, Kaitila I, Savilahti E. Susceptibility to infections and in vitro immune functions in cartilage-hair hypoplasia. *Eur J Pediatr.* 1998;157:816–820.

186. Castigli E, Irani AM, Geha RS, et al. Defective expression of early activation genes in cartilage-hair hypoplasia (CHH) with severe combined immunodeficiency (SCID). *Clin Exp Immunol.* 1995;102:6–10.

187. Pierce GF, Polmar SH. Lymphocyte dysfunction in cartilage hair hypoplasia. II: evidence for a cell cycle specific defect in T cell growth. *Clin Exp Immunol.* 1982;50:621.

188. van der Burgt I, Haraldsson A, Oosterwijk JC, et al. Cartilage hair hypoplasia, metaphyseal chondrodysplasia type McKusick: description of seven patients and review of the literature. *Am J Med Genetics.* 1991;41:371–380.

189. Kooijman R, van der Burgt CJ, Weemaes CM, et al. T cell subsets and T cell function in cartilage-hair hypoplasia. *Scand J Immunol.* 1997;46:209–215.

190. Francomano CA, Trojak JE, McKusick VA. Cartilage-hair hypoplasia in the Amish: increased susceptibility to malignancy. *Am J Hum Genetics.* 1983;35:89A.

191. Steele RW, Britton HA, Anderson CT, et al. Severe combined immunodeficiency with cartilage-hair hypoplasia: in vitro response to thymosin and attempted reconstitution. *Pediatr Res.* 1976;10:1003–1005.

192. Berthet F, Siegrist CA, Ozsahin H, et al. Bone marrow transplantation in cartilage-hair hypoplasia: correction of the immunodeficiency but not the chondrodysplasia. *Eur J Pediatr.* 1996;155:286–290.

193. Frank MD. Complement in the pathophysiology of human disease. *N Engl J Med.* 1987;316:1525.

194. Ross SC, Densen P. Complement deficiency states and infection: epidemiology, pathogenesis and consequences of neisserial and other infections in an immune deficiency. *Medicine (Baltimore).* 1984;63:243–273.

195. Ugazio AG, Maccario R, Notarangelo LD, et al. Immunology of Down syndrome: a review. *Am J Med Genetics.* 1990;7:204–212.

196. Kondo N, Otoyoshi F, Ori S, et al. Long term study of the immunodeficiency of Bloom's syndrome. *Acta Paediatr Scand.* 1992;81:86–90.

197. Chandra RK. Acrodermatitis enteropathica: zinc levels and cell-mediated immunity. *Pediatrics.* 1980;66:789–791.

198. van Wouwe JP. Clinical and laboratory diagnosis of acrodermatitis enteropathica. *Eur J Pediatr.* 1989;149:2–8.

199. Sweetman L, Nyhan WL. Inheritable biotin-treatable disorders and associated phenomena. *Annu Rev Nutr.* 1986;6:317–343.

200. Girot R, Hamet M, Perignon JL, et al. Cellular immune deficiency in two siblings with hereditary orotic aciduria. *N Engl J Med.* 1983;308:700–704.

201. Alvarado CS, Livingstone LR, Jones ME, et al. Uridine-responsive hypogammaglobulinemia and congenital heart disease in a patient with hereditary orotic aciduria. *J Pediatr.* 1988;113:867–871.

202. Kaikov Y, Wadsworth LD, Hall CA, et al. Transcobalamin II deficiency: case report and review of the literature. *Eur J Pediatr.* 1991;150:841–843.

203. Hitzig WH, Dohmann U, Pluss JJ, et al. Hereditary transcobalamin II deficiency: clinical findings in a new family. *J Pediatr.* 1974;85:622–628.

204. Hill HR. Biochemical, structural, and functional abnormalities of polymorphonuclear leukocytes in the neonate. *Pediatr Res.* 1987;22:375–382.

205. Etzioni A. Neutrophil function in the newborn— a review. [Review]. *Isr J Med Sci.* 1994;30:328–330.

206. Christensen RD. Neutrophil kinetics in the fetus and neonate. *Am J Pediatr Hematol Oncol.* 1989;11:215–223.

207. McIntosh N, Kempson C, Tyler RM. Blood counts in extremely low birthweight infants. *Arch Dis Child.* 1988;63:74–76.

208. Schelonka RL, Yoder BA, des Jardins SE, et al. Peripheral leukocyte count and leukocyte indexes in healthy newborn term infants [see comments]. *J Pediatr.* 1994;125:603–606.

209. Xanthou M. Leucocyte blood picture in healthy full-term and premature babies during neonatal period. *Arch Dis Child.* 1979;45:242–249.

210. Manroe BL, Weinberg AG, Rosenfeld CR, et al. The neonatal blood count in health and disease, I: neutrophilic cells. *J Pediatr.* 1979;95:89–98.

211. Wheeler JG, Chauvenet AR, Johnson CA, et al. Neutrophil storage pool depletion in septic, neutropenic neonates. *Pediatr Infect Dis J.* 1984;3:407–409.

212. Erdman SH, Christensen RD, Bradley PP, et al. Supply and release of storage neutrophils: a developmental study. *Biol Neonate.* 1982;41:132–137.

213. Weinberg AG, Rosenfeld CR, Manroe BL, et al. Neonatal blood cell count in health and disease. II: values for lymphocytes, monocytes, and eosinophils. *J Pediatr.* 1985;106:462–466.

214. Wright WC Jr, Ank B, Herbert J, Stiehm ER. Decreased bactericidal activity of leukocytes of stressed newborn infants. *Pediatrics.* 1975;56:579–584.

215. Masuda K, Kinoshita Y, Kobayashi Y. Heterogeneity of Fc receptor expression in chemotaxis and adherence of neonatal neutrophils. *Pediatr Res.* 1989;25:6–10.

216. Anderson DC, Rothlein R, Marlin SD, et al. Impaired transendothelial migration by neonatal neutrophils: abnormalities of Mac-1 (CD11b/CD18)-dependent adherence reactions. *Blood.* 1990;76:2613–2621.

217. McEvoy LT, Zakem-Cloud H, Tosi MF. Total cell content of CR3 (CD11b/CD18) and LFA-1 (CD11a/CD18) in neonatal neutrophils: relationship to gestational age. *Blood.* 1996;87:3929–3933.

218. Jones DH, Schmalstieg FC, Dempsey K, et al. Subcellular distribution and mobilization of Mac-1 (CD11b/CD18) in neonatal neutrophils. *Blood.* 1990;75:488–492.

219. Cairo MS, VandeVen C, Toy C, et al. GM-CSF primes and modulates neonatal PMN motility: up-regulation of C3bi (Mo1) expression with alteration in PMN adherence and aggregation. *Am J Pediatr Hematol Oncol.* 1991;13:249–257.

220. Yasui K, Masuda M, Matsuoka T, et al. Abnormal membrane fluidity as a cause of impaired functional dynamics of chemoattractant receptors on neonatal polymorphonuclear leukocytes: lack of modulation of the receptors by a membrane fluidizer. *Pediatr Res.* 1988;24:442–446.

221. Yin HS, Stossel TP. Control of cytoplasmic actin gelsol transformation by gelsolin, a calcium-dependent regulatory protein. *Nature.* 1979;281:583.

222. Harris MC, Shalit M, Southwick F. Diminished actin polymerization by neutrophils from newborn infants. *Pediatr Res.* 1992;33:27–31.

223. Miller ME. Phagocyte function in the neonate: selected aspects. *Pediatrics.* 1979;64(suppl):709.

224. Kamran S, Usmani SS, Wapnir RA, et al. In vitro effect of indomethacin on polymorphonuclear leukocyte function in preterm infants. *Pediatr Res.* 1992;33:32–35.

225. Tono-oko T, Nakayama M, Uehara H, et al. Characteristics of impaired chemotactic function in cord blood leukocytes. *Pediatr Res.* 1979;13:148–151.

226. Klein RB, Fischer TJ, Gard SE, et al. Decreased mononuclear and polymorphonuclear chemotaxis in human newborns, infants, and young children. *Pediatrics.* 1977;60:467–472.

227. Yegin O. Chemotaxis in childhood. *Pediatr Res.* 1983;17:183–187.

228. Fontan G, Lorente F, Garcia Rodriguez MC, et al. In vitro human neutrophil movement in umbilical cord blood. *Clin Immunol Immunopathol.* 1981;20:224–230.

229. Laurenti F, Ferro R, Marzetti G, et al. Neutrophil chemotaxis in preterm infants with infections. *J Pediatr.* 1980;96:468–470.

230. Anderson DC. Abnormal mobility of neonatal polymorphonuclear leukocytes: relationship to impaired redistribution of surface adhesion sites by chemotactic factor or colchicine. *J Clin Invest.* 1981;68:863.

231. Yoder M., Polin R. The immune system. In: Fanaroff AA, Martin RJ, eds. *Neonatal-Perinatal Medicine: Diseases of the Fetus and Infant.* St. Louis, Mo: CV Mosby Co; 1992:587–619.

232. Jones, DH. Subcellular distribution and mobilization of MAC-1 (CD11b/CD18) in neonatal neutrophils. *Blood*. 1990;75:488.

233. Sacchi F. Abnormality in actin polymerization associated with defective chemotaxis in neutrophils from neonates. *Int Arch Allergy Appl Immunol*. 1987;84:32.

234. Maeda M, van Schie RC, Yuksel B, et al. Differential expression of Fc receptors for IgG by monocytes and granulocytes from neonates and adults. *Clin Exp Immunol*. 1996;103:343–347.

235. Falconer AE, Carr R, Edwards SW. Impaired neutrophil phagocytosis in preterm neonates: lack of correlation with expression of immunoglobulin or complement receptors. *Biol Neonate*. 1995;68:264–269.

236. Forman ML, Stiehm ER. Impaired opsonic activity but normal phagocytosis in low-birth-weight infants. *N Engl J Med*. 1969;281:926.

237. Xanthou M. Phagocytosis and killing ability of *Candida albicans* by blood leucocytes of healthy term and preterm babies. *Arch Dis Child*. 1975;50:72.

238. Harris MC. Phagocytosis of group B streptococcus by neutrophils from newborn infants. *Pediatr Res*. 1983;17:358.

239. Matoth Y. Phagocytic and ameboid activities of the leukocytes in the newborn infant. *Pediatrics*. 1952;9:748.

240. Shigeoka AO. Functional analysis of neutrophil granulocytes from healthy, infected and stressed neonates. *J Pediatr*. 1979;95:454.

241. Cocchi P, Marianelli L. Phagocytosis and intracellular killing of *Pseudomonas aeruginosa* in premature infants. *Helv Paediatr Acta*. 1967;1:110.

242. Anderson DC, Pickering LK, Feigin RD. Leukocyte function in normal and infected neonates. *J Pediatr*. 1974;85:420–425.

243. Mills EL, Thompson M, Bjorksten B, et al. The chemiluminescence response and bactericidal activity of polymorphonuclear neutrophils from newborns and their mothers. *Pediatrics*. 1979;63:429–434.

244. Driscoll MS, Thomas VL, Ramamurthy RS, et al. Longitudinal evaluation of polymorphonuclear leukocyte chemiluminescence in premature infants. *J Pediatr*. 1990;116:429–434.

245. Ambruso DR, Altenburger KM, Johnston RB. Defective oxidative metabolism in newborn neutrophils: discrepancy between superoxide anion and hydroxyl radical generation. *Pediatrics*. 1979;64:722–725.

246. Frenck RW, Buescher ES, Vadhan-Raj S. The effects of recombinant human granulocyte-macrophage colony stimulating factor on in vitro cord blood granulocyte function. *Pediatr Res*. 1989;26:43–48.

247. Bortolussi R, Howlett S, Rajaraman K, et al. Deficient priming activity of newborn cord blood-derived polymorphonuclear neutrophilic granulocytes with lipopolysaccharide and tumor necrosis factor-alpha triggered with formyl-methionyl-leucyl-phenylalanine. *Pediatr Res*. 1993;34:243–248.

248. Qing G, Rajaraman K, Bortolussi R. Diminished priming of neonatal polymorphonuclear leukocytes by lipopolysaccharide is associated with reduced CD14 expression. *Infect Immunol*. 1995;63:248–252.

249. Dossett JH, Williams RC, Quie PG. Studies on interaction of bacteria, serum factors and polymorphonuclear leukocytes in mothers and newborns. *Pediatrics*. 1996;44:49.

250. Al-Hadithy H, Addison IE, Goldstone AH, et al. Defective neutrophil function in low-birth-weight, premature infants. *J Clin Pathol.* 1981;34:366–370.

251. Becker ID, Robinson OM, Bazan TS, et al. Bactericidal capacity of newborn phagocytes against group B beta-hemolytic streptococci. *Infect Immunol.* 1981;34:535–539.

252. Oseas R, Lehrer RI. A micromethod for measuring neutrophil candidacidal activity in neonates. *Pediatr Res.* 1978;12:828–829.

253. Yoder MC, Hassan NF, Douglas SD. Mononuclear phagocyte system. In: Polin R, Fox W, eds. *Fetal and Neonatal Physiology.* Philadelphia, Pa: WB Saunders; 1992:1438–1461.

254. Speer CP, Gahr M, Wielenga JJ, et al. Phagocytosis-associated functions in neonatal monocyte-derived macrophages. *Pediatr Res.* 1988;24:213–216.

255. Raghunathan R, Miller ME, Everett S, et al. Phagocyte chemotaxis in the perinatal period. *J Clin Immunol.* 1982;2:242–245.

256. Marwitz PA, Van Arkel Vigna E, Rijkers GT, et al. Expression and modulation of cell surface determinants on human adult and neonatal monocytes. *Clin Exp Immunol.* 1988;72:260–266.

257. Speer CP. Phagocyte function. In: Ogra PL, ed. *Neonatal Infections: Nutritional and Immunologic Interactions.* Orlando, Fla: Grune & Stratton; 1984:21–36.

258. Schuit KE, Powell DA. Phagocytic dysfunction in monocytes of normal newborn infants. *Pediatrics.* 1980;65:501–504.

259. Marodi L, Leijh PC, van Furth R. Characteristics and functional capacities of human cord blood granulocytes and monocytes. *Pediatr Res.* 1984;18:1127–1131.

260. Mardódi L, Káposzta R, Campbell DE, et al. Candidacidal mechanisms in the human neonate: impaired IFN-γ activation of macrophages in newborn infants. *J Immunol.* 1994;153:5643–5649.

261. Stiehm ER, Sztein MB, Steeg PS, et al. Deficient DR antigen expression on human cord blood monocytes: reversal with lymphokines. *Clin Immunol Immunopathol.* 1984;30:430–436.

262. Hoffman AA. Presentation of antigen by human newborn monocytes to maternal tetanus toxoid-specific T-cell blasts. *J Clin Immunol.* 1981;1:217.

263. Kurnick J. Long term maintenance of HLA-D restricted T cells specific for soluble antigens. *Scand J Immunol.* 1980;11:131.

264. Zlabinger GJ, Mannhalter JW, Eibl MM. Cord blood macrophages present bacterial antigen (Escherichia coli) to paternal T cells. *Clin Immunol Immunopathol.* 1983;28:405–412.

265. Wilmott RW, Harris MC, Haines KM, et al. Interleukin-1 activity from human cord blood monocytes. *Diagn Clin Immunol.* 1987;5:201–204.

266. Peters AM, Bertram P, Gahr M, et al. Reduced secretion of interleukin-1 and tumor necrosis factor-alpha by neonatal monocytes. *Biol Neonate.* 1993;63:157–162.

267. Schibler KR, Liechty KW, White WL, et al. Defective production of interleukin-6 by monocytes: a possible mechanism underlying several host defense deficiencies of neonates. *Pediatr Res.* 1992;31:18–21.

268. Yachie A, Takano N, Yokoi T, et al. The capacity of neonatal leukocytes to produce IL-6 on stimulation assessed by whole blood culture. *Pediatr Res.* 1990;27:227–233.

269. Schibler KR, Trautman MS, Liechty KW, et al. Diminished transcription of interleukin-8 by monocytes from preterm neonates. *J Leukoc Biol.* 1993;53:399–403.

270. Rowen JL, Smith CW, Edwards MS. Group B streptococci elicit leukotriene B4 and interleukin-8 from human monocytes: neonates exhibit a diminished response. *J Infect Dis.* 1995;172:420–426.

271. Winkelstein JA. The complement system in the fetus and newborn. In: Polin R, Fox W, eds. *Fetal and Neonatal Physiology.* Philadelphia, Pa: WB Saunders; 1992:1470–1476.

272. Berger M. Complement deficiency and neutrophil dysfunction as risk factors for bacterial infection in newborns and the role of granulocyte transfusion in therapy. *Rev Infect Dis.* 1990;12(suppl 4):S401–S409.

273. Zilow G, Zilow EP, Burger R, et al. Complement activation in newborn infants with early onset infection. *Pediatr Res.* 1993;34:199–203.

274. McCracken GH, Eichwald HF. Leukocyte function and the development of opsonic and complement activity in the neonate. *Am J Dis Child.* 1971;121:120–126.

275. Tenuvuo J, Pruitt KM. Relationship of the human salivary peroxidase system to oral health. *J Oral Pathol.* 1984;13:573–584.

276. Anderson DC, Hughes BJ, Edwards MS, et al. Impaired chemotaxogenesis by type III group B streptococci in neonatal sera: relationship to diminished concentration of specific anticapsular antibody and abnormalities of serum complement. *Pediatrics.* 1983;17:496–502.

277. Gathings WE, Kubagawa H, Cooper MD. A distinctive pattern of B cell immaturity in perinatal humans. *Immunol Rev.* 1981;57:107–126.

278. Gathings WE, Lawton AR, Cooper MD. Immunofluorescent studies of the development of pre-B cells, B lymphocytes and immunoglobulin isotype diversity in humans. *Eur J Immunol.* 1977;7:804–810.

279. Kubagawa H, Gathings WE, Levitt D, et al. Immunoglobulin isotype expression of normal pre-B cells as determined by immunofluorescence. *J Clin Immunol.* 1982;2:264–269.

280. Asma GEM, Langlois van den Bergh R, Vossen JM. Development of pre-B and B lymphocytes in the human fetus. *Clin Exp Immunol.* 1984;56:407–414.

281. Bofill M, Janossy G, Janossa M, et al. Human B cell development, II: subpopulations in the human fetus. *J Immunol.* 1985;134:1531–1538.

282. Campana D, Janossy G, Bofill M, et al. Human B cell development, I: phenotypic differences of B lymphocytes in the bone marrow and peripheral lymphoid tissue. *J Immunol.* 1985;134:1524–1530.

283. Nahmias A, Stoll B, Hale E, et al. IgA-secreting cells in the blood of premature and term infants: normal development and effect of intrauterine infections. *Adv Exp Med Biol.* 1991;310:59–69.

284. Edwards JA, Durant BM, Jones DB, et al. Differential expression of HLA class II antigens in fetal human spleen: relationship of HLA-DP, DQ, and DR to immunoglobulin expression. *J Immunol.* 1986;137:490–497.

285. Antin JH, Emerson SG, Martin P, et al. Leu-1+ (CD5+) B cells. A major lymphoid subpopulation in human fetal spleen: phenotypic and functional studies. *J Immunol.* 1986;136:505–510.

286. Bastian JF, Ruedi JM, MacPherson GA, et al. Lymphocyte ecto-5'-nucleotidase activity in infancy: increasing activity in peripheral blood B cells precedes their ability to synthesize IgG in vitro. *J Immunol.* 1984;132:1767–1772.

287. Durandy A, de Saint Basile G, Lisowska-Grospierre B, et al. Undetectable CD40 ligand expression on T cells and low B cell responses to CD40 binding agonists in human newborns. *J Immunol.* 1995;154:1560–1568.

288. Miyawaki T, Kubagawa H, Butler VP, et al. Ig isotypes produced by EBV-transformed B cells as a function of age and tissue distribution. *J Immunol.* 1988;140:3887–3892.

289. Konowalchuk J, Speirs JI, Perelmutter L. Immunoglobulin properties of Epstein-Barr virus transformed human umbilical cord and adult peripheral blood lymphocytes. *Cell Immunol.* 1982;67:190–196.

290. Miyawaki T, Moriya N, Nagaoki T, et al. Maturation of B-cell differentiation ability and T-cell regulatory function in infancy and childhood. *Immunol Rev.* 1981;57:63–87.

291. Pittard WB, Miller KM, Sorensen RU. Perinatal influences on in vitro B lymphocyte differentiation in human neonates. *Pediatr Res.* 1985;19:655–658.

292. Knutsen AP, Buckley RH. Immunoglobulin synthesis by cord and maternal blood mononuclear cells and their effect on synthesis by normal adult cells. In: Seligmann M, Hitzig W, eds. *Primary Immunodeficiencies.* New York, NY: Elsevier North-Holland Inc; 1980:13–22.

293. Miyagawa Y, Sugita K, Komiyama A, et al. Delayed in vitro immunoglobulin production by cord lymphocytes. *Pediatrics.* 1980;65:497–500.

294. Hayward AR, Lawton AR. Induction of plasma cell differentiation of human fetal lymphocytes: evidence for functional immaturity of T and B cells. *J Immunol.* 1977;119:1213–1217.

295. Ito S, Lawton AR. Response of human B cells to *Staphylococcus aureus* Cowan I: T- independent proliferation and T-dependent differentiation to immunoglobulin secretion involve subsets separable by rosetting with mouse erythrocytes. *J Immunol.* 1984;133:1891–1895.

296. Miller KM, Pittard WB, Sorensen RU. Cord blood B cell differentiation. *Clin Exp Immunol.* 1984;56:415–424.

297. Punnonen J, Aversa GG, Vandekerckhove B, et al. Induction of isotype switching and Ig production by CD5+ and CD10+ human fetal B cells. *J Immunol.* 1992;148:3398–3404.

298. Rothberg RM. Immunoglobulin and specific antibody synthesis during the first weeks of life of premature infants. *J Pediatr.* 1969;75:391–399.

299. Ballow M, Cates KL, Rowe JC, et al. Development of the immune system in very low birth weight (less than 1500 g) premature infants: concentrations of plasma immunoglobulins and patterns of infections. *Pediatr Res.* 1986;9:899–904.

300. Buckley RH, Dees SC, O'Fallon WM. Serum immunoglobulins. I: levels in normal children and in uncomplicated childhood allergy. *Pediatrics.* 41:600–611, 1968.

301. Hanson LÅ, Carlsson B, Dahlgren U, et al. The secretory IgA system in the neonatal period. *Ciba Found Symp.* 1979;77:187–204.

302. Bridges RA, Condie RM, Zak SJ, Good RA. The morphologic basis of antibody formation development during the neonatal period. *J Lab Clin Med.* 1959;53:331–336.

303. Girard JP, de Kalbermatten A. Antibody activity in human duodenal fluid. *Eur J Clin Invest.* 1970;1:188–195.

304. Cohen AB, Goldberg S, London RL. Immunoglobulins in nasal secretions of infants. *Clin Exp Immunol.* 1970;6:735–760.

305. Hawworth JC, Dilling L. Concentration of γA-globulin in serum, saliva and nasopharyngeal secretions of infants and children. *J Lab Clin Med.* 1966;67:922–933.

306. Burgio GR, Lanzaveccia A, Plebani A, et al. Ontogeny of secretory immunity: levels of secretory IgA and natural antibodies in saliva. *Pediatr Res.* 1980;14:1111–1114.

307. Burgio GR, Ugazio AG, Notarangelo LD. Immunology of the neonate. *Curr Opin Immunol.* 1990;2:770–777.

308. van Furth R, Schuit HR, Hijmans W. The immunological development of the human fetus. *J Exp Med.* 1965;122:1173–1186.

309. Gill TJ, Repetti CF, Metlay LA, et al. Transplacental immunization of the human fetus to tetanus by immunization of the mother. *J Clin Invest.* 1983;72:987–996.

310. Mellander L, Carlsson B, Hanson LÅ. Secretory IgA and IgM antibodies to *E. coli* O and poliovirus type I antigens occur in amniotic fluid, meconium and saliva from newborns. *Clin Exp Immunol.* 1986;63:555–561.

311. Halsey N, Galazka A. The efficacy of DTP and oral poliomyelitis immunization schedules initiated from birth to 12 weeks of age. *Bull World Health Organ.* 1985;63:1151–1169.

312. Osborn JJ, Dancis J, Julia JF. Studies of the immunology of the human newborn infant, 1: age and antibody production. *Pediatrics.* 1952;9:736–744.

313. Kurikka S, Kayhty H, Peltola H, et al. Neonatal immunization: response to *Haemophilus influenzae* type b-tetanus toxoid conjugate vaccine. *Pediatrics.* 1995;95:815–822.

314. Makela PH, Peltola H, Kayhty H, et al. Polysaccharide vaccines of group A *Neisseria meningiditis* and *Haemophilus influenzae* type b: a field trial in Finland. *J Infect Dis.* 1977;136(suppl):S43–50.

315. Anderson P, Smith DH, Ingram DL, et al. Antibody of polyribophosphate and *Haemophilus influenzae* type b in infants in children: effect of immunization of polyribophosphate. *J Infect Dis.* 1977;136(suppl):S57–62.

316. Robbins JB, Parke JC, Schneerson R, et al. Quantitative measurement of "natural" and immunization-induced *Haemophilus influenzae* type b capsular polysaccharide antibodies. *Pediatr Res.* 1973;7:103–110.

317. Cates KL, Goetz C, Rosenberg N, et al. Longitudinal development of specific and functional antibody in very low birth weight premature infants. *Pediatr Res.* 1988;23:14–22.

318. Holt PG. Postnatal maturation of immune competence during infancy and childhood. *Pediatr Allergy Immunol.* 1995;6:59–70.

319. Wilson CB, Lewis DB, English BK. T cell development in the fetus and neonate. *Adv Exp Med Biol.* 1991;310:17–27.

320. McDuffie M, Hayward AR. T-cell development. In: Polin R, Fox W, eds. *Fetal and Neonatal Physiology.* Philadelphia, Pa: WB Saunders; 1992:1427–1438.

321. Lobach DF, Haynes BF. Ontogeny of the human thymus during fetal development. *J Clin Immunol.* 1987;7:81–97.

322. Hofman FM, Modlin RL, Bhoopat L, et al. Distribution of cells bearing the tac antigen during ontogeny of human lymphoid tissue. *J Immunol.* 1985;134:3751–3755.

323. Kay HEM, Doe J, Hockley A. Response of human foetal thymocytes to phytohemagglutinin (PHA). *Immunology.* 1970;18:393–396.

324. Stites DP, Carr MC, Fudenberg HH. Ontogeny of cellular immunity in the human foetus: development of responses to phytohemagglutinin and to allogeneic cells. *Cell Immunol.* 1974;11:257–271.

325. Papiernik M. Correlation of lymphocyte transformation and morphology in the human fetal thymus. *Blood.* 1970;36:470–479.

326. Toivanen P, Uksila J, Leino A, et al. Development of mitogen responding T cells and natural killer cells in the human fetus. *Immunol Rev.* 1981;57:89–105.

327. Rayfield LS, Brent L, Rodeck CH. Development of cell-mediated lympholysis in human foetal blood lymphocytes. *Clin Exp Immunol.* 1980;42:561–570.

328. Notarangelo LD, Panina P, Imberti L, et al. Neonatal T4+ lymphocytes: analysis of the expression of 4B4 and 2H4 antigens. *Clin Immunol Immunopathol.* 1988;46:61–67.

329. Maccario R, Chirico G, Mingrat G, et al. Expression of CD45R0 antigen on the surface of resting and activated neonatal T lymphocyte subsets. *Biol Neonate.* 1993;64:346–353.

330. Miles EA, Warner JA, Lane AC, et al. Altered T lymphocyte phenotype at birth in babies born to atopic parents. *Pediatr Allergy Immunol.* 1994;5:202–208.

331. Morita CT, Parker CM, Brenner MB, et al. TCR usage and functional capabilities of human gamma delta T cells at birth. *J Immunol.* 1994;153:3979–3988.

332. Fuleihan R, Ahern D, Geha RS. Decreased expression of the ligand for CD40 in newborn lymphocytes. *Eur J Immunol.* 1994;24:1925–1928.

333. Brugnoni D, Airo P, Graf D, et al. Ineffective expression of CD40 ligand on cord blood T cells may contribute to poor immunoglobulin production in the newborn. *Eur J Immunol.* 1994;24:1919–1924.

334. Zola H, Fusco M, Weedon H, et al. Reduced expression of the interleukin-2-receptor γ chain on cord blood lymphocytes: relationship to functional immaturity of the neonatal immune response. *Immunology.* 1996;87:86–91.

335. Saito S, Morii T, Umekage H, et al. Expression of the interleukin-2 receptor gamma chain on cord blood mononuclear cells. *Blood.* 1996;87:3344–3350.

336. Moretta A, Valtorta A, Chirico G, et al. Lymphocyte subpopulations in preterm infants: high percentage of cells expressing P55 chain of interleukin-2 receptor. *Biol Neonate.* 1991;59:213–219.

337. Gerli R, Bertotto A, Spinozzi F, et al. Thymic hormone modulation of CD38 (T10) antigen on human cord blood lymphocytes. *Clin Immunol Immunopathol.* 1987;45:323–332.

338. Griffiths-Chu S, Patterson JAK, Berger CL, et al. Characterization of immature T cell subpopulations in neonatal blood. *Blood.* 1984;64:296–300.

339. Maccario R, Ferrari FA, Siena S, et al. Receptors for peanut agglutinin on a high percentage of human cord-blood lymphocytes: phenotype characterization of peanut-positive cells. *Thymus.* 1981;2:229–237.

340. Zola H, Fusco M, MacArdle PJ, et al. Expression of cytokine receptors by human cord blood lymphocytes: comparison with adult blood lymphocytes. *Pediatr Res.* 1995;38:397–403.

341. Erkeller-Yuksel FM, Deneys V, Yuksel B, et al. Age-related changes in human blood lymphocyte subpopulations. *J Pediatr.* 1992;120:216–222.

342. The European Collaborative Study: age-related standards for T lymphocyte subsets based on uninfected children born to human immunodeficiency virus 1-infected women. *Pediatr Infect Dis J.* 1992;11:1018–1026.

343. Raes M, Alliet P, Gillis P, et al. Lymphocyte subpopulations in healthy newborn infants: comparison of cord blood values with values five days after birth. *J Pediatr.* 1993;123:465–467.

344. Kontny U, Barrachina C, Habermehl P, et al. Distribution of lymphocyte surface antigens in healthy neonates. *Eur J Pediatr.* 1994;153:257–259.

345. Slukvin II, Chernishov VP. Two-color flow cytometric analysis of natural killer and cytotoxic T-lymphocyte subsets in peripheral blood of normal human neonates. *Biol Neonate.* 1992;61:156–161.

346. Yanase Y, Tango T, Okumura K, et al. Lymphocyte subsets identified by monoclonal antibodies in healthy children. *Pediatr Res.* 1986;20:1147–1151.

347. Carr MC, Stites DP, Fudenberg HH. Cellular immune aspects of the human fetal-maternal relationship. I: in vitro response of cord blood lymphocytes to phytohemagglutinin. *Cell Immunol.* 1972;5:21–29.

348. Ceppellini R, Bonnard GD, Coppo F, et al. Mixed leukocyte cultures and HL-A antigens. I: reactivity of young fetuses, newborns and mothers at delivery. *Transplantation Proc.* 1971;3:58–70.

349. Pirenne H, Aujard Y, Eliaafari A, et al. Comparison of T cell functional changes during childhood with the ontogeny of CDw29 and CD45RA expression on CD4$^+$ cells. *Pediatr Res.* 1992;32:81–86.

350. Stern DA, Hicks MJ, Martinez FD, et al. Lymphocyte subpopulation number and function in infancy. *Dev Immunol.* 1992;2:175–179.

351. Montagna D, Moretta A, Marconi M, et al. In vivo activated cord blood lymphocytes express high affinity interleukin-2 receptor: evaluation of their responsiveness to in vitro stimulation with recombinant interleukin-2. *Biol Neonate.* 1992;62:385–394.

352. Gerli R, Bertotto A, Crupi S, et al. Activation of cord T lymphocytes, I: evidence for a defective T cell mitogenesis induced through the CD2 molecule. *J Immunol.* 1989;142:2583–2589.

353. Bertotto A, Gerli R, Lanfrancone L, et al. Activation of cord T lymphocytes, II: cellular and molecular analysis of the defective response induced by anti-CD3 monoclonal antibody. *Cell Immunol.* 1990;127:247–259.

354. Papadogiannakis N, Johnson SA, Olding LB. Monocyte regulated hyporesponsiveness of human cord blood lymphocytes to OKT3 Mo-Ab-induced mitogenesis. *Scand J Immunol.* 1986;23:91–99.

355. Hassan J, Reen DJ. Interleukin-1 augments the diminished interleukin-2 mRNA expression and proliferative response of neonatal T lymphocytes to anti-CD2 antibodies. *Scand J Immunol.* 1994;39:597–601.

356. Bussel JB, Cunningham-Rundles S, LaGamma EF, et al. Analysis of lymphocyte proliferative response subpopulations in very low birth weight infants and during the first 8 weeks of life. *Pediatr Res.* 1988;23:457–462.

357. Leino A, Ruuskanen O, Kero P, et al. Depressed phytohemagglutinin and concanavalin A responses in premature infants. *Clin Immunol Immunopathol.* 1981;19:260–267.

358. Noyes BE, Kurland G, Orenstein DM, et al. Experience with pediatric lung transplantation. *J Pediatr.* 1994;124:261–268.

359. Herrod HG, Cooke RJ, Valenski WR, et al. Evaluation of lymphocyte phenotype and phytohemagglutinin response in healthy very low birth weight infants. *Clin Immunol Immunopathol.* 1991;60:268–277.

360. Kavelaars A, Zijlstra J, Bakker JM, et al. Increased dexamethasone sensitivity of neonatal leukocytes: different mechanisms of glucocorticoid inhibition of T cell proliferation in adult and neonatal cells. *Eur J Immunol.* 1995;25:1346–1351.

361. Olding LB, Oldstone MBA. Lymphocytes from human newborns abrogate mitosis of their mother's lymphocytes. *Nature.* 1974;249:161–162.

362. Unander AM, Olding LB. Ontogeny and postnatal persistence of a strong suppressor activity in man. *J Immunol.* 1981;127:1182–1186.

363. Miyawaki T, Moriya N, Nagaoki T, et al. Mode of action of humoral suppressor factor derived from pokeweed mitogen-stimulated cord T cells on adult B cell differentiation. *J Immunol.* 1981;126:282–285.

364. Rodriguez MA, Bankhurst AD, Ceuppens JL, et al. Characterization of the suppressor cell activity in human cord blood lymphocytes. *J Clin Invest.* 1981;68:1577–1585.

365. Hayward AR, Merrill D. Requirement for OKT8+ suppressor cell proliferation for suppression by human newborn T cells. *Clin Exp Immunol.* 1981;45:468–474.

366. Yachie A, Miyawaki T, Nagaoki T, et al. Regulation of B cell differentiation by T cell subsets defined with monoclonal OKT4 and OKT8 antibodies in human cord blood. *J Immunol.* 1981;127:1314–1317.

367. Papadogiannakis N, Johnsen S-A, Olding LB. Human fetal/neonatal suppressor activity: relation between OKT phenotypes and sensitivity to prostaglandin E₂ in maternal and neonatal lymphocytes. *Am J Reprod Immunol Microbiol.* 1985;9:105–110.

368. Jacoby DR, Oldstone MBA. Delineation of suppressor and helper activity within the OKT4-defined T lymphocyte subset in human newborns. *J Immunol.* 1983;131:1765–1770.

369. Cheng H, Delespesse G. Evaluation of the functional maturity of newborn T8⁺ suppressor cells and the resistance of newborn lymphocytes to suppression. *Am J Reprod Immunol Microbiol.* 1986;11:1–5.

370. Cheng H, Delespesse G. Human cord blood suppressor T lymphocytes, II: characterization of inducer of suppressor cells. *Am J Reprod Immunol Microbiol.* 1986;11:39–43.

371. Morito T, Bankhurst AD, Williams RC. Studies of human cord blood and adult lymphocyte interactions with in vitro immunoglobulin production. *J Clin Invest.* 1979;64:990–995.

372. Dwyer JM, Johnson C. Comparative analysis of the suppression by cord blood mononuclear cells of adult and neonatal lymphocytes. *Cell Immunol.* 1983;81:81–87.

373. Papadogiannakis N, Johnsen S-A, Olding LB. Strong prostaglandin associated suppression of the proliferation of human maternal lymphocytes by neonatal lymphocytes linked to T versus T cell interactions and differential PGE$_2$ sensitivity. *Clin Exp Immunol.* 1984;61:125–134.

374. Johnsen S-A, Olding LB, Westberg NG, et al. Strong suppression by mononuclear leukocytes from human newborns on maternal leukocytes: mediation by prostaglandins. *Clin Immunol Immunopathol.* 1982;23:606–615.

375. Papadogiannakis N, Johnsen SA. Mitogenic action of phorbol ester TPA and calcium ionophore A23187 on human cord and maternal/adult peripheral lymphocytes: regulation by prostaglandin E$_2$. *Clin Exp Immunol.* 1987;70:173–181.

376. Splawski JB, Lipsky PE. Cytokine regulation of immunoglobulin secretion by neonatal lymphocytes. *J Clin Invest.* 1991;88:667–677.

377. Bryson YJ, Winter HS, Gard SE, et al. Deficiency of immune interferon production by leukocytes of normal newborns. *Cell Immunol.* 1980;55:191–200.

378. Miyawaki T, Seki H, Taga K, et al. Dissociated production of interleukin-2 and immune (gamma) interferon by phytohemagglutinin stimulated lymphocytes in healthy infants. *Clin Exp Immunol.* 1985;59:505–511.

379. Frenkel L, Bryson YJ. Ontogeny of phytohemagglutinin-induced gamma interferon by leukocytes of healthy infants and children: evidence for decreased production in infants less than 2 months of age. *J Pediatr.* 1987;111:97–100.

380. Lewis DB, Yu CC, Meyer J, et al. Cellular and molecular mechanisms for reduced interleukin 4 and interferon-gamma production by neonatal T cells. *J Clin Invest.* 1991;87:194–202.

381. Taylor S, Bryson YJ. Impaired production of gamma-interferon by newborn cells in vitro is due to a functionally immature macrophage. *J Immunol.* 1985;134:1493–1497.

382. Burchett SK, Corey L, Mohan KM, et al. Diminished interferon-gamma and lymphocyte proliferation in neonatal and postpartum primary herpes simplex virus infection. *J Infect Dis.* 1992;165:813–818.

383. Stephens S, Duffy SW, Page C. A longitudinal study of gamma-interferon production by peripheral blood mononuclear cells from breast- and bottle-fed infants. *Clin Exp Immunol.* 1986;65:396–400.

384. Wu CY, Demeure C, Kiniwa M, et al. IL-12 induces the production of IFN-gamma by neonatal CD4 T cells. *J Immunol.* 1993;151:1938–1949.

385. Watson W, Oen K, Ramdahin R, et al. Immunoglobulin and cytokine production by neonatal lymphocytes. *Clin Exp Immunol.* 1991;83:169–174.

386. Hassan J, Reen DJ. Reduced primary antigen-specific T-cell precursor frequencies in neonates is associated with deficient interleukin-2 production. *Immunology.* 1996;87:604–608.

387. Winter HS, Gard SE, Fischer TJ, et al. Deficient lymphokine production of newborn lymphocytes. *Pediatr Res.* 1983;17:573–578.

388. Uksila J, Lassila O, Hirvonen T, et al. Development of natural killer cell function in the human fetus. *J Immunol.* 1983;130:153–156.

389. Ueno Y, Miyawaki T, Seki H, et al. Differential effects of recombinant human interferon-gamma and interleukin 2 on natural killer cell activity of peripheral blood in early human development. *J Immunol.* 1985;135:180–184.

390. Phillips JH, Hori T, Nagler A, et al. Ontogeny of human natural killer (NK) cells: fetal NK cells mediate cytolytic function and express cytoplasmic CD3ε,δ proteins. *J Exp Med.* 1992;175:1055–1066.

391. Antonelli P, Stewart W, Dupont B. Distribution of natural killer cell activity in peripheral blood, cord blood, thymus, lymph nodes, and spleen and the effect of in vitro treatment with interferon preparation. *Clin Immunol Immunopathol.* 1981;19:161–169.

392. Kaplan J, Shope TC, Bollinger RO, et al. Human newborns are deficient in natural killer activity. *J Clin Immunol.* 1982;2:350–355.

393. Uksila J, Lassila O, Hirvonen T. Natural killer cell function of human neonatal lymphocytes. *Clin Exp Immunol.* 1982;48:649–654.

394. Lubens RG, Gard SE, Soderberg-Warner M, et al. Lectin-dependent T-lymphocyte and natural killer cytotoxic deficiencies in human newborns. *Cell Immunol.* 1982;74:40–53.

395. Sancho L, de la Hera A, Casas J, et al. Two different maturational stages of natural killer lymphocytes in human newborn infants. *J Pediatr.* 1991;119:446–454.

396. Abo T, Miller CA, Balch CM. Characterization of human granular lymphocyte subpopulations expressing HNK-1 (Leu-7) and Leu-11 antigens in the blood and lymphoid tissues from fetuses, neonates, and adults. *Eur J Immunol.* 1984;14:616–623.

397. Sancho L, Martinez C, Nogales A, et al. Reconstitution of natural-killer-cell activity in the newborn by interleukin-2. *N Engl J Med.* 1986;314:57–58.

398. Hallberg A, Malström P. Natural killer cell activity and antibody-dependent cellular cytotoxicity in newborn infants. *Acta Paediatr Scand.* 1982;71:431–436.

399. Xanthou M, Mandyla-Sfagou H, Economou-Mavrou C, et al. Cytotoxicity of lymphocytes in the newborn. *Arch Dis Child.* 1981;56:377–381.

400. Montagna D, Maccario R, Ugazio AG, et al. Natural cytotoxicity in the neonate: high levels of lymphokine activated killer (LAK) activity. *Clin Exp Immunol.* 1988;71:177–181.

401. Munoz AI, Limbert D. Skin reactivity to *Candida* and streptokinase-streptodornase antigens in normal pediatric subjects: influence of age and acute illness. *J Pediatr.* 1977;91:565–568.

402. Kniker WT, Lesourd BM, McBryde JL, et al. Cell-mediated immunity assessed by Multitest CMI skin testing in infants and preschool children. *Am J Dis Child.* 1985;139:840–845.

403. Antall PM, Meyerson H, Kaplan D, et al. Selective anti-polysaccharide antibody deficiency associated with peripheral blood CD5[+] B-cell predominance. *J Allergy Clin Immunol.* 1999;103:637–641.

404. Semple JW, Siminovitch KA, Mody M, et al. Flow cytometric analysis of platelets from children with the Wiskott-Aldrich syndrome reveals defects in platelet development, activation and structure. *Br J Haematol.* 1997;97:747–754.

405. Azzolina LS, Stevanoni G, Tridente G. DNA analysis of stimulated lymphocytes by automatic sampling for flow cytometry. *Cytometry.* 1988;9:508–511.

406. Allsopp CEM, Nicholls SJ, Langhorne J. A flow cytometric method to assess antigen-specific proliferative responses of different subpopulations of fresh and cryopreserved human peripheral blood mononuclear cells. *J Immunol Methods.* 1998;214:175–186.

407. Simms PE, Ellis TM. Utility of flow cytometric detection of CD69 expression as a rapid method for determining poly- and oligoclonal lymphocyte activation. *Clin Diagn Lab Immunol.* 1996;3:301–304.

408. Maino VC, Suni MA, Ruitenberg JJ. Rapid flow cytometric method for measuring lymphocyte subset activation. *Cytometry.* 1995;20:127–133.

409. Mardiney M III, Brown MR, Fleisher TA. Measurement of T-cell CD69 expression: a rapid and efficient means to assess mitogen- or antigen-induced proliferative capacity in normals. *Cytometry.* 1996;26:305–310.

410. Biselli R, Matricardi PM, D'Amelio R, et al. Multiparametric flow cytometric analysis of the kinetics of surface molecule expression after polyclonal activation of human peripheral blood T lymphocytes. *Scand J Immunol.* 1992;35:439–447.

411. Fleisher TA, Dorman SE, Anderson JA, et al. Detection of intracellular phosphorylated STAT-1 by flow cytometry. *Clin Immunol.* 1999;90:425–430.

412. Collins DP, Luebering BJ, Shaut DM. T-lymphocyte functionality assessed by analysis of cytokine receptor expression, intracellular cytokine expression, and femtomolar detection of cytokine secretion by quantitative flow cytometry. *Cytometry.* 1998;33:249–255.

413. North ME, Webster ADB. Primary defect in CD8[+] lymphocytes in the antibody deficiency disease (common variable immunodeficiency): abnormalities in intracellular production of interferon-gamma (IFN-g) in CD28[+] ('cytotoxic')and CD28[-] ('suppressor') CD8[+] subsets. *Clin Exp Immunol.* 1998;111:70–75.

414. Hatam L, Schuval S, Bonagura VR. Flow cytometric analysis of natural killer cell function as a clinical assay. *Cytometry.* 1994;16:59–68.

415. Flieger D, Gruber R, Schlimok G, et al. A novel non-radioactive cellular cytotoxicity test based on the differential assessment of living and killed target and effector cells. *J Immunol Methods.* 1995;180:1–13.

416. Goldberg JE, Sherwood SW, Clayberger C. A novel method for measuring CTL and NK cell-mediated cytotoxicity using annexin V and two-color flow cytometry. *J Immunol Methods.* 1999;224:1–9.

12

Lymphocyte Immunophenotyping and Human Immunodeficiency Virus (HIV) Infection

John L. Carey, III
David F. Keren

Clinical Overview

In 1981, there appeared in *The New England Journal of Medicine* 2 separate reports of young gay men presenting with unusual opportunistic infections and/or Kaposi sarcoma.[1,2] These articles were the ominous harbingers of the HIV epidemic. In the ensuing decade, medical science identified the etiologic agent (human immunodeficiency virus [HIV]) of the acquired immune deficiency syndrome (AIDS), as well as its molecular biology, primary modes of infection, pathogenesis, and clinical presentations. During this time, HIV has become the global pandemic of the twentieth century and beyond. In 1998, the United Nations estimated that 33.4 million persons worldwide are infected with HIV, including over a million children under 15 years of age.[3]

Despite criticism about slow progress, never before in the history of medicine has such intensive worldwide investigative effort yielded so much information and knowledge about an infectious disease in so short a time. Clearly, the AIDS pandemic will continue to consume huge amounts of health care resources for the next several decades. The judicious use of flow cytometry and molecular techniques will be a key to instituting and evaluating the effectiveness of medications that are rapidly emerging to combat this disease.

HIV Infection: Pathogenesis and Clinical Spectrum

HIV is a member of the Lentivirus subfamily of retroviruses. These viruses are widely distributed in nature, being found in sheep, horses, cattle, nonhuman primates, goats, and cats.[4-7] Typically, they cause latent infections affecting primarily the central nervous system and cells of the immune system. They contain an RNA genome and reverse transcriptase, an enzyme that transcribes viral RNA into proviral DNA. The latter is integrated into host cell DNA, and is subsequently transcribed into viral RNA during cell division. Essential viral proteins are then synthesized for assembly into new virions.

HIV is spread by sexual contact, exposure to blood or blood products and body fluids, and vertical transmission from mother to child.[4] As of December 31, 1997, over 640,000 cases of AIDS in the United States had been reported to the Centers for Disease Control and Prevention (CDC).[8] In December 1999, UNAIDS estimated 44,000 new HIV infections in North America in 1999. For most countries of the world, the number of women infected is approximately equal to the number of men. However, in the United States, homosexuals/bisexuals and intravenous drug users are the major groups at risk. Nonetheless, heterosexually acquired HIV infection has increased from 8.5% to 17.5% between 1991 and 1996.[8] This trend is especially apparent among minority populations. In 1996, the CDC reported that the number of adults with AIDS among non-Hispanic blacks and Hispanics exceeded those among non-Hispanic whites for the first time.[9,10] By 1997, 66% of reported cases of AIDS occurred among blacks or Hispanics, while only 33% occurred in whites.[10]

When the virus is transmitted through genital exposure, data from studies in rhesus monkeys indicate that the virus first enters Langerhans cells in the lamina propria.[11] The virus can be found in regional lymph nodes within about 2 days and may be cultured from the bloodstream as early as 5 days after initial exposure.[11,12] When the virus is transmitted by means of direct inoculation (eg, intravenous drug use, contaminated blood, or needle stick) or when there are tears in the mucosa, it has immediate access to the systemic circulation.

The initial binding of the virus is due to the attachment of the gp120 envelope protein to the CD4 molecule.[6] Immunoprecipitation studies have shown intimate association of the CD4 molecule with the gp120 viral envelope glycoprotein, which, in conjunction with the gp41 envelope protein, is thought to facilitate cell entry. Once attached, the virus gains access to the cell through interaction with a chemokine coreceptor: CCR5 for macrophage-tropic strains of HIV-1 and CXCR4 for T lymphocyte-tropic strains of HIV-1.[13,14] Indeed, individuals who have deletions of the *CCR5* gene may have a higher, although

Table 12-1
Frequency of Symptoms and Findings Associated with Acute HIV-1 Infection

Symptom or Finding	Percentage of Patients
Fever	> 80-90
Fatigue	> 70-90
Rash	> 40-80
Headache	32-70
Lymphadenopathy	40-70
Pharyngitis	50-70
Nausea, vomiting, or diarrhea	30-60
Night sweats	50
Asceptic meningitis	24
Oral ulcers	10-20
Genital ulcers	5-15
Thrombocytopenia	45
Leukopenia	40
Elevated hepatic enzyme levels	21

Reprinted with permission from Kahn JO, Walker BD. Acute human immunodeficiency virus type 1 infection. N Engl J Med. *1998;339:33-39.*

not absolute, resistance to HIV-1 compared with individuals with the wild-type *CCR5* gene.[15-17]

Whether the virus is acquired through genital or percutaneous exposure, a viremia occurs within a few days. At that time, the patient often displays symptoms of fever, rash, fatigue, lymphadenopathy, headache, and myalgia (**Table 12-1**).[11] Some patients may also demonstrate oral and gastrointestinal symptoms, including nausea, vomiting, diarrhea, pharyngitis, and oral ulcers.[18] A minority of patients will exhibit central nervous system symptoms of aseptic meningitis or, rarely, encephalitis.[19,20] After establishment of infection by the virus, it becomes integrated into the host as proviral DNA.

During the acute stage of viremia, high levels of viral RNA, often exceeding a million copies per milliliter, are present in the peripheral blood. Within approximately 9 months of infection, the plasma HIV RNA levels drop to a baseline plateau that may be used to predict the risk of disease progression.[21] Whereas HIV RNA can be amplified from many fluids, the viral loads in non-blood fluids (saliva, semen, cerebrospinal fluid and cervical-vaginal lavage fluid) are generally lower than those in plasma.[22] The recent CDC guidelines recommend that 2 HIV RNA plasma values be obtained within 1 to 2 weeks of each other at this point in the infection (baseline, 6 to 9 months after infection) to

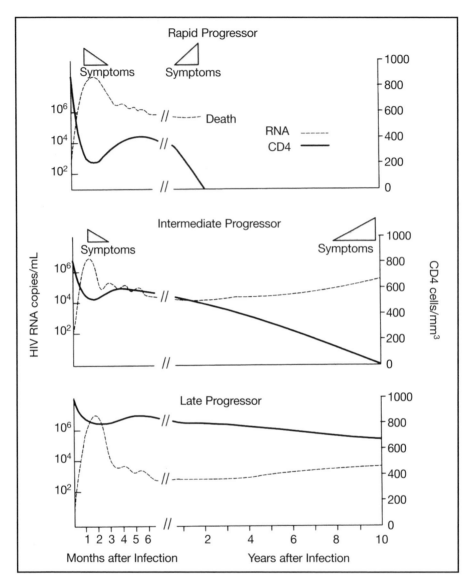

Figure 12-1
Generalized time course of HIV infection and disease. Reprinted with permission from
MMWR Morb Mortal Wkly Rep. 1998;47:34.

optimize the accuracy of the baseline measurement.[23,24] In **Figure 12-1**, the generalized time course of HIV infection and disease is demonstrated for 3 situations: rapid progressor, intermediate progressor, and late progressor.[23]

The acute illness is followed in 2 to 4 weeks by host production of antibodies to a number of viral proteins, including p24, p31, gp41, gp120, and gp160.

This immune response to the virus forms the basis for the screening and confirmatory tests for HIV antibody. After seroconversion, if no antiviral therapy is given, there occurs a progressive loss of $CD4^+$ T lymphocytes in 4 defined stages.[25] First, in the 12 to 18 months after seroconversion, there is a decline in $CD4^+$ lymphocytes from approximately $1000/mm^3$ to about $600/mm^3$. Second, this is followed by a relatively stable period with little change in circulating $CD4^+$ cells that may last for years. In the third stage the patient undergoes a rapid loss of $CD4^+$ lymphocytes to levels less than $200/mm^3$, presaging frank AIDS. In the fourth stage inexorable cell loss occurs until death.

Active viral replication is triggered by T-cell activation by a number of factors, including antigens, cytokines, mitogens, and heterologous viral cofactors. Production of viral particles is cytolytic for the $CD4^+$ lymphocyte, and depletion of these cells is the hallmark of HIV disease.[23,26] Although the exact mechanism of cell death is not well understood, it is known that both HIV-infected and uninfected cells are killed, possibly by some recruitment phenomenon. HIV-infected CD4 lymphocytes might also be rendered more susceptible to superinfection by other viral pathogens (eg, cytomegalovirus, hepatitis B virus, or herpes virus). When CD4 cells are infected by HIV, they experience a loss of several cell receptors, including CD4 and HLA class 1.[27] Furthermore, expression of a molecule associated with lymphocyte trafficking, CD62L, is also lost during HIV infection.[28] This loss may interfere with homing of CD4 lymphocytes into lymph nodes.

Whatever the mechanism, when sufficient numbers of these major effectors of the immune system are depleted, manifestations of cellular immune deficiency appear. The profound immunodeficiency that results renders the host susceptible to a myriad of opportunistic infectious organisms and several unusual neoplasms, particularly Kaposi sarcoma and non-Hodgkin lymphomas of the B-cell type. Although cellular immune defenses are most severely affected, there is good evidence that humoral immunity is also disrupted. B lymphocytes exhibit poor proliferative response to mitogens and to soluble antigens. Paradoxically, patients typically manifest marked polyclonal increases in immunoglobulins, presumably because of loss of the suppressor subset among CD4 lymphocytes, which normally exert control over B cells to prevent unbridled production of immunoglobulin.

The $CD4^+$ lymphocyte count is an indicator of the damage present in the immune system.[29-31] Indeed, it may be preferable to HIV RNA levels in individuals in whom the clinical course is at variance with the viral load. Palumbo et al[30] found that in children plasma RNA and $CD4^+$ lymphocyte counts are independent predictors of the clinical course of the child's disease. The progression-free survival (PFS) of the children in their study could be predicted by a combination of the baseline CD4$^+$ lymphocyte count and the child's age (**Figure 12-2**). In the children 16 to 18 years of age, 99% of those who had CD4$^+$ lymphocyte counts of greater than 500 had 2 years' PFS, whereas the youngest group of children studied (< 30 months) had lower PFS (see **Figure 12-2**). Greenough et al[32] report a case in which CD4 T-cell counts declined despite an undetectable viral load. Although some reports have noted occasional long-term HIV survivors with CD4 cell counts of less than 200/mm^3, these individuals usually have relatively low HIV RNA viral loads.[33] Such studies point out the necessity of performing regular quantitative evaluations of both the HIV-1 RNA levels and the CD4 cell counts to estimate the current state of the immune system.

Therapy and Monitoring of HIV

Therapy

Recently, aggressive use of newly available therapeutic agents has resulted in a dramatic decrease in the development of AIDS among HIV-infected individuals. In addition, this application of multidrug therapy on a large scale has produced a decrease in the death rate attributable to HIV infection.[34-36] By comparing the risk of death of patients from 1990 to 1993 versus those treated from July 1995 to July 1997, Detels et al[36] documented that the relative survival time improved to 1.21 ($P < .05$), correlating with the introduction of aggressive antiretroviral therapy. The CDC reported a 12% decline in new AIDS cases between 1996 and 1997.[9] There was a further dramatic reduction in HIV-related deaths from 31,130 in the US in 1996 to 16,685 in 1997.[37]

Some investigators urge caution because of the lack of data on long-term use of the multidrug regimens for long periods of time beginning in patients with early HIV disease.[38] However, the combined benefits of elevating the CD4 counts and the greater chance of preventing viral genetic evolution or slowing the development of drug-resistant strains of HIV are powerful arguments for early use of these medications. Even authors who advocate the early use of these drugs stress the importance of using them in motivated patients who understand the importance of compliance with the dosage regimen.[39] The complications of the medications, the complex regimens, and the cost of the drugs are all factors in the current treatment of this disease.[40] Although ideally the cost of care would not be a factor, the estimated cost of $12,000 to $20,000 a year in 1998 is not attainable for all patients.[41] In developing countries, such as in sub-Saharan Africa, where the rate of infection may be 10% or more of the population, one estimate is that only approximately $10 per year per patient is spent for HIV care.[42]

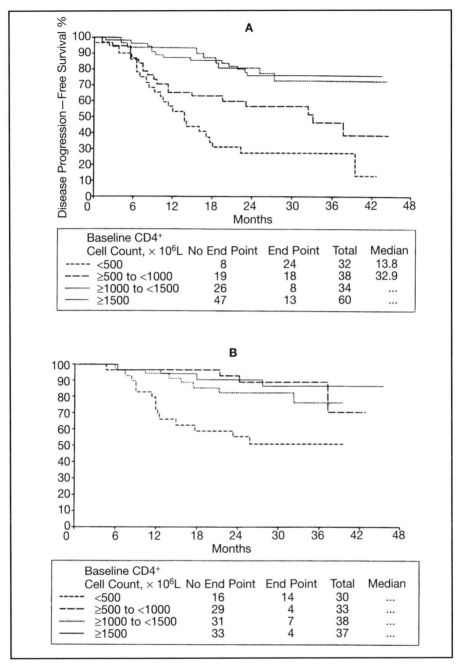

Figure 12-2

Disease progression in children on the basis of CD4 counts. **A.** Children 3 months to less than 12 months. **B.** Children 12 months to less than 30 months. Reprinted with permission from Palumbo PE, Raskino C, Fiscus S, et al. Predictive value of quantitative plasma HIV RNA and CD4+ lymphocyte count in HIV-infected infants and children. *JAMA.* 1998;279:756-761.

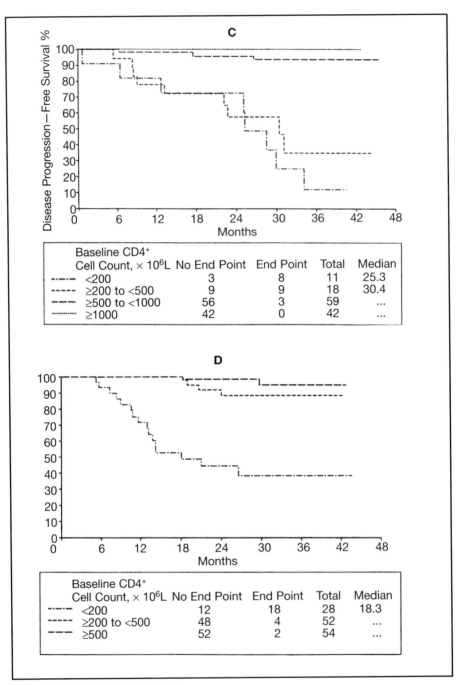

Figure 12-2 (continued)

Disease progression in children on the basis of CD4 counts. **C.** Children 30 months to less than 6 years. **D.** Children 6 years to 18 years. Reprinted with permission from Palumbo PE, Raskino C, Fiscus S, et al. Predictive value of quantitative plasma HIV RNA and CD4+ lymphocyte count in HIV-infected infants and children. *JAMA.* 1998;279:756-761.

Despite enormous effort by several groups of investigators worldwide, the near-term (within 5 to 10 years) prospect of the development of an AIDS vaccine is poor at the time of this writing.[43,44] This reflects the extreme mutability of HIV, the presence of a multitude of genetic variants in each infected individual, and the resultant rapid evolution of variants able to escape immune surveillance.

There are now a wide variety of drugs available to combat HIV infection, and the number is growing quickly. They may be grouped into 3 broad categories: nucleoside reverse transcriptase inhibitors, nonnucleoside reverse transcriptase inhibitors, and protease inhibitors. Before the availability of HIV viral load testing and the numerous therapeutic agents available today, treatment was generally withheld until the patient had symptoms of opportunistic infections and/or until the CD4$^+$ lymphocyte count fell to $500/mm^3$ or less.[45,46] Today, a much more aggressive approach is continuing to evolve.[23,47-49] These reports urge aggressive use of multidrug therapy to lower the viral count in the plasma. Patient compliance is stressed to decrease the likelihood of development of drug-resistant strains.

HIV Quantitation and Mutational Analysis

HIV has considerable genetic variability. Several subtypes have been characterized and are useful in epidemiologic studies.[50] Although techniques are available to determine genotype and phenotype with regard to designing best treatment with therapeutic agents, the use of these techniques to predict drug resistance has not become part of the routine analysis at the time of this writing. However, several groups and laboratories have demonstrated correlation of specific genetic forms of HIV with resistance to certain drugs. Unfortunately, the role of resistance testing in clinical management of these patients is uncertain.[51] This uncertainty reflects the high rate of mutability of this virus, the large number (over a million) of mutant forms of the virus in individual patients at any point in time, and the ability of current tests to examine only a few of the predominant strains in the patient. This type of testing is a rapidly evolving field the most recent international AIDS Society-USA Panel recommendation is that drug resistance testing is recommended in helping to guide the choice of new drug therapy when there has been treatment failure and that it should be considered even in treatment-naïve patients (though the panel did not "firmly recommend" it in this setting).[52]

CD4 T-cell Quantitation

The current definition of clinical AIDS includes a patient with positive serology for HIV who has less than 200 CD4[+] lymphocytes per cubic millimeter of whole blood.[53] This definition reflects the changes that occur as the disease progresses. Early in the course of the disease, as CD4 cells are destroyed, there is a marked increase in the number of CD8[+] lymphocytes to twice the normal values or more. Examination of peripheral blood smears at this time reveals the presence of atypical lymphocytes. The increase in CD8 cells tends to offset the loss of CD4 cells, and therefore the total number and percentage of T lymphocytes may be little changed from normal. This CD8 lymphocytosis persists for the course of the disease until the very late stages. At that time, lymphopenia occurs when the CD8 cells also disappear.[54]

There is a strong association between CD4[+] lymphocyte counts and development of opportunistic infections, progression to AIDS, and eventually death **(Figure 12-3)**.[55-58] Indeed, by means of multivariate analysis, CD4 cell lymphocyte count is a key parameter in predicting clinical outcome.[56] Other markers, such as beta-2-microglobulin or neopterin levels, that were once suggested as providing useful adjunctive information[5,59] have fallen into disuse now that HIV viral load studies are readily available. CD4 counts remain of great importance because they provide an independent factor to estimate the degree of immune suppression and to predict mortality.[60]

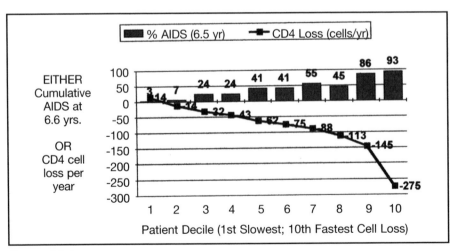

Figure 12-3
Relationship of clinical outcome and rate of CD4[+] T-cell decline in HIV-infected individuals. Data from Sheppard H, Lang W, Ascher MS, et al. The characterization of non-progressors: long-term HIV-1 infection with stable CD4+ T-cell levels. *AIDS*. 1993;7:1159-1166.

Pneumocystis carinii pneumonia (PCP) is the most frequent and one of the most life-threatening infections in HIV-infected persons, occurring in up to 80% of patients.[25] In adults, mortality from first episodes of PCP ranges from 5% to 20%, and reinfections are common.[61] Immunosuppressed patients, including those who are HIV infected, have benefited from PCP prophylaxis in clinical trials.[62,63] Given the high rate of morbidity and mortality associated with PCP, it is important to identify those patients who would benefit most from prophylactic therapy. The number of CD4$^+$ lymphocytes in the peripheral blood correlates strongly with, and can help define risk for, PCP. For example, in a study by Masur et al,[2] a CD4$^+$ cell count of less than 200/mm^3 or less than 20% of lymphocytes was highly predictive for development of PCP. In their retrospective study 93% of cases of PCP occurred among patients with less than 200 CD4$^+$ cells/mm^3. In adults receiving newer combination antiretroviral treatment, Furrer et al[64] reported that stopping PCP primary prophylaxis may be safe, as long as the patients have sustained CD4 counts of at least 200 cells/mm^3 and 14% or more of the total lymphocytes.

In infants and young children PCP is a much more serious infection, and mortality for first infection approaches 60%.[65] CD4 lymphocyte counts are superior to CD19 lymphocyte counts or serum immunoglobulin G levels in predicting the risk of bacterial infection in children.[66] However, a number of studies of HIV-infected children have shown that PCP develops in young patients with CD4 counts at much higher levels than in adult patients.[65,67] This is probably because studies of normal children have shown baseline CD4 levels of 2 to 3 times those of healthy adults (**Table 12-2**),[68,69] and significant depletion of CD4 cells can occur and still leave normal circulating levels by adult standards. The problem is compounded in the pediatric population because HIV infection

Table 12-2
Age-related differences in T-lymphocyte subsets

Marker	Age (y)				
	< 1	1 to < 3	3 to < 5	5 to 13	> 13
CD4	3810 ± 2570*	2094 ± 1527	1798 ± 1372	1104 ± 616	998 ± 616
CD8	1614 ± 1131	1019 ± 990	1003 ± 779	865 ± 530	485 ± 328
CD3	5026 ± 2996	2971 ± 2188	2641 ± 1739	1890 ± 872	1664 ± 772

Pediatric data from Denny TN, Niyen P, Skuza C, et al. Age related changes of lymphocyte phenotypes in healthy children [abstract]. Pediatr Res. 1990;27:155A. Adult data from Warde Medical Laboratory, Ann Arbor, MI. Data are expressed as mean values (± 2 SD).

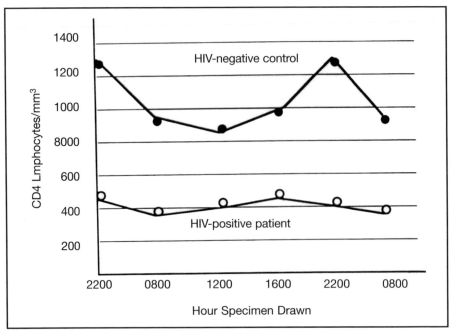

Figure 12-4
Diurnal variation of CD4[+] lymphocytes. Data from Malone JL, Simms TE, Gray CG, et al. Sources of variability in repeated T-helper lymphocyte counts from human immunodeficiency virus type 1-infected patients: total lymphocyte count fluctuations and diurnal cycle are important. *J Acquir Immun Defic Syndr.* 1990;3:144-151.

is more difficult to diagnose in the perinatal period because the screening tests used to detect antibodies to the virus will measure maternal antibody, which crosses the placenta, rather than *de novo* host antibody in response to HIV infection. On the basis of studies of adult patients with PCP, the CDC recommends PCP prophylaxis for children when CD4 counts fall below 200/mm³.[61,70] However, because of the issues discussed above, some authorities recommend initiating PCP prophylaxis for all HIV-infected pediatric patients under 1 year of age, regardless of the CD4 count.[65]

Studies of the absolute numbers of CD4 cells show a diurnal variation (**Figure 12-4**). There is a nadir in the morning and peak in the late evening. During the peak, counts can be twice those of the nadir.[71] This variation has been demonstrated in HIV-infected persons, as well as in seronegative control subjects, although the variation in the former is blunted in comparison with the control population (**Figure 12-5**). The variation is largely attributable to fluctuations in the percentage of lymphocytes in the white blood cell differential.[72]

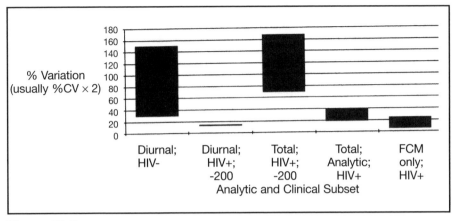

Figure 12-5
Total variation of CD4$^+$ lymphocytes. Data from Hoover DR, Graham NMH, Chen B, et al. Effect of CD4+ cell count measurement variability on staging HIV-1 infection. *J Acquir Immune Deficic Syndr.* 1992;5:794-802.

CD8 T-cell Quantitation

The striking proliferation of CD8$^+$ T lymphocytes begins during the acute stage of HIV infection and persists to the end stage of the disease. Study of these activated and proliferating CD8 cells may lead to an increased understanding of the pathobiology of HIV disease and possibly to additional markers of prognostic significance. For example, studies of CD8 T-cell subsets in 4 groups of homosexual men who were seronegative, recently seropositive, remotely seropositive, or who had AIDS showed a marked progressive increase in CD8$^+$ cells that coexpressed CD38 and HLA-DR (markers of T-cell activation).[25] This immune activation is interpreted as an immunologic response to the viral infection and may represent the host's attempt to kill and clear the HIV.

Further evidence to support this hypothesis came from another study of HIV-infected homosexuals with AIDS-related complex and AIDS. A significant increase in CD8$^+$/CD11b$^-$ T lymphocytes was seen in the infected groups compared with healthy seronegative homosexual and heterosexual control subjects.[73] The CD8$^+$/CD11b$^-$ subset of T lymphocytes is known to have cytotoxic function.[74,75] Although an increase in this subset may be associated with a poor clinical outcome,[25] Musey et al[76] demonstrated that during early HIV infection, the memory T-cytotoxic cells with reactivity for HIV envelope proteins are related to a slower rate of decline in CD4$^+$ T lymphocytes. This corroborates the earlier work of Bouscarat et al,[77] who found relative preservation of CD4$^+$ T-lymphocyte counts in patients with expanded populations of activated CD8 cells. Clearly, complex changes in the CD8 T-lymphocyte compartment occur as the course of HIV infection plays out, and immune dysfunction resulting from infection by HIV is likely a consequence of alteration of more than just the CD4$^+$ subset of T lymphocytes. Additional study of these cells and other subsets may yield important information about the pathophysiology of AIDS that could have prognostic implications and help determine strategies for development of antiretroviral drugs or vaccines.

Traditional Flow Cytometric Lymphocyte Quantitation

Accuracy and precision in measuring lymphocyte subsets require meticulous attention to quality control. Instrument characteristics, reagent antibody specificity, type of anticoagulant, specimen storage, method of specimen preparation, gating criteria, and normal diurnal variation of lymphocyte subsets all affect the laboratory results.[78-81]

Preanalytic Processing

It is recommended that whole blood staining and lysis methods for specimen preparation always be used. Density gradient separation methods can cause selective loss of the CD8 subset. Density gradient techniques are also difficult in pediatric cases because very small specimen volumes may be used. In addition, specimens should be stored at room temperature because storage at 4°C can result in selective loss of CD4 lymphocytes.[82,83] Obviously, freezing will destroy the specimen. Furthermore, in extremely hot weather conditions, an insulated container with an ice pack (but *not* dry ice) may be used to keep the overall temperature within the container near room temperature (64°F to 72°F).[84,85]

The specimen should be processed within 48 hours from the time it is obtained from the patient. Specimens should be examined as soon as they arrive in the laboratory. They should be rejected if there is evidence of hemolysis or if the anticoagulation is inadequate (clot visible).[85] The authors prefer the use of ACD-Solution B-treated whole blood. Blood anticoagulated with either heparin or ethylenediamine tetraacetic acid is acceptable, but use such blood within 30 hours of the drawing time.

Because instrument characteristics can vary significantly and subtle variations in the CD4 subset are known to occur in certain ethnic groups (eg, blacks and Asians), each laboratory should establish its own reference range of normal values by using 50 to 100 healthy control subjects. Each laboratory should decide which of the recommended antibody panels and analytic protocols it wishes to use, adhering to suggested gating and quality control checks (see below). Each run should include a quantitative control run in parallel with routine patient samples.

Acquisition and Analysis

Antibody Panels

Several different panels have been recommended for enumeration of CD4[+] and CD8[+] T lymphocytes using flow cytometry, depending on the laboratory's capability.[85] Antibodies to CD3 are preferable to those against other pan-T-cell antigens for the enumeration of total T cells. In particular, the use of anti-CD2 reagents for this purpose is discouraged because natural killer (NK) cells may also express the CD2 antigen, and overestimation of T-cell numbers by as much as 10% may result.[78] Note that dual-color reagents are used where feasible because most antigens are not lineage-specific, and therefore antibodies directed toward them may react with more than one type of cell. Furthermore, multiparametric analysis yields more information than single-parameter histograms and allows for dissection of lymphocyte subsets that may share common epitopes.

Two different panels have been recommended for laboratories making use of 2-color monoclonal antibody panels. The first time a patient has immunophenotyping performed, the CDC guidelines recommend that a complete panel (**Table 12-3**) be used. Whether this panel results in a clinically relevant improvement in accuracy has not been demonstrated. According to the CDC guidelines, it is acceptable to use a simpler panel in individuals who have been previously evaluated by the comprehensive panel shown. The abbreviated panel includes CD3/CD4, CD3/CD8, and CD45/CD14 and may be attractive in reducing reagent and labor costs, as well as providing a faster turnaround time. CD4 counts obtained by 2 single-tube methods with either CD3/CD4/CD8 or CD4 (including an isotype control) did not provide clinically different data from those obtained by use of the original CDC-recommended, 6-tube, 2-color panel.[86] In situations of limited resources, Sherman et al[86] suggest these simpler panels as useful alternatives.

Table 12-3

Recommended 2-Color Panel of Monoclonal Antibodies for Evaluation of HIV-Infected Patients

Reagent	Purpose
Isotype control	Background fluorescence
CD45/CD14	Lymphocyte gate
CD3/CD4	CD4$^+$ T lymphocytes
CD3/CD8	CD8$^+$ T lymphocytes
CD3/CD19	Total T and B lymphocytes
CD3/CD16 and/or CD56	T lymphocytes and NK cells

Modified from Centers for Disease Control and Prevention. 1997 Revised guidelines for performing CD4+ T-cell determinations in persons infected with human immunodeficiency virus (HIV). MMWR Morb Mortal Wkly Rep. 1997;46 (No. RR-2):1-29.

In the 2-color CDC panel, several quality control checks are used. First and foremost is the use of the CD45/CD14 tube. This should be applied to establish appropriate light scatter gating (**Figures 12-6 and 12-7**).[78,87,88] This allows the laboratory to maintain accuracy by ensuring the following:

- the vast majority of lymphocytes are included in the gate (ideally > 95% but at least > 90%); and
- the contamination of the lymph gate by nonlymphoid cells is minimized (ideally < 5% but no more than 15%).

Should either the minimum recovery and/or purity not be attainable, the sample should be restained and analyzed or a new sample requested. In addition, if the purity is less than 95% but greater than 85%, the lymphocyte subset quantities should be corrected for this excess contamination (**Figure 12-6**).

Three other quality control checks are available from the comprehensive 2-color panel. The first is the variability of the CD3$^+$ T cells in each tube. This range should be no more than 3% among the 4 tubes that contain this marker. Secondly, the sum of the T (mean percentage CD3$^+$), B (percentage CD19$^+$CD3$^-$), and NK cells (CD16$^+$CD56$^+$CD3$^-$) should be ± 5% of the lymphoid purity (see above and **Figures 12-6 and 12-7**, p 488). Lastly, the sum of the CD4 percentage and the CD8 percentage should equal approximately 95% ± 5% of the total T lymphocytes (CD3). Of course, the patient's clinician should be aware of the use and theoretic limitations of the abbreviated panel.[85]

The inclusion of CD3 in these tubes greatly enhances the accuracy of T and non-T quantitation (**Figure 12-8**, p 490). This is because the T subset and NK markers are also present on other blood cells.

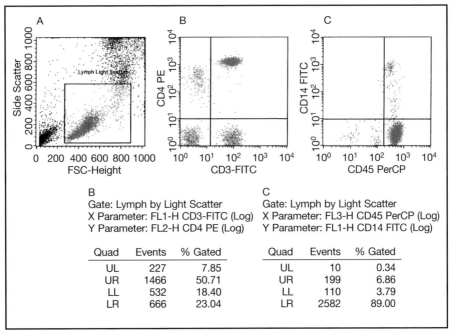

Quad	Events	% Gated
UL	227	7.85
UR	1466	50.71
LL	532	18.40
LR	666	23.04

B
Gate: Lymph by Light Scatter
X Parameter: FL1-H CD3-FITC (Log)
Y Parameter: FL2-H CD4 PE (Log)

C
Gate: Lymph by Light Scatter
X Parameter: FL3-H CD45 PerCP (Log)
Y Parameter: FL1-H CD14 FITC (Log)

Quad	Events	% Gated
UL	10	0.34
UR	199	6.86
LL	110	3.79
LR	2582	89.00

Figure 12-6
Lymphocyte Gate Purity (Specificity)

Two tubes of whole blood are stained with CD3 FITC/CD4 PE and CD45 PerCP/CD14 FITC, respectively, then light scatter and immunofluorescence data acquired on the flow cytometer. The total number of true lymphocytes is determined by setting a large light scatter gate around the lymphocyte cluster (panel A; "Lymph Light Scatter" region — indicated by red color). From this, the bivariant plots gated cell immunofluorescence of CD3/CD4 (Panel B) and CD45 / CD14 (panel C) are generated. In the latter, a quandrant is drawn around the cluster that contains only the brightest CD45+ and CD14 negative lymphs.

The number of cells in this lower right quadrant (LR) of Panel C is the number of true lymphocytes in the "Lymph Light Scatter" gate (= 2582 cells). Hence the purity or specificity of the "Lymph Light Scatter" gate is 89.0% (= # cells in LR Quadrant of panel C / # cells in "Lymph Light Scatter" gate, or 2582/2901). Since the purity is less than 95%, the %CD4 result must be corrected by dividing the %CD4 by the purity (51% / 0.89) in order to correct for non-lymphoid cell contamination. The latter is primarily due to inclusion of monocytes, which appear as the CD3− CD4^{dim+} cluster in the UL quandrant of panel B, and the CD45$^{bright+}$ CD14$^{bright+}$ cluster in the UR quandrant of panel C.

For CD4$^+$ T cells, the inclusion of CD3 allows the analyst to clearly define CD4$^+$/CD3$^+$ T cells from CD4$^+$ (dim)/CD3$^-$ monocytes. Because monocyte clusters are close to lymphocyte clusters in either light scatter or CD45/side scatter (SSC) gating plots, there will usually be a residual number of monocytes contaminating the gate.

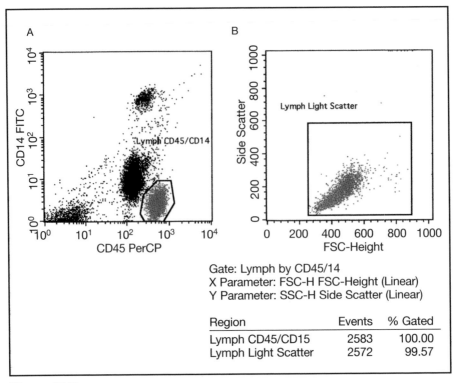

Gate: Lymph by CD45/14
X Parameter: FSC-H FSC-Height (Linear)
Y Parameter: SSC-H Side Scatter (Linear)

Region	Events	% Gated
Lymph CD45/CD15	2583	100.00
Lymph Light Scatter	2572	99.57

Figure 12-7
Lymphocyte Gate Recovery (Sensitivity)
The sensitivity of the "Lymph Light Scatter" gate (see Figure 12-6 panel A and panel B in this Figure) for true lymphocytes (the recovery) is determined using the tube stained with CD45 PerCP and CD14 FITC. The CD45bright+ CD14- cluster is assumed to define all lymphocytes, and a gate is drawn about it (Panel A, "Lymph CD45/14" – indicated by red color). The light scatter of only these cells is then displayed in panel B. The recovery of the "Lymph Light Scatter" gate is then calculated by determining the percentage of the CD45bright+ CD14- cluster that fall into this gate (99.7%).
This high recovery is a result of the overly large light scatter gate, and, hence a low purity (see figure 12-6). The recovery is only marginally decreased (still > 95%) and purity increased to > 95% if the "Lymph Light Scatter" gate is drawn more closely about the lymph cluster in Panel A Figure 12-6. Please see text for further details.

In calculating CD8+ T cells, one should use a dual-color CD3/CD8 reagent and report only those cells that coexpress the CD3 and CD8 antigens (CD3+CD8+). This is because NK cells, which are CD3−, may express CD8 in low antigen density, and including them in the CD8+ calculation would spuriously reduce the CD4:CD8 ratio.[90]

Table 12-4

Recommended 3-Color Panel of Monoclonal Antibodies for Evaluation of HIV-Infected Patients*

A Reagent	Purpose
CD3/CD4/CD45	Gating on lymphocytes by using CD45 and side light scatter; measure CD3⁺CD4⁺ T cells
CD3/CD8/CD45	Gating on lymphocytes by using CD45 and side light scatter; measure CD3⁺CD8⁺ T cells
CD3/CD19/CD45†	Gating on lymphocytes by using CD45 and side light scatter; measure CD19⁺ B cells

B‡ Reagent	Purpose
Isotype control	Background fluorescence
CD3/CD4/CD8	CD4⁺ and CD8⁺ T lymphocytes
CD3/CD19/CD16 and/or CD56	Total T, NK, and B lymphocytes

*Modified from Centers for Disease Control and Prevention. 1997 Revised guidelines for performing CD4+ T-cell determinations in persons infected with human immunodeficiency virus (HIV). MMWR Morb Mortal Wkly Rep. 1997;46 (No. RR-2):1-29.
†Recommended in specimens from children.
‡This panel may be used for systems determining absolute cell numbers directly from the flow cytometer, with percentage determinations calculated from the absolute numbers.

To define NK cells, the inclusion of CD3 is necessary because the NK markers CD16 and CD56 are also expressed at low levels on a minority of T cells. Thus true NK cells are CD3⁺/CD16⁺ (and/or CD56⁺).

As far as B-cell quantitation is concerned, CD3 is needed if one uses CD20 as the B-cell marker. Like the NK markers, CD20 is dimly expressed on a variably small minority of T cells.[91] Although this limitation does not extend to CD19, the tradition of including CD3 for other quality control reasons has led to the retention of CD3/CD19 combinations.

Many laboratories now take advantage of 3-color monoclonal antibody panels (**Table 12-4** and **Figures 12-9**, p 491 **and 12-10**, p 492).[92] These allow a more efficient accurate gating of lymphocytes, thus obviating the need for the additional reagents and labor costs associated with the 2-color panels. Most laboratories use the 3-color panel, which adds CD45 to the CD3/CD4, CD3/CD8, and (in the case of pediatric samples) CD3/CD19 tubes (see **Table 12-4, A**). By gating on CD45 and side light scatter, the specific lymphocyte populations can be enumerated.

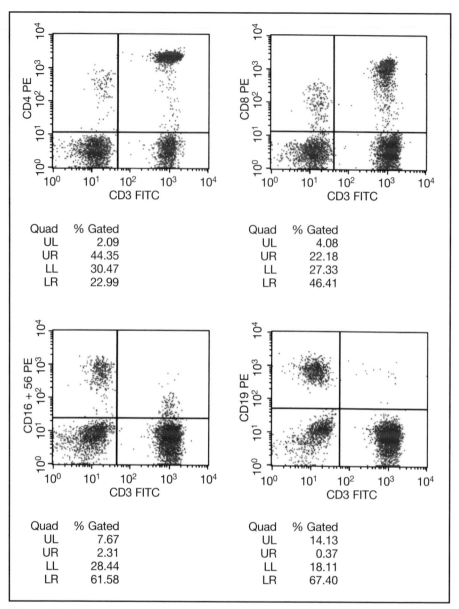

Figure 12-8

Two-color lymphocyte subset quantitation from analytic gating set by fluorescence purity and recovery technique. Lymphocyte subset quantitation is performed from the same sample as was gated in Figure 12-6. Although not shown, an isotype-matched control was initially analyzed, and quadrant gates were set per CDC guidelines. These were then subtly adjusted to reflect variation in background immunofluorescence in each tube, as judged by the predominant negative cluster in the lower right quadrant of each bivariant plot. The data shown is not corrected for purity and would need to be divided by 0.87 (eg, the true percentage of CD4+ T cells is 44%/0.87 = 51%). If the purity was 0.95 or less, then this correction would not be needed.

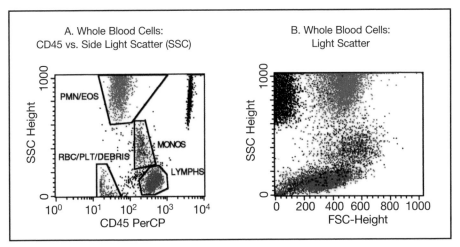

Figure 12-9

Three-color lymphocyte gating technique.[92] Very good lymphocyte recovery and gating purity can be obtained by replacing the forward light scatter parameter with CD45. Typically, true lymphocytes can be unambiguously identified at the brightest CD45+ cluster with low side light scatter/SSC (lymph region indicated in red). The neutrophil and eosinophil (PNM/EOS, indicated in fuchsia) cluster is distinct by having a dimmer CD45 intensity and much higher side light scatter. Erythrocytes, platelets, and debris (RBC/PLT/DEBRIS, indicated in blue) typically are CD45− and have low side light scatter. Monocytes usually have a subtly dimmer CD45 intensity with a mild, yet distinctly higher, side light scatter. Typically, the CD45/side scatter gate for lymphocytes gives greater than 95% recovery and purity. Hence, the need to check for purity or recovery and the CD45/CD14 tube is not needed. For similar reasons, the various lymphosum checks are not indicated.

An alternative 3-color panel makes use of CD3/CD19/CD16 (or CD56) in one tube and CD3/CD4/CD8 in another, along with an isotype control (see **Table 12-4, B**, p 489).[85] These 3-color combinations are useful with cytometers that directly measure lymphocyte concentrations and allow fewer tubes with resultant labor efficiency. Lastly, 4-color monoclonal antibody panels have been used. Typically, CD45 is added to the tube containing CD3/CD4/CD8. As with the 3-color methods, the gating is performed on CD45 with side light scatter to identify the lymphocytes. The recommended second tube would contain CD45/CD3/CD19/CD16 (or CD56).[85]

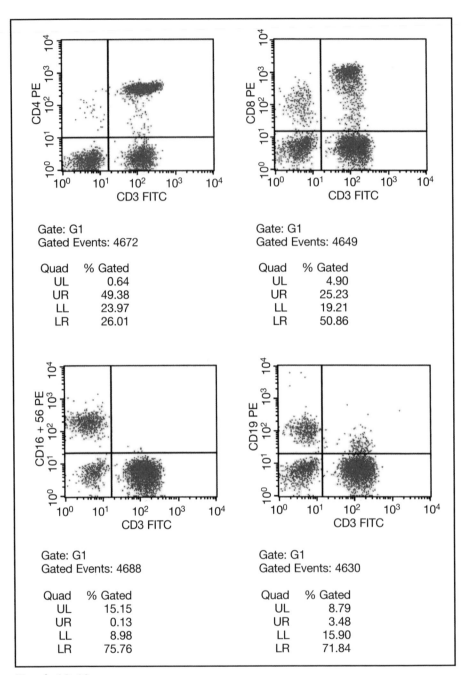

Figure 12-10

Three-color lymphocyte subset quantitation. The 4 bivariant plots are obtained by CD45/side scatter gating (see Figure 12-9). The quadrants were set by means of cluster gating and not by using isotype controls. The sample for these aliquots is the same as for Figures 12-6 and 12-7. Note that the various percentage CD values are essentially the same as the corrected values from Figure 12-8.

Alternative Methods of Lymphocyte Immunophenotyping

Rationale

Advantages
Precision and Accuracy

There is a considerable degree of imprecision associated with lymphocyte subset quantitation by traditional multiplatform analysis (see **Figure 12-5**, p 483). However, only 40% to 50% of this is due to the analytic component, as measured by the traditional 2-platform flow cytometry/hematology analyzer method.[91] The implication of this lack of precision for an individual patient undergoing routine treatment is, at best, uncertain. For the evaluation of large groups of patients with HIV, particularly those undergoing experimental treatment protocols, greater analytic precision can translate into better and/or faster resolution of better therapies with fewer patients.

Cost

As discussed above, the method first advocated by the CDC used 6 tubes and required extensive, often manual, quality control checks. In addition, the quantitation of total lymphocytes required a separate complete blood count (CBC) along with either an automated or manual CBC. The labor costs associated with this are considerable. The subsequent CDC recommendations for T-cell quantitation (CD45/side light scatter gating) and observations by others of the lack of need for isotyped negative controls were certainly more streamlined (2 to 4 tubes without need for purity and recovery quality control checks) than the earlier method. However, a CBC with differential was still required.[85]

Workflow and Integration

A related issue is specimen workflow and integration of laboratory testing and reporting. The above methods require 2 to 3 different analytic procedures and in many cases are done in different laboratories. This results in an awkward delivery of specimen samples (often necessitating 2 separate blood samples) and delayed acquisition and reporting of data. The overall effect of this is to raise the direct and indirect costs and somewhat lower the quality and timeliness of the blood T-cell subset quantitation.

Limitations of Alternative Technologies
Flow CD4 Cost Marginalized

The transfer of a flow-based T-subset quantitation to an alternative technology may not result in cost savings. Indeed, the overall cost may go up. Most intermediate-to-large flow laboratories also perform immunophenotypic analysis of lymphomas and leukemias. Although such services may be obtained from regional vendors, the timeliness of such data and clinical-pathologic correlation make it attractive enough for most laboratories to retain this service. As such, when T-cell quantitation is removed, the savings are initially only marginal (eg, cytometer and related labor costs remain). Furthermore, the new CD4 testing site will have to establish its own proficiency testing and quality control costs.

Effect on Existing Laboratory Testing

If the existing flow laboratory implements the new technology, there will be an increase in analytic effort. This may be partially offset by reductions in effort expended to ensure performance and incorporation of CBC and differential count results. The transfer of testing to a new platform will result in an increase in labor and overall cost. The new testing may also compete with the performance of existing tests on a shared platform (eg, hematology analyzer). This potentially may compromise the timely performance of such tests, particularly in a STAT (rapid turnaround) or high-volume test laboratory.

Methods

Single-platform Cytometry Methods
Standard Flow Cytometers

Several systems have been presented in the literature and/or are available commercially for absolute CD4 counts on standard flow platforms.[93,94] Flow-based systems include the TruCount from Becton-Dickinson (San Jose, CA), Flow Count® from Coulter (Fullerton, CA), and the ImmunoCount™ from Ortho (Raritan, NJ). The methods all use multiparameter 3-color flow cytometry. Briefly, this is a *no-wash* stain, lyse, and fix system with a 3-color panel using CD45/side scatter gating. A precise amount of whole blood is added to the TruCount tubes. The latter contain a calibrated number of beads, which, given the amount of blood and reagents added, will give back a true concentration of beads. By using the Attractors software, the various immunofluorescence cell and bead clusters can be quantitated as the percentage of lymphocytes. By comparing the number of beads with the number of cells counted, a simple ratio can be used to multiply the beads' concentration to directly calculate a particular cell concentration. The concentrations are determined either by comparing the ratio of CD4$^+$ cells to internal bead standards of known concentration or to a precise volume containing a given number of CD4$^+$ cells (**Figure 12-11**, pp 496-497).

The technology is modestly more complex than the traditional method. The sample requirements are the same, and hence the transport window is identical. Because of modifications and/or entirely new instruments, most cytometers used for absolute counts have the ability to process batches ranging from several dozen to over 100 samples. This feature alone may make this quite attractive to larger laboratories. Accuracy with the alternative methods is excellent and, on average, probably somewhat better than accuracy with the traditional method, particularly when manual differentials are used. Minimal detection levels are quite good. The authors have been able to measure down to 10 cells/microliter (with coefficients of variation of 20%). Precision (within-run tube-to-tube variation in CD4 fraction and concentration) is likewise quite good, ranging from 2% to 5%.

Only a modest amount of additional training is required to learn these techniques, which should not be a challenge to the skilled technologists running cytometers. Along with automated loading and analysis, many vendors have automated preanalytic staining and/or use no-wash techniques. All of this translates into significant reductions in hands-on labor and overall turnaround time for large-volume laboratories. As a corollary, cost is often reduced. The target laboratories for such instruments include those with large volumes of CD4 testing or ones with a need for other on-site flow assays (eg, substantial number of leukemia/lymphoma samples).

Standard Hematology Analyzers

Methods are available to perform CD4 enumeration on standard hematology analyzers.[95] This may be attractive to laboratories with relatively few requests for CD4 enumeration. Examples of such analyzers include the Technicon H*1 and the Immuno-VCS technology from Coulter. The former makes use of immunoperoxidase staining, whereas the latter uses immunobeads to measure the fraction and concentration of CD4$^+$ cells. Both methods require some manual preanalytic handling to stain the sample.

Although the technology is complex, the hematology analyzers are much more self-contained than the bench-top cytometer. The technique for performing the analysis is similar to that involved in performing a routine CBC. Although batch size is potentially large, the manual preanalytic handling and/or the need to switch into a batch mode on the instrument probably limits throughput somewhat. Accuracy and precision are excellent. Reliable minimum detection levels are 30 cells/microliter.

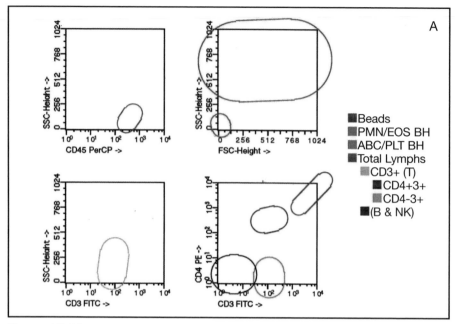

Figure 12-11

Automated CD4+ T-cell quantitation with absolute counts. In A, a blank analysis template for CD4+ T-cell quantitation is shown. There are 4 bivariant plots (CD45/side scatter [SSC]; forward scatter/side scatter [FSC/SSC], CD3/side scatter [SSC], and CD3/CD4). In each, there are 1 or more analysis regions or cluster gates. These are colored and labeled per the legend in the lower right. In B (p 497), the listmode data from a tube stained with CD3/CD4/CD45 is shown in the template. Note that during acquisition, a gating threshold was set using CD45/side scatter, such that most CD45⁻ cells (erythrocytes and platelets) were excluded from the list mode data set. What remains are the 3 major cellular clusters and the bead cluster in the upper right part of the CD45/side scatter plot. In C (p 497), the data is automatically analyzed. First, cells with light scatter are clearly not true lymphocytes (neutrophils, eosinophils, residual erythrocytes, and debris) and are eliminated electronically by using so-called "black hole clusters" in the forward scatter/side scatter plot. Next, the analytic regions in the other 3 bivariant plots are moved by the program to optimally include the target cell clusters. Quality control checks are included so that only cells with the light scatter and immunofluorescence of true lymphocytes are included in the final count. These and the beads show as colored clusters, with the residual nonlymphoid cells being gray. From these cell counts, the percentage of lymphocytes and absolute concentrations can be directly calculated by the program and display (in this case at the bottom of the page).

As mentioned above, considerable training is required to perform CD4 analysis on hematology analyzers, although much of the technique is similar to performing routine testing. Depending on the degree of preanalytic preparation and instrument modification, hands-on time is similar to that found with the

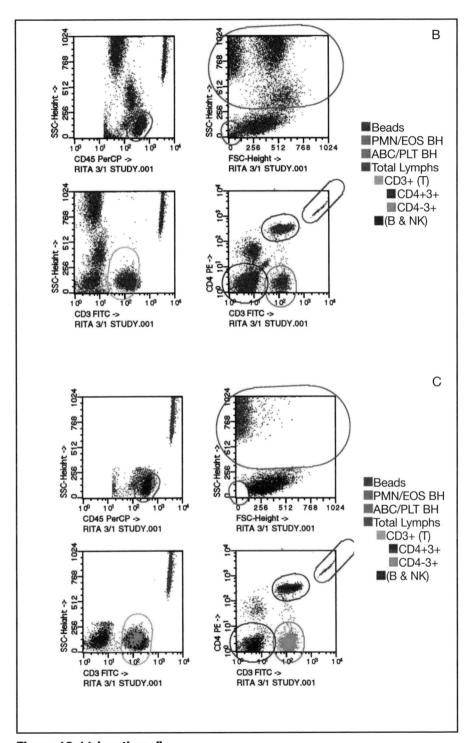

traditional method. Depending on the reduction in laboratory and flow cytometer costs from the use of the hematology analyzer, there will be a reduction in total laboratory costs. A target laboratory for this methodology would be those with low levels of CD4 assays and no other need for non-CD4 flow assays.

Manual Methods
Microtiter Plate Technologies

An alternative method to perform immunophenotyping that has been put forth in the last 5 years is based on microtiter plate immunoassay analysis.[96,97] The relative simplicity and large batch sizes make this method particularly attractive for higher volume laboratories.

Zymune is a microtiter-type assay developed by Zynaxis (Malvern, PA). It uses both magnetic and fluorescence immunobeads to separate and detect CD4 antigen-positive cells. Although CD3 is not measured, discrimination of CD4+ lymphocytes from monocytes is possible because of the greater density of CD4 antigen on the former lymphocytes. Vendor-supplied standards allow the conversion of fluorescence intensity signal into CD4 concentrations.

The technology is less complex than traditional cytometry. The specimen transport window is about the same as that for traditional cytometry. Batch size is modestly increased over that of traditional cytometry. Although accuracy is excellent, precision is in the range of 11% to 12%. Minimum detection is 50 cells/microliter.

Training requires a relative amount of skill, particularly for critical pipetting steps in the assay. Hands-on time and overall turnaround time is quite short for a standard batch of 12 samples ($\leq$ 45 minutes). Cost may be lower than that of routine flow cytometry, depending on the number of samples and turnaround requirements. The target laboratory would be one with moderate numbers of CD4 samples and no other need for non-CD4 flow cytometry.

The TRAX method is probably the most unique method of enumerating CD4. It is an enzyme-linked immunosorbent assay (ELISA)-based assay manufactured by T Cell Diagnostics (Woburn, MA). It does not count CD4+ T cells per se; rather, it measures solubilized cellular CD4 protein by means of an immunoassay and converts the signal to cell concentration through vendor-supplied standards.[98]

The TRAX hardware is simpler to use than either the traditional or absolute count flow cytometry. Furthermore, the plate reader may be used for other ELISA assays. One advantage of the TRAX system is that the lysates can be refrigerated and held for up to 3 days before analysis. If the lysate is stored at –70°C, it is stable for up to 12 months. This, along with the microtiter format, allows for large batch sizes. Beside the economies of scale it enables, this method may help minimize between-run or between-laboratory imprecision. The time to analyze each batch (96 samples) is about 4 hours. The accuracy is good, and precision is competitive with the absolute count flow methods. The minimum detectable CD4 count is 86 cell/microliter. This relatively low sensitivity, however, may be of concern to clinicians who prefer a cutoff of 50 cells for prognostication.

For the TRAX assay, training is less complex than with traditional cytometry. Furthermore, if the laboratory already performs a substantial number of ELISA assays, the marginal increase in complexity is low. Hands-on time and overall turnaround time is reduced compared with that of traditional flow cytometry, particularly for large batch sizes. Cost is also reduced. The ideal target laboratory for this assay is one with dozens to hundreds of samples per day and no other need for flow cytometry. Laboratories with smaller but still significant daily CD4 volumes may wish to investigate this technology as long as there is no need for non-CD4 flow cytometry.

The most recent of the alternative methods developed to enumerate CD4+ and CD8+ lymphocytes is the modified whole blood Capcellia immunoenzymatic method. An earlier version of this assay required a centrifugation step and a Ficoll-Paque gradient.[99] The new assay differs from its predecessors by beginning with a purification step that separates T lymphocytes from the remainder of the leukocytes by using anti-CD2-coated magnetic beads.[100] The T cells attached to the beads adhere to microtiter wells (because of the presence of magnets beneath the wells), and the nonadherent cells are readily aspirated. Wells containing the T cells are then reacted with either anti-CD4 or anti-CD8 monoclonal antibody conjugated with peroxidase. After a brief 20-minute incubation at room temperature, the wells are washed, and the substrate (3,3',5,5'-tetramethylbenzidine) is added to the wells. The reaction is stopped with sulfuric acid, and the absorbance is correlated with a calibration curve to determine the CD4 and CD8 lymphocyte count. In comparison with the standard flow cytometric technique, the Capcellia assay gives an impressive r^2 of 0.95 for CD4 lymphocytes and a somewhat less impressive 0.81 for CD8 lymphocytes.[100] The assay has an impressive sensitivity of 15 CD4 lymphocytes/microliter. For sites where flow cytometry is not used for other functions, such as leukemia/lymphoma immunophenotyping, this assay may prove to be a workable alternative.

None of the alternative methods has replaced the diversity of flow cytometry for evaluating patients infected with HIV. However, at the writing of the previous edition of this book, the same was true for reticulocyte analysis, which is now typically performed by using routine hematology analyzers. It would be prudent to keep a close watch as these methods evolve.

References

1. Gottlieb MS, Schroff R, Schanker HM, et al. *Pneumocystis carinii* pneumonia and mucosal candidiasis in previously healthy homosexual men: evidence of a new acquired cellular immunodeficiency. *N Engl J Med.* 1981;305:1425-1431.

2. Masur H, Michelis MA, Greene JB, et al. An outbreak of community-acquired *Pneumocystis carinii* pneumonia: initial manifestation of cellular immune dysfunction. *N Engl J Med.* 1981;305:1431-1438.

3. UNAIDS. Report on the Global HIV/AIDS Epidemic. 1998.

4. Greene WC. The molecular biology of human immunodeficiency virus type 1 infection. *N Engl J Med.* 1991;324:308-317.

5. Hsiung GD. Perspectives on retroviruses and the etiologic agent of AIDS. *Yale J Biol Med.* 1987;60:505-514.

6. Fauci AS. The human immunodeficiency virus: infectivity and mechanisms of pathogenesis. *Science.* 1988;239:617-622.

7. Smith RD. The pathobiology of HIV infection. A review. *Arch Pathol Lab Med.* 1990;114:235-239.

8. Centers for Disease Control and Prevention. *HIV/AIDS surveillance report 1997.* Atlanta, Ga: Centers for Disease Control and Prevention; 1997: 1-44.

9. Centers for Disease Control and Prevention. Update: trends in AIDS incidence, deaths, and prevalence—United States, 1996. *MMWR Morb Mortal Wkly Rep.* 1997;76:156-173.

10. Dobkin JF. U.S. AIDS: the minority becomes the majority. *Infect Med.* 1995;12:18.

11. Kahn JO, Walker BD. Acute human immunodeficiency virus type 1 infection. *N Engl J Med.* 1998;339:33-39.

12. Spira AI, Marx PA, Patterson BK, et al. Cellular targets of infection and route of viral dissemination after an intravaginal inoculation of simian immunodeficiency virus into rhesus macaques. *J Exp Med.* 1996;183:215-225.

13. O'Brien TR, Goedert JJ. Chemokine receptors and genetic variability. Another leap in HIV research [editorial]. *JAMA.* 1998;279:317-318.

14. Dragic T, Litwin V, Allaway GP, et al. HIV-1 entry into CD4+ cells is mediated by the chemokine receptor CC-CKR5. *Nature.* 1996;381:667-673.

15. Samson M, Libert F, Doranz BJ, et al. Resistance to HIV-1 infection in Caucasian individuals bearing mutant alleles of the CCR5 chemokine receptor gene. *Nature.* 1996;382:722-725.

16. Biti R, French R, Young J, et al. HIV-1 infection in an individual homozygous for the CCR5 deletion allele. *Nat Med.* 1997;3:252-253.

17. Balotta C, Bagnarelli P, Violin M, et al. Homozygous delta 32 deletion of the CCR5 chemokine receptor gene in an HIV-1 infected patient. *AIDS.* 1997;11:F67-F71.

18. Schneider T, Ullrich R, Zeitz M. Immunopathology of human immunodeficiency virus infection in the gastrointestinal tract. *Springer Semin Immunopathol.* 1997;18:515-533.

19. Price RW, Brew B, Sidtis J, et al. The brain in AIDS: central nervous system HIV-1 infection and AIDS dementia complex. *Science.* 1988;239:586-592.

20. Johnson RT, McArthur JC, Narayan O. The neurobiology of human immunodeficiency virus infections. *FASEB J.* 1988;2:2970-2981.

21. Mellors JW, Rinaldo CR Jr, Gupta P, et al. Prognosis in HIV-1 infection predicted by the quantity of virus in plasma. *Science.* 1996;272:1167-1170.

22. Shepard RN, Schock J, Robertson K, et al. Quantitation of human immunodeficiency virus type 1 RNA in different biological compartments. *J Clin Micro.* 2000;38:1414-1418.

23. Centers for Disease Control and Prevention. Report of the NIH panel to define principles of therapy of HIV infection and guidelines for the use of antiretroviral agents in HIV-infected adults and adolescents. *MMWR Morb Mortal Wkly Rep.* 1998;47(No.RR-5):1-82.

24. Lefrere J, Roudot-Thoraval F, Mariotti M, et al. The risk of disease progression is determined during the first year of human immunodeficiency virus type 1 infection. *J Infect Dis.* 1998;177:1541-1548.

25. Giorgi JV, Detels R. T-cell subset alterations in HIV-infected homosexual men: NAID Multicenter AIDS Cohort Study. *Clin Immunol Immunopathol.* 1989;52:10-18.

26. Wei X, Ghosh SK, Taylor ME, et al. Viral dynamics in human immunodeficiency virus type 1 infection. *Nature.* 1995;373:117-122.

27. Schwartz O, Marechal V, Legall S, et al. Endocytosis of major histocompatibility complex class I molecules is induced by the HIV-1 Nef protein. *Nat Med.* 1996;2:338-342.

28. Marodon G, Landau NR, Posnett DN. Altered expression of CD4, CD54, CD62L, and CCR5 in primary lymphocytes productively infected with the human immunodeficiency virus. *AIDS Res Hum Retroviruses.* 1999;15:161-171.

29. Stein DS, Korvick JA, Vermund SH. CD4+ lymphocyte cell enumeration for prediction of clinical course of human immunodeficiency virus disease: a review. *J Infect Dis.* 1992;165:352-363.

30. Palumbo PE, Raskino C, Fiscus S, et al. Predictive value of quantitative plasma HIV RNA and CD4+ lymphocyte count in HIV-infected infants and children. *JAMA.* 1998;279:756-761.

31. Vlahov D, Graham N, Hoover D, et al. Prognostic indicators for AIDS infectious disease death in HIV-infected injection drug users. Plasma viral load and CD4+ cell count. *JAMA.* 1998;279:35-40.

32. Greenough TC, Sullivan JL, Desrosiers RC. Declining CD4 T-cell counts in a person infected with nef-deleted HIV-1. *N Engl J Med.* 1999;340:236-237.

33. Keet IPM, Janssen M, Veugelers PJ, et al. Longitudinal analysis of CD4 T cell counts, T cell reactivity and human immunodeficiency virus type 1 RNA levels in persons remaining AIDS-free despite CD4 cell counts < 200 for > 5 years. *J Infect Dis.* 1997;176:665-671.

34. Palella FJ Jr, Delaney KM, Moorman AC, et al. Declining morbidity and mortality among patients with advanced human immunodeficiency virus infection. *N Engl J Med.* 1998;338:853-860.

35. Temesgen Z, Wright AJ. Recent advances in the management of human immuno-deficiency virus infection. *Mayo Clin Proc.* 1997;72:854-859.

36. Detels R, Munoz A, McFarlane G, et al. Effectiveness of potent antiretroviral therapy on time to AIDS and death in men with known HIV infection duration. *JAMA.* 1998;280:1497-1503.

37. Centers for Disease Control and Prevention, National Center for Health Statistics. *National vital statistics report.* Vol. 47. Atlanta, Ga: Centers for Disease Control and Prevention; 1997.

38. Burman WJ, Reves RR, Cohen DL. The case for conservative management of early HIV disease. *JAMA.* 1998;280:93-95.

39. Walker BD, Basgov N. Treat HIV-1 infection like other infections—treat it. *JAMA.* 1998;280:91-93.

40. Volberding PA, Deeks SG. Antiretroviral therapy for HIV infection. Promises and problems. *JAMA.* 1998;279:1343-1344.

41. Bozzette SA, Berry SH, Duan N, et al. The care of HIV-infected adults in the United States. *N Engl J Med.* 1998;339:1897-1904.

42. Hirschel B, Francioli P. Progress and problems in the fight against AIDS. *N Engl J Med.* 1998;338:906-908.

43. Wainberg MA. Global perspective from International AIDS Society President Mark Wainberg [interview]. *JAMA.* 1998;280:1811-1813.

44. Tsoukas CM, Raboud J, Bernard NF, et al. Active immunization of patients with HIV infection: a study of the effect of VaxSyn, a recombinant HIV envelope subunit vaccine, on progression of immunodeficiency. *AIDS Res Hum Retroviruses.* 1998;14:483-490.

45. Fischl MA, Richman DD, Grieco MH, et al. The efficacy of Azidothymidine (AZT) in the treatment of patients with AIDS and AIDS-related complex. A double-blind, placebo-controlled trial. *N Engl J Med.* 1987;317:185-191.

46. Volberding PA, Lagakos SW, Koch MA, et al. Zidovudine in asymptomatic human immunodeficiency virus infection. A controlled trial in persons with fewer than 500 CD4-positive cells per cubic millimeter. *N Engl J Med.* 1990;322:941-949.

47. Ndaler JP, Oehler RL, Holt D. Update of antiretroviral therapy for HIV infection. *Infect Med.* 1998;15:113-116.

48. Havlir DV, Marschner IC, Hirsch MS, et al. Maintenance antiretroviral therapies in HIV-infected subjects with undetectable plasma HIV RNA after triple-drug therapy. *N Engl J Med.* 1998;339:1261-1268.

49. Temesgen Z, Wright AJ. Recent advances in the management of human immunodeficiency virus infection. *Mayo Clin Proc.* 1997;72:854-859.

50. Brodine SK, Mascola JR, McCutchan FE. Genotypic variation and molecular epidemiology of HIV. *Infect Med.* 1997;14:739-748.

51. Carpenter CCJ, Fischi MA, Hammer SM, et al. Antiretroviral therapy for HIV infection in 1998. Updated recommendations of the international AIDS society—USA panel. *JAMA.* 1998;280:78-86.

52. Hirsch MS, Brun-Vezinet F, D'Aquila RT, et al. Antiretroviral drug resistance testing in adult HIV-1 infection. Recommendations of an international AIDS society—USA Panel. *JAMA* 2000;283:2417-2426.

53. Chang SW, Katz MH, Hernandez SR. The new AIDS case definition. Implications for San Francisco. *JAMA*. 1992;267:973-975.

54. Giorgi JV, Nishanian JPG, Schmid I, et al. Selective alterations in immunoregulatory lymphocyte subsets in early HIV (human T-lymphotropic virus type III/lymphadenopathy-associated virus) infection. *J Clin Immunol*. 1987;7:140-150.

55. Phillips AN, Lee CA, Elford J, et al. Serial CD4 lymphocyte counts and development of AIDS. *Lancet*. 1991;337:389-392.

56. Eyster ME, Ballard JO, Gail MH, et al. Predictive markers for the acquired immunodeficiency syndrome (AIDS) in hemophiliacs: persistence of p24 antigen and low T4 cell count. *Ann Intern Med*. 1989;110:963-969.

57. Yarchoan R, Venzon DJ, Pluda JM, et al. CD4 count and the risk for death in patients infected with HIV receiving antiretroviral therapy. *Ann Intern Med*. 1991;115:184-189.

58. Sheppard H, Lang W, Ascher MS, et al. The characterization of non-progressors: long-term HIV-1 infection with stable CD4+ T-cell levels. *AIDS*. 1993;7:1159-1166.

59. Hofmann B, Wang Y, Cumberland WG, et al. Serum beta2-microglobulin level increases in HIV infection: relation to seroconversion, CD4 T-cell fall and prognosis. *AIDS*. 1990;4:207-214.

60. Mofenson LM, Harris DR, Rich K, et al. Serum HIV-1 p24 antibody, HIV-1 RNA copy number and CD4 lymphocyte percentage are independently associated with risk of mortality in HIV-1-infected children. *AIDS*. 1999;13:31-39.

61. Centers for Disease Control and Prevention. Guidelines for PCP prophylaxis. *MMWR Morb Mortal Wkly Rep*. 1989;38(Suppl S-5):1-9.

62. Fischl MA, Dickinson GM, La Voie L. Safety and efficacy of sulfamethoxazole and trimethoprim chemoprophylaxis for *Pneumocystis carinii* pneumonia in AIDS. *JAMA*. 1988;259:1185-1189.

63. Hughes WT, Rivera GK, Schell MJ, et al. Successful intermittent chemoprophylaxis for *Pneumocystis carinii* pneumonitis. *N Engl J Med*. 1987;316:1627-1632.

64. Furrer H, Egger M, Opravil M, et al. Discontinuation of primary prophylaxis against *Pnemocystis carinii* pneumonia in HIV-1-infected adults treated with combination antiretroviral therapy. *N Engl J Med*. 1999;340:1301-1306.

65. Leibovitz E, Rigaud M, Pollack H, et al. *Pneumocystis carinii* pneumonia in infants infected with the human immunodeficiency virus with more than 450 CD4 lymphocytes per cubic millimeter. *N Engl J Med*. 1990;323:531-533.

66. Betensky RA, Calvelli T, Pahwa S. Predictive value of CD19 measurements for bacterial infections in children infected with human immunodeficiency virus. *Clin Diagn Immunol*. 1999;6:247-253.

67. Kovacs A, Frederick T, Church J, et al. CD4 T-lymphocyte counts and *Pneumocystis carinii* pneumonia in pediatric HIV infection. *JAMA*. 1991;265:1698-1703.

68. Denny TN, Niyen P, Skuza C, et al. Age related changes of lymphocyte phenotypes in healthy children [abstract]. *Pediatr Res*. 1990;27:155A.

69. Yanase Y, Tango T, Okumura K, et al. Lymphocyte subsets identified by monoclonal antibodies in healthy children. *Pediatr Res*. 1986;20:1147-1151.

70. Centers for Disease Control and Prevention. Guidelines for PCP prophylaxis. *MMWR Morb Mortal Wkly Rep*. 1991;40(no. RR-2):1-13.

71. Malone JL, Simms TE, Gray CG, et al. Sources of variability in repeated T-helper lymphocyte counts from human immunodeficiency virus type 1-infected patients: total lymphocyte count fluctuations and diurnal cycle are important. *J Acquir Immun Defic Syndr.* 1990;3:144-151.

72. Taylor JMG, Fahey JL, Detels R, et al. CD4 percentage, CD4 number, and CD4:CD8 ratio in HIV infection: which to choose and how to use. *J Acquir Immun Defic Syndr.* 1989;2:114-124.

73. Stites DP, Casavant CH, McHugh TM, et al. Flow cytometric analysis of lymphocyte phenotypes in AIDS using monoclonal antibodies and simultaneous dual immunofluorescence. *Clin Immunol Immunopathol.* 1986;38:161-177.

74. Clement LT, Dagg MK, Landay A. Characterization of human lymphocyte subpopulations: alloreactive cytotoxic T-lymphocyte precursor and effector cells are phenotypically distinct from Leu2+ suppressor cells. *J Clin Immunol.* 1984;4:395-402.

75. Formenti SC, Turner RR, de Martini RM, et al. Immunophenotypic analysis of peripheral blood leukocytes at different stages of HIV infection. An analysis of asymptomatic, ARC, and AIDS populations. *Am J Clin Pathol.* 1989;92:300-307.

76. Musey L, Hughes J, Schacker T, et al. Cytotoxic T-cell responses, viral load, and disease progression in early human immunodeficiency virus type 1 infection. *N Engl J Med.* 1997;337:1267-1274.

77. Bouscarat F, Levacher-Clergeot M, Dazza M, et al. Correlation of CD8 lymphocyte activation with cellular viremia and plasma HIV RNA levels in asymptomatic patients infected by human immunodeficiency virus type 1. *AIDS Res Hum Retroviruses.* 1996;12:17-24.

78. Landay A, Ohlsson-Wilhelm B, Giorgi JV. Application of flow cytometry to the study of HIV infection. *AIDS.* 1990;4:479-497.

79. Muirhead KA, Wallace PK, Schmitt TC, et al. Methodological considerations for implementation of lymphocyte subset analysis in a clinical reference laboratory. *Ann NY Acad Sci.* 1986;468:113-127.

80. Shield CF III, Marlett P, Smith A, et al. Stability of human lymphocyte differentiation antigens when stored at room temperature. *J Immunol Methods.* 1983;62:347-352.

81. Ritchie AWS, Oswald I, Micklem HS, et al. Circadian variation of lymphocyte subpopulations: a study with monoclonal antibodies. *BMJ.* 1983;286:1773-1775.

82. Dzik WH, Neckers L. Lymphocyte subpopulations altered during blood storage. *N Engl J Med.* 1983;309:435-436.

83. Weiblen BJ, Debell K, Valeri CR. "Acquired immunodeficiency" of blood stored overnight. *N Engl J Med.* 1983;309:793.

84. Paxton H, Bendele T. Effect of time, temperature, and anticoagulant on flow cytometry and hematological values. *Ann NY Acad Sci.* 1993;677:440-443.

85. Centers for Disease Control and Prevention. 1997 Revised guidelines for performing CD4+ T-cell determinations in persons infected with human immunodeficiency virus (HIV). *MMWR Morb Mortal Wkly Rep.* 1997;46 (No. RR-2):1-29.

86. Sherman GG, Galpin JS, Patel JM, et al. CD4+ T cell enumeration in HIV infection with limited resources. *J Immunol Methods.* 1999;222:209-217.

87. Loken MR, Brosnan JM, Ault K. Establishing optimal lymphocyte gates for immunophenotyping by flow cytometry. *Cytometry*. 1990;11:453-459.

88. Schenker EL, Hultin LE, Bauer KD, et al. Evaluation of a dual color flow cytometry immunophenotyping panel in a multicenter quality assurance program. *Cytometry*. 1993;14:307-317.

89. Gebel HM, Anderson JE, Gottschalk LR, et al. Determination of helper-suppressor T-cell ratios. *N Engl J Med*. 1987;316:113.

90. Quintanilla-Martinez L, Preffer F, Rubin D, et al. CD20+ T-cell lymphoma: neoplastic transformation of a normal T-cell subset. *Am J Clin Pathol*. 1994;102:483-489.

91. Hoover DR, Graham NMH, Chen B, et al. Effect of CD4+ cell count measurement variability on staging HIV-1 infection. *J Acquir Immune Defic Syndr*. 1992;5:794-802.

92. Nicholson, JK, Hubbard M, Jones BM. Use of CD45 fluorescence and side-scatter characteristics for gating lymphocytes when using the whole blood lysis procedure and flow cytometry. *Cytometry*. 1996;26:16-21.

93. Schnizlein-Bick CT, Spritzler J, Wilkening CL, et al. Evaluation of TruCount absolute-count tubes for determining CD4 and CD8 cell numbers in human immunodeficiency virus-positive adults. *Clin Diag Lab Immunol*. 2000;7:336-343.

94. Reimann KA, O'Gorman MRG, Sprtzler J, et al. Multisite comparison of CD4 and CD8 T-lymphocyte counting by single- versus multiple-platform methodologies: evaluation of Beckman Coulter Flow-Count Fluorospheres and the tetraONE system. *Clin Diag Lab Immunol*. 2000;7:344-351.

95. Hudson JC, Brunhouse RF, Garrison C, et al. Lymphocyte subset determination using a hematology analyzer. *Cytometry*. 1995;22:150-153.

96. Denny TN, Jensen BD, Louzao AG, et al. Evaluation of the Zymmune TM CD4/CD8 immunoassay method for measuring absolute CD4+ and CD8+ lymphocyte levels: results in adults and pediatric specimens [abstract]. *Natl Conf Hum Retroviruses Relat Infect*. 1995;124:12.

97. Denny T, Jensen B, Garcia A, et al. CD4+/CD8+ subset immunoassay in HIV+ adults and children [abstract]. *Int Conf AIDS*. 114;10:161.

98. Saah AJ, Spruill C, Hoover DR, et al. Helper T-lymphocyte count. TRAx CD4 test kit versus conventional flow cytometry. *Arch Pathol Lab Med*. 1997;121:960-962.

99. Carriere D, Fontaine C, Berthier AM, et al. Two-site enzyme immunoassay of CD4 and CD8 molecules on the surface of T lymphocytes from healthy subjects and HIV-1 infected patients. *Clin Chem*. 1994;40:30-37.

100. Carriere D, Vendrell JP, Fontaine C, et al. Whole blood Capcellia CD4CD8 immunoassay for enumeration of CD4+ and CD8+ peripheral T lymphocytes. *Clin Chem*. 1999;45:92-97.

13

Clinical Utility of Flow Cytometry in Allogeneic Transplantation

Robert A. Bray
Howard M. Gebel

Introduction

The application of flow cytometric techniques to assess multiple parameters related to the care of transplant recipients has witnessed enormous growth during the past decade. Currently, flow cytometry is one of the most valuable clinical tools available to transplant professionals. Of the numerous flow-based assays available for the care, management, and analysis of patients receiving transplants, the foremost application in organ transplantation is the flow cytometric detection of alloantibodies. The major advantage of flow cytometry in this application is its ability to detect circulating alloantibodies at levels too low to be detected by other, less sensitive methods. Because even low levels of pretransplant antibodies can significantly affect the incidence of early rejection episodes, as well as overall graft survival, antibody detection with flow cytometry is now a critical component in donor-recipient selection for kidney, kidney-pancreas, and heart allografts at numerous transplant centers.

Our initial discussions will outline the historical perspective of antibody detection in transplantation and then move to more current applications of flow cytometry in transplantation. In so doing, we will discuss the clinical rationale for antibody detection and touch on some of the critical technical aspects of this methodology. It is hoped that the reader will gain an appreciation for the clinical relevance of flow cytometric antibody detection in transplantation and an understanding of how this methodology can best be applied and interpreted.

Historical Perspective

A negative crossmatch result between donor lymphocytes and recipient serum has long been recognized as the single best predictor of short-term graft function. In its initial configuration, the crossmatch assay was a leukoagglutination test. This assay was neither particularly sensitive nor reproducible and soon gave way to a complement-dependent cytotoxicity (CDC) assay. This assay made use of lymphocytes obtained from a potential donor that were mixed with serum from the putative recipient. After an initial incubation, a source of complement was added, usually rabbit serum, and cell death was determined. The scoring was entirely visual and relied on the trained eye of the technologist to discern cell death. Cell death was assessed by the uptake of a vital dye (eg, trypan blue, eosin, or ethidium bromide). Clinically, the cytotoxic crossmatch was the gold standard for organ allocation.

In an elegant study by Patel and Terasaki[1] in 1969, a retrospective analysis of renal allograft recipients revealed that kidneys were nonfunctional within 48 hours after transplantation in 80% of recipients with detectable antidonor lymphocyte antibodies. In contrast, less than 5% of patients with undetectable antidonor antibodies exhibited such so-called hyperacute rejection. From that moment, pretransplant crossmatch assays became mandatory.

Nonetheless, in that study there were patients who experienced graft loss but whose crossmatch results were negative. Although cytotoxic crossmatching did reduce the incidence of hyperacute rejection, accelerated (antibody-mediated) graft loss still occurred among some recipients, even though the donor crossmatch was negative. To reduce the risk of this type of rejection, a more sensitive crossmatch technique using antihuman globulin (AHG) was developed.[2] AHG crossmatching significantly improved graft survival[3] not only by detecting low levels of antibody but also by detecting antibodies that apparently did not or could not fix complement. These noncomplement-fixing antibodies were termed *cytotoxicity negative-adsorption positive (CYNAP)*.[4] As a result of the advances in cytotoxicity crossmatching, hyperacute rejection has been virtually eliminated, and episodes of accelerated rejection have been significantly reduced among donor-recipient pairs with negative AHG-CDC crossmatch results.

However, certain patients (eg, multiparous women, multitransfused patients, and patients awaiting a second transplant) still experienced episodes of accelerated vascular rejection and/or early graft loss, presumably attributable to low-level alloantibodies. These observations led to the development of the flow cytometric crossmatch (FCXM). Garovoy et al[5] began categorizing patients into defined risk groups on the basis of their FCXM results. Subsequent studies demonstrated that accelerated rejection occurred among patients whose pre-transplant anti-HLA antibodies were undetectable with the standard CDC assay but were detected using flow cytometry. Numerous studies have since documented that patients who underwent transplantation based on a flow cytometry-negative crossmatch enjoyed better graft survival than those who underwent transplantation based on cytotoxicity crossmatching alone.[6-16] This fact is particularly true for high-risk patients.[15-16] Therefore, for many centers, flow cytometry crossmatching has become the gold standard of practice.

Flow Cytometry Crossmatching

Since its initial description,[5] many investigators have reported that the FCXM detects alloantibodies that correlate with poor graft outcome, particularly in high-risk patients, such as those who are highly sensitized or who have received a previous allograft.[6-17] Among such patients, at least in certain centers, a negative cytotoxicity crossmatch result with a positive FCXM result is a contraindication to transplantation. Initially developed as a single-color immunofluorescence assay, the FCXM has undergone numerous reconfigurations.[18-20] Currently, the most common FCXM design involves a multicolor format (**Figure 13-1**). This multiparameter approach permits simultaneous detection of major histocompatibility complex (MHC) alloantibodies binding to T cells (anti-class I) and/or B cells (anti-class I and/or class II).

From a methodological standpoint, the FCXM is rather straightforward. However, there are some distinct methodological aspects that must be addressed. The preferred method is outlined in **Figure 13-2.** First, the selection of the *reporter* antibody is of critical importance. In the flow crossmatch, immunoglobulin G (IgG) anti-HLA antibody is the immunoglobulin class that is of clinical importance in transplantation. Therefore, the use of a specific anti-IgG is critical. This reagent should be titered and should not cross-react with immunoglobulins from other species, specifically mouse, horse, or rabbit.

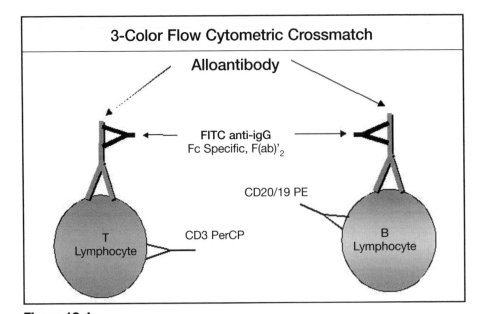

Figure 13-1

Three-color flow cytometric crossmatch assay. Anti-HLA antibody (alloantibody) binding to T cells and B cells is detected using a 3-color method. Fluorescein-conjugated goat anti-human IgG is used as the reporter to detect the binding of alloantibody. Simultaneously, a phycoerythrin-conjugated anti-CD20 or CD19 and a peridinin-chlorophyll-protein (PerCP)-conjugated anti-CD3 monoclonal antibody are added. Analysis is performed by acquiring lymphocyte-gated events and backgating on either CD3 (T cells) or CD20 (B cells) and assessing the level of fluorescence of the reporter anti-IgG.

Mouse, horse, and rabbit immunoglobulins are the basis for several anti-rejection therapies (eg, OKT3 and anti-lymphocyte globulin) and can interfere with the detection of alloantibodies. Next, the actual staining procedure also presents a few areas of concern. Of equal importance are the concentration of cells used and the quantity of serum tested. Because the ultimate sensitivity of this assay is dependent on these 2 parameters, great care should be taken to ensure that both serum volume and cell concentrations are constant. In opposition to classical immunophenotyping, where the primary antibody is always in excess, the primary antibody (ie, the patient's serum) used in the FCXM may contain limited quantities of alloantibody. Hence, the approach in the FCXM is to optimize for low levels of antibody. As shown in **Figure 13-3,** the actual serum/cell ratio is significantly different from that of classic cytotoxicity. In effect, the FCXM is being performed at an equivalent dilution of 1:4 or greater. However, the FCXM is still more sensitive than standard or antiglobulin-enhanced cytotoxicity. Lastly, the actual analysis of the data is important. It is recommended that multiple gate sets be used to ensure analysis of the correct cell type. An example of a suggested gating strategy is shown in **Figure 13-4.**

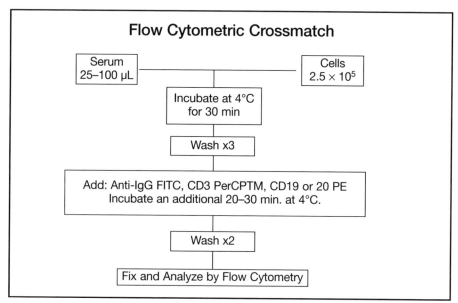

Figure 13-2
Diagram depicting the method for performing the flow cytometric crossmatch assay.

Serum/Cell Ratios		
Method	Volume of Serum	# of Cells
Cytotoxicity	1μL	2,000 cells
Flow Cytometry Equivalent	10 μL 100 μL	20,000 cells 200,000 cells
Flow Cytometry Actual	25–50 μL	2.5×10^5–1×10^6 cells

Result = 1:4 or greater dilution equivalent

Figure 13-3
Although shown to be more sensitive than the cytotoxicity assay, the flow cytometric crossmatch assay actually uses a serum/cell ratio that is less than that for the cytotoxicity assay. Care should be taken to ensure that this aspect of the test is well controlled within the laboratory. That is, all technologists should follow a standard protocol and perform accurate cell counts.

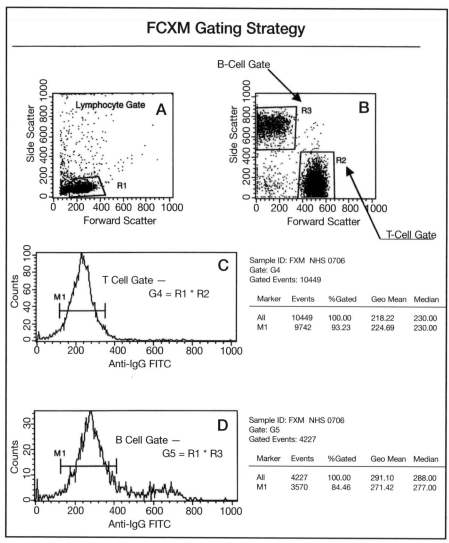

Figure 13-4
The gating algorithm used to set up the flow cytometric crossmatch. This gating structure is required to ensure that one analyzes only T cells and/or B cells. Note that gates G4 and G5 are logical gates.

Interpretation of the FCXM is the most complicated and subjective aspect of this method. In order for the crossmatch result to be considered positive, the fluorescence intensity of the test serum must significantly exceed that of the negative control. The 2 important aspects of the previous statement are "significantly exceed" and "negative control." Both of these issues are intimately related. Significance is usually assessed as an increase in fluorescence that is at least 3 standard deviations (SDs) above the mean of the negative control. The assumption is that the negative control will always approximate the background fluorescence of the patient's serum. The problem with this assumption is that it assumes that background fluorescence is constant. This is not always the case. What then would be the best negative control? By definition, the best negative control would be the patient's own serum, with only anti-HLA antibody, if present, removed. Currently, this is neither possible nor practical. Therefore, laboratories use a well-characterized pool or single-donor control serum that approximates average background fluorescence. Because using a negative control serum with too high or too low background fluorescence can result in false-negative or false-positive results, respectively, extreme care must be taken in the selection of this control serum. Optimally, this serum should be devoid of anti-HLA antibody and should exhibit a consistent and reproducible reactivity with a variety of different cell types. This aspect of the flow crossmatch is arguably the most important and the one that laboratories must devote significant effort to in order to provide appropriate testing results.

Once an appropriate negative control serum is obtained and validated, it is time to determine what will be considered a positive result. There are 2 basic approaches for determining a positive value. One approach is based on comparing the fluorescence value of the test serum with the value of the negative control and using statistics to determine whether there is a significant difference between the two. The second approach establishes a fluorescence cutoff point based exclusively on patient outcome data. In this approach, a laboratory would assess transplant outcome and then compare patient and graft survival with the observed changes in fluorescence between the test and control sera. The laboratory would then determine what would be considered a positive value in terms of clinically relevant outcomes.[21] The clinical outcome is of importance when determining a cutoff point because the type of patient transplanted (high-risk vs low-risk), as well as the immunosuppressive regimen used at a particular center are interrelated and can affect outcome. Therefore, each center should determine its own cutoff values. In practice, although most laboratories choose to the former approach for determining a positive value, laboratories should always correlate the results of any laboratory test with the clinical outcome. For the sake of discussion, we will address only the statistical measurement of fluorescence and the determination of a mathematically positive result.

For the statistical evaluation of the crossmatch assay, there are at least 3 acceptable ways to determine a statistically positive result: (1) channel displacement, (2) linear ratio, and (3) semiquantitative fluorescence measurements with molecules of equivalent soluble fluorochrome (MESFs). Representative examples are shown in **Figure 13-5.** The statistical approach that is taken is

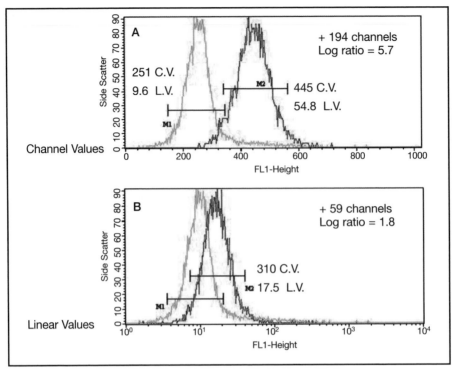

Figure 13-5
This figure illustrates how the flow cytometric crossmatch is calculated. Histograms **A** and **B** illustrate a comparison between a test sample (dark tracing) and the negative control (light tracing). Histogram **A** illustrates a strong positive reaction and histogram **B** illustrates a weak reaction. For both examples, the channel values (C.V.) and linear values (L.V.) are shown. For both examples, the channel displacement and the fluorescence ratio are calculated and shown.

entirely up to the individual laboratory and dependent on the desired end result. The 2 main applications of flow cytometric crossmatching are to generate a result that can be reported as positive or negative and to assess changes in antibody levels during therapy for rejection. For determining a positive or negative result, any of the 3 approaches are satisfactory. However, linear ratio and MESFs do provide a more quantitative assessment of antibody levels. It is critical, however, not to interchange these methods. For example, with channel displacement, the negative channel value is subtracted from the positive result to produce a *channel shift* or *displacement*. For linear values, the linear value of the positive result is divided by the value for the negative result to produce a fluorescence ratio. This ratio indicates the fold increase in fluorescence over background. Therefore it would not be correct to subtract linear values nor would it be appropriate

Table 13-1

Associations Offering Proficiency Testing Programs and/or Accreditation in Flow Cytometry Crossmatching

Agency	Proficiency Testing Program	Accreditation
ASHI[*]	Yes	Yes
CAP[†]	Yes	Yes[††]
SEOPF[‡]	Yes	Yes[**]

[*]ASHI = The American Society for Histocompatibility and Immunogentics, Lenexa, KS, 66285; (913) 541-0009.
[†]CAP = College of American Pathologists, 325 Waukegan Rd., Northfield, IL 60093; (800) 323-4040
[‡]SEOPF = The Southeastern Organ Procurement Foundation, Richmond, VA, 23235; (804) 323-9890.
[¶]Joint PT program between ASHI and CAP.
[**]Offers accreditation in flow cytometry but not crossmatching.
[††]Uses ASHI accreditation for credentialing.

to calculate a ratio of channel values. The third approach, with MESFs, actually calibrates the instrument by converting channel values to a fluorescence measurement on the basis of a set of fluorescence standards. To determine a positive result, one merely determines the number of fluorescence molecules over background that constitutes a statistically significant difference.

For some applications, it may be useful to assess in a semi-quantitative manner whether antibody levels are declining, increasing, or remaining stable. In situations in which a patient is experiencing a humoral (antibody-mediated) rejection episode and the antirejection therapy is directed toward reducing antibody levels, either linear values or MESFs are preferred approaches for exacting a quantitative assessment of antibody levels. For any of the above instances, it is incumbent on the laboratory personnel to maintain proper quality control of all reagents. At present, no commercial kits are available to support flow cytometric crossmatching, although all of the necessary reagents are commercially available.

Over the past decade, flow cytometry has been shown to be the most sensitive method for detecting alloantibodies and has emerged as an invaluable tool in the assessment of potential solid organ allograft recipients. Because low levels of antibody may significantly affect overall graft survival, it is not surprising that a prospective FCXM is now recognized as a key laboratory procedure in the selection of allograft recipients. Except for zero-antigen mismatched renal allografts, a negative crossmatch result between donor cells and recipient serum is the principal criterion for solid organ allocation. For this reason, it is imperative that laboratories performing flow cytometric crossmatching adopt standardized methods and participate in appropriate quality control and proficiency testing programs. At present, several organizations provide standards and/or proficiency testing programs for the flow cytometric crossmatch (**Table 13-1**).

Panel-reactive Antibody Analysis

The success of the FCXM in improving graft survival has led to a dilemma. The observation that cytotoxicity-negative/FCXM-positive crossmatch results are associated with decreased early graft survival created the desire to identify such at-risk patients before a final crossmatch. As a standard practice, HLA laboratories perform routine (monthly) assessments of antibody levels (antibody screening) in patients awaiting solid organ transplantation. From the results of these ongoing assessments, clinicians and surgeons have a measure of a patient's probability for obtaining a crossmatch-negative organ. Until recently, the routine screening of patient sera for anti-HLA antibodies used a panel of 30 to 60 HLA-typed individuals as targets in a cytotoxicity assay. Referred to as panel-reactive antibody (PRA) analysis, this screening test has 2 useful applications. First, the percentage of PRA, representing the number of positive reactions in the panel, indicates the percentage of allograft donors likely to have a positive crossmatch result with a given patient's serum. Hence, an individual whose PRA value was 75% would be expected to have a positive crossmatch result with approximately 75% of all potential organ donors, whereas an individual with a PRA value of 0% would be expected to have a negative crossmatch result with all donors. Clearly, the higher the PRA, the greater the likelihood that a final crossmatch result will be positive with any given donor. In fact, among patients whose PRA levels are 100%, a negative crossmatch result would be rare, except when the donor was HLA-identical to the recipient. Second, a detailed analysis of PRA reactivity can identify which HLA antigens are the targets of the alloantibody. This information can then be used prospectively to aid in the selection of the most appropriate donor-recipient combination. For example, a renal transplant recipient with a PRA value of 35% and specificity of anti-HLA-A1 would be excluded from crossmatching with any HLA-A1-positive donor. Because most organ donors are prospectively HLA-typed, information regarding the specificity of a patient's HLA antibody is very helpful in directing the organ to the most appropriate recipient. Hence, excluding such anti-A1 antibody-bearing individuals from consideration for transplant significantly aids organ allocation and reduces cold ischemia time.

Although the overall goal of PRA testing is to provide predictive crossmatch information for a given donor-recipient combination, the predictive value of this test is best achieved when (1) the HLA types of the donor and potential recipient are known, (2) *all* anti-HLA antibodies in a given recipient are identified, and (3) the PRA test and the final crossmatch assay are performed by methods with comparable sensitivity. However, the ability to detect one or more anti-HLA antibodies in a patient's serum is a function of the sensitivity of the test used. Presently, although nearly 50% of all HLA laboratories in North America use flow cytometry as their final crossmatch method, only a handful of these institutions use cytometry to perform routine screening of patient sera. Most laboratories perform PRA testing using a cytotoxic or enzyme-linked immunosorbent assay (ELISA)-based method. The sensitivity differences between flow cytometry and these other procedures can result in an underestimation of the alloantibody present in any given patient and an increased frequency of unanticipated positive final crossmatch results.[22-50] Selecting patients on the basis of a perceived lack of HLA antibody only to experience a positive final crossmatch result is costly both financially and psychologically. In many instances patients have endured a long wait for a transplant and/or traveled long distances to the transplant center and incurred significant hardships in making themselves available for transplantation. In an effort to reduce the occurrence of these types of events, prospective screening of transplant recipient sera with flow cytometry is recommended.

Flow Cytometric PRA

The flow cytometric PRA (FC-PRA) is not a new concept. The first report of an FC-PRA was made by Cicciarelli et al[23] in 1992. Moreover, it has long been proposed that crossmatching and antibody screening should be performed using methods with similar sensitivities.[24] The logistic problems involved in performing a FC-PRA are not trivial and have delayed its development as a routine test. Nevertheless, several groups have attempted to develop methods for routine antibody screening using cytometry.[25,26] The first attempt at this method used a single pool of 10 cells of known but differing HLA types.[23] This pool was tested for reactivity against only patient T cells. Although this method appeared to work, it had many drawbacks. First, specificity could not be assigned with a pool of cells. Second, a meaningful PRA value could not be attained because there were only 10 cells. Third, monospecific antibody reactivity was difficult to detect unless the antibody was of a high titer. The pool worked best when the antibody titer was high or the specificity was quite broad. Although a positive or negative result could be attained with this method, the level of sensitivity, although improved, did not match that of the flow cytometric crossmatch assay. This technique was subsequently modified.[25] Briefly, the modified test relied on a pool of 8 cells in which each individual cell was selected for its expression of a specific HLA cross-reactive group (CREG) antigen. Although individual specificities could not be discerned, the PRA values attained correlated somewhat with cytotoxic PRA values.

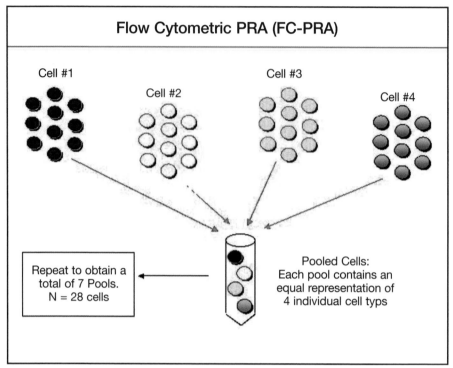

Figure 13-6

Schematic representation of how the cell-based flow cytometric panel-reactive antibody is constructed.

More recently, the authors have developed and implemented a method that incorporates aspects of both of the above methods.[27] Our method uses 7 pools of cells wherein each pool contains 4 cells (**Figure 13-6**). Each cell is selected on the basis of the CREG antigens they expressed,[4] and the pools are constructed to contain only members of a single A-locus or B-locus CREG (**Table 13-2**). Using this approach, a meaningful PRA can be obtained and antibody reactivity can be clustered into CREGs (frequently with unique private specificities identified). Furthermore, this method has the added potential of testing individual cells from a given pool to clearly identify distinct private HLA specificities. Hence this form of flow cytometric PRA screening not only can confirm the presence of an alloantibody but can also provide a meaningful PRA value and identify HLA specificities. A sample analysis is shown in **Figures 13-7** and **13-8** (p 520).

The authors' data with this FC-PRA method has shown a significant increase in sensitivity over the AHG-enhanced cytotoxicity assay (**Table 13-3**, p 521).[28,29] In this comparison we observed a correlation of 86% between AHG-PRA and our CREG FC-PRA. Only one sample had positive results for the AHG-PRA and

Table 13-2

Cell-based Flow Cytometric PRA Pools

POOL	Private HLA Antigens	CRGEs*
4	A2, A24; B13, B44	2C, 12C
	A2, A28; B44, B60	2C, 12C
	A68, A23; B44, B49	2C, 12C
	A2, A2; B45, B50	2C, 12C
5	A68, A69; B7, B7	2C, 7C
	A24, A24; B7, B56	2C, 7C
	A2, A28; B27, B49	2C, 7C
	A2, A28; B27, B60	2C 7C

*CREG = cross-reactive group.

Example of 2 of the FC-PRA pools. Pool 4 contains 4 cells that share A-locus A2 CREG antigens and B-locus B12 CREG antigens. Pool 5 contains 4 cells that share A-locus A2 CREG antigens and share B-locus antigens of the B7 CREG. Therefore, if a patient's serum reacted with both pools, the most likely specificity would be the A2 CREG. However, if a patient's serum reacted with either pool 4 or pool 5, one could assign the appropriate specificity.

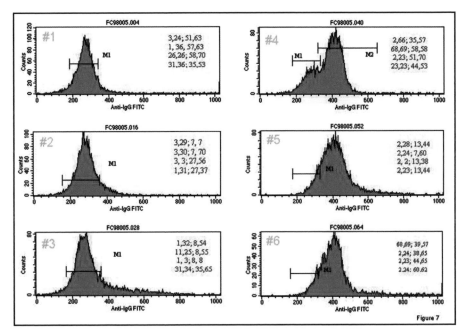

Figure 13-7

Representative example of the flow cytometric panel-reactive antibody analysis from a patient with an anti-A2, A28 antibody. The region labeled M1 indicates the boundaries of the negative control. The class I HLA types of each of the 4 cells contained within the pool is indicated in the top right corner of each histogram. As the data indicate, pools 1 to 3 are negative, and pools 4 to 6 are positive. Pools 4 to 6 contain A2 or A28 (A68, A69) antigens. The exception is pool 4, which has one apparently negative cell. The negative cell was shown to be cell 4, which is homozygous for A23 and does not possess A2 or A28 (A68, A69).

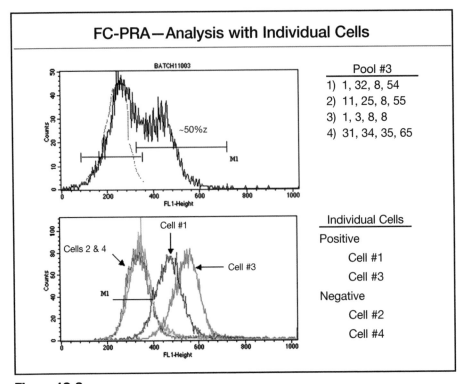

FC-PRA—Analysis with Individual Cells

BATCH11003

~50%z

M1

FL1-Height

Cell #1

Cells 2 & 4

Cell #3

M1

FL1-Height

Pool #3
1) 1, 32, 8, 54
2) 11, 25, 8, 55
3) 1, 3, 8, 8
4) 31, 34, 35, 65

Individual Cells
Positive
    Cell #1
    Cell #3
Negative
    Cell #2
    Cell #4

Figure 13-8

Example of cell-based flow cytometric panel-reactive antibody analysis. **A.** A representative pool and the associated channel displacements. In this example, approximately 50% of the total events are considered positive. Because there are only 4 cells per pool, the results reflect 2 positive cells and 2 negative cells. **B.** The combined results from staining of the 4 individual cells from the pool. Cells 1 and 3 are positive, and cells 2 and 4 are negative. From these data, it can be determined that the predominant HLA specificity is directed against HLA A1 (the common HLA antigen shared between cells 1 and 3).

negative results for the FC-PRA. This sample contained a true anti-HLA antibody of the IgM class. In contrast, 25 (15%) of 180 of the samples had positive results for the FC-PRA but negative results for the AHG-PRA. All the patients in this group had a history of sensitizing events (eg, pregnancies, multiple transfusions, or previous transplant). Thus, our FC-PRA is more sensitive in detecting IgG anti-HLA antibodies and more closely approximates the final flow cytometric crossmatch result.

Although this method can work quite well, it has several drawbacks. First, it requires viable cells. Second, a significant amount of technician time must be devoted to the preparation and maintenance of these pools. Third, significant quality control is required to validate the pools. Lastly, the method is somewhat expensive and time consuming to perform. STAT testing is not possible with

Table 13-3
Comparison Between AHG-CDC* and FC-PRA†

AHG-CDC	FC-PRA	N (%)
Negative	Negative	77 (43)
Positive	Negative	10 (5)
Negative	Positive	25 (15)
Positive	Positive	68 (38)

Comparison between antiglobulin-enhanced cytotoxicity PRA (AHG-PRA) and flow cytometric PRA (FC-PRA) using cell pools. The data illustrate that the AHG-PRA and the FC-PRA had an agreement of 81%. However, the FC-PRA identified 15% more positive reactions than the AHG-PRA. In addition, of the 68 samples where AHG and FC were in agreement, the average PRA value for the FC-PRA was approximately 35% to 40% greater. This indicates that the FC-PRA not only identified antibodies not detected in the AHG-PRA but can identify additional specificities even when the AHG-PRA result is positive. Of the 10 samples that were AHG-positive/FC-negative (5%), 9 samples were either not reproducible or contained IgM-autoreactive (ie, non-HLA) antibodies. Only one sample possessed a true IgM anti-HLA antibody.
*AHG-CDC = antiglobulin-enhanced, complement-mediated ,cytotoxicity assay.
†FC-PRA = flow cytometric panel-reactive antibody.

this method. Therefore, alternative technologies are required to move flow cytometric PRA testing into the routine clinical laboratory.

Microparticle Flow Cytometric PRA

Although they represent a significant improvement over cytotoxicity assays, cell-based flow PRAs are quite cumbersome and costly to perform. More importantly, however, serum reactivity with lymphocytes does not always guarantee that such antibodies are truly HLA-specific. Lymphocytes express a multitude of cell surface molecules in addition to MHC antigens. Additionally, patients awaiting transplantation may have an autoimmune disease, such as systemic lupus erythematosus, as the underlying cause of their renal failure. In such situations, these patients can have autoreactive antibodies either as a result of their disease or from treatments for their disease. Thus, as the sensitivity of cell-based assays increases, so too does the possibility for detecting non-HLA antibodies that would not be a contraindication for transplantation. Recently, however, several methods have been developed to help ascertain whether antilymphocyte reactivity (either T-cell or B-cell reactivity) is due to anti-HLA antibody. One approach is a more classical ELISA-based method that uses purified or captured HLA antigen. However, a newer and more promising approach makes use of flow cytometry and microparticle technology. This approach involves a solid-phase assay with microparticles coated exclusively with class I or class II MHC proteins. Although the sensitivity of this microparticle assay far exceeds that of cytotoxic assays, and it is slightly more sensitive than ELISA-based assays, a more important aspect of this method is that the specificity of any antibodies detected in this fashion is unequivocally anti-MHC.

Recently, descriptions of this new approach to routine flow cytometric PRAs have been published.[26,30] In addition to being more specific and sensitive, the microparticle assay uses small amounts of serum (25-100 microliters) and is quite rapid to perform. A bead-based flow PRA can be completed in less than 90 minutes. Hence this assay is truly a STAT flow PRA. The microparticle assay is quite simple to perform. In brief, the microparticles are incubated with the patient's serum, washed, and then stained with a fluoresceinated anti-IgG. Analysis is performed using flow cytometry. Two types of bead-based assays are available: FlowPRA I and II is a screening assay, and Flow Specific Beads (both from One Lambda, Inc, Canoga, CA) are used to identify HLA specificity. The FlowPRA I and II screening beads are designed as a quick screening tool. These beads can simultaneously detect the presence of class I and/or class II antibodies. The Flow Specific Beads are designed to identify the anti-HLA specificity. There are slight differences between these 2 assays. The screening beads are comprised of unstained beads that are coated with class I antigen and red-stained beads that are coated with class II antigens. The importance of this distinction is that the 2 beads can be run simultaneously to test for the presence of class I and/or class II antibody. A sample analysis is shown in **Figures 13-9** and **13-10.** Data from the authors' laboratories have shown a good correlation with cytotoxicity. More importantly, however, this solid-phase PRA assay is more sensitive than cytotoxicity assays and appears to approach cell-based cytometry for the detection of alloantibodies (**Figure 13-11**, p 525).

The microparticle flow cytometric PRA has many advantages, including reporting an appropriate PRA value, confirming specificity for HLA antigen, being simple to perform, and being capable of simultaneously determining class I and/or class II reactivity. The ability to detect class II antibody is of particular clinical importance. In the past it has been nearly impossible to detect class II antibody unless the patient possessed only high-titer class II antibody. For patients who possessed class I antibody, cumbersome absorptions with platelets were necessary to remove class I antibody before one could test for class II antibody. In our studies we have shown that among patients with a detectable class I antibody, an average of more than 80% also possess class II antibodies. From a clinical standpoint, the importance of class II antibodies has been somewhat controversial, although the consensus is that class II antibodies are detrimental in solid organ transplantation.[31-33]

Although microparticle flow cytometric PRA is simple to perform and (for the most part) to interpret, there are a few issues that require additional discus-

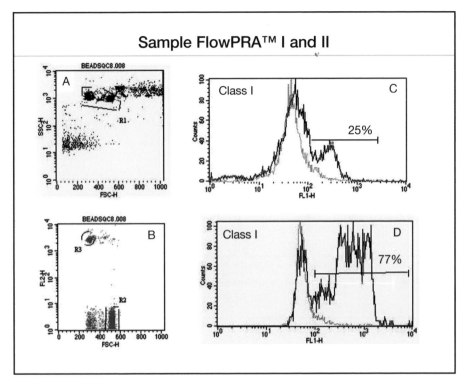

Figure 13-9

Example of the FlowPRA I and FlowPRA II. Beads containing either HLA class I or HLA class II can be run simultaneously to identify the presence of anti-HLA antibody. **A.** The forward scatter versus side scatter of the bead mixture. The class I and class II beads are easily separable by slight scatter properties. An analysis gate (R1) can be placed around both bead populations. **B.** The forward scatter versus FL-2 plot of beads gated from R1 in **A.** As shown, the class II beads (R3) can also be separated from the class I beads (R2) by means of FL-2 fluorescence and size because the class II beads are both smaller and impregnated with a red fluorescent dye. **C** and **D.** Examples of positive results for both class I and class II antibodies. In this example the patient possesses antibodies against class I and class II HLA antigens.

sion. First, although negative and positive controls are provided by the manufacturer, it is recommended that each laboratory use an in-house negative control as well. A second concern is how the actual analysis is performed. The screening beads are a mixture of 30 individual beads. If a single bead is positive, then only 3% of the total events should be positive. However, more important than the number of positive events is the architecture of the positive staining. If indeed a single bead is positive, then there should be a discernible and discrete peak that contains approximately 3% of the total events collected. Mere baseline noise that reaches 3% is not sufficient to be considered positive. A third issue is fluctuation in baseline staining. As mentioned in the discussion about

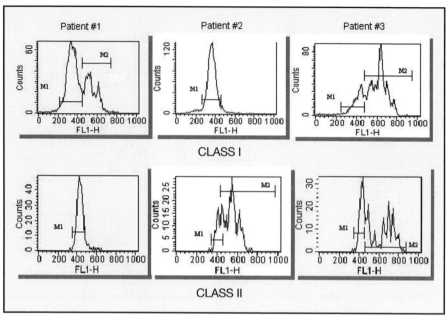

Figure 13-10

Histograms from 3 patients whose sera were evaluated with the FlowPRA I and II beads. Patient 1 is an individual with only class I antibodies. Patient 2 is an individual with only class II antibodies. Patient 3 possesses both types of antibodies.

FCXM, the negative control is a critical element for evaluating whether a serum will have a positive or negative result; the microparticle assay is no different. A negative control should be selected that produces consistent and reproducible staining for both class I and class II beads. When evaluating a patient's serum, the architecture of the test peak with respect to the negative peak is critical. Note that even though the microparticles are specific for HLA antibody, the amount of nonspecific background staining can vary and may reflect differences in the total immunoglobulin level of a patient's serum. Fourth, some samples may produce indeterminant staining (ie, alterations in staining architecture that are suggestive of antibody but not conclusive). In **Figure 13-12**, we illustrate a few examples of potentially misleading staining patterns. In these instances, the use of a cell-based assay or ELISA may provide additional information. Alternatively, repeating the test with greater quantities of serum may provide more convincing results regarding the presence or absence of anti-HLA antibody. Finally, one must remember that all reactivities should not be considered alone but in the context of the patient being tested. Unanticipated results should be investigated and, whenever possible, confirmed by additional testing.

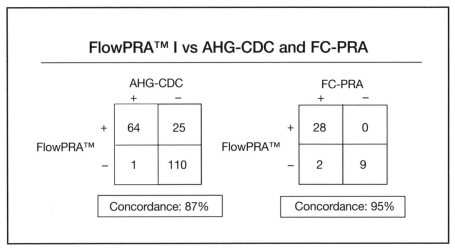

FlowPRA™ I vs AHG-CDC and FC-PRA

	AHG-CDC				FC-PRA	
	+	−			+	−
FlowPRA™ +	64	25		FlowPRA™ +	28	0
FlowPRA™ −	1	110		FlowPRA™ −	2	9

Concordance: 87%   Concordance: 95%

Figure 13-11

Comparison among antihuman globulin panel-reactive antibody analysis, FlowPRA I bead assay, and cell-based flow cytometric panel-reactive antibody analysis. As shown, the concordance was 87% between the FlowPRA I assay and the antiglobulin-enhanced, complement-mediated, cytotoxicity assay. However, FlowPRA I identified 25 (12.5%) more samples with positive reactions. The one sample that had a positive result for antihuman globulin and a negative result for FlowPRA was shown to contain a true IgM anti-HLA antibody. In addition (although this is not shown), FlowPRA produced higher panel-reactive antibody values (25% higher) than the antihuman globulin panel-reactive antibody, indicating that it detected additional antibody. A comparison between FlowPRA and the cell-based flow cytometric panel-reactive antibody showed good correlation (95%). Only 2 samples had positive results with cells but negative results with beads. Both of these samples were low-titer anti-HLA antibody from patients with a history of sensitization.

Once anti-HLA reactivity has been determined, the specificity beads can be used. Although quite similar in design to the screening beads, the specificity beads are designed to identify distinct HLA specificities within the patient's serum. Specificity is determined by using 4 pools of beads, with each pool consisting of 8 individual beads. Within each pool, one bead is unstained and 7 beads are labeled with various levels of red fluorescence. With this format, the reactivity of individual beads can then be assessed. Because each bead represents the class I or class II HLA antigens derived from a single cell line, antibody specificity can generally be assigned on the basis of the observed reactivity patterns. An example of a specificity derived from the Flow Specific Beads is shown in **Figures 13-13** (p 527) and **13-14** (p 528).

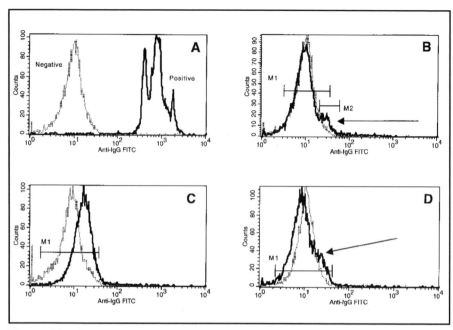

Figure 13-12
Some examples of difficult FlowPRA I bead results. Histogram **A** illustrates examples of a negative and positive control. For all histograms, the dotted line indicates the negative control. In histogram **B**, the arrow points to a small peak observed in the test sample. The peak is actually within the bounds of the negative marker (M1); however, it does represent true anti-HLA antibody at a low titer. These results show staining with a weak anti-B44, B45 antibody. Three cells in the pool had positive results for these antigens, and the resulting positive percentage was approximately 12%. Histogram **C** illustrates a staining pattern observed in a sample from a nonsensitized male subject. The peak architecture is similar to that of the negative control but is shifted significantly to the right, suggesting the presence of an antibody. However, further testing showed that this individual did not have HLA antibody, and the peak shift is most likely caused by a high total serum immunoglobulin concentration. Histogram **D** illustrates a small "shoulder" on the test serum *(arrow)* that is also within the bounds of the negative control (M1). Further testing did identify an anti-HLA antibody in this serum.

Future Applications in Clinical Transplantation

When an organ transplant is performed, the immune system of the recipient is unaware that the allograft has life-saving benefits. Dictated by thousands of years of evolution, the unfortunate consequence is immune-mediated rejection of the foreign material.[34] We are just beginning to understand some of the mechanisms that contribute to graft rejection, tolerance, and long-term graft survival. Clearly, low levels of preformed antibody that can be detected only with flow

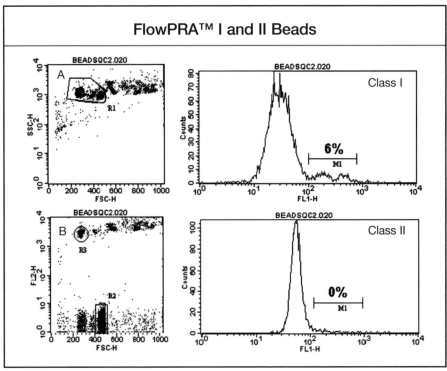

Figure 13-13

Testing a patient's serum with a defined anti-HLA antibody. FlowPRA I and II bead reactivity is shown. As shown, this patient demonstrated a PRA value of 6%, which indicates that 2 beads had positive results from the pool.

cytometry can portend a poorer prognosis. However, antibodies are only half of the immune equation. Cell-mediated immune responses make up the other contingent of our immune armamentarium. In general, the initiation of an immune response occurs when recipient T cells are activated by donor alloantigens. Specifically, antigen-specific receptors on recipient T lymphocytes engage alloantigenic peptide fragments and transduce cytoplasmic signals.[35] This interaction leads to the production of cytokines. Cytokines are a large family of signaling proteins including interleukins (IL1-IL20), colony-stimulating factors (eg, granulocyte-macrophage colony-stimulating factor), growth factors (eg, vascular endothelial cell growth factor [VEGF]), tumor necrosis factors (eg, TNF-alpha), interferons (eg, INF-gamma), and chemokines (eg, regulated upon activation normal T cells expressed and resected [RANTES]).[36,37] Cytokines regulate cell function in autocrine, paracrine, and/or endocrine fashion, binding to cells with their specific cell surface receptors and initiating a cascade of intra-

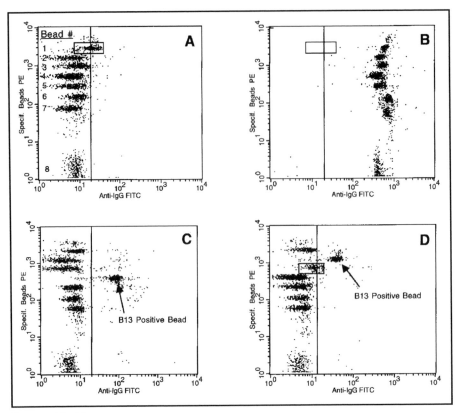

Figure 13-14
This figure shows how specificity was determined with the FlowPRA Specific Beads. Plots **A** and **B** show a negative and positive control from one bead combination. Plots **C** and **D** show that both beads that demonstrated a positive reaction bore the B13 antigen. Therefore, the specificity of the antibody is anti-B13.

cellular signaling. In the posttransplant period, the production of certain cytokines appears to promote the clonal expansion and differentiation of alloantigen-specific T lymphocytes. These activated and specific cells migrate to the allograft, where they are directly or indirectly involved in the rejection process.[38] Newer studies are beginning to explore how and to what extent different cytokines mediate allograft responses.[39] Studies suggest that analysis of specific cytokine patterns in cells isolated from allograft recipients may identify patients at risk for development of acute and/or chronic rejection or patients who may be at risk for development of immune tolerance of their grafts.

This approach requires the assessment of cytokine production at the single cell level. Such assessments can provide information regarding the efficacy of immunosuppressive therapy.[40] Tests for intracellular cytokine production can be performed using either anticoagulated whole blood or isolated mononuclear cells.[41] Because cytokine production by normal resting cells is, at best, minimal, a supraphysiologic in vitro stimulus (eg, mitogens or calcium ionophores) must be incorporated to establish the ability of the target cells to synthesize cytokines. A complicating factor is that once synthesized, cytokines are rapidly exported from the cells through the Golgi apparatus. Therefore, cytokine transport must be inhibited (eg, with monensin [Sigma, St Louis, MO] or brefeldin-A [A.G. Scientific, Inc, San Diego, CA]). The inhibition of cytokine transport results in the intracellular accumulation of cytokines and facilitates their detection.

Detection of intracellular cytokines is performed with flurochrome-conjugated anticytokine antibodies. The assay is typically performed in a 2- or 3-color format in which a fluorochrome-conjugated antibody directed to a known surface marker (eg, CD3 or CD20) is used to identify the target cell of interest. Target cell membranes must be permeabilized (eg, treated with saponinin [Sigma, St Louis, MO], a glycoside that forms reversible pores in the cell membrane) in order for the labeled anticytokine antibodies to penetrate the cells and bind to the intracellular cytokines. Numerous positive and negative controls must be incorporated into each assay to ensure that the experimental conditions were appropriate. Several approaches can be applied, such as the purchase of a commercial source of prescreened activated and fixed cells to document the reliability of the fluorochrome-conjugated anticytokine reagents. Alternatively, frozen cells from donors previously documented to produce the cytokine or cytokines of interest can be used to document activation conditions. Generally, fresh cells from a walk-in panel of healthy control subjects will suffice to document activation conditions. There are 3 different types of negative controls[42,43] that should be incorporated into each assay: (1) target cells should be stained with a fluorochrome-conjugated irrelevant isotype control antibody; (2) the fluorochrome-conjugated anticytokine antibody should be preincubuated with recombinant cytokine (blocking); or (3) target cells should be preincubated with unconjugated antibody before staining with the fluorochrome-conjugated anticytokine antibody. Individually or collectively, these controls allow the investigator to distinguish specific from nonspecific intracellular staining. An example of intracellular cytokine staining is shown in **Figure 13-15**.

A major limitation of the current intracellular assays is that unstimulated cells (at least from peripheral blood) do not have detectable levels of intracellular cytokines. Therefore, the only way cytokines can be detected in peripheral blood samples is through in vitro activation. Clearly, this adds an artificial component to the testing that is difficult to standardize and could explain the high degree of intertest and intratest variability. Additionally, the configuration of the intracellular cytokine assay only determines what percentage of a given cell pop-

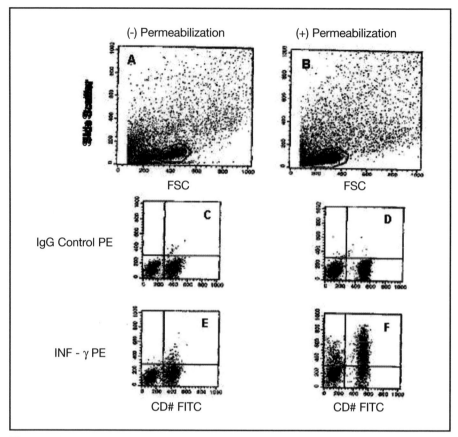

Figure 13-15

The effect of permeabilization solution on cellular light scatter properties, cell surface antigen staining, and intracellular cytokine staining. **A** and **B** are the forward scatter and side scatter profiles of normal human peripheral blood mononuclear cells cultured in media for 6 hours. Cells in **A** were not permeabilized, whereas cells in **B** were permeabilized with media containing saponinin (0.1%) before antibody staining. Note: Although no difference is detected between permeabilized and nonpermeabilized samples of nonactivated cells, forward and/or side light scatter properties of cells incubated with different biologic activators may be altered. **C-F** represent lymphocyte gated cells from **A** or **B** after activation with phorbol myristate acetate (50 ng/mL) plus ionomycin (1 mmol/L) for 6 hours. **C** and **E** are activated cells that were not permeabilized, and **D** and **F** represent activated cells that were permeabilized before antibody staining. **C** and **D** are negative controls (consisting of a phycoerythrin-conjugated irrelevant antibody isotype matched to the phycoerythrin-conjugated anticytokine antibody) to assess background staining. **E** and **F** were stained with phycoerythrin-conjugated anti-IFN-gamma. Cells in quadrant 2 (the upper right quadrant) represent CD3-positive cells that demonstrate coexpression of intracellular IFN-gamma. Note: Although the permeabilization solution did not alter the expression of CD3 on the surface of these cells, some biologic activators may down-regulate the expression of certain surface antigens.

ulation produces the cytokine or cytokines under study and is unable to quantify the amount of cytokine per cell. Because polymorphisms in cytokine genes (eg, those encoding for TNF-alpha, INF-gamma, and IL-10) differentiate individuals as high or low producers, it is feasible that a high producer with a small percentage of cells producing TNF-alpha might have a higher risk of rejection than a low producer with twice as many TNF-alpha-producing cells. New generation assays will need to consider these observations.

In addition to intracellular cytokine staining, several additional approaches have been used as means for predicting long-term survival. One such mechanism is described as *donor-specific hyporesponsiveness.*[44] In this mechanism it is proposed that solid organ recipients have a specific lack of responsiveness to donor antigens but remain completely responsive to third-party cells. Although a major aspect of this mechanism is cellular, it is certainly conceivable that a humoral component (ie, an antibody) may be used to indicate individuals who do not exhibit donor-specific hyporesponsiveness. In such a situation, the detection of antidonor antibodies in the posttransplant period may have significance in identifying these individuals. Several recent publications have indicated that anti-donor antibodies are harbingers of poor outcome in renal transplantation.[45,46] These studies showed that classifying patients on the basis of their posttransplant development of HLA antibody clearly identified a group with an unfavorable clinical outcome. Therefore, clinical studies now support posttransplant monitoring for antibody production because early detection of antibody may be useful in designing specific protocols to treat an ongoing rejection episode or to thwart an impending rejection. Hence these newer flow cytometric methods for performing rapid, sensitive, and specific antibody identification may become useful in the routine monitoring of patients after solid organ transplantation. Moreover, because cytometry can perform a semiquantitative assessment of antibodies, it would be possible to monitor therapy. Clinical decisions can then be made on the basis of the success or failure of antibody-reducing therapies. One such promising therapy uses intravenous immunoglobulin to essentially neutralize circulating alloantibody.[47] Flow cytometric assays may be key in identifying patients in whom this therapy will be successful, as well as following the clinical course of treatment.

In summary, the future of cytometry in transplantation appears quite optimistic because cytometry remains the most sensitive method for detecting antidonor antibodies either before or after transplant.

Summary

Flow cytometry in solid organ transplantation has evolved significantly since the initial description of the flow cytometric crossmatch assay by Garovoy et al[5] in 1983. The flow cytometric crossmatch assay represents the most sensitive test for antidonor antibody available today and has become a standard method in many histocompatibility laboratories. Reports from many laboratories have clearly demonstrated the clinical utility of the flow crossmatch in predicting early graft failure and increased risk for rejection episodes. For retransplant and highly sensitized individuals, a negative flow cytometric crossmatch result predicts graft survival comparable with that of nonsensitized primary transplant recipients. However, the increased sensitivity of the flow crossmatch has been as much a hindrance as it has been an advantage. For example, although proficiency testing for the FCXM exists, there is no standardized protocol or method. Although concordance between laboratories is good, it has not routinely reached a 90% consensus, particularly for samples which contain low levels of antibody. However, efforts by national transplant organizations, such as the American Society for Histocompatibility and Immunogenetics and the Southeastern Organ Procurement Foundation, are beginning to address these issues.

Until recently, it has not been feasible to perform routine PRA testing of patient sera using cytometric techniques. Therefore, discordance often occurred between cytotoxic PRA testing and the final flow cytometric crossmatch assay. The labor-intensive flow crossmatch was much too costly and time-consuming to be performed on a large scale as a means for PRA testing. As a result, patients were deemed "antibody negative" by less sensitive techniques. In some instances patients were called in for transplant only to find out that the final crossmatch result was positive, as determined by flow cytometry. Such an occurrence can also put the organ at risk by increasing its ischemia time while a more compatible recipient is sought. An additional issue has recently arisen in that recent reports have suggested not performing a final crossmatch for those patients deemed "antibody negative."[48,49] However, these centers used only cytotoxicity PRA testing for all their assumptions. Unfortunately, our data would suggest that up to 25% of these patients still possess anti-HLA antibody. Hence, such antibody-negative individuals may actually experience a positive crossmatch result if the assays are performed with flow cytometry. Therefore our position is that a patient should be deemed "antibody negative" only if the results of flow cytometric assays are negative.[50]

As we have demonstrated above, newer flow cytometric approaches that may help in organ allocation. PRA testing with cell pools or microparticles has significantly streamlined many logistic considerations and thereby made it possible to perform routine screening with flow cytometry. This improvement has distinct advantages to the transplant community in terms of organ allocation and financial considerations. First, routine screening can now be performed with the same level of sensitivity as the final crossmatch and PRA values can now better reflect a patient's potential to obtain a negative FCXM result. Second, better specificity determinations will assist in optimizing appropriate organ allocation. Third, the use of microparticle assays permits the rapid and simultaneous detection of class I and class II antibodies, a determination that was difficult, if not impossible, to perform in the past. Lastly, these collective approaches will reduce organ ischemia time and expedite transplantation to the most appropriate recipient, which will result in overall reduced costs to transplant centers. An added benefit of these assays may be in the posttransplant period, during which rapid and specific monitoring may affect posttransplant treatment protocols. Because of the specificity and rapid turnaround time of microparticle assays, real-time decisions can be made with regard to patient treatment options. The underlying assumption is that if a humoral rejection episode can be detected early and before clinical manifestations appear, more organs may be spared, or at least their survival may be extended.

In conclusion, the flow cytometric approaches we have described here are only the beginning of a continued effort to improve patient and graft survival through cutting-edge laboratory methods. As these methods evolve, the HLA community will be able to provide state-of-the-art cytometric testing for all patients awaiting transplantation.

Case Studies

Case 13-1

History

A 52-year-old man awaiting his first renal transplant is being considered for a cadaveric transplantation. In cytotoxicity assays, this patient demonstrated a PRA of 0%. His history is significant for multiple (more than 10) blood transfusions. The donor being considered is a complete HLA mismatch with the patient. The crossmatch results are shown below.

Serum Date	Method	Crossmatch Results T cell/B cell
12-5-98	Cytotoxicity	NEG/NEG
	Flow cytometry	NEG/POS

Does the B cell-positive result present a contraindication for transplantation?

Interpretation

This case is not an uncommon occurrence in the transplant laboratory. A patient with a history of potentially sensitizing events presents for transplant as an "unsensitized" individual based on a cytotoxic PRA. Upon testing by flow cytometry, a B cell-positive result is obtained. B cell-positive results can be due to either a class II antibody or a weak class I antibody. In this case, 2 additional pieces of information were helpful in making the decision regarding transplantation. First, the microparticle PRA value was also 0%, indicating that this patient did not possess a class I or class II antibody. Second, the autologous crossmatch (ie, the patient's cells tested against his own serum) was also B cell-positive. Hence, the combined information led to the determination that the B cell-positive result was not a contraindication to transplant.

History

A 48-year-old woman and mother of 2 children is in need of a kidney transplant. The HLA types of the patient and her 2 children are given below.

Patient: HLA A2, A26; B44, B62; Bw4; DR4, DR7
Son: HLA A1, A2; B7, B44; Bw4, Bw6; DR4, DR14
Daughter: HLA A1, A26; B7, 62; Bw4, Bw6; DR7, DR14

The son, who is medically eligible, wishes to donate a kidney to his mother. Cross-matches are performed between the mother and her son and the results are shown below.

Serum Date	Method	Crossmatch Results T cell/B cell
11-10-95	Cytotoxicity	NEG/NEG
	Flow cytometry	NEG/POS
12-14-96	Cytotoxicity	NEG/NEG
	Flow cytometry	NEG/POS
1-5-96	Cytotoxicity	NEG/NEG
	Flow cytometry	NEG/POS

The autologous crossmatches for all 3 serum dates were negative. PRA by cytotoxicity demonstrates a value of 0% against a 60-cell panel. However, a flow cytometric PRA using microparticles demonstrates a value of 0% for class I and 66% for class II. Should transplantation be recommended? What would be the cause of the high flow cytometric PRA?

Interpretation

Like the patient in Case 13-1, this patient presents with a history significant for sensitization and a positive B cell crossmatch with her son. Unlike the patient in Case 13-1, this individual has clear evidence of a class II HLA antibody. Although the specificity was not determined, the mismatched antigen from her pregnancies was DR14, which is also associated with DR52 (DRB3). Hence, the most likely specificity for this antibody is DR14, DR52 (DRB3). In this instance, the decision was made not to treat this individual with a transplant because the antibody reactivity appears specific for an HLA antigen(s) to which she has been sensitized. Subsequent analysis by flow cytometry did prove that the specificity was anti-DR14 and DR52.

Case 13-3

History

A 42-year-old man is awaiting his second renal transplant. Presently, he is experiencing chronic rejection of his first renal allograft. A related donor has become available and the patient wishes to be considered for retransplantation.

HLA typing data:

Patient:	A2, A3; B60, B62; DR1, DR4
Donor 1:	A2, Axx; B44, Bxx; DR4, DR4
Potential 2nd donor:	A2, Axx; B44, B62; DR4, DRxx

Abbreviations: xx = undetermined; most likely represents homozygosity for a HLA antigen.

HLA antibody screening results:

Serum date	Cytotoxicity	FlowPRA Class I/II
5 / 2000	Negative	0%/0%

(See Figure 13-16a)

Crossmatch results:

Donor	Method	Results (T / B cell)
Self	Cytotoxicity	Neg/Neg
	Flow cytometry	Neg/Neg
Donor 1	Cytotoxicity	Neg/Neg
	Flow cytometry	Pos/Pos
Donor 2	Cytotoxicity	Neg/Neg
	Flow Cytometry	Pos/Pos

(See Figure 13-16b)

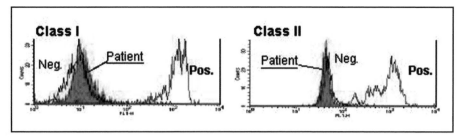

Figure 13-16a
Microparticle FlowPRA™

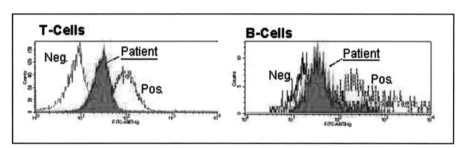

Figure 13-16b
Flow Cytometric Crossmatch

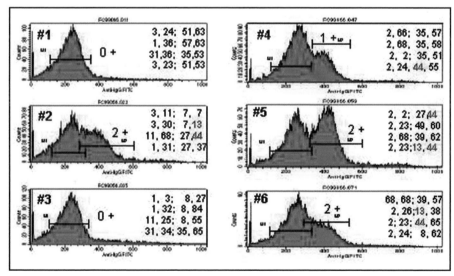

Figure 13-16c
Cell-Based Flow PRA

Although the crossmatches were positive, the fact that the microparticle FlowPRA was negative suggested that the crossmatch results were due to a non-HLA antibody. Hence, the crossmatches could be considered irrelevant and not a contraindication for transplantation.

Interpretation

Unfortunately, this turned out not to be the case. Additional testing using a cell-based flow cytometric PRA clearly demonstrated the presence of an HLA specific antibody directed against the B44 antigen (**Figure 13-16c**, p 537). HLA B44 was one of the mismatched antigens from the first transplant that was also present in the second potential donor. Hence, the positive crossmatch was a contraindication for transplantation. The explanation for the discrepancy is most likely a conformational change in the B44 protein that is attached to the microparticle. Therefore, processing the HLA antigen and adhering it to a plastic bead either altered or eliminated the epitope recognized by this antibody. In any solid-phase assay it is important to confirm that the immunologic reactivity of all clinically relevant epitopes are maintained. The manufacturer of the microparticles has since corrected this problem.

References

1. Patel R, Terasaki PI. Significance of the positive crossmatch test in kidney transplantation. *N Engl J Med.* 1969;280:735-739.

2. Fuller TC, Phelan D, Gebel HM, et al. Antigenic specificity of antibody reactive in the antiglobulin-augmented lymphocytotoxicity test. *Transplantation.* 1982;34:24-29.

3. Fuller TC, Cosimi AB, Russell PS. Use of antiglobulin reagent for detection of low levels of alloantibody-improvement of allograft survival in presensitized recipients. *Transplant Proc.* 1978;10:460-466.

4. Rodey GE, Fuller TC. Public epitopes and the antigenic structure of the HLA molecules. *Crit Rev Immunol.* 1987;7:229-267.

5. Garovoy MR, Rheinschmilt MA, Bigos M, et al. Flow cytometry analysis: a high technology crossmatch technique facilitating transplantation. *Transplant Proc.* 1983;15:1939-1941.

6. Cook DJ , Terasaki PI, Iwaki Y. An approach to reducing early kidney transplant failure with a positive flow cytometric crossmatch. *Clin Transplant.* 1987;1:253-260.

7. Thistlewaite, JR, Buckingham M, Stuart JK, et al. T cell immunofluorescence flow cytometry crossmatch results in cadaver donor renal transplantation. *Transplant Proc.* 1987;19:722-724.

8. Lazda VA, Pollack R, Mozes, MF, et al. The relationship between flow cytometry crossmatch results and subsequent rejection episodes in cadaver renal allograft rejection. *Transplantation.* 1988;45:562-569.

9. Talbot D, Givan Al, Shenton BK, et al. Relevance of a more sensitive crossmatch assay to renal transplantation. *Transplantation.* 1989;47:552-558.

10. Mahoney RJ, Ault KA, Given SR, et al. The flow cytometric crossmatch and early renal transplant loss. *Transplantation.* 1990;49:527-535.

11. Karuppan SS, Ohlman S, Moller E. The occurrence of cytotoxic and non-complement fixing antibodies in the crossmatch serum of patients with early rejection episodes. *Transplantation.* 1992;54:839-843.

12. Ogura K, Terasaki RI, Johnson C, et al. The significance of a positive flow cytometric crossmatch test in primary renal transplantation. *Transplantation.* 1993;56:294-298.

13. Talbot D, White M, Shenton BK, et al. Flow cytometric crossmatching in renal transplantation—the long-term outcome. *Transpl Immunol.* 1995;3:352-355.

14. Scornik JC. Detection of alloantibodies by flow cytometry: Relevance to clinical transplantation. *Cytometry.* 1995;22:259-263.

15. Nelson PW, Eschliman P, Shield CF, et al. Improved graft survival in cadaveric renal retransplantation by flow crossmatching. *Arch Surg.* 1996;131:599-603.

16. Bryan CF, Baier KA, Nelson PW, et al. Long-term graft survival is improved in cadaveric renal retransplantation by flow cytometric crossmatching. *Transplantation.* 1998;66:1827-1832.

17. Przybylowski P, Balogna M, Radovancevic B, et al. The role of flow cytometry-detected IgG and IgM anti-donor antibodies in cardiac allograft recipients. *Transplantation.* 1999;67:258-262.

18. Bray RA, Lebeck LL, Gebel HM. The flow cytometric crossmatch: dual-color analysis of T cell and B cell reactivities. *Transplantation.* 1989;48:834-840.

19. Bray RA. Flow cytometry crossmatching for solid organ transplantation. *Methods Cell Biol.* 1994;41:103-119.

20. Scornik JC, Bray RA, Pollack MS, et al. Multi center evaluation of the flow cytometric T-cell crossmatch: results from the American Society of Histocompatibility and Immunogenetics-College of American Pathologists proficiency testing program. *Transplantation.* 1997;63:252-257.

21. Lefor WM, Ackerman JR, Alveranga DY, et al. Flow cytometric crossmatching and primary cadaver kidney outcome: reliance of T and B cell targets, historic sera and autologous controls. *Clin Transplant.* 1996;10:601-606.

22. Bray RA. The clinical utility of flow cytometry in the histocompatibility laboratory. *Clin Immunol Newslett.* 1996;16:10-14.

23. Cicciarelli J, Helstab K, Mendez R. Flow cytometric PRA, a new test that is highly correlated with graft survival. *Clin Transplant.* 1992;63:159-164.

24. Fuller TC. Monitoring of HLA alloimmunization. Analysis of HLA alloantibodies in the serum of prospective transplant recipients. *Clin Lab Med.* 1991;11:551-570.

25. Shroyer TW, Deierhoi MH, Mink CA, et al. A rapid flow cytometric assay for HLA antibody detection using a pooled cell panel covering 14 serological cross reacting groups. *Transplantation*. 1995;59:626-630.

26. Pei R, Wang G, Tarsitani C, et al. Simultaneous HLA class I and class II antibodies screening with flow cytometry. *Hum Immunol*. 1998;59:313-322.

27. Bray RA, Chapman PT, Sinclair DA, et al. The flow cytometric PRA: evaluation of antibody reactivity and specificity using cell pools based on CREGs. *Hum Immunol*. 1996;49(suppl 1):106.

28. Bray RA, Foulks C, Wilmoth L, et al. Comparison between antiglobulin-enhanced cytotoxicity, flow cytometry and GTI quick screen for the detection of HLA alloantibody. *Hum Immunol*. 1997;55(suppl 1):74.

29. Bray RA, Sinclair DA, Wilmoth-Hosey, et al. Significance of the flow cytometric PRA (FC-PRA) in the evaluation of patients awaiting renal transplantation. *Hum Immunol*. 1998;59(suppl 1):121.

30. Bray RA, Cook DJ, Gebel HM. Flow cytometric detection of HLA allo-antibodies using class I coated microparticles. Hum *Immunol*. 1997;55(suppl 1):36.

31. Ghasemian SR, Light JA, Sasaki TA, et al. Hyperacute rejection from antibody against class II HLA antigens. *Clin Transplant*. 1998;12:569-71.

32. Schonemann C, Groth J, Leverenz S, et al. HLA class I and class II antibodies: monitoring before and after kidney transplantation and their clinical relevance. *Transplantation*. 1998;65:1519-1523.

33. Bittencourt MC, Rebibou JM, Saint-Hillier Y, et al. Impaired renal graft survival after a positive B-cell flow cytometric crossmatch. *Nephrol Dial Transplant*. 1998;13:2059-2064.

34. Rosenberg AS, Singer A. Cellular basis of skin allograft rejection: an in vivo model of immune-mediated tissue destruction. *Annu Rev Immunol*. 1992;10:333-358.

35. Weiss A, Littman DR. Signal transduction by lymphocyte antigen receptors. *Cell*. 1994;76:263-274.

36. Curfs JH, Meis JF, Hoogkamp-Korstanje JA. A primer on cytokines: sources, receptors, effects, and inducers. *Clin Microbiol Rev*. 1997;10:742-780.

37. Mantovani A. The chemokine system: redundancy for robust outputs. *Immunol Today*. 1999;20:254-257.

38. Nickerson P, Steurer W, Steiger J, et al. Cytokines and the Th1/Th2 paradigm in transplantation. *Curr Opin Immunol*. 1994;6:757-764.

39. Zhai Y, Ghobrial RM, Busuttil RW, et al. Th1 and Th2 cytokines in organ transplantation: paradigm lost? *Crit Rev Immunol*. 1999;19:155-172.

40. van den Berg AP, Twilhaar WN, Mesander G, et al. Quantitation of immunosuppression by flow cytometric measurement of the capacity of T cells for interleukin-2 production. *Transplantation*. 1998;65:1066-1071.

41. Gebel HM, Ortegel JW, Tambur AR. Flow cytometric post-transplant monitoring: intracellular cytokine production. In: *ASHI Procedure Manual*. Lenexa, Kan: The American Society for Histocompatibility and Immunogentics; 1999.

42. Prussin C, Metcalfe D. Detection of intracytoplasmic cytokine using flow cytometry and directly conjugated anti-cytokine antibodies. *J Immunol Methods.* 1995;188:117-128.

43. Hutchinson IV, Pravica V, Perrey C, et al. Cytokine gene polymorphisms and relevance to forms of rejection. *Transplant Proc.* 1999;31:734-736.

44. Reinsmoen NL, Matas AJ. Evidence that improved late renal transplant outcome correlates with the development of in vitro donor antigen-specific hyporeactivity. *Transplantation.* 1993;55:1017-1023.

45. Christiaans MHL, Overhof-de Roos R, Nieman F, et al. Donor-specific antibodies after transplantation by flow cytometry. *Transplantation.* 1998;65:427-433.

46. Kimball P, Rhodes C, King A, et al. Flow crossmatching identifies patients at risk for postoperative elaboration of cytotoxic antibodies. *Transplantation.* 1998;65:444-446.

47. Jordan SC, Quartel AW, Czer LSC, et al. Post transplant therapy using high-dose human immunoglobulin (intravenous gammaglobulin) to control acute humoral rejection in renal and cardiac allograft recipients and potential mechanism of action. *Transplantation.* 1998;66:800-805.

48. Kerman RH, Susskind B, Ruth J, et al. Can an immunologically, nonreactive potential allograft recipient undergo transplantation without a donor-specific crossmatch? *Transplantation.* 1998;66:1833-1835.

49. Matas AJ, Sutherland DE. Kidney transplantation without a final crossmatch. *Transplantation.* 1998;66:1835-1837.

50. Gebel HM, Bray RA. Sensitization and sensitivity: defining the unsensitized patient. *Transplantation.* 2000;69:1370-1374.

14

Clinically Useful Nontraditional Applications of Flow Cytometry

Tom Huard
Jerry Katzmann
Bruce H. Davis

Introduction

The number of nontraditional applications of flow cytometry has grown since the last version of this text. Although many new techniques have been developed, their use in the routine clinical setting has been tempered by such formidable issues as managed care, reductions in reimbursements from Medicare and other providers, corporate compliance, medical necessity, and the overall "doing more with less" phenomenon that has been prevalent in health care management. This has resulted in the development of specialized "centers of excellence," where some of the more esoteric assays have been incorporated into testing algorithms. Nevertheless, some of the new techniques have made their way to community-based laboratories and have become more routine and cost-effective.

This chapter will attempt to highlight several of these formerly nontraditional applications that have been accepted as essential for comprehensive medical care and can be done in a practical way in almost any clinical laboratory (**Table 14-1**). The focus of this chapter will be on methods regarding the biology of the red blood cell. Several other applications, not discussed here, have been described in other sections of this text. A brief section on HLA-B27 analysis has also been included in this chapter.

Table 14-1
Some Examples of Nontraditional Applications of Flow Cytometry

Analysis of platelet activation
Detection of anti-platelet antibodies
Thrombopoiesis assessment
Evaluation of heparin-induced thrombocytopenia
Detection of apoptosis
Cell proliferation analysis
Evaluation of intracellular cytokines
HLA phenotype analysis
HLA cross-match assays
In situ hybridization assays
Dendritic cell quantification
Stem cell quantification
Evaluation of mitochondrial activity
Detection of fetal-maternal hemorrhage
Evaluation of paroxysmal nocturnal hemoglobinuria
Determination of multidrug resistance
Microbial detection
Chromosome analysis
Neutrophil function analysis
Ca^{2+} immobilization detection
Telomerase activity analysis

Flow Cytometry in Red Blood Cell Antigen-Antibody Detection Assays

Assays of red blood cell (RBC) biology have become important parameters of patient management (**Table 14-2**). These are important for managing difficult pregnancies, bleeding disorders, transfusion-dependent therapies, coagulopathies, and autoimmune diseases. Classical laboratory approaches to RBC analysis and anti-RBC antigen screening have depended on relatively crude in vitro agglutination reactions. The use of flow cytometry in monitoring RBCs has added significant advantages with respect to sensitivity, quantitation, reproducibility, and accuracy of results. Although flow cytometry assays of RBC antigen expression and function are currently being performed in only a few specialized centers, these relatively simple techniques are now available for the routine immunohematology-blood bank laboratory.

An initial obstacle to the use of flow cytometry to assay RBCs has been the exquisite sensitivity of RBCs to agglutination. Analysis by means of flow cytometry is dependent on interrogation of single cells by a laser beam, and therefore even modest agglutination could lead to erroneous assumptions. As outlined in **Table 14-3,** there are multiple techniques to ensure that RBC analysis is performed at the single-cell level.[1-5] Mechanical agitation has been the hallmark method for this approach, but Garratty and others[3,4,6] have shown that weak fixation in glutaraldehyde or formaldehyde is superior.

Another feature of RBCs, which is also common to platelets, is their relatively small size and lack of nuclear density. This presents a unique problem in that the background autofluorescence and light scatter characteristics are often difficult to distinguish from background signals. This obstacle can be overcome by increases in gain, photomultiplier tube (PMT) voltages, and careful color compensation. In addition, use of multiparameter analysis (eg, 3- or 4-color

Table 14-2
Applications/Disease Associations for Flow Cytometric Analysis of Red Blood Cells

Alloimmunization during childbirth
Autoimmune hemolytic anemia
Transfusion-related reactions
Congenital chimerism-mosaicism
Erythrocyte phenotyping
Bone marrow engraftment
Classification in myelodysplastic syndrome
Fetal-maternal hemorrhage
Sickle cell disease

Table 14-3
Methods to Prevent Red Blood Cell Agglutination

Vortex specimen
Transfer through small-bore needle (26-29 gauge)
Glutaraldehyde fixation
Formaldehyde fixation
Formaldehyde and sodium dodecylsulfate treatment
Dimethylsuberimidate
Dithiothreitol
2-Mercaptoethanol
Use of Fab-2 fragments of antibody

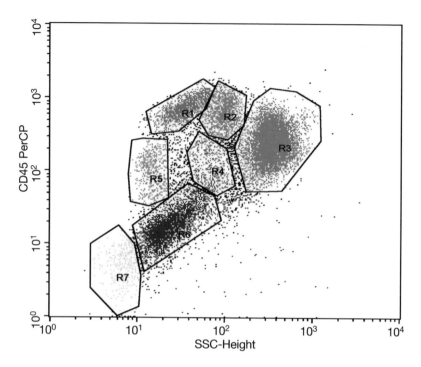

Figure 14-1

Two-parameter dot plot of a patient's bone marrow showing the selective gating of multiple cellular elements, including the red blood cell compartment.
Abbreviations: R1 = mature lymphocytes; R2 = monocytes; R3 = mature granulocytes; R4 = myeloblasts; R5 = lymphoid precursors (hematogones and B lymphoblasts); R6 = RBC compartment (eg, red blood cells, reticulocytes, platelets, megakaryocytes); R7 = debris.

fluorescence coupled with forward and 90° light scatter) can help to segregate the RBC compartment (**Figure 14-1**).[7,8]

Flow cytometry analysis of RBCs has been applied in multiple ways to study clinically important parameters of RBC biology.[1-6] As outlined in **Table 14-4,** these include assays with the potential to monitor cytoplasmic immunoglobulins bound to the RBC membrane, to detect specific membrane-associated RBC antigens, and to detect allogenic RBCs in patients after transfusion, bone marrow transplantation, or a traumatic event such as fetal-maternal hemorrhage (FMH) or a sickle-cell episode.

Because of the unique agglutination-prone nature of RBCs, multiple detection methods have been used (**Table 14-5**).[1-9] Fab'-2 fragments of antibodies to RBC components that are directly conjugated with fluorescent dyes (fluorescein

Table 14-4

Specific Uses of Flow Cytometry for Red Blood Cells

Detection of RBC-bound immunoglobulins (ie, IgG, IgA, and IgM)

Detection of RBC-bound complement proteins (ie, C3, C4, CR1, CD55, CD 59, and CD71)

Quantitation of RBC-bound immunoglobulins (ie, IgG, IgM, and IgA)

Detection of blood group antigens (ie, Rh-CDE, ABO, Le, Kell)

Zygosity analysis, congenital and acquired

Detection of circulating Anti-Rh, ABO antibodies

Detection of immunoglobulin subclasses (ie, IgG1, 2, 3, and 4)

Detection of intracellular nucleotides (ie, nucleated RBCs and reticulocytes)

Detection of intracellular proteins (ie, fetal hemoglobin)

Table 14-5

Antibody-mediated Detection of Red Blood Cell–associated Problems

Direct fluorescent antibody conjugates

Indirect second antibody fluorescent conjugates

Tertiary immunoconjugates: biotin-avidin antibody complexes

---

isothiocyanate and phycoerythrin) offer the best way to detect cell surface molecules, such as immunoglobulin G (IgG), without induction of agglutination. Alternative methods include using an indirect approach with a fluorescent-labeled second antibody, usually directed against IgG, IgA, or IgM. In addition, some investigators use an amplification system similar to routine immunohisto-chemistry, which makes use of biotin-avidin complexes to enhance the sensitivity of the detection assay. The latter approach, however, is often associated with higher background fluorescence and spontaneous cellular agglutination. Monoclonal antibodies have been used successfully to detect both cell surface and intracellular RBC antigens, for example, CD55 and CD59 in paroxysmal nocturnal hemoglobinuria (PNH)[10] and hemoglobin F (Hgb-F) in adult and fetal RBCs.[11]

The direct agglutination test (DAT) has been the primary assay for the detection of RBC-associated binding of immunoglobulins. This assay is relatively inexpensive and reliable and has been used extensively in cases of autoimmune hemolytic anemia (AIHA). This usually entails using anti-human IgG, IgA, or IgM to detect membrane-bound immunoglobulins. Although the sensitivity of the test may be relatively good, for most cases of AIHA, detecting

100 to 200 molecules of IgG per cell, it has been shown that gross differences in sensitization concentrations have very little effect on subsequent agglutination.[12] In fact, 2- to 4-fold differences in IgG concentration per cell have very little effect on subsequent DAT results. The recent advent of quantitative flow cytometry has the significant advantage of quantitating the relative amount of immunoglobulin bound to each RBC at very low levels of expression (< 30 molecules per cell).[13] This has lead to the discovery of significant immunoglobulin expression on RBCs from patients with hemolysis but a negative DAT result.[14,15] This has been shown for cases in which warm reactive immunoglobulins are bound to RBCs and do not usually yield effective DAT results.[16]

It remains controversial as to whether the amount of RBC-bound immunoglobulin can be used to determine a clinical risk for in vivo hemolysis to occur,[1] but it has been shown that aging RBCs[17] and RBCs from patients with active hemolysis harbor high concentrations of cell-bound immunoglobulins. This may be a more complicated phenomenon, involving not only antigen densities[18] but also distribution patterns on the cell surface. It is well known that certain Rh antigens are clustered on the cell membrane, and this feature of antigen distribution could have a profound effect on secondary events leading to hemolysis.[19-21]

The quantitation of cell surface molecules using flow cytometry is a complex technique. Issues of calibration and standardization are crucial for results to be accurate and reproducible.[22-24] The use of fluorescent beads impregnated with fluorochrome at concentrations similar to what would be expected on a per-cell basis have been successfully used to study this phenomenon.[24] Essential to this process is the accurate measurement of the fluorochrome/protein ratio for each antibody or protein being used. This area of flow cytometry application is being extensively studied, especially in the analysis of cell activation in immunodeficient patients. This technique is by no means routine but has great potential to become an important addition to the multiparameter applications of flow cytometry.

The threshold for sensitivity of using flow cytometry applications in detecting potential hemolytic disease is much lower than that for the traditional DAT assay.[6] As shown in **Table 14-6**, both the sensitivity (defined as the lowest reported limit of detection of allogenic RBCs) and reproducibility (defined as the percentage coefficient of variation [CV] of assay-assay variation) are significantly better with flow cytometry.[6,25-27]

These data highlight one of the advantages that flow cytometry measurements of RBC antigen expression and protein interactions may have over conventional methodologies. This subject has recently been reviewed in detail[6] and poses great potential for transfer to the routine clinical laboratory.

Table 14-6
Sensitivity and Reproducibility in Detection of Mixed Allogenic Red Blood Cells

Test	Conjugate	Sensitivity	Intra Assay Variability
DAT	Direct	0.1–3%	10–24% CV
FC	Direct	0.1–0.5%	8–14% CV
FC	Indirect	0.01–0.3%	6–10% CV

Detection of Fetal Hemoglobin in Maternal-fetal Hemorrhage

Another important application of flow cytometry in RBC biology is the detection of intracellular markers of RBC maturation and function.[11,28-38] One of the most recent advances has been in the detection of fetal hemoglobin (Hgb-F).[11,31,32]

The detection of Hgb-F is of critical importance in the diagnosis and management of several medical disorders, including Rh-D incompatibilities (FMH), sickle cell disease, dyserythropoeisis, myelodysplastic syndrome, thalassemias, hemolytic anemias, and others. Methods for measurement of Hgb-F have been relatively crude with respect to clinical sensitivity and quantitation (**Table 14-7**).

The most important clinical use for detection of fetal components has been in the treatment and prevention of FMH.[28] FMH usually occurs during pregnancy, with increasing volumes during fetal development that can result in allosensitization of the maternal immune cells after parturition. This can lead to life-threatening autoimmune sequelae for any subsequent pregnancies (eg, erythroblastosis fetalis). Sensitization occurs in the highest frequency subsequent to incompatibilities between an Rh(-) mother and an Rh(+) fetus (the so-called D-antigen mismatches).[33] As the fetal RBCs penetrate the maternal circulation, they can induce anti-Rh (D antigen)-specific antibodies that can

Table 14-7
Assay for Fetal Hemoglobin

RBC agglutination (D^{mu} test)
RBC acid elution (Kleihauer-Betke)
RBC rosette formation
Hemoglobin electrophoresis
High-performance liquid chromatography
Anti-Hgb-F and anti-D antigen with flow cytometry

lead to hemolysis in subsequent pregnancies. Detection of fetal cells or Hgb-F is an essential part of the management of these patients,[34-36] who are treated with anti-Rh globulin preparations, such as RhoGam (Ortho Systems, Raritan, NJ). Hence assay sensitivity and specificity is a critical factor in that process.

The most well-characterized assay for Hgb-F used throughout the world has been the Kleihauer-Betke acid elution method.[37] Agglutination assays have also been popularized. These techniques fail in good clinical reproducibility with very high CVs (up to nearly 90%). Enzyme immunoassay methods have also been evaluated but lack the necessary specificity and sensitivity for determining low levels of fetal RBC contamination of the maternal circulation.[38,39] Flow cytometry methods have been applied to this field by using antibodies to Rh-D antigens.[40-44] These methods can reliably detect low levels of allogeneic RBCs in maternal circulation (0.1%) and aid in the diagnosis of potential maternal alloimmunization. This has also been used to help determine the necessity and dosage of anti-Rh antibody therapy (Rho-GAM).

One of the drawbacks of this method is that it is not necessarily fetal cell specific. A more recent approach has been developed with flow cytometry used to detect cells containing Hgb-F.[11,45-49] This approach was enhanced by the development of a HbF-specific monoclonal antibody.[11] This assay has proven to be very sensitive, capable of detecting less than 0.1% fetal RBCs, with precision considerably superior to that of other methods (CVs < 15%). Comparison with other standard methods, including the Kleihauer-Betke test, have shown excellent correlation.[11,31,32] In a recent study of 150 blood donors, including patients with hemoglobinopathies and persistent Hgb-F, this method reliably detected as low as 0.02% of fetal Hgb-F–containing cells.[11]

A unique aspect to the detection of fetal RBCs by this method is the pretreatment regimen to make permeable the RBCs for hemoglobin detection.[11] For this, the cells are fixed in 0.05% glutaraldehyde for 10 minutes at room temperature, followed by a brief incubation in a nonionic detergent (0.1% Triton-X 100). This is followed by staining with a fluorochrome-conjugated anti-Hgb-F at a saturating concentration. Light scatter thresholds are set to trigger the collection of fluorescent events, thus eliminating small particles (eg, bare nuclei, platelets) from the analysis. Specific gating is based on dual-parameter fluorescence with autofluorescent cells (ie, white blood cells) excluded from the Hgb-F–containing populations (**Figure 14-2**).

This technique allows for significant separation of adult and fetal RBCs, as well as adult F cells. F cells are red cells that have Hgb-F as a minor hemoglobin content and are normally present as less than 3% of the red cell population. F cells can be increased in anemia or other causes of increased hematopoiesis, as well as being increased as a result of genetic variations. The precision and

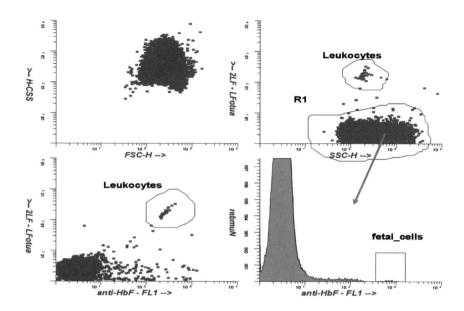

Figure 14-2
Flow cytometric detection of fetal RBCs with anti-hemoglobin F antibody (Caltag Laboratories, Burlingame, CA).

sensitivity are significantly improved with this flow cytometric approach, with CVs of less than 7.5% over a range of fetal RBCs of 0% to 5.4%, and in counting F cells.[11]

This method has also been applied to other clinical conditions. The monoclonal antibody to Hgb-F can also recognize adult cells with abnormal Hgb-F expression (**Figure 14-3**).[32] This has important implications in patients with sickle cell disease, for example, which in crisis or pretreatment may demonstrate elevated levels of circulating Hgb-F and F cells. Additionally, F cells may be of potential value in the prognostic evaluation of patients with myelodysplasia or thalassemia.

Another important caveat of this technique is the incorporation of control cells known to contain intracellular Hgb-F.[11] As part of this method, blood specimens known to contain 1% to 5% fetal cord blood RBCs or stabilized fetal RBC control material are used as a means of identifying the region for specific fetal RBC gating. This has provided a better measure of fetal cells than the traditional isotype control samples, which are often misleading because of nonspecific cytoplasmic binding of antibody. The ability to control this assay has additionally been facilitated by the recent FDA clearance of a stabilized control suitable

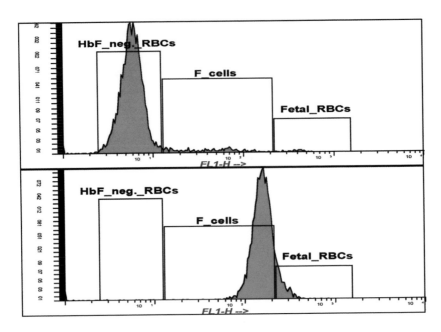

Figure 14-3
F-cell counting with an anti-hemoglobin F antibody technique shown in a normal pregnant individual with some fetal red blood cells also present *(top)* and in an individual with homocellular-type hereditary persistence of hemoglobin F *(bottom)*.

for all assays of fetomaternal hemorrhage detection, called Fetaltrol™ and manufactured by Trillium Diagnostics (Portland, Maine). This selective control is useful, and this approach should be advocated for other applications of flow cytometry (eg, PNH evaluation).

Flow Cytometry in the Diagnosis of Paroxysmal Nocturnal Hemoglobinuria

PNH is an acquired chronic disorder affecting RBC survival and hematopoiesis.[50-52] The disease is thought to arise from a clonal proliferation of abnormal precursor cells, resulting in mature cells that are exquisitely susceptible to in vivo hemolysis. The cause of the disease is not fully understood, but perturbations of the function of normal bone marrow cells are suspected. The

Table 14-8
Glycosylphosphatidylinositol-associated proteins

Acetylcholinesterase

Leukocyte alkaline phosphatase

Decay-accelerating factor (CD55)

Membrane inhibitor of reactive lysis (CD59)

Homologous restriction factor (C8-binding protein)

Lymphocyte function–associated antigen (CD58)

5' ectonucleotidase

Low-affinity IgG Fc receptor (CD16)

Urokinase-type plasminogen activator

Endotoxin-binding protein receptor (CD14)

GPI-anchored glycoprotein (CD48)

GPI-sialoglycoprotein (CD24)

---

disease is often associated with other bone marrow-derived diseases, such as myelodysplastic syndrome, aplastic anemias, and even acute leukemia.

The primary clinical manifestation of PNH is the increased susceptibility of the RBCs to in vivo hemolysis.[51,52] This is mediated by enhanced binding and activation of complement proteins on the RBC membrane.[53] This occurs as a consequence of the loss of specific abnormal glycosylphospholipids from the cell membrane.[54]

In normal RBCs many membrane-bound molecules are anchored to the membrane by means of a glycosylphosphatidylinositol (GPI) moiety.[51-56] This moiety serves as a transmembrane molecule to adhere these proteins to the cell membrane and serves to communicate with the intracellular compartment. Several of the proteins anchored by means of a GPI moiety are crucial to the regulation or inactivation of complement proteins (**Table 14-8**).[51,52] In PNH somatic mutations in GPI synthesis lead to incomplete molecules incapable of anchoring protein to the cell membrane.[57] This is thought to occur from an error in early GPI synthesis, resulting in GPI molecules of terminal mannosyl residues. This defect appears to be in the X-linked gene encoding for phosphatidylinositol glycan A.[58,59] Transfection of affected cells with a construct capable of transcribing functional phosphatidylinositol glycan A protein has been shown to correct the defect.[60-64]

The GPI-associated proteins primarily responsible for susceptibility to complement-dependent RBC hemolysis are DAF and membrane inhibitor of reactive lysis (MIRL; CD55 and CD59, respectively).[65,66] Each has a unique regulatory influence on the complement cascade. DAF (CD55) functions as a catalyst to enhance the dissociation or decay of the C3 convertases (C4b2a or C3bBb) from the cell membrane.[65] This reduces the amount of C3 activation and, ultimately, the concentration of the terminal membrane attack complexes of

Table 14-9

Assays for the Diagnosis of Paroxysmal Nocturnal Hemoglobinuria

Sucrose hemolysis (sugar-water test)
Acid hemolysin test (HAM test)
Acetylcholinesterase activity
Leukocyte alkaline phosphatase activity
Urine hemosiderin
Reticulocyte count
Immunophenotyping of blood cells

the complement cascade that are generated. Deficiencies in GPI expression lead to a loss of CD55 membrane antigens and result in increased C3 complexes bound to the cell.[67]

MIRL (CD59) plays a more prominent role in PNH. This antigen functions to inhibit the interaction between C8 and C9 in the membrane attack complex in the terminal phase of complement activation.[68] Whereas deficiencies in CD55 do not always correlate with in vivo hemolysis and hemoglobinuria, the loss of CD59 is almost always associated with a high degree of hemolysis and the production of RBCs with the most sensitivity to in vitro complement-dependent hemolysis.[69,70] This phenomenon can be corrected with insertion of exogenous CD59.[51,71]

There are multiple assays to detect PNH in patients with clinical symptoms (**Table 14-9**). The primary algorithm should include screening tests, such as the sugar-water test and the acid hemolysin (HAM) test, to determine any increase in complement-dependent lysis. In addition, the primary algorithm should always include assays to detect hemoglobinuria and hemosiderin, which are almost always found in true PNH.[51,52]

The sugar-water test is dependent on in vitro activation of complement in the presence of autologous RBCs.[72] Many different factors can be used to activate complement in vitro (**Table 14-10**). In this test, sucrose in an isotonic buffer is used. PNH-affected RBCs, when incubated in sucrose with autologous serum, will lyse more readily than normal RBCs. Visual detection of the release of hemoglobin is used as the endpoint for a positive reaction. This is a subjective determination, and false-positive results are common. Patients with myelodysplastic syndrome, megaloblastic anemia, other forms of hemolytic anemia (eg, AIHA), or even acute leukemia may have a positive reaction as well.[73]

The low-end threshold for the minimal number of PNH-affected cells is not well defined. This sensitivity is dependent on (1) the relative amount of affected cells in the circulation, (2) the relative amount of GPI loss, and (3) the concen-

Table 14-10
Factors for In Vitro Activation of Complement

Lower pH (eg, HAM test)

Lower ionic strength (sugar-water test)

Exogenous protein activators (cobra venom factor)

Increase in divalent cations (mgH)

Sensitization with specific antibodies (anti-ABO)

Sensitization with exogenous immunoglobulin (cold agglutination)

tration of complement in the serum. The expression of this sensitivity is thought to be triphasic, with at least 3 subpopulations defined: those that lyse readily with only a small amount of complement (PNH III), those with moderate release of hemoglobin (PNH II), and those requiring relatively high concentrations of complement (PNH I). The expression of these subsets in patients with PNH may vary widely, as will the concentration of functional complement proteins, limiting the sensitivity of this assay.[51,74,75]

It is recommended that a positive reaction in the sucrose hemolysis test be confirmed with the HAM test.[52] This test is more specific in that few other RBC abnormalities will give a positive reaction. Patients with hereditary erythroblastic multinuclearity with acidified serum can exhibit positive hemolysis but not in the presence of autologous serum. Although the HAM test may be more specific than the sugar-water test, interpretation is still subjective and the sensitivity is restricted, with small populations of PNH-affected cells sometimes going undetected.[51]

The advent of flow cytometry as a diagnostic tool in PNH has enabled the specific detection and quantitation of GPI-linked proteins.[10,76-80] This has the distinct advantage of detecting pertinent surface antigens on multiple cell populations in addition to detection of very minute subpopulations at a level considered to be rare events (eg, < 0.1%). The primary target molecules used today are antibodies to DAF (CD55) and MIRL (CD59) (**Figure 14-4a**). Many investigators also include CD14 and CD16 in this diagnostic scheme (**Figure 14-4b**, p 558). Those antigens are distributed in varying densities on multiple cellular elements in the bone marrow and circulation, including RBCs, lymphocytes, granulocytes, monocytes, platelets, megakaryocytes, reticulocytes, and stem cells. Flow cytometry offers significant advantage in that these populations can be selectivity gated to assess their relative involvement in GPI-linked protein deficiencies. This is especially important in regard to the monitoring and management of patients with PNH because deficiencies in GPI-linked proteins may

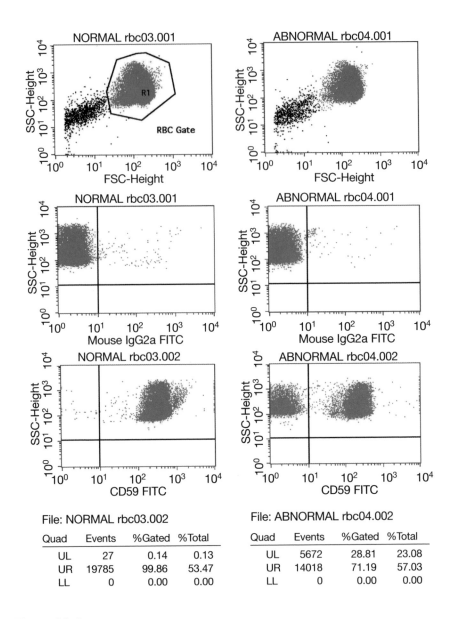

Figure 14-4a

Use of glycosylphosphatidylinositol-linked proteins in the detection of paroxysmal noctur-nal hemoglobinuria in human red blood cells. Note loss of antibody reactivity to CD59 in patient with paroxysmal nocturnal hemoglobinuria.

have significantly different physiologic effects on the clinical complications of PNH. For example, patients with PNH are much more susceptible to perturba-tions of hemostasis. This is thought to be directly related to platelet expression

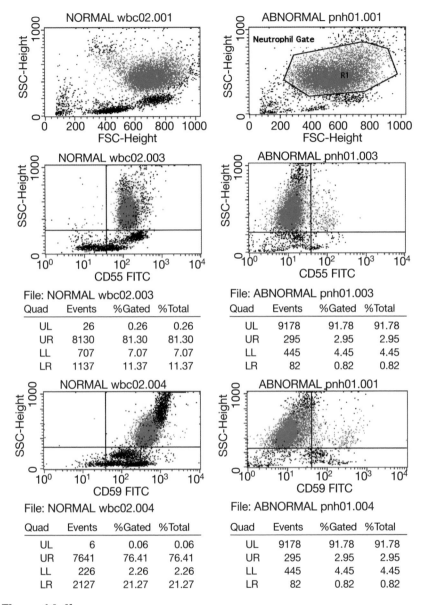

Figure 14-4b

Use of glycosylphosphatidylinositol-linked proteins in the detection of paroxysmal nocturnal hemoglobinuria human white blood cells. Note change in antibody reactivity to CD55 and CD59 in patients with paroxysmal nocturnal hemoglobinuria.

of GPI-linked proteins. In addition, many of these patients may experience deep vein thrombosis, such as in the Budd-Chiari syndrome. Detection of PNH-affected platelets by means of flow cytometry could serve to provide evidence for prophylactic anticoagulation or thrombolytic treatment. This is made possible by the selective gating and multiparameter capabilities of the flow cytometer (**Figure 14-4, a and b**).

Sequential testing of patients with PNH is crucial in following disease progression or response to therapy. This is important because the disease appears to be episodic, and the presence of detectable PNH-affected cells may fluctuate dramatically with diurnal, disease-based, and treatment-based variations.[51,52] It is well known, for example, that PNH can have profound effects on hematopoiesis and RBC turnover. Multiparameter staining with antibodies to GPI-linked proteins and thiazole orange for newly formed reticulocytes has been reported as a way to monitor hematopoietic cycles and response to erythropoietin therapy. This capability is unique to flow cytometry.

The high sensitivity of flow cytometry to identify rare events is another advantage in the management of patients with PNH. This is especially important because many patients with PNH must undergo multiple transfusions to restore cellular elements (eg, platelets in thrombocytopenic patients) or hemoglobin (for profound hemolysis and hemoglobinuria). In addition, the multiparameter gating and analysis afforded flow cytometry is useful in determining the prevalence of disease in concert with engraftment after bone transplantation that may be required for some patients.

Data interpretation of immunophenotyping results for cell subpopulations in patients with PNH is complex. There is no consensus to date as to criteria specific for diagnosis. This is complicated by the episodic nature of PNH, therapeutic modalities, and the lack of clinical correlations with the intensities of GPI-linked antigen expression and disease status. This is also complicated by the fact that genetic polymorphisms and somatic mutations can influence epitope-antibody binding (eg, CD16 variants) in several GPI-linked proteins.[79] Nevertheless, flow cytometry offers the most comprehensive mechanism to study these events and devise strategies of management for patients with PNH to prevent or predict untoward clinical complications.

Detection of Immature Red Blood Cells

The detection of immature forms of RBCs (nucleated [n]RBCs and reticulocytes) is an important feature in the management of patients with severe anemia. This would include patients with other diseases in which complications from the disease process or treatment protocols may influence erythropoiesis (**Table 14-11**).[81-87]

Table 14-11

Clinical Conditions Requiring Measurements of Immature Red Blood Cell Fraction

Aplastic anemia

Iron deficiency

B_{12} deficiency

Folate deficiencies

Megaloblastic anemia

Myelodysplastic syndrome

Autoimmune hemolytic anemia

Hemorrhage

Occult bleeding or hemolysis

Posttransfusion monitoring

Postchemotherapy monitoring

Post-bone marrow transplantation

Specific drug therapy (eg, erythropoietin)

PNH

The stress induced during these conditions on the hematopoietic function of the bone marrow and other tissue sites of erythropoietic activity (eg, liver and spleen) leads to the extravasation of immature forms of RBCs into the circulation. These forms are relatively unstable (mean half-life, 1-3 days) because maturation proceeds at a relatively rapid rate. Nevertheless, monitoring of the presence of these forms, quantitation, and determination of relative maturity can help to define bone marrow hematopoietic function, disease severity and classification, and rapid response to therapeutic intervention.[88,89]

The maturation sequence of the RBC life span is dependent on the enucleation of primitive RBC precursors (normoblasts). Early release of stress erythrocytes from the bone marrow results in a systemic rise in nRBCs rich in both DNA and RNA. These rapidly enucleate (most before leaving the marrow), and the resultant reticulated RBC (reticulocyte) is essentially void of DNA but retains remnant RNA molecules. This process is accompanied by many other changes to the immature RBC (**Table 14-12**).[88] Assays for many of these components are available; however, they are usually impractical to implement for cost-effective applications. In addition, some require functional assays for molecular characterization and are difficult to incorporate into a routine clinical laboratory algorithm.

Most current applications for detection of the immature forms of RBCs with flow cytometry are dependent on the detection of residual DNA or RNA by using fluorescent dyes with high binding affinities for nucleotides.[90,91] Some examples are shown in **Table 14-13**. These dyes have relatively high binding

Table 14-12

Components of Red Blood Cells Associated with Maturation

Cellular enucleation

Loss of intracellular DNA

Presence of reticulated RNA

Change in intracellular enzyme activity (eg, G6PD)

Loss of membrane antigens (eg, transferrin receptor CD71)

Alterations in membrane phospholipids

Increase in circulating RBC proteins (eg, CD71)

Changes in form and quantity of heme

Presence of specific intracellular moieties (eg, glycophorin A)

Table 14-13

Common Dyes Used to Detect Immature Red Blood Cells

Acridine orange

Auramine-O

Ethidium bromide

Propidium iodide

Thiazole orange

coefficients for nucleic acid, and emissions are not usually influenced by other intracellular components of the RBC (eg, hemoglobin). The most widely accepted dyes currently available for detection of nRBC or reticulocytes are propidium iodide and thiazole orange. These form relatively stable complexes with intracellular nucleotides and emit with high intensities at wavelengths enabling accurate separation of background autofluorescent noise from specific signals of detection (**Figure 14-5**). Most of these reagents suffer from a lack of specificity because almost all will bind both RNA and DNA moieties.

The real advantage of using flow cytometry or other automated methods to detect immature RBCs in the circulation over the manual counting method is in the flexibility of using a multiparameter approach to analysis.[8] This allows for specific analysis of subpopulations of cells with differences in light scatter characteristics (size and granularity) and specific fluorescence (see **Figure 14-5**). In addition, it significantly improves the precision and sensitivity of detection of relatively small populations, with average CVs of less than 10% and sensitivities of less than 0.1%, compared with CVs as high as 40% by manual counting.[91-97]

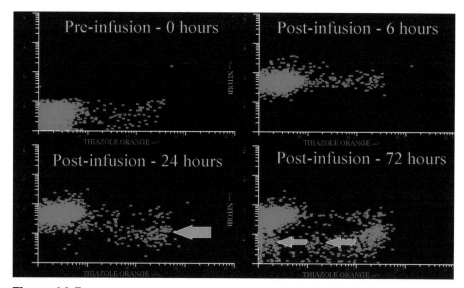

Figure 14-5

Detection of immature red blood cells (reticulocytes) by using flow cytometry with thiazole orange. The red cells are labeled with biotin at 0 hours and detected by means of avidin-fluorescein isothiocyanate. As shown in the *lower right histogram*, the first reticulocytes released from the bone marrow (biotin negative) have a high level of RNA and thiazole orange staining. These cells mature during the subsequent 48 hours. Data provided by Ken Ault, Portland, ME.

The traditional flow cytometry assay for immature RBCs makes use of a single-parameter analysis to plot cell number versus log fluorescent intensity of thiazole orange-stained whole blood preparations.[91] Reticulocytes are identified as having a mean fluorescence intensity of 0.5 to 1.0 log higher than the autofluorescence of normal mature RBCs. Large numbers of cells can be analyzed in a very short time (seconds), with gating parameters usually set for collection of at least 50,000 RBCs. This enables detection of very low numbers of reticulocytes in peripheral blood samples, with an accurate dynamic measurement range of 0.2% to 30% reticulocytes. By determination of the RBC count measured on a clinical hematology analyzer from the same sample, the total reticulocyte count can be determined (**Table 14-14**). This can also be corrected for significant fluctuations in hematocrit levels to yield an accurate assessment of erythropoiesis.

Fluorescence-based reticulocyte analysis also allows for a reporting of the fraction of immature reticulocytes (IRF).[7,97-102] The IRF is a measurement of those reticulocytes being most recently produced by the bone marrow and recognized by the high levels of RNA-related fluorescence (see **Figure 14-5**). The IRF allows for therapeutic monitoring of patients undergoing changes in

Table 14-14
Typical Normal Ranges for Circulating Reticulocytes

Parameter	Normal Range	Dynamic Range
% Reticulocytes	0.2–2%	0.2–30% of RBC
Absolute Reticulocyte Count	$28–120 \times 10^9$/L	$5.5–750 \times 10^9$/L

Table 14-15
Clinical Utility of Immature Reticulocyte Fraction

Clinical condition	Reticulocyte count	IRF
Aplastic anemia/crisis	Low	Low
Hypoplastic anemia	Low	Low
BM regeneration	Low	High/WNL
Chronic disease	Low/WNL	WNL
Iron deficiency	Low/WNL	High
Thalassemia	WNL/high	WNL/high
Folate/B_{12} deficiency	Low/WNL	High
Myelodysplasia	Any level	WNL/high
Hemolytic anemia	High	High
Blood loss/anoxia	WNL/high	high

Abbreviations: BM = bone marrow; WNL = within normal limits.

erythropoiesis and provides the basis for better classification of anemias (**Table 14-15**).[99,102]

Other markers have been used to evaluate the presence and relative concentration of immature RBCs. Two such markers are the transferrin receptor (CD71) and glycophorin A.[103-106] The transferrin receptor is a transmembrane protein that serves as the primary mechanism for iron transport to the intracellular compartment. CD71 is expressed in the cell membrane of reticulocytes. After the binding of iron, the cell is stimulated, and endocytosis of the receptor-ligand complex ensues. Under hemostatic conditions, the reticulocytes can be recognized by the binding of fluorescent antibody to CD71.[103-105] The CD71⁺ reticulocytes represent cells within the immature reticulocyte fraction by all automated methods of fluorescence-based reticulocyte counting. This has been applied to detection of immature RBCs in the bone marrow of patients with myelodysplastic syndrome. Although this approach has the potential to detect circulating reticulocytes, it is limited by the fact that (1) it is influenced by membrane turnover during iron-induced endocytosis and (2) that most other cells also express some level of CD71. Glycophorin A likewise has been used as a cell surface marker for detecting immature RBCs.[30,106] It is a transmembrane sialoglycoprotein that is associated with the expression of blood group antigens (MNS). Glycophorin A is expressed at the early erythroblast stage and is therefore a potential target to detect RBC precursors in the circulation. As with CD71, this marker has not been shown to have good clinical utility in monitoring patients with anemia but has shown promise in bone marrow analysis of myelodysplasia. Identification by means of nucleic acid measurement remains the primary method of choice for reticulocyte detection and quantitation.

Detection of HLA-B27

Although not related to RBC biology, detection of HLA-B27 by flow cytometry has made strides into the routine clinical setting. This section is intended as a brief update of that assay, which is no longer considered a nontraditional test. Because another chapter in this book discusses HLA antigen detection as it relates to transplantation screening, this chapter includes material on HLA-B27 detection as it relates to disease states.

As reviewed in the last edition of this book, the association between HLA expression and specific disease states is well documented, although its significance is controversial. In general, predisposition to disease positively correlates with certain HLA genotypes or genotype groups.[109] HLA genotypes from all classes, including HLA-A, B, C, and D series, have been implicated in certain pathogenic states. One example that illustrates the strong correlation between HLA expression and disease potential is the expression of HLA-B27. This genotype is associated with the development of a group of seronegative arthropathies, including ankylosing spondylitis (AS) and Reiter's syndrome (RS) (**Table 10-8**).[10,113,119-121] From 85% to 95% of the patients with AS exhibit cell surface expression of HLA-B27, compared with a frequency of 4% to 8% in the normal population. HLA-B27 expression is also highly associated with RS (79%), acute anterior uveitis (52%), and juvenile rheumatoid arthritis (25%). Although the majority of individuals (80%) who express HLA-B27 do not manifest these diseases, determination of the HLA-B27 phenotype or genotype in patients with high familial risk factors for AS, or in those patients exhibiting clinical symptoms of the "unspecified" seronegative arthropathies, may help confirm a suspected diagnosis that has not been confirmed by other criteria.

Table 14-16

Association of HLA-B27 with Ankylosing Spondylitis

Population	Parameter	Disease Association (%)
Normal (whites)	HLA-B27+	4–8
Normal (blacks)	HLA-B27+	2–4
HLA-B27+ (all races)	With ankylosing spondylitis	20
HLA-B27+ (all races)	Without ankylosing spondylitis	80
Ankylosing spondylitis (whites)	HLA-B27+	85–95
Ankylosing spondylitis (blacks)	HLA-B27+	57
Reiter's syndrome	HLA-B27+	79
Acute anterior uveitis	HLA-B27+	52

The causative relationship between HLA-B27 expression and disease activity is not yet clear. Current hypotheses are that the molecule could serve as a receptor-like ligand for an unknown etiological element (eg, virus, Klebsiella, environmental toxin), or that it is merely closely genetically linked to another gene involved in the disease.[109,111] The strong familial association of HLA-B27 expression supports the concept of some direct involvement. There are no significant racial or gender preferences in the expression of HLA-B27, although the incidence of AS is higher in males, and the expression of HLA-B27 is lower in blacks without evidence of disease. There is no known predilection for any of the B27 genetic variants or altered epitopes (M1 or M2) for patients with AS or other related diseases. At least one report, however, has identified a subset of AS patients with HLA-C (W1 or W2) antigens without the expression of HLA-B27.[112] Because HLA-CW1 and 2 are commonly associated with HLA-B27 and usually segregate together, the researchers postulated that the putative gene(s) involved in AS or other unspecified spondylitis may reside within the same coding region.

The classical assay for determining the HLA-B27 phenotype has been lymphocytotoxicity.[111-115] Although this is still an important method for serologic determination of the phenotype, recent advances in molecular diagnostics have enabled gene sequencing (so-called PCR-SSP) that provides a complete description of the HLA-ABC genotype. These methods are very time-consuming, expensive, and labor-intensive and are generally applied in the transplant setting to determine donor-recipient histocompatibility (as is reviewed in another chapter of this textbook). A more practical approach for determining disease associations has been the use of flow cytometry for rapid determination of the HLA-B27 phenotype.[117-124]

A simplified flow cytometric assay for HLA-B27 has been devised using fluorochrome-conjugated monoclonal antibodies directed at the B27 epitope.

Early versions of this technique required cell isolation by buffy coat preparations or Ficoll-Hypaque cell separation.[116-118] More recently, improvements in antibody specificity have enabled this technique to be performed with unseparated whole blood specimens.[125-129] To briefly review the technique, small aliquots of peripheral blood (100 ul) are incubated with FITC-conjugated anti-HLA-B27 for 10 to 30 minutes at room temperature and in the dark. An isotype-matched, FITC-conjugated, irrelevant monoclonal antibody is used as a control. This represents a change from previous assays, which required antibodies to HLA framework domains as a control for specificity (see previous edition of this text). After several brief washes, cells are analyzed on the flow cytometer as a single parameter of FITC-fluorescence based on lymphocyte gating (see **Figure 14-6**). Data from the mean peak channel of fluorescence is then calculated to determine the qualitative expression of HLA-B27 (ie, "positive" or "negative").

The clinical cut-off used to indicate a positive B27 phenotype is dependent on the antibody and method used. Most methods use a mean peak fluorescence channel number for positive reactions.[124-128] The peak fluorescence intensity will vary significantly between HLA-B27 positive individuals.[128,130] Comparison with an isotype control is useful to determine the relative amount of autofluorescence, which can vary with cell activation (see **Figure 14-6**).

The fluorescence intensity can be reported as the channel exhibiting the maximum amount of fluorescence of the FITC-histogram (ie, peak channel number), the mean channel of the fluorescent histogram, or the median channel of the fluorescent histogram.[124-128] All reports are dependent on a Gaussian distribution of fluorescent cells passing through the laser of the flow cytometer. In cases where this distribution is skewed due to population heterogeneity or disequilibrium of expression of the B27 antigen, a geometric mean channel number of the fluorescent histogram can be used. An example of using the mean peak channel is shown in **Figure 14-6.** For this example, HLA-B27 expression was based on setting a gate on the lymphoid cells in the peripheral blood from an HLA-B27-negative and an HLA-B27-positive patient. The authors' laboratory uses reference range values of a mean peak channel number < 70 for negative, 70-95 for indeterminate specimens, and > 95 for positive specimens. These values were established by testing patients with variant HLA-B27 expression and confirmed by lymphocytotoxicity. Most HLA-B27-negative patients have a mean peak channel of fluorescence of < 40, and most HLA-B27-positive patients have a mean peak channel of fluorescence of > 130 (with many > 200).

The gating strategy used to identify the population of cells that will be used for HLA-B27 antigen analysis can make a significant difference in the relative proportion and staining intensity of HLA-B27-positive cells in a sample. Some

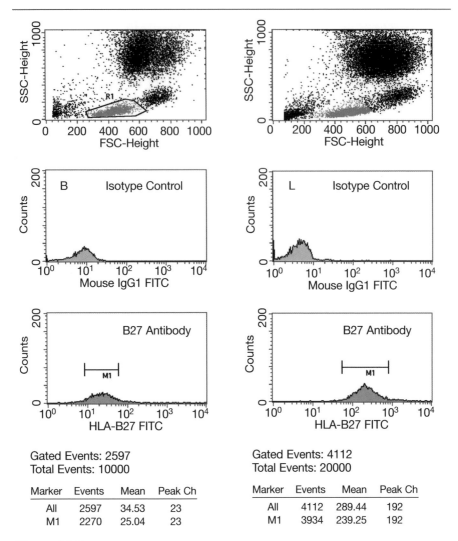

Figure 14-6
Illustration of an HLA-B27-negative (a, b, c) and an HLA-B27-positive (d, e, f) patient. The monoclonal antibody used was clone FD705. Negative = a mean peak channel < 70; Indeterminate = a mean peak channel of 71-95; Positive = a mean peak channel > 95. In this example, the B27-negative patient had a mean peak channel of 25 (peak = 23) (c); the B27-positive patient had a mean peak channel of 235 (mean = 192) (f).

methods use gating of the lymphoid cells using 2-parameter dot plots of forward versus right-angle light scatter (as in **Figure 14-6**).[125,131-133] Other methods advocate a combination of lymphocyte gating based on light scatter to identify the lymphocytes and a secondary gate that selects only the CD-3 positive T-cells for analysis.[126-128,130] Both strategies have advantages; the former is more cost-effective because not as many antibodies are required, and the latter is able to reduce background autofluorescence and the amount of cross-reactivity. Because the relative fluorescence of HLA-B27 can vary between individuals, cell types, states of cell activation, and allele expression, the quantitation of fluorescence must be validated through lymphocytotoxicity or PCR-SSP genotyping by each individual laboratory in order to determine a reliable reference or cut-off range.[116,128,133-135] Chen et al have used the number of molecules of equivalent soluble fluorochrome (MESF) expressed on cells rather than the mean channel number as a determinant for B27-positivity.[130] This process entails using inert beads with known amounts of fluorescent molecules to standardize the fluorescent intensity. Software is also commercially available (by such suppliers as Becton-Dickinson) which automatically calculates the percent-positive cells based on calibration to an internal standard of fluorescent beads.[126] All these techniques have shown relatively good correlation with lymphocytotoxicity, and range in clinical sensitivity from 95%-97%.

Antibody specificity is also a concern when doing HLA-B27 assays by flow cytometry. Most antibodies for detecting B27 have some cross-reactivity to other HLA-B determinants (see **Table 14-17**); these are known as the *cross-reactive groups* (CREGs).[128,131-133] The most common known cross-reactivities of HLA-B27 antibodies are to CREGs of HLA-B7, and consist of cross-reactive epitopes from HLA-B7, B13, B22, B40, B41, B42, B44, B47, B48, and B57. The most problematic cross-reactivities because of their relatively high frequencies in the population are B7, B44, and B57. In addition, some antibodies react differently with allelic variants of HLA-B27 antigen (see **Table 14-17**).[133,134] These cross-reactivities usually result in intermediate increases in fluorescent intensity, which can be mistakenly interpreted as positive reactions (see **Figure 14-7a and b**).

The cross-reactivity of HLA-B27 antibodies with other HLA-B antigenic determinants and the varied reactivity with allelic variants of B27 antigens are dependent on the clone of HLA-B27 antibody that is used (**Table 14-17**).[128,131-133] For example, clone HLA-ABC-m3 is known to recognize epitopes on both HLA-B27 and HLA-B7 molecules, while clone FD705 may react with B27 and B44. Clone FD705 may not react with allelic variant 2708.[133,134] These differences in antibody specificity can result in equivocal or even false-positive and false-negative reactions (see **Figure 14-7a and b**). For this reason, most laboratories have established an equivocal or indeterminate range of mean peak channel fluorescence values, which require some other method for verification. The authors' indeterminate range (ie, "gray zone") is a mean peak channel fluorescence of 71-95; any results in this range are verified as HLA-B27-positive or -negative by lymphocytotoxicity.

Table 14-17

Cross-Reactive Epitopes and Allele Associations of Monoclonal Antibodies to HLA-B27

HLA-B7 (CREG) or Other Related Antigen	Monoclonal Antibody Clone			
	FD705	ABC-m3	GS145.2	FH1503
7	-	+	+	+
13		+		
22		+	+	
27	+	+	+	+
37	+	+	+	
39			+	
41			+	
42		+		
44	+	+	+	-
55			+	
57	+			
60				
62				
73		+		

HLA-B27 Allele				
2701	+			
2702	+/-	+	+	
2703	+	+/-	+	
2704	+		+	
2705	+	+	+	
2706	+	+	+	
2707	+			
2708	-	+		

A practical approach to eliminating false-positive HLA-B27 results is to use multiple monoclonal antibodies to determine whether the reactivity is specific.[128,132-134] This is much less expensive and much more rapid than relying on lymphocytotoxicity or DNA sequencing. An example is shown in **Figure 14-7a and b.** Two different B27 antibodies were used to verify B27 specificity in 3 patients with varying HLA haplotypes. This approach was able to correctly identify 2 patients who could have been incorrectly classified as HLA-B27-positive. Clone FD705 is known to react with CREGs of B27 and B44, while clone FH1453 is known to react with B7 and B27. Patients with the B7 or B44 antigen can be eliminated as false-positives by this approach. The use of multiple antibodies is common among labs doing HLA-B27 determinations, and has been used to correctly identify > 97% of HLA-B27-positive patients as part of an

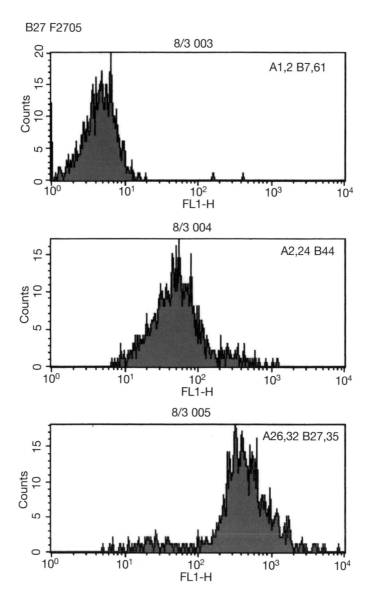

Figure 14-7a

Illustration of monoclonal anti-HLA-B27 (clone F2705) cross-reactivity with other related epitopes (eg, B44). Note lack of cross-reactivity with HLA-B7. (Data provided by Jar-How Lee, PhD [dip. ABHI] and Rui Pei, PhD, One-Lambda, Inc., Canoga Park, CA.)

international quality assurance study.[133] This approach is supported by the American Society for Histology and Immunology and the College of American Pathologists (ASHI/CAP).

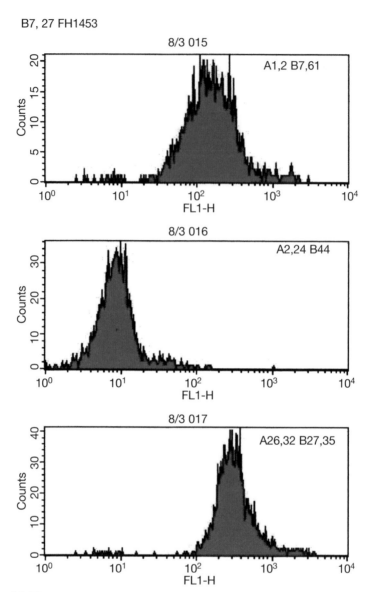

B7, 27 FH1453

Figure 14-7b

Illustration of monoclonal anti-HLA-B27 (clone FD 1453) cross-reactivity with other related epitopes (eg, B7). Note lack of cross-reactivity with HLA-B44. (Data provided by Jar-How Lee, PhD [dip. ABHI] and Rui Pei, PhD, One-Lambda, Inc., Canoga Park, CA.)

With the availability of multiple antibodies and varied criteria for cut-off ranges in flow cytometric HLA-B27 assays, quality control and quality assurance issues are important factors in implementing HLA-B27 testing routinely in the clinical laboratory.[133,135] Positive, negative, or isotope control specimens should always be used for comparison with patient results. These are easily obtainable from human patients, and antigenic expression is relatively stable in cryopreserved lymphocytes. Participation in external proficiency testing surveys is also available through ASHI/CAP in the USA and the Foundation of Quality Control in Medical Immunology (SKMI) and the Belgian Association for Cytometry (BUC/ABC) in Europe. Review of ASHI/CAP performance results indicates that most labs and methods can correctly identify B27-positive individuals; however, reporting of false-positive and false-negative results is not uncommon.[135] This point was echoed in a recent review by Levering et al of an external quality assurance program in the Netherlands for HLA-B27 phenotyping by flow cytometry.[133] While there was excellent concordance (95%) among the 36-47 participating labs in the reporting of HLA-B27-positive patients, there were sufficient false-positive results in the HLA-B27-negative specimens to cause alarm (53-70% concordance). Use of the multiple B27 antibody approach proved to significantly improve the concordance for these samples and reduce the level of false reporting. The conclusion of all the participants in this study was that HLA-B27 typing by flow cytometry can be significantly improved by (1) application of quantitative parameters to standardize the distinction between relatively dim (cross-reactive) and strong (true-positive) signals, (2) complete documentation of the reactivity of all defined HLA-B27 alleles, and (3) rigorous analysis of the cross-reactive patterns of the available monoclonal anti-HLA-B27 antibodies with HLA antigens other than B27.[133] Reliance on lymphocytotoxicity and molecular typing should also always be considered for result verification.

The advent of microarray technology and other rapid assays for molecular sequencing may provide many new advances in clinical diagnosis in the future. Because DNA sequencing is becoming the ultimate, "gold standard" assay in HLA genotyping for transplant biology, development of these techniques may also become a valuable approach to HLA-B27 screening and analysis. Given the variations between HLA-B27 assays currently being used in flow cytometry, molecular analysis may provide a more definitive method of analysis, especially in cases of questionable positivity. This approach could also identify allelic variants that could be incorrectly classified with current flow cytometric methods. Until such advances are made available, however, flow cytometry remains an economical, rapid, and accurate approach for the majority of patients requiring HLA-B27 phenotyping.

Summary

The incorporation of new methodologies into laboratories performing routine flow cytometric assays is difficult to accomplish. Issues regarding standardization of methods, quality control, proficiency testing, and reimbursements limit the easy transfer of new technologies. The assays described in this chapter have significant potential to meet the criteria necessary for routine testing. Quality control suggestions were indicated, and guidelines have been proposed for all aspects of RBC biology and HLA-B27 assessment.[107,108,133,135] The next wave of potential applications will certainly involve issues of molecular diagnosis and cytokine immunobiology. The future is bright for growth and development in exploitation of flow cytometry technologies for use in clinical diagnosis.

References

1. Van der Meulen FW, de Bruin HG, Goosen PCM, et al. Quantitative aspects of the destruction of red cells sensitized with IgG1 autoantibodies: an application of flow cytometry. *Br J Haematol.* 1980;46:47-56.

2. Nance SJ, Garratty G. Application of flow cytometry to immunohematology. *J Immunol Methods.* 1987;101:127-131.

3. Garratty G, Arndt P. Applications of flow cytometry to transfusion science. *Transfusion.* 1995;35:157-178.

4. Berneman ZN, van Bockstaele DR, Uyttenbroeck WM, et al. Flow cytometric analysis of erythrocyte blood group A antigen density profile. *Vox Sang.* 1991;61:265-274.

5. Freedman J, Lazarus AH. Applications of flow cytometry in transfusion medicine. *Transfusion Med Rev.* 1995;9:87-109.

6. Garratty G, Arndt PA. Applications of flow cytofluorometry to red blood cell immunology. *Cytometry.* 1999;38:259-267.

7. Davis BH. Immature reticulocyte fraction (IRF): by any name, a useful clinical parameter of erythropoietic activity. *Lab Hematol.* 1996;2:2-8.

8. Tsuji T, Sakata T, Hamaguchi Y, et al. New rapid flow cytometric method for the enumeration of nucleated red blood cells. *Cytometry.* 1999;37:291-301.

9. De Man AJM, Foolen WJG, van Dijk, et al. A fluorescent microsphere method for the investigation of erythrocyte chimaerism after allogeneic bone marrow transplantation using antigenic differences. *Vox Sang.* 1988;55:37-41.

10. Hall SE, Rosse WF. The use of monoclonal antibodies and flow cytometry in the diagnosis of paroxysmal nocturnal hemoglobinuria. *Blood.* 1996;87:5332-5340.

11. Davis BH, Olsen S, Bigelow NC, et al. Detection of fetal red cells in fetomaternal hemorrhage using fetal hemoglobin monoclonal antibody by flow cytometry. *Transfusion.* 1998;38:749-756.

12. Garratty G. The significance of IgG on the red cell surface. *Transfusion Med Rev.* 1987;1:47-57.

13. Garratty G. Effect of cell-bound proteins on the in vivo survival of circulating blood cells. *Gerontology.* 1991;37:68-94.

14. Garratty G. Factors affecting the pathogenicity of red cell auto- and alloantibodies. In: Nance SJ, ed. *Immune Destruction of Red Blood Cells.* Arlington, Va. American Association of Blood Banks; 1989:109-169.

15. Garratty G. Autoimmune hemolytic anemia. In: Garratty G, ed. *Immunobiology of Transfusion Medicine.* New York, NY: Dekker; 1993:493-521.

16. Garratty G, Arndt P, Domen R, et al. Severe autoimmune hemolytic anemia associated with IgM warm autoantibodies directed against determinants on or associated with glycophorin A. *Vox Sang.* 1997;72:124-130.

17. Magnani M, Papa S, Rossi L, et al. Membrane-bound immunoglobulin increase during red blood cell aging. *Acta Haematol (Basel).* 1988;79:127-132.

18. Nicholson G, Lawrence A, Ala FA, et al. Semi-quantitative assay of D antigen site density by flow cytometry analysis. *Transfusion Med.* 1991;1:87-90.

19. Petz LD, Yam P, Wilkinson L, et al. Increased IgG molecules bound to the surface of red blood cells of patients with sickle cell anemia. *Blood.* 1984;64:301-304.

20. Green GA. Autologous IgM, IgA, and complement binding to sickle erythrocytes in vivo. Evidence for the existence of dense sickle cell subsets. *Blood.* 1993;82:985-992.

21. Garratty G, Nance SJ. Correlation between in vivo hemolysis and the amount of red cell-bound IgG measured by flow cytometry. *Transfusion.* 1990;30:617-621.

22. Austin EB, McIntosh Y, Hodson C, et al. Anti-D quantification by flow cytometry: an alternative to the Autoanalyser? *Transfusion Med.* 1995;5:203-208.

23. Christensson M, Bremme K, Shanwell A, et al. Flow cytometric quantitation of serum anti-D in pregnancy. *Transfusion.* 1996;36:500-505.

24. Hilden, J-O, Backteman K, Nilsson J, et al. Flow-cytometric quantitation of anti-D antibodies. *Vox Sang.* 1997;72:172-176.

25. Nelson M, Popp H, Forsyth C, et al. Rapid quantitation of mixed red cell populations using flow cytometry. *Clin Lab Haematol.* 1996;18:207-213.

26. Blanchard D, Bruneau, V, Bernard D, et al. Flow cytometry analysis of dual red blood cell populations after bone marrow transplantation. *Br J Haematol.* 1995;89:741-747.

27. Wagner FF, Flegel WA. Analysis by flow cytometry of chimerism after bone-marrow transplantation and erythrocyte antigen density. In: Gutensohn K, Sonneborn HH, Kuhnl P, eds. *Aspects of the Flow-Cytometric Analysis of Red Blood Cells.* Heidelberg, Germany: Clin Lab Publications; 1997:95-103.

28. Sebring E, Polesky H. Fetomaternal hemorrhage: incidence, risk factors, time of occurrence, and clinical effects. *Transfusion*. 1990;30:344-357.

29. Nelson M, Zarkos K, Popp H, et al. A flow-cytometric equivalent of the Kleihauer test. *Vox Sang*. 1998;75:234-241.

30. Lloyd-Evans P, Guest AR, Austin EB, et al. Use of a phycoerythrin-conjugated anti-glycophorin A monoclonal antibody as a double label to improve the accuracy of FMH quantification by flow cytometry. *Transfusion Med*. 1999;9:155-160.

31. Campbell TA, Ware RE, Mason M. Detection of hemoglobin variants in erythrocytes by flow cytometry. *Cytometry*. 1999;35:242-248.

32. Chen JC, Bigelow N, Davis BH. Novel and simplified method for the flow cytometric determination of F cells. *Cytometry*. 2000. Submitted for publication.

33. Cohen F, Zeuler WW, Gustafson DC, et al. Mechanisms of isoimmunization. I. The transplacental passage of fetal erythrocytes in homospecific pregnancies. *Blood*. 1964;23:621-646.

34. Polesky H, Sebring E. Evaluation of methods for detection and quantitation of fetal cells and their effect on RhIgG usage. *Am J Clin Pathol*. 1981;76:525-529.

35. Sebring E, Polesky H. Detection of fetal maternal hemorrhage in Rh immune globulin candidates. A rosetting technique using enzyme-treated Rh^2 indicator erythrocytes. *Transfusion*. 1982;22:468-471.

36. Bayliss KM, Kueck BD, Johnson ST, et al. Detecting fetomaternal hemorrhage: a comparison of five methods. *Transfusion*. 1991;31:303-307.

37. Kleihauer E, Braun H, Betke K. Demonstration of fetal hemoglobin in erythrocytes of a blood smear. *Klin Wochenschr*. 1957;35:637-638.

38. Riley J, Ness P, Taddie S, et al. Detection and quantitation of fetal maternal hemorrhage utilizing an enzyme-linked antiglobulin test. *Transfusion*. 1982;22:472-474.

39. Greenwalt TJ, Dumaswala UJ, Domino MM. The quantification of fetomaternal hemorrhage by an enzyme-linked antibody test with glutaraldehyde fixation. *Vox Sang*. 1992;63:268-271.

40. Nance SJ, Nelson JM, Arndt PA, et al. Quantitation of fetal-maternal hemorrhage by flow cytometry. A simple and accurate method. *Am J Clin Pathol*. 1989;91:288-292.

41. Nelson M, Popp H, Horky K, et al. Development of a flow cytometric test for the detection of D-positive fetal cells after fetomaternal hemorrhage and a survey of the prevalence in D-negative women. *Immunohematology*. 1994;10:55-59.

42. Lloyd-Evans P, Kumpel BM, Bromelow I, et al. Use of a directly conjugated monoclonal anti-D (BRAD-3) for quantification of fetomaternal hemorrhage by flow cytometry. *Transfusion*. 1996;36:432-437.

43. Bianchi D, Zickwolf G, Yih M, et al. Erythroid-specific antibodies enhance detection of fetal nucleated erythrocytes in maternal blood. *Prenat Diagn*. 1993;13:293-300.

44. Johnson PR, Tait RC, Austin EB, et al. Flow cytometry in diagnosis and management of large fetomaternal hemorrhage. *J Clin Pathol*. 1995;48:1005-1008.

45. Thorpe SJ, Thein SL, Sampietro M, et al. Immunochemical estimation of haemoglobin types in red blood cells by FACS analysis. *Br J Haematol*. 1994;87:125-132.

46. Zheng YL, Demaria M, Zhen D, et al. Flow sorting of fetal erythroblasts using intracytoplasmic anti-fetal haemoglobin: preliminary observations on maternal samples. *Prenat Diagn.* 1995;15:897-905.

47. Demaria M, Zheng Y, Zhen D, et al. Improved fetal nucleated erythrocyte sorting purity using intracellular antifetal hemoglobin and Hoechst 33342. *Cytometry.* 1996;25:37-45.

48. Navenot JM, Muller JY, Blanchard D. Expression of blood group i antigen and fetal hemoglobin in paroxysmal nocturnal hemoglobinuria. *Transfusion.* 1997;37:291-297.

49. Bromilow IM, Dugguid JK. Measurement of feto-maternal haemorrhage: a comparative study of three Kleihauer techniques and two flow cytometry methods. *Clin Lab Haematol.* 1997;19:137-142.

50. Rosse WF. Paroxysmal nocturnal hemoglobinuria. In: *Clinical Immunohematology: Basic Concepts and Clinical Applications.* Oxford: Blackwell Scientific Publications; 1990:593.

51. Rosse WF. Paroxysmal nocturnal hemoglobinuria. In: Hoffman R, Benz, EJ, Shattil SJ, et al, eds. *Hematology: Basic Principles and Practice.* 2nd ed. New York, NY: Churchill Livingstone; 1995:370-381.

52. Beutler E. Paroxysmal nocturnal hemoglobinuria. In: Beutler E, Lichtman MA, Coller BS, Kipps TJ, eds. *Williams Hematology.* 5th ed. New York, NY: McGraw-Hill; 1995:252-256.

53. Rosse WF, Dacie JV. Immune lysis of normal human and paroxysmal nocturnal hemoglobinuria (PNH) red blood cells. I. The sensitivity of PNH red cells to lysis by complement and specific antibody. *J Clin Invest.* 1966;45:736-748.

54. Rosse WF. Phosphatidylinositol-linked proteins and paroxysmal nocturnal hemoglobinuria. *Blood.* 1990;75:1595-1601.

55. Low MG, Finean JB. Release of alkaline phosphatase from membranes by a phosphatidylinositol-specific phospholipase C. *Biochem J.* 1977;167:281-284.

56. Auditore JV, Hartmann RC, Flexner JM, et al. The erythrocyte acetylcholinesterase enzyme in paroxysmal nocturnal hemoglobinuria. *Arch Pathol.* 1960;69:534-543.

57. Hirose S, Rav L, Prince GM, et al. Synthesis of mannosylglucosaminylinositol phospholipids in normal but not paroxysmal nocturnal hemoglobinuria cells. *Proc Natl Acad Sci USA.* 1992;89:6025-6029.

58. Takeda J, Miyata T, Kawagoe K, et al. Deficiency of the GPI anchor caused by a somatic mutation of the PIG-A gene in paroxysmal nocturnal hemoglobinuria. *Cell.* 1993;73:703-711.

59. Miyata T, Takeda J, Iida Y, et al. The cloning of PIG-A, a component in the early step of GPI-anchor biosynthesis. *Science.* 1993;259:1318-1320.

60. DeGasperi R, Thomas LJ, Sugiyama E, et al. Correction of a defect in mammalian GPI anchor biosynthesis by a transfected yeast gene. *Science.* 1990;250:988-991.

61. Norris J, Hall S, Ware RE, et al. Glycosyl-phosphatidylinositol anchor synthesis in paroxysmal nocturnal hemoglobinuria: partial or complete defect in an early step. *Blood.* 1994;83:816-821.

62. Bessler M, Mason PJ, Hillmen P, et al. Paroxysmal nocturnal hemoglobinuria (PNH) is caused by somatic mutations in the PIG-A gene. *EMBO J.* 1994;13:110-117.

63. Miyata T, Yamada N, Iida Y, et al. Abnormalities of PIG-A transcripts in granulocytes from patients with paroxysmal nocturnal hemoglobinuria. *N Engl J Med.* 1994;330:249-255.

64. Ware RE, Rosse WF, Howard TA. Mutations within the Piga gene in patients with paroxysmal nocturnal hemoglobinuria. *Blood.* 1994;83:2418-2422.

65. Nicholson-Weller A, March JP, Rosenfeld SI, et al. Affected erythrocytes of patients with paroxysmal nocturnal hemoglobinuria are deficient in the complement regulatory protein, decay accelerating factor. *Proc Natl Acad Sci USA.* 1983;80:5066-5070.

66. Holguin MH, Wilcox LA, Bernshaw NJ, et al. Relationship between the membrane inhibitor of reactive lysis and the erythrocyte phenotypes of paroxysmal nocturnal hemoglobinuria. *J Clin Invest.* 1989;84:1387-1394.

67. Shichishima T, Terasawa T, Saitoh Y, et al. Diagnosis of paroxysmal nocturnal haemoglobinuria by phenotypic analysis of erythrocytes using two-color flow cytometry with monoclonal antibodies to DAF and CD59/MACIF. *Br J Haematol.* 1993;85:378-386.

68. Rollins SA, Zhao J, Ninomiya H, et al. Inhibition of homologous complement by CD59 is mediated by a species-selective recognition conferred through binding to C8 within C5b-8 or C9 within C5b-9. *J Immunol.* 1991;146:2345-2351.

69. Merry AH, Rawlinson VI, Uchikawa M, et al. Studies on the sensitivity to complement-mediated lysis of erythrocytes (Inab phenotype) with a deficiency of DAF (decay accelerating factor). *Br J Haematol.* 1989;73:248-253.

70. Yamashina M, Ueda E, Kinoshita T, et al. Inherited complete deficiency of 20-kilodalton homologous restriction factor (CD59) as a cause of paroxysmal nocturnal hemoglobinuria. *N Engl J Med.* 1990;323:1184-1189.

71. Wilcox LA, Ezzell JL, Bernshaw NJ, et al. Molecular basis of the enhanced susceptibility of the erythrocytes of paroxysmal nocturnal hemoglobinuria to hemolysis in acidified serum. *Blood.* 1991;78:820-829.

72. Hartmann RC, Jenkins DE Jr. The "sugar-water" test for paroxysmal nocturnal hemoglobinuria. *N Engl J Med.* 1965;275:155-157.

73. Hartmann RC. Diagnostic specificity of the sucrose hemolysis test for paroxysmal nocturnal hemoglobinuria. *Blood.* 1970;35:462-475.

74. Rosse WF. Variations in the red cells in paroxysmal nocturnal hemoglobinuria. *Br J Haematol.* 1973;24:327-342.

75. Rosse WF, Hoffman S, Campbell M, et al. The erythrocytes in paroxysmal nocturnal hemoglobinuria of intermediate sensitivity to complement lysis. *Br J Haematol.* 1991;79:99-107.

76. Schubert J, Alvarado M, Uciechowski P, et al. Diagnosis of paroxysmal nocturnal haemoglobinuria using immunophenotyping of peripheral blood cells. *Br J Haematol.* 1991;79:487-492.

77. Van der Schoot CE, Huizinga TW, van't Veer Korthof ET, et al. Deficiency of glycosyl-phosphatidylinositol-linked membrane glycoproteins of leukocytes in paroxysmal nocturnal hemoglobinuria, description of a new diagnostic cytofluorometric assay. *Blood.* 1990;76:1853-1859.

78. Nagakura S, Nakakuma H, Horikawa K, et al. Expression of decay-accelerating factor and CD59 in lymphocyte subsets in healthy individuals and paroxysmal nocturnal hemoglobinuria patients. *Am J Hematol.* 1993;43:14-18.

79. Nebe CT. Paroxysmal nocturnal hemoglobinuria: clinical aspects and flow cytometric analysis. In: Gutensohn K, Sonneborn HH, Kuhnl P, eds. *Aspects of the Flow-Cytometric Analysis of Red Blood Cells.* Heidelberg, Germany: Clin Lab Publications; 1997:81-94.

80. Navenot JM, Muller JY, Blanchard D. Investigation of the survival of paroxysmal nocturnal hemoglobinuria red cells through the immunophenotyping of reticulocytes. *Transfusion.* 1998;88:337-342.

81. Schwartz FO, Stanbury F. Significance of nucleated red blood cells in peripheral blood. *JAMA.* 1954;154:1339-1340.

82. Cline M, Berlin N. The reticulocyte count as an indicator of the rate of erythropoiesis. *Am J Clin Pathol.* 1963;39:121-128.

83. Hillman R, Finch C. Erythropoiesis: normal and abnormal. *Semin Hematol.* 1967;4:327.

84. Hillman R. Characteristics of marrow production and reticulocyte maturation in normal man in response to anemia. *J Clin Invest.* 1969;48:443-453.

85. Weick JK, Hagedorn AB, Linman JW. Leukoerythroblastosis: diagnostic and prognostic significance. *Mayo Clin Proc.* 1974;49:110-113.

86. Van Assendelft OW. Anemia and polycythemia. Interpretation of laboratory tests and differential diagnosis. In: Koepke JA, ed. *Laboratory Hematology.* New York, NY: Churchill-Livingstone, Inc; 1984:865-901.

87. Tarallo P, Humbert J-C, Mahassen P, et al. Reticulocytes: biological variations and reference limits. *Eur J Haematol.* 1994;53:11-15.

88. Houwen B. Reticulocyte maturation. *Blood Cells.* 1992;18:167-186.

89. Watanabe K, Kawai Y, Takeuchi K, et al. Reticulocyte maturity as an indicator for estimating qualitative abnormality of erythropoiesis. *J Clin Pathol.* 1994;47:736-739.

90. Gilmer PR Jr, Koepke JA. The reticulocyte. An approach to definition. *Am J Clin Pathol.* 1976;66:262-267.

91. Hanson CA. Reticulocyte analysis by flow cytometry. In: Keren DF, Hanson CA, Hurtubise PE, eds. *Flow Cytometry and Clinical Diagnosis.* Chicago, Ill: ASCP Press; 1994:368-389.

92. Davis BH, Bigelow NC. Flow cytometric reticulocyte quantification using thiazole orange provides clinically useful reticulocyte maturity index. *Arch Pathol Lab Med.* 1989;113:684-689.

93. Spanish Multicenter Study Group for Hematologic Recovery. Flow cytometric reticulocyte quantification in the evaluation of hematologic recovery. *Eur J Haematol.* 1995;53:293-297.

94. Kanold J, Bezou M, Coulet M, et al. Evaluation of erythropoietic/hematopoietic reconstitution after BMT by highly fluorescent reticulocyte counts compares favorably with traditional peripheral blood cell counting. *Bone Marrow Transplant.* 1993;11:313-318.

95. ICSH expert Panel on Cytometry. Guidelines for the evaluation of blood cell analyzers including those used for differential leukocyte and reticulocyte counting and cell marker applications. *Clin Lab Haematol.* 1994;16:157-62.

96. Weber N, Mast BJ, Houwen B. Performance evaluation of hematology analyzers: an outline for clinical laboratory testing. *Sysmex J Int.* 1995;5:103-113.

97. Paterakis G, Kossivas L, Kendall R, et al. Comparative evaluation of the erythroblast count generated by three-color fluorescence flow cytometry, the Abbott CELL-DYN 4000 hematology analyzer, and microscopy. *Lab Hematol.* 1998;4:64-70.

98. Davis BH, Bigelow NC. Automated reticulocyte analysis: clinical practice and associated new parameters. *Hematol Oncol Clin North Am.* 1994;8:617-630.

99. Davis BH, Ornvold K, Bigelow NC. Flow cytometric reticulocyte maturity index: a useful laboratory parameter of erythropoietic activity in anemia. *Cytometry.* 1995;22:35-39.

100. Davis BH, Bigelow NC, Van Hove L. Immature reticulocyte fraction (IRF) and reticulocyte counts: comparison of CELL-DYN 4000, Sysmex R-3000, thiazole flow cytometry, and manual counts. *Lab Hematol.* 1996;2:144-150.

101. Davis BH. Immature reticulocyte fraction: a clinically useful laboratory parameter by any other name. *Lab Hematol.* 1996;2:2-8.

102. Davis BH, Bigelow NC, Van Hove L, et al. Evaluation of automated reticulocyte analysis with immature reticulocyte fraction as a potential outcomes indicator in anemia of chronic renal failure. *Lab Hematol.* 1998;4:169-175.

103. Bianchi D, Yih M, Zickwolf G, et al. Transferrin receptor (CD71) expression on circulating mononuclear cells during pregnancy. *Am J Obstet Gynecol.* 1994;170:202-206.

104. Himmelfarb J, Connerney M, Mitchell J, et al. Increased transferrin receptor expression on reticulocytes is an early indicator of response to erythropoietin. *Lab Hematol.* 1995;1:105-111.

105. Bianchi DW, Klinger KW, Vadnais TJ, et al. Development of a model system to compare cell separation methods for the isolation of fetal cells from maternal blood. *Prenat Diagn.* 1996;16:289-298.

106. Rasamoelisolo M, Czerwinski M, Bruneau V, et al. Fine characterization of a series of new monoclonal antibodies directed against glycophorin A. *Vox Sang.* 1997;72:185-191.

107. Koepke JA, Broden PN, Corash L, et al. Methods for reticulocyte counting (flow cytometry and supravital dyes). Approved guideline; 1997. *NCCLS Document No. H44-A* 17(15), NCCLS, Wayne, PA.

108. Chen JC, Bigelow NC, Davis BH. Proposed flow cytometric reference method for erythroid F cell counting. *Cytometry.* 2000;42:239-246.

109. Svejgaard A. HLA and disease. In: Rose NR, Friedman HF, Fahey JL, eds. *Manual of Clinical Laboratory Immunology.* 3rd ed. Washington, DC: ASM; 1986.

110. Kahn MA, Skosey JL. Ankylosing spondylitis and related spondyloarthropathies. In: Sampter, Talmadge, Frank, et al, eds. *Immunological Diseases*, 4th ed. Boston: Little, Brown and Co; 1988.

111. Brewerton DA, Caffrey M. Hart FD, et al. Ankylosing spondylitis and HL-A 27. *Lancet.* 1973;1:904-907.

112. Schlosstein L, Terasaki PI, Bluestone R, et al. High association of HL-A antigen, W27, with ankylosing spondylitis. *N Engl J Med.* 1973;288:704-7109.

113. Svejgaard A, Platz P, Ryder LP. HLA and disease 1982 – a survey. *Immunol Rev.* 1983;70:193-218.

114. Duquesnoy RJ, Kosin F. HLA-B27, CW1 and CW2 in seronegative spondyloarthritis. *Tissue Antigens.* 1989;10:188.

115. Terasaki PI, McClelland JD. Microdroplet assay of human serum cytotoxins. *Nature.* 1964;204:998-1000.

116. Bonnaud G, Aupetit C, et al. Optimisation of HLA-B27 testing by association of flow cytometry and DNA typing. *Clin Rheumatol.* 1999;18:23-27.

117. Albrecht J, Muller HAG. HLA-B27 typing by use of flow cytometry. *Clin Chem.* 1987;33:1619-1623.

118. Shapira D, Sullivan J, Hooper K. HLA-B27 typing using flow cytometry. *Cytometry.* 1991;5:79. Abstract 398B.

119. Alexander T. HLA B-27 identification by indirect immunofluorescence. *Procedure Manual.* Akron, OH: Akron City Hospital; 1990.

120. Sumida SE, Hansen J, Lefor W. Evaluation of a direct immunofluorescence test for HLA-B27. *Proceedings of the 5th Medical Laboratory Immunology Symposium*, Abst. MS-8, Williamsburg, VA 1987.

121. Kemple K, Bluestone R. The histocompatability complex and rheumatic diseases. *Med Clin North Am.* 1977;61:331.

122. Trucco M, dePetris S, Garotta G, et al. Quantitative analysis of cell surface HLA structures by means of monoclonal antibodies. *Hum Immunol.* 1980;3:233.

123. McGuigan LE, Geczy AF, Edmonds JP. The immunopathology of ankylosing spondylitis—a review. *Semin Arthritis Rheum.* 1985;15:81.

124. Pei R, Arjomand-Shamsai, et al. A monospecific HLA-B27 fluorescein isothiocyanate-conjugated monoclonal antibody for rapid, simple, and accurate HLA-B27 typing. *Tissue Antigens.* 1993;41:200-203.

125. Orr K, Glen TD, Alfa M. Utilization of commercial antisera and flow cytometry in HLA-B27 typing. *Cytometry.* 1994;18:17-20.

126. Hulstaert F, Albrecht J, Hannet I, et al. An optimized method for routine HLA-B27 screening using flow cytometry. *Cytometry.* 1994;18:21-29.

127. Lingenfelter B, Fuller TC, Hartung L et al. HLA-B27 screening by flow cytometry. *Cytometry.* 1995;22:146-149.

128. Neumuller J, Schwartz DWM, Dauber E, et al. Evaluation of four monoclonal antibodies against HLA-B27 for their reliability in HLA-B27 typing with flow cytometry (FC): comparison with the classic microlymphocytotoxic test (MLCT*). Cytometry.* 1996;26:209-215.

129. Horsburgh T, Martin S, Robson AJ. The application of flow cytometry to histo-compatibility testing. *Transpl Immunol.* 2000;8:3-15.

130. Chen JC, Davis BH, Bigelow NC, et al. Flow cytometric HLA-B27 typing using CD3 gating and molecules of equivalent soluble fluorochrome (MESF) quantitation. *Cytometry.* 1996;26:286-292.

131. Ward AM, Nikaein A. Comparison of monoclonal antibodies for flow cytometric analysis of HLA-B27 antigen. *Cytometry.* 1995;22:65-69.

132. Hoffmann J, Janssen W. HLA-B27 phenotyping with flow cytometry: further improvement by multiple monoclonal antibodies. *Clin Chem.* 1997;43:1975-1981.

133. Levering W, van den Beemd R, te Marvelde JG, et al. External quality assessment of flow cytometric HLA-B27 typing. *Cytometry.* 2000;42:95-105.

134. Coates E, Darke C. Routine HLA-B27 typing by flow cytometry: differentiation of the products of HLA-B*2702, B*2705, and B*2708. *Eur J Immunogenet.* 1998;25:29-37.

135. Warzynski MJ. HLA-B27 testing: mean channels, QC, and surveys. *Cytometry.* 1997;30:208-211.

15

Enumeration of CD34+ Stem Cells

J. Philip McCoy, Jr.

Introduction

The hematopoietic pluripotent stem cell is of increasing interest to both researchers and clinicians as it gains therapeutic application. Stem cells, derived from bone marrow, peripheral blood, and even cord blood, are being used extensively in stem cell transplantation therapy for a wide variety of malignant and nonmalignant diseases. The success of engraftment and the prompt reconstitution of the hematopoietic system has been linked to the number of stem cells used for transplantation. Therefore there is a need for accurate stem cell enumeration to obtain effective, reproducible, clinical results. Before immunophenotyping studies, the most widely accepted method of stem cell enumeration was accomplished through in vitro colony-forming methods, including the commonly used granulocyte-macrophage colony-forming unit.[1,2] In general, these studies were time-consuming, variable, and expensive to perform. Therefore flow cytometric enumeration of stem cells, which is capable of rapid detection of infrequent types of cells, became a highly desirable assay to develop.[3] One key to the flow cytometric detection and enumeration of hematopoietic stem cells was the discovery of the appropriate antigen or antigens that uniquely distinguished stem cells from other hematopoietic and nonhematopoietic cells.

What is a Stem Cell?

The term *stem cell* is generally used to identify hematopoietic cells capable of reconstituting the immune system of an immunocompromised host. The most primitive hematopoietic stem cell, referred to as the pluripotent stem cell, is capable of both self-replication and of yielding mature cells in all hematopoietic lineages.[4] Later, more mature stem cells are also present, and these are the progenitors for cells of more limited predetermined lineages. This distinction between the ultimate pluripotent stem cell and later, more mature stem cells has been and remains the source of much controversy. Often, the term *CD34+ cell* is used as a synonym for the term *stem cell*. As will be discussed further below, caution must be used when doing this because these 2 terms are not synonymous but rather overlapping. Indeed, although enumeration of CD34+ cells is today the standard for stem cell counting, several investigators have reported a pluripotent stem cell that is CD34−.[5,6]

Sources of Hematopoietic Stem Cells

Human hematopoietic pluripotent stem cells may be found in numerous sites throughout the body. For stem cell transplantation, the common sources of stem cells include bone marrow, (mobilized) peripheral blood, and umbilical cord blood. Historically, bone marrow has been the primary source of stem cells for therapeutic applications. Although bone marrow is still widely used as a source of stem cells, other sources are becoming favored for transplantation because of a number of factors, not the least of which is the discomfort of marrow procurement. Recently, blood from the umbilical cord has been demonstrated to contain pluripotent stem cells capable of engraftment into immunocompromised hosts.[7-9] In general, bone marrow contains higher percentages of CD34+ cells than do the other 2 sources of stem cells. Pluripotent stem cells in normal peripheral blood are infrequent, necessitating the mobilization of these cells in peripheral blood through the use of cytokines, such as granulocyte colony-stimulating factor.[10,11] The immunophenotypes of stem cells from these 3 sources differ in certain aspects. Cord blood and mobilized peripheral blood stem cells express more myeloid antigens and fewer B-lymphoid antigens than do stem cells from bone marrow; however, all 3 sites contain similar proportions of immature progenitor cells, as estimated by lack of expression of CD38 and HLA-Dr.[12,13] Fritsch et al[12] suggest that because of the higher proportions of myeloid progenitor cells in umbilical cord blood and mobilized peripheral blood, between 1.4- and 2.2-fold higher numbers of stem cells should be transplanted from bone marrow vis a vis cord or peripheral blood.

Factors Affecting CD34+ Stem Cell Enumeration

A number of technical factors can influence the enumeration of CD34+ cells, leading to variable results not only between institutions but also within an institution if rigid protocols are not followed. These include the use of a lysing reagent, washing of the specimen, the type of monoclonal antibody used, the type of fluorochrome used, gating procedures, the way in which isotype controls are to be used, the number of cells to analyze, and live-dead cell discrimination.[14-22] Given the numbers of factors that can influence CD34+ cell enumeration, it is not surprising that substantial variation of stem cell counting occurs among laboratories. This variation has been documented in several interinstitutional studies.[23-25]

Antibodies Identifying Stem Cells

Although other monoclonal antibodies (MAbs), such as AC133,[26] have been reported to identify hematopoietic stem cells, the gold standard of MAbs for the identification of stem cells is clearly CD34, which was first described by Civin et al.[27] This does not preclude, however, that one or several of the alternative antibodies may become a widely accepted reagent for stem cell enumeration in the future. CD34 is a cluster designation; that is, multiple MAbs having similar, but not identical, specificities may be termed CD34 clones. Not all clones of CD34 antibodies are identical, because different epitopes are recognized by different clones. CD34 clones may be divided into 3 classes on the basis of the resistance of the reactive epitopes to enzyme digestion, as demonstrated in **Table 15-1**. In general, class II and class III CD34 antibodies are preferred for enumeration of stem cells because class I antibodies depend on carbohydrate residues and terminal sialic acid moieties for binding, and these are variably present on CD34 molecules.[28,29]

As will be discussed subsequently, there is some debate as to whether a single MAb is sufficient to identify the pluripotent stem cell. Although some investigators use additional antibodies or dyes, such as CD45 or LDS-751, to enhance gating,[2,15,24,30-32] still other investigators assert the need to use more

Table 15-1

Classes of CD34 Monoclonal Antibodies

Class	Examples	Enzyme sensitivity
I	MY10, B1.3C5, 12.8, ICH3, Imm133, Imm409	Sialic acid and *Pasteurella haemolytica* glycoprotease
II	QBEND10	*Pasteurella haemolytica* glycoprotease
III	TUK3, 115.2, 581, 8G12, HPCA-2, BIRMA-K3	None

than just CD34 to truly define pluripotent stem cells. Examples of this include $CD34^+CD38^-$ populations and $CD34^-CD38^-$ populations,[5,6] both of which have been reported to contain more primitive pluripotent progenitor cells than $CD34^+$ populations.

Fluorochromes and Their Effect on Stem Cell Enumeration

The accuracy of stem cell detection is not only affected by the choice of MAb but also by the selection of which fluorochrome is conjugated to the MAb. Historically, there has been some debate concerning whether both $CD34^{dim}$ and $CD34^{bright}$ populations should be included in the enumeration of stem cells. Fluorochromes such as phycoerythrin (PE) are much brighter (ie, have a better quantum yield) than other common fluorochromes, such as fluorescein isothiocyanate (FITC) and peridinin chlorophyll protein. Thus the resolution of 2 populations of stem cells, bright and dim, for CD34 may become the discrimination between positive and negative populations if a fluorochrome with a lower quantum yield is conjugated to CD34. With this in mind, the standard practice, originating from the guidelines for CD34 enumeration issued from the International Society of Hematotherapy and Graft Engineering (ISHAGE) is to use only PE-conjugated CD34 antibodies for stem cell counting.[32] This has proven to be a reasonable standard for all multiparameter flow cytometric methods for CD34 enumeration. By standardizing this parameter, the relative importance of bright versus dim CD34 cells may be gleaned from interinstitutional studies.

Methods of Stem Cell Enumeration

A variety of methods making use of CD34 are used for the enumeration of stem cells in the clinical environment. A number of articles are present in the literature describing methods for CD34 enumeration which are used in various individual laboratories but have yet to be adopted as consensus methods. These will not be discussed because (1) they are too numerous for comprehensive inclusion in this text, and (2) a selective inclusion would only reflect the bias of this author. An abbreviated list of methods, other than consensus protocols, is given in **Table 15-2**.[33-35]

Consensus Protocols

Why use consensus protocols? Several studies have documented that wide variability was observed in CD34 enumeration among institutions if different procedures were used; this is discussed further in the "Standardization and Quality Assurance" section of this text. Because successful engraftment of stem cells after transplantation has been shown to be dependent on the number of CD34$^+$ cells transplanted, the development of uniform therapeutic protocols requires uniformity in counting stem cells. A list of the most common consensus protocols and commercial techniques is given in **Table 15-3**. Each of these is derived from interinstitutional studies designed to minimize variation in CD34$^+$ cell counts among different laboratories, while at the same time making use of methodologies that are readily implemented in the clinical laboratory.

Table 15-2
Methods for CD34$^+$ Stem Cell Enumeration

Authors	Protocol	Reference
Sandhaus et al	CD34 staining only; processed within 4 hours; 250,000 events collected	33
Hubl et al	Modified ProCount; addition of CD38 and a nucleic acid dye	31
Roscoe et al	Uses 2 FITC-CD34 MAbs and multiple PE-labeled MAbs to identify lineage-committed cells	34
Venditti et al	Uses specific commercial software	35

Table 15-3

Protocols and Techniques for CD34+ Stem Cell Enumeration

Protocol-Technique	MAbs and dyes used	Number of events collected
ISHAGE	CD34 (class II or III for PE, class III for FITC), CD45	75,000 CD45+
SIHON	CD34, CD14, CD66e, LDS-751	50,000 nucleated
Milan	CD34	50,000 gated
ProCount*	CD34 (class III), CD45, nucleic acid dye	Variable (driven by statistics)
IMAGN2000 STELLer†	CD34 (class III)	Counting of fluorescent cells within a defined volume
Stem-kit‡	CD34, CD45 (modified ISHAGE)	75,000 CD45+

*Trademark of Becton Dickinson, Inc, San Jose, CA.
†Trademark of Biometric Imaging, Inc, Mountain View, CA.
‡Trademark of Beckman Coulter, Miami, FL (for research use only).

ISHAGE

ISHAGE published guidelines for CD34+ cell determination in 1996.[32] These guidelines were specifically designed to meet the following criteria: simplicity, high sensitivity, accuracy, reproducibility, and speed. These guidelines were comprehensive in nature, addressing every aspect of CD34+, from specimen collection to antibody selection to gating to data storage. Portions of these guidelines have been readily accepted, such as using only the brightest fluorochromes (eg, PE) for conjugation to CD34, whereas other recommendations have been more controversial, such as the gating strategy,[15,17,36] the use of isotype controls,[17,33] and the identification of which clones of CD34 are acceptable for use.[19,20] The enumeration of CD34 in this protocol uses CD34 and CD45, but no other antibodies or dyes, in a 4-parameter study. (The other parameters are forward and side light scatter.) Only CD34 class II and III antibodies may be used in this procedure. The data analysis involves the use of four 2-parameter dot plots and a Boolean gating strategy, as demonstrated in **Figure 15-1**. A minimum of 75,000 CD45+ events with at least 100 CD34+ cells should be collected according to these guidelines. Absolute counts are determined by using parallel determination of total leukocyte count and differential on an automated hematology analyzer. This protocol is being validated by a multi-institutional study in North America.

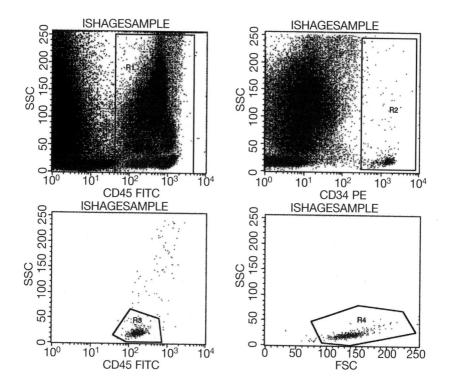

Figure 15-1

ISHAGE protocol for CD34+ stem cell enumeration. A series of 4 sequential gates are used to precisely gate stem cells. Plot 1 *(upper left)* displays the initial CD45 versus side light scatter gate. Here all events, except those that are CD45−, are included in the gate (gate 1, R1). Plot 2 *(upper right)* displays CD34 and side light scatter of cells from gate 1. This gate (gate 2, R2) should be set wide enough to include all potential CD34+ cells. Plot 3 *(lower left)* displays CD45 versus side light scatter staining of the cells meeting the criteria of gates 1 and 2. A gate set in this dot plot (gate 3, R3) excludes cells with high CD45 expression or with high side light scatter. Plot 4 *(lower right)* displays the forward versus side light scatter of cells meeting the criteria of gates 1, 2, and 3. A gate (gate 4, R4) is set to include only the cells with light scatter characteristics of stem cells.

MILAN

The MILAN protocol is also known as the Milan-Mulhouse protocol; a modified version is known as the Milan-Nordic protocol. These are modifications of a procedure first described by Siena et al[2] in which CD34, CD33, forward light scatter, and side light scatter were used to characterize hematopoietic stem cells. The modified versions of this protocol do not examine CD33. In these protocols (original Siena and the modified version), gating of the stem cells is accomplished through the use of CD34 staining versus side light scatter

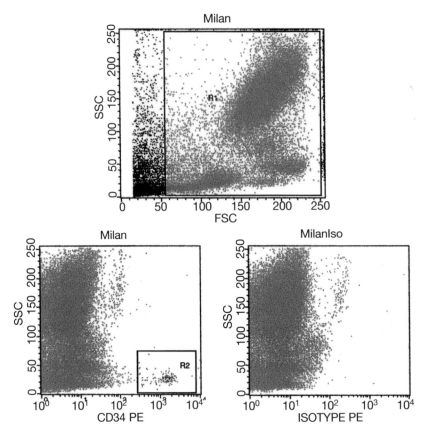

Figure 15-2

Milan protocol for CD34+ stem cell enumeration. Plot 1 *(top)* displays the forward and side light scatter pattern of the specimen. A wide gate (gate 1, R1) is set to include all events other than debris or other small particles. Plot 2 *(lower left)* displays the CD34 versus side light scatter staining of the cells within gate 1. A gate (gate 2, R2) is set to exclude CD34⁻ cells and cells with high side light scatter. Plot 3 *(lower right)* displays staining observed with an isotype control of the cells within gate 1. This serves as a control in this protocol.

(Figure 15-2). In the Milan-Mulhouse modification, an additional gate is set to exclude debris on the basis of forward light scatter. As with the ISHAGE protocol, an isotype control is used, and absolute CD34 counts depend on concomitant absolute leukocyte counts and differentials performed on a hematology analyzer. In contrast to ISHAGE, only 50,000 events need to be collected for analysis. The CD34 MAb used in this protocol is the class III clone HPCA-2 conjugated to PE. This procedure was modified and widely evaluated by 24 laboratories of the Nordic Myeloma Study Group.[37]

SIHON

SIHON, the Foundation for Immunophenotyping in Hemato-Oncology of the Netherlands, in conjunction with the Foundation for Quality Control in Medical Immunology, the Foundation for Quality Control of Hospital Laboratories, and the Belgian Association for Cytometry, evaluated a standard protocol to replace the numerous local protocols of participating institutions. This protocol differs from the 2 described above in that it uses (1) a nucleic acid stain, LDS-751, to identify nucleated cells and (2) CD14 and CD66e, both conjugated to PE, to eliminate monocytes and myeloid cells, which may nonspecifically bind antibody, from the analysis gate. **Figure 15-3** illustrates the gating used in this protocol. As originally published,[24] this procedure uses FITC-conjugated CD34 and PE-conjugated reagents against monocytes and myeloid cells; however, SIHON modified this procedure to use CD34 conjugated to PE (as found in other consensus protocols) and CD14 and CD66e conjugated to FITC.[17] This method required analysis of 50,000 nucleated cells, which is in contrast to the higher number required by ISHAGE. Isotype controls are used in this protocol.

Commercial Protocols and Products

Imagn2000 STELLer

The Imagn2000 STELLer system (Biometric Imaging, Mountain View, CA) for CD34 enumeration uses automated microvolume fluorimetry to obtain absolute counts.[38] Although the method uses fluorescently tagged CD34, this procedure is unlike flow cytometric assays for stem cell enumeration. The stained specimen is analyzed within a capillary by using a laser that scans a portion of it to detect fluorescent cells. Thus a precise volume of specimen is analyzed, eliminating the need for a secondary cell count to derive absolute concentrations. The kit uses Cy5 as the dye conjugated to a class III CD34 MAb. The kit also includes an isotype-matched nonspecific antibody and beads as controls. In an evaluation of this method, Sims et al[39] reported that this was the most simple and rapid methodology among the 3 tested (ProCount and TruCount being the other 2 methodologies). These investigators noted potential shortcomings of the STELLer method to be (1) the inability to quantitate CD34 counts over 2000/mL, (2) the lack of capacity to examine CD34 subsets, and (3) the lack of percentages and absolute counts.

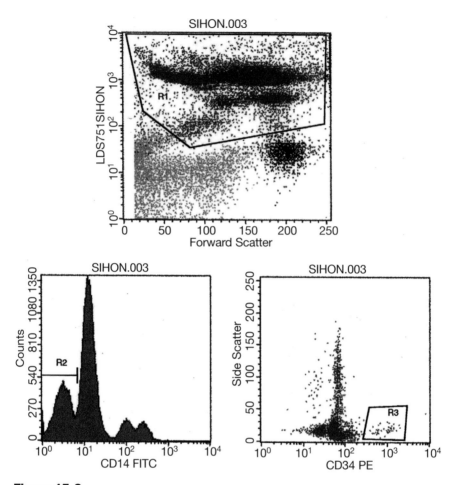

Figure 15-3

SIHON protocol for CD34+ stem cell enumeration. Plot 1 *(top)* displays the forward light scatter pattern and LDS-751 uptake (nucleic acid content) of the specimen. A wide gate (gate 1, R1) is set to include the LDS-751 bright cells, which are the nucleated cells in the specimen. Plot 2 *(lower left)* displays CD14 staining (CD14 + CD66e is preferred) of the cells within gate 1. A gate (gate 2, R2) is set to exclude cells staining for CD14 (and preferably CD66e). Plot 3 *(lower right)* displays the CD34 versus side light scatter staining of the cells within gates 1 and 2. A gate (gate 3, R3) is set on the CD34+ low side light scatter cells.

ProCount

The ProCount kit (BD Immunocytometry Systems, San Jose, CA) is a commercial product based on the system described by Chen et al.[30] This system uses a nucleic acid dye, peridinin chlorophyll protein-CD45, and PE-CD34 to enumerate stem cells. An isotype control is also used to detect nonspecific binding. The specimen and reagents are added to special tubes preloaded with a known quantity of microbeads. This permits calculation of absolute numbers of stem cells. Gating involves identifying nucleated cells with the nucleic acid dye, low side scatter, and CD45 positivity. In a manual mode 60,000 nucleated events are collected, while in a software-driven mode the number of events collected varies according to statistical precision. In their assessment of stem cell enumeration methodologies, Sims et al[39] found the ProCount system to be rapid, simple, and reproducible. Caveats included the need to dilute some specimens, cumbersome initial gating, and quality control issues related to defective tubes.

STEM-Kit

The STEM-Kit (Beckman-Coulter, Hialeah, FL) is a commercial kit for CD34$^+$ stem cell enumeration based on a modification of the ISHAGE guidelines.[40] In this kit, FITC-CD45 and PE-CD34 are used in conjunction with fluorescent microbeads to obtain absolute CD34$^+$ stem cell counts. Additionally, a third fluorescent stain, such as 7-amino actinomycin D, may be used to assess cell viability. An isotype control is not included for assessment of nonspecific binding, but a control consisting of a competitive blocking with unlabeled CD34 is provided (termed *an isoclonic control*). As with the ProCount system, the STEM-KIT was found to be rapid, simple, and reproducible.[40]

Standardization and Quality Assurance

Intrinsic to any clinical assay is the need for standardization and quality assurance. The protocols described above are attempts to standardize stem cell enumeration. Several studies have examined the variability in stem cell counts among different laboratories, each using their own unique protocols.[15,23,41,42] Gratama et al[17] have summarized many of the interlaboratory studies and have shown that the interlaboratory coefficient of variation (CV) for CD34$^+$ enumeration frequently exceeds 100%. Collectively, these data indicate an urgent need for standardization of counting procedures if therapeutic protocols are based on transplantation of precise numbers of stem cells. Indeed, the same data summarized by Gratama et al demonstrates that, in general, interlaboratory CVs are much less when strict protocols (eg, ProCount and SIHON) are adhered to. The need for a consensus standardized protocol for CD34$^+$ cell enumeration is widely recognized; however, there remains great debate as to which protocol, if any, should be universally adopted.[36,43,44]

While awaiting a universal consensus protocol for stem cell enumeration, steps are being taken to more rigidly control the quality of this testing. For example, a stem cell standard is now commercially available (Stem-trol, Beckman-Coulter). Farley et al[45] presented valuable recommendations for intralaboratory quality control. The College of American Pathologists has initiated proficiency testing for laboratories that perform CD34[+] cell enumeration, and German laboratories have developed an interlaboratory stem cell testing survey.[46] Measures such as these should aid in reducing the interinstitutional variation in CD34[+] cell enumeration and make such testing more useful in clinical decisions about the number of these cells required to successfully engraft an individual.

Summary and Conclusions

Clearly, there is no universal agreement on exactly how stem cell enumeration should be performed. In fact, there may not be such agreement for some time to come. For the clinical flow cytometrist, this is not an unusual situation. Today there is little consensus or uniformity of practice in many aspects of immunophenotyping of leukemias and lymphomas. Nonetheless, leukemia immunophenotyping is an important and useful application of flow cytometry in the clinical environment. Similarly, the lack of a single, universal, consensus protocol should not deter laboratories from performing high-quality stem cell enumeration.

Although many areas of controversy remain in stem cell enumeration, there appear to be areas of general agreement. These include the following:

- The use of class III CD34 antibodies if possible. These clones tend to pose the fewest technical problems for identifying all CD34[+] cells.
- The use of PE as the fluorochrome conjugated to CD34. As one of the brightest fluorochromes available, its consistent use will permit investigators and clinicians to coherently discuss the significance of bright CD34 populations versus dim CD34 populations.

Counting high numbers of cells to obtain statistically meaningful numbers of rare events. The precise number varies from protocol to protocol, and the question of whether these are gated events is unanswered. Probably a minimum of 50,000 events, exclusive of debris, is the absolute minimum to acquire in specimens, such as peripheral and cord blood. With the ease of mass data storage, collection of 100,000 events is quite reasonable and offers a greater security that the CD34$^+$ cell count is accurate.

There also appear to be areas of possible agreement, including the following:

- Single-platform analysis (eg, bead counting) to obtain absolute counts. The use of beads or other methods to achieve absolute counts by a single technique appears to reduce the interinstitutional variability. This is highly valued in group studies and in the construction of interinstitutional therapeutic protocols. As with CD4 enumeration for HIV monitoring, the introduction of a second method, such as cell counting on a hematology analyzer, introduces additional variables and thus increases the CVs in multicenter studies.
- Viability assessment. This is not universally accepted as a necessary component of CD34 enumeration procedures.[33] Clearly, it is reasonable to propose that counting viable CD34$^+$ cells rather than all CD34$^+$ cells is more pertinent to successful engraftment. However, this has not been widely documented in clinical studies.

Finally, there are areas of little agreement, such as the following:

- Lysing of red blood cells and its effect on CD34$^+$ cell enumeration. Several studies have demonstrated that lysing reagents, as well as density gradient separation, have an effect on the stem cell count,[14,16] yet there is no consensus on what is the preferred method of preparation. Despite the studies demonstrating the effect of red cell lysis on stem cell enumeration,[22] many consensus protocols, such as the ISHAGE and Milan protocols,[18,32,37] use lysing reagent to remove erythrocytes.
- Gating strategies for CD34$^+$ stem cells. Various protocols use either light scatter, DNA stains, or CD45 as gating parameters. A good case can be made for each of these approaches, and therefore no overall consensus has been reached.
- Isotype controls—if and how to use them. Although many current protocols call for the use of isotype controls, many investigators agree that they are of little practical use and are somewhat misleading if used as the sole criteria for setting gates or analysis quadrants.[18,33,40] One alternative that appears attractive is the control used in the STEM-KIT, which consists of an excess of unlabeled CD34 to block binding by labeled CD34.[40]

In summary, the enumeration of hematopoietic stem cells is continuing to evolve and mature as a clinical assay. An awareness of the many pitfalls involved in the flow cytometric detection of relatively rare events is a seminal step in devising a precise, reproducible, and widely acceptable assay. Although universal consensus remains elusive for an overall method for CD34$^+$ stem cell determination, agreement on the items listed above and the implementation of proficiency surveys is leading to more uniform and better quality clinical assessment of stem cells. Perhaps the greatest controversy remains in the hands of the research scientists: whether a better marker than CD34 can be developed for identification of the most primitive, omnipotent, hematopoietic stem cell.

References

1. Moore MAS, Williams N, Metcalf D. In vitro colony formation by normal and leukemic human hematopoietic cells. Characterizaton of the colony forming cells. *J Natl Cancer Inst.* 1973;56:603-628.

2. Siena S, Bregni M, Brando B, et al. Flow cytometry for clinical estimation of circulating hematopoietic progenitors for autologous transplantation in cancer patients. *Blood.* 1991;77:400-409.

3. Sutherland DR. Assessment of peripheral blood stem cell grafts by CD34+ cell enumeration: toward a standardized flow cytometric approach. *J Hematother.* 1996;5:209-210.

4. Morrison SJ, Uchida N, Weissman IL. The biology of hematopoietic stem cells. *Ann Rev Cell Dev Biol.* 1995;11:35-71.

5. Bhatia M, Bonnet D, Wang JCY, et al. Repopulating capacity of primitive human hematopoietic cells following ex vivo expansion. *J Exp Med.* 1997;186:1-6.

6. Goodell MA, Rosenzweig M, Kim H, et al. Dye efflux studies suggest that hematopoietic stem cells expressing low or undetectable levels of CD34 antigen exist in multiple species. *Nature Med.* 1997;3:1337-1345.

7. Wagner JE, Broxmeyer HE, Byrd RL, et al. Transplantation of umbilical cord blood after myeloablative therapy: analysis of engraftment. *Blood.* 1992;72:1874-1881.

8. Hogan CJ, Shpall EJ, McNulty O, et al. Engraftment and development of human CD34+ enriched cells from umbilical cord blood in NOD/LtSz-scid/scid mice. *Blood.* 1997;90:85-96.

9. Weber-Nordt RM, Schott E, Finke J, et al. Umbilical cord blood: an alternative to the transplantation of bone marrow stem cells. *Cancer Treat Rev.* 1996;22:381-391.

10. Anderlini P, Korbling M. The use of mobilized peripheral blood stem cells from normal donors for allografting. *Stem Cells.* 1997;15:9-17.

11. Dreger P, Glass B, Uharek L, et al. Allogeneic peripheral blood progenitor cells: current status and future directions. *J Hematother.* 1996;5:331-337.

12. Fritsch G, Stimpfl M, Kurz M, et al. The composition of CD34 subpopulations differs between bone marrow, blood, and cord blood. *Bone Marrow Transplant.* 1996;17:169-178.

13. Steen R, Tjonnfjord GE, Egeland T. Comparison of the phenotype and clonogenecity of normal CD34+ cells from umbilical cord blood, granulocyte colony-stimulating factor-mobilized peripheral blood, and adult human bone marrow. *J Hematother.* 1994;3:253-262.

14. Cassens U, Gutensohn K, Garritsen H, et al. The influence of different erythrocyte lysing procedures on flow cytometric determination of CD34+ cells in umbilical cord blood transplants. *Transfusion Med.* 1998;8:111-118.

15. Chang A, Ma DDF. The influence of flow cytometric gating strategy on the standardization of CD34+ cell quantitation: an Australian multicenter study. *J Hematother.* 1996;5:605-616.

16. Fritsch G, Printz D, Stimpfl M, et al. Quantification of CD34+ cells: comparison of methods. *Transfusion.* 1997;37:775-784.

17. Gratama JW, Orfao A, Barnett D, et al. Flow cytometric enumeration of CD34+ hematopoietic stem and progenitor cells. *Cytometry.* 1998;34:128-142.

18. Marti GE, Johnsen H, Sutherland R, et al. A convergence of methods for a worldwide standard for CD34+ cell enumeration [letter]. *J Hematother.* 1998;7:105-109.

19. Sutherland DR, Anderson L, Keeney M, et al. RE: QBEnd10 (CD34) antibody is unsuitable for routine use in the ISHAGE CD34+ cell determination assay [letter]. *J Hematother.* 1996;5:601-603.

20. Weinberg DS, Benjamin RJ. QBEnd10 (CD34) antibody is unsuitable for routine use in the ISHAGE CD34+ cell determination assay [letter]. *J Hematother.* 1996;5:599-600.

21. Knape CC. Standardization of absolute CD34 cell enumeration [letter]. *J Hematother.* 1996;5:211-212.

22. Menendez P, Rodriguez A, Lopez-Berges, MC, et al. Comparison between a lyse-and-then-wash method and a lyse-non-wash technique for the enumeration of CD34+ hematopoietic progenitor cells. *Cytometry.* 1998;34:264-271.

23. Brecher ME, Sims L, Schmitz J, et al. North American multicenter study on flow cytometric enumeration of CD34+ hematopoietic stem cells. *J Hematother.* 1996;5:227-236.

24. Gratama JW, Kraan J, Levering W, et al. Analysis of variation in results of CD34+ hematopoietic progenitor cell enumeration in a multicenter study. *Cytometry.* 1997;30:109-117.

25. Lowdell MW, Bainbridge DR. External quality assurance for CD34 cell enumeration—results of a preliminary national trial. *Bone Marrow Transplant.* 1996;17:849-853.

26. Yin AH, Miraglia S, Zanjani ED, et al. AC133, a novel marker for human hematopoietic stem and progenitor cells. *Blood.* 1997;90:5002-5012.

27. Civin C, Strauss LC, Brovall C, et al. Antigenic analysis of hematopoiesis III. A hematopoietic progenitor cell surface antigen defined by a monoclonal antibody raised against KG1a cells. *J Immunol.* 1984;133:157-165.

28. Serke S, Abe Y, Kirsch A, et al. Phenotyping of peripheral blood hemopoietic progenitor cells—in vitro cultures using CD34+/CD33- immunomagnetic purging. *Eur J Haematol.* 1991;47:361-366.

29. Sutherland DR, Keating A. The CD34 antigen: structure, biology, and potential clinical applications. *J Hematother.* 1992;1:115-129.

30. Chen CH, Lin W, Shye S, et al. Automated enumeration of CD34+ cells in peripheral blood and bone marrow. *J Hematother.* 1994;3:3-13.

31. Hubl W, Iturraspe J, Martinez GA, et al. Measurement of absolute concentration and viability of CD34+ cells in cord blood and cord blood product using fluorescent beads and cyanine nucleic acid dyes. *Cytometry.* 1998;34:121-127.

32. Sutherland DR, Anderson L, Keeney M, et al. The ISHAGE guidelines for CD34+ cell determination by flow cytometry. *J Hematother.* 1996;5:213-226.

33. Sandhaus LM, Edinger MG, Tubbs RR, et al. A simplified method for CD34+ cell determination for peripheral blood progenitor cell transplantation and correlation with clinical engraftment. *Exp Hematol.* 1998;26:73-78.

34. Roscoe RA, Rybka WB, Winkelstein A, et al. Enumeration of CD34+ hematopoietic stem cells for reconstitution following myeloablative therapy. *Cytometry.* 1994;16:74-79.

35. Venditti A, Buccusano F, Del Poeta G, et al. Multiparametric analysis for the enumeration of CD34+ cells from bone marrow and stimulated peripheral blood. *Bioorg Med Chem Lett.* 1998;1:67-70.

36. Johnsen HE. Toward a worldwide standard for CD34+ enumeration? [letter]. *J Hematother.* 1997;6:83-84.

37. Johnsen HE, Knudsen LM. Nordic flow cytometry standards for CD34+ cell enumeration in blood and leukapheresis products: report from the Second Nordic Workshop. *J Hematother.* 1996;5:237-245.

38. Read EJ, Kunitake ST, Carter CS, et al. Enumeration of CD34+ hematopoietic progenitor cells in peripheral blood and leukapheresis products by microvolume fluorimetry: a comparison to flow cytometry. *J Hematother.* 1997;6:291-301.

39. Sims LC, Brecher ME, Gertis K, et al. Enumeration of CD34-positive stem cells: evaluation and comparison of three methods. *J Hematother.* 1997;6:213-226.

40. Keeney M, Chin-Yee I, Weir K, et al. Single platform flow cytometric absolute CD34+ cell counts based on the ISHAGE guidelines. *Cytometry.* 1998;34:61-70.

41. Chin-Yee I, Anderson L, Keeney M, et al. Quality assurance of stem cell enumeration by flow cytometry. *Cytometry.* 1997;30:296-303.

42. Lumley MA, McDonald DF, Czarnecka HM, et al. Quality assurance of CD34+ cell estimation in leucapheresis products. *Bone Marrow Transplant.* 1996;18:791-796.

43. Chabannon C, Moatti JP, Maraninchi D. Will CD34+ standardization solve all problems related to cell therapy? [letter]. *J Hematother.* 1997;6:439-440.

44. Sutherland DR, Anderson L, Keeney M, et al. Toward a worldwide standard for CD34+ enumeration? [letter]. *J Hematother.* 1997;6:85-89.

45. Farley TJ, Rooney W, Kuhns E, et al. An intralaboratory quality control program for quantitation of CD34+ cells by flow cytometry. *J Hematother.* 1997;6:303-308.

46. Serke S, Huhn D. Circulating CD34-expressing cells: German Proficiency Testing Survey. *J Hematother.* 1998;7:37-43.

16

Leukocyte Functional Assays by Flow Cytometry

Jeffrey S. Warren

Introduction

The localized clinical features of inflammation have been recognized for nearly 5,000 years, and the importance of the inflammatory response in host defense has been recognized for hundreds of years. Recognition that leukocytic phagocytes participate in host defense occurred in the late nineteenth century with the observations by Elie Metchnikoff and Theodore Leber that phagocytes accumulate at sites of injury and that leukocytes are capable of tropic migration (chemotaxis), respectively.[1] Specific knowledge of the molecular mechanisms of leukocyte adhesion and phagocyte-mediated microbial killing has existed for a period of only 3 to 4 decades. Beginning with the 1954 description by Janeway et al[2] of hypergammaglobulinemia and severe recurrent soft tissue infections in patients who would ultimately bear the diagnosis of chronic granulomatous disease (CGD), a variety of clinical syndromes characterized by leukocyte dysfunction have been described. The modern techniques of biochemistry, cell culture, monoclonal antibody production, and recombinant DNA technology, coupled with the ability to manipulate the genotypes of experimental animals, have led to our current understanding of the nature of many disorders of leukocyte function. It should be emphasized that each of the entities described in this chapter is rare. Despite their infrequency, disorders of leukocyte function are often considered in the differential diagnosis of patients with recurrent infections. Important insights into leukocyte function have been gained from understanding such experiments of nature. This chapter will present overviews of the biology of leukocyte-endothelial adhesion, leukocyte adhesion deficiency I (LAD I), and other even less prevalent disorders of leukocyte adhesion. This chapter will also provide an overview of oxidative and nonoxidative phagocyte-mediated microbicidal mechanisms and related disorders of phagocyte function (eg, chronic granulomatous disease). These entities are relevant to a textbook of clinical flow cytometry because LAD disorders, CGD, and related disorders of leukocyte function lend themselves to diagnostic evaluation by means of flow cytometry.

Leukocyte Adhesion Deficiency and Related Disorders

Biology of Leukocyte-Endothelial Adhesion

In vitro experimental observations, coupled with animal studies and clinical investigations, have led to our current understanding of the mechanisms that orchestrate leukocyte adhesion and recruitment.[3] Directed movement of leukocytes from the lumen of a blood vessel to the interstitial space is called extravasation and includes the processes of margination, rolling, and adhesion. Extravasation also encompasses diapedesis and chemotaxis, the movement of leukocytes out of the vascular space and up a chemical gradient, respectively. The focus of this section is rolling and adhesion, which can be viewed as relatively weak, transient, leukocyte-endothelial adhesion interactions and stronger, more protracted, leukocyte-endothelial adhesive interactions, respectively.[3] Although much has been learned about leukocyte binding to extracellular matrix molecules, to high endothelial venules (in lymphocyte homing), and to each other, these processes will not be addressed. The hemodynamic changes that occur early in acute inflammation result in a decreased flow rate accompanied by a decrease in wall shear stress, increased vascular permeability that leads to hemoconcentration, and an increase in the displacement of leukocytes from the central laminar flow of red blood cells to the luminal surface of the vessel wall. Individual leukocytes tumble or roll along the endothelial surface until they finally stick, spread, and exit the vascular lumen through interendothelial

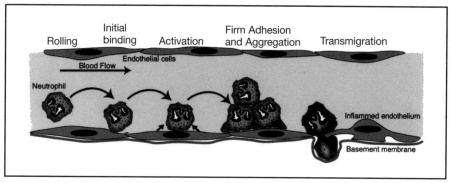

Figure 16-1

Leukocyte-endothelial adhesive interactions. Marginated leukocytes engage in low-affinity, selectin-mediated, rolling adhesive interactions with endothelial cells. As the leukocytes and endothelial cells become activated by locally produced cell surface and soluble mediators, the cells engage in high-affinity, immunoglobulin superfamily-mediated, adhesive interactions.

Adapted from: Butcher EC. Leukocyte-endothelial cell recognition: three (or more) steps to specificity and diversity. *Cell.* 1991;67:1033–1036; Bevilacqua MP, Nelson RM. Selectins. *J Clin Invest.* 1993;91:379–387; Tedder TF, Steeber DA, Chen A, et al. The selectins: vascular adhesion molecules. *FASEB J.* 1995;9:866–873; Springer TA. Traffic signals for lymphocyte recruitment and leukocyte emigration: the multistep paradigm. *Cell.* 1994;76:301–314; and Hynes RO. Integrins: versatility, modulation, and signaling in cell adhesion. *Cell.* 1992;69:11–25.

junctions. Although the array and the timing of expression of leukocyte and endothelial adhesion molecules vary, neutrophils, monocytes, lymphocytes, basophils, and eosinophils use the same route. In turn, the arrays, and in some cases the functions, of complementary adhesion molecules expressed on leukocytes and endothelial cells are directed by locally produced cell surface and soluble mediators (**Figure 16-1**). The most important leukocyte-endothelial adhesion molecules fall primarily within 4 families. These include the selectins, the integrins, members of the immunoglobulin superfamily, and a series of mucin-like glycoproteins.[3]

After a series of functional identifications (and the development of a complex nomenclature) through the 1980s, the 3 known members of the selectin family (E-, P-, and L-selectin) were identified at the DNA level in 1989.[4] In addition to several other homologous structural features, selectins contain an N-terminal, extracellular, carbohydrate-binding domain that is similar to that found in many mammalian lectins.[4] All 3 selectins are involved in leukocyte-endothelial adhesive interactions. These include the following: P-selectin

(CD62P), previously called PADGEM or GMP140; E-selectin (CD62E), previously called ELAM-1; and L-selectin (CD62L), previously called MEL-14, LECAM-1, or LAM-1.[4,5] P-selectin is expressed by endothelium and platelets, E-selectin exclusively by endothelium, and L-selectin by most types of leukocytes. Through their N-terminal lectin-like domains, selectins bind to sialylated oligosaccharides (eg, sialyl Lewis^X), which are components of several mucin-like glycoproteins (eg, GlyCAM-1, CD34, P-selectin glycoprotein ligand 1 [PSGL-1], and E-selectin ligand 1 [ESL-1]).[4,5] Although the selectins participate in the relatively weak, rolling, adhesive interactions that occur between leukocytes and endothelial cells, they vary substantially with respect to their regulation.[5]

Among a number of adhesion molecules within the immunoglobulin superfamily are intercellular adhesion molecule (ICAM) 1, 2, and 3 and vascular cell adhesion molecule 1 (VCAM-1).[6] ICAM-1, -2, and -3 exhibit important differences in structure, tissue distribution, and regulation.[6] Although all 4 ICAMs bind to lymphocyte function-associated antigen 1 (LFA-1, see below), they vary in their interactions with other adhesion molecules. The most important VCAM-1 binding interaction is with the integrin very late antigen 4 (VLA-4, see below).

Integrins are transmembrane heterodimers that each contain a structurally homologous beta chain, include one of a variety of alpha chains, and are involved in a number of cell-cell and cell-matrix binding interactions.[7] The most important integrins involved in leukocyte-endothelial binding are LFA-1 (CD11a/CD18) and macrophage antigen 1 (Mac-1; CD11b/CD18), which bind primarily to ICAM-1. Along with p150,95 (CD11c/CD18) and the recently discovered alpha$_d$beta$_2$[8], these beta$_2$ or leukocyte integrins are expressed only on leukocytes. The distribution of beta$_2$ integrins among subsets of leukocytes differs.[9] In addition, beta$_2$ integrins participate in several adhesion-related functions other than binding to endothelium.[9] The integrins, alpha$_4$beta$_1$ (VLA-4) and alpha$_4$beta$_7$, which both bind VCAM-1 and fibronectin, as well as, in the case of alpha$_4$beta$_7$, the mucosal vascular addressin cell adhesion molecule, are also important in leukocyte-endothelial binding.

A series of mucin-like glycoproteins serve as counterreceptors or selectin ligands.[10] Although this group of adhesion molecules is less well defined than those discussed above, it appears that selectins, through their lectin and epidermal growth factor domains, bind to a series of glycoproteins and proteoglycans (GlyCAM-1, CD34, ESL-1, and PSGL-1) and mucosal addressin cell adhesion molecule-1 (MadCAM-1) through sialylated and fucosylated tetrasaccharides related to the sialylated Lewis^X blood group.[10]

Rolling leukocyte-endothelial adhesive interactions occur rapidly and can withstand the low wall shear stress that occurs in the blood flow conditions of an incipient inflammatory response.[3-6] P-selectin, which is stored in intracytoplasmic endothelial granules (Weibel-Palade bodies), is translocated to the endothelial surface within minutes after exposure of the endothelium to mediators, such as thrombin, histamine, and platelet-activating factor. In contrast, E-selectin expression requires new protein synthesis, which occurs within 1 to 2 hours after exposure of endothelium to such mediators as IL-1beta and TNF-alpha. As alluded to above, the complementary leukocyte receptors for P-selectin include sialyl Lewis^X moieties on PSGL-1, and for E-selectin, these include sialyl Lewis^X moieties on ESL-1 and PSGL-1. P-selectin and E-selectin are particularly important in the early binding of neutrophils, hence their critical roles in acute inflammation. L-selectin is expressed by leukocytes and binds to L-selectin ligands (GlyCAM-1, CD34, and other less well-characterized ligands) on endothelial cells. The rolling phase of leukocyte-endothelial adhesion is transient (minutes) because L-selectin is rapidly shed from leukocytes, P-selectin is internalized by endothelial cells, and locally produced soluble sialyl Lewis^X interferes with selectin-mediated cell binding.[3-6]

Firm leukocyte-endothelial adhesive interactions are dependent on leukocyte integrins (LFA-1 and Mac-1) and complementary ICAM-1 molecules, which, before endothelial activation, are expressed at low levels on the surface of endothelial cells.[3] A necessary step in both LFA-1/ICAM-1 and Mac-1/ICAM-1 binding is either a C5a-induced, leukotriene B$_4$-induced, platelet-activating factor-induced, or IL-8-induced conformational change in LFA-1 (and Mac-1), which then exhibits high-affinity binding to ICAM-1.[6,7] LFA-1/ICAM-1 and Mac-1/ICAM-1 interactions occur over a longer time period than do selectin-mediated interactions and are important in the binding of all types of leukocytes, whereas VLA-4/VCAM-1 and alpha$_4$beta$_7$/VCAM-1 interactions are especially important in the adhesion of chronic inflammatory cells (lymphocytes, monocytes, and eosinophils). It should be clear from the foregoing discussion that the spatial, temporal, and cellular composition characteristics of leukocyte recruitment are tightly regulated. The critical features include hemodynamic changes, endothelial activation, rolling adhesive interactions, changes in leukocyte adhesion molecule avidity, firm adhesion, and ultimately transmigration, a step that requires both endothelial ICAM-1/leukocyte integrin interactions and platelet endothelial cell adhesion molecule (PECAM-1)/PECAM-1 interactions. PECAM-1 is (CD31) an immunoglobulin superfamily member that is found on both leukocytes and endothelial cells (near interendothelial junctions) and engages in homophilic proadhesive interactions.[11] The human leukocyte adhesion defects can be best understood in terms of the basic biology of leukocyte-endothelial adhesion. These entities lend themselves to clinical diagnosis by virtue of the dependence of leukocyte-endothelial adhesion on cell surface proteins, which in turn can be quantified by using flow cytometry.

Human Leukocyte Adhesion Defects

Leukocyte Adhesion Deficiency I

Leukocyte adhesion deficiency I is an autosomal recessive disorder in which a mutation in the gene (*ITGB2*) that encodes the beta$_2$ integrin subunit CD18 results in markedly reduced expression of the leukocyte integrins.[12,13] Expression of intact heterodimeric alpha-beta$_2$ surface molecules requires the biosynthesis of beta$_2$ subunits.[14] Accordingly, defects in CD18 biosynthesis result in reduction or absence of LFA-1, Mac-1, and p150,95. Severity of the clinical manifestations of LAD I is in general directly related to the degree of CD11/CD18 deficiency.[12,13] Patients in whom leukocytes express less than 1% of normal surface beta$_2$ integrin levels experience early, frequent, and severe infectious complications, whereas patients in whom leukocytes exhibit 2.5% to 30% of normal expression have less serious complications. The former group of patients is designated the *severe deficiency phenotype,* and the latter is designated the *moderate deficiency phenotype.*[15] Nearly 200 patients with LAD I have been studied, and a large number of mutations in *ITGB2* have been described.[13,16] These include a variety of point mutations, splicing defects, and even a gross chromosomal deletion (21q22.1-3).[13,16] In 1997, a patient with "LAD I variant" was described.[17] This patient exhibited the clinical manifestations of LAD I but expressed normal CD11/CD18 levels. In this case the beta$_2$ integrins were nonfunctional.

Although the genetic basis for LAD I was not defined until 1987,[12,13] patients with this syndrome were recognized in the 1970s.[18] Leukocyte functional defects and the absence of a high-molecular-weight neutrophil membrane glycoprotein in patients with this disorder were described during the 1970s and 1980s.[19,20] Patients with LAD I experience recurrent bacterial and fungal infections from birth.[12,13] Indolent, expanding, necrotic, skin and mucous membrane lesions are characteristic. A prominent clinicopathologic feature is the absence of pus. Many patients experience delayed separation of the umbilical cord after birth and many have omphalitis. Common infectious pathogens include *Staphylococcus aureus*, gram-negative enterics, and *Candida* species. Most patients exhibit marked elevations in circulating white blood cell counts, and pronounced gingivitis and periodontitis are common in patients who live into childhood.

These distinctive clinical features are highly suggestive of LAD I. A variety of beta$_2$ integrin-dependent leukocyte functional defects have been characterized,[20,21] but definitive diagnosis rests on the demonstration, by means of flow cytometry, of a marked reduction in leukocytic cell surface CD18 expression (**Figure 16-2**).[13] It is critical that appropriately handled normal control blood be

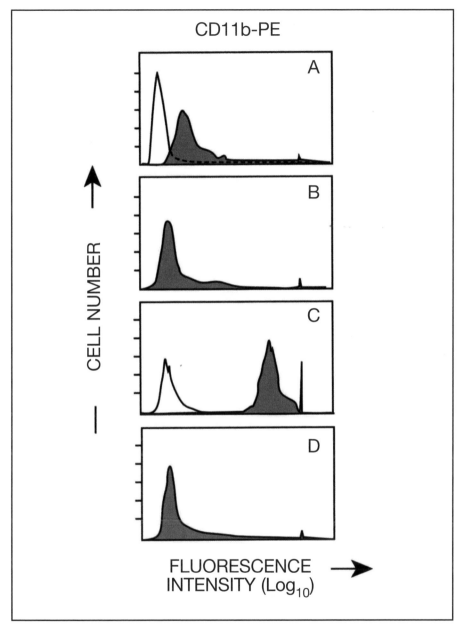

Figure 16-2

Diagnosis of CD11/CD18 glycoprotein deficiency (LAD I) by using indirect immunofluorescence flow cytometric analysis. Comparison of unstimulated **(A)** and phorbol ester-stimulated normal control **(C)** neutrophils reveals a marked increase in cell surface CD11b expression. Comparison of unstimulated **(B)** and phorbol-stimulated **(D)** neutrophils from a patient with the severe phenotype of LAD I reveals markedly reduced expression of CD11b in unstimulated cells **(B)** and no increase in cell surface expression after stimulation **(D)**. In this study cells were analyzed with phycoerythrin-labeled monoclonal antibody.

collected for diagnostic studies. LAD I carriers are almost always asymptomatic and express approximately 50% of normal CD18 concentrations. Prenatal diagnosis is possible because fetal leukocytes normally express CD18 by 20 weeks' gestation.[22] Finally, DNA sequence analysis may be appropriate in both postnatal and prenatal diagnostic circumstances.[13] Patients with the moderate deficiency phenotype usually respond well to assiduous management of infectious lesions and prompt use of antibiotics. Severely affected patients are treated with bone marrow transplantation and will doubtlessly be strong candidates for gene therapy.[23]

Leukocyte Adhesion Deficiency II (Rambon-Hasharon Syndrome)

Leukocyte adhesion deficiency II, also known as the Rambon-Hasharon syndrome, is believed to be an autosomal recessive disorder attributable to an incompletely characterized fucose biosynthetic defect, which results in the absence of sialyl Lewis^X and other fucosylated selectin ligands.[13] Two unrelated patients, both male subjects of Arabic descent, have been described.[24,25] These individuals both exhibit the rare Bombay blood group phenotype (h/h, absence of the H antigen) and have been found to be Lewis a- and b-negative nonsecretors. All of these biochemical abnormalities are explained by a defect in fucosylation of glycoconjugates. However, given that several different nonlinked transferases are responsible for fucosylation of these different structures and that alpha$_2$-fucosyltransferase, which is required for H-antigen synthesis, is functional, it is believed that there is a general defect in fucose production.[13,26] Additional experimental data suggest that there is a defect in the *de novo* pathway of L-fucose production.[27] This biosynthetic pathway is not unique to hematopoietic cells, perhaps explaining the more generalized abnormalities (growth and mental retardation) that occur in LAD II.

Both patients were born after normal pregnancies and at birth exhibited normal height and weight.[24,25] In contrast to patients with LAD I, there was no delay in umbilical cord separation. Both patients exhibit a distinctive facial appearance and have had recurrent cellulitis, pneumonia, periodontitis, and otitis media. As in patients with LAD I, these patients do not form pus and exhibit very high circulating neutrophil counts. The 2 described patients have experienced less severe disease than seen in typical patients with severe deficiency LAD I.

In practical reality LAD II is very unlikely to be encountered. Nevertheless, LAD II has provided important insight into the biology of leukocyte-endothelial adhesion and should be a consideration in a patient with recurrent infections, leukocytosis, and both mental and growth retardation. These patients exhibit the Bombay blood group phenotype, and flow cytometry can be used, with appropriate controls, to document the absence of sialyl Lewis^X expression on the surface of leukocytes.

Mac-1 (CD11b/CD18) and L-selectin Abnormalities in the Neonate

Phagocytic cells are believed to play a particularly important role in neonatal host defense because of the immaturity of the immune system.[28] Several deficits in neonatal neutrophil function have been well characterized and are believed to be at least in part attributable to reduced upregulation and/or functional activation of Mac-1 and reduced cell surface expression of L-selectin.[29] Although neonates clearly exhibit increased susceptibility to a number of infectious diseases, the biologic importance of isolated neutrophil Mac-1 and L-selectin defects is somewhat unclear because the functional abnormalities and reductions in expression of these adhesion molecules are commonly observed in healthy neonates. It is important to understand this caveat when evaluating the host defense system of a newborn.

Neutrophils from neonates exhibit reduced in vitro chemotactic responses to C5a and bacterially derived formyl peptides, abnormalities that are especially pronounced in premature infants.[29] Neutrophils from neonates exhibit reduced upregulation of Mac-1 expression and a subnormal increase in functional Mac-1-mediated neutrophil-endothelial binding.[28,29] Neutrophils from neonates also bind less well to endothelial cells under conditions of wall shear stress that favor selectin-dependent cell binding.[28,29] Finally, these neutrophils express relatively low levels of L-selectin. It is unclear whether the low levels of L-selectin expression are the result of excessive shedding or reduced production.

Mac-1 deficiency and L-selectin deficiency can be demonstrated by using flow cytometry.[29] Again, a more compelling argument for clinical importance can be made when age-matched positive control cells are also analyzed and when the interpretation of the results are held in proper clinical context.

Specific Granule Deficiency

The precise molecular basis of specific granule deficiency is unknown but appears to be the result of a regulatory defect in hematopoietic gene expression.[29-32] Neutrophils exhibit abnormal nuclear morphology and are either completely or nearly completely devoid of specific granules and their contents.[32]

Specific granules contain a variety of proteins that are involved in host defense. These include lactoferrin, lysozyme, and Mac-1. Deficiency of Mac-1 results in defective adhesion to endothelium. Although not emphasized in the section that reviewed the biology of leukocyte-endothelial adhesion, Mac-1 also functions as the iC3b complement receptor CR3. Neutrophils deficient of specific granules exhibit defective adhesion, chemotaxis, and intracellular microbicidal activities. The fundamental defect or defects result in more pervasive abnormalities than a deficiency of neutrophil-specific granules in that these patients also lack azurophilic granule defensins and possess abnormal platelet alpha granules and eosinophil-specific granules.[29]

Patients with specific granule deficiency have recurrent and severe bacterial (*Staphylococcus aureus*, *Pseudomonas aeruginosa*, and gram-negative enterics) and fungal (*Candida* species) infections of the skin, mucous membranes, and lungs. The diagnosis, suggested by the history and abnormal neutrophil morphology, is supported by data from leukocyte functional assays (eg, formyl peptide-induced specific granule release assay) and flow cytometry (reduced or absent CD11b/CD18 [Mac-1]).[29]

Disorders of Phagocyte Killing

Microbicidal Mechanisms of Phagocytic Cells

Phagocytic leukocytes are capable of killing and degrading microorganisms through a variety of pathways.[33] Phagocytosis, as well as a variety of other cell surface, receptor-mediated, activation processes, stimulates a burst in oxygen consumption, glucose oxidation through the hexose monophosphate shunt, and glycogenolysis. The respiratory burst results in the generation of several species of reactive oxygen intermediates (ROIs), which can kill microorganisms (and can contribute to tissue damage). Defects in ROI generation can lead to increased susceptibility to infectious diseases. Several of these disorders can be diagnosed by using flow cytometry.

Oxygen-independent Mechanisms

Leukocytes (neutrophils, monocytes, macrophages, and eosinophils) vary in their content of microbicidal peptides, proteins, and enzymes.[33] Oxygen-independent microbicidal mediators include such substances as lactoferrin, an iron-binding protein that interferes with iron-dependent bacterial metabolism; lysozyme, an enzyme that hydrolyzes muramic acid-N-acetylglucosamine bonds found in the glycopeptide walls of bacteria; bactericidal permeability-increasing protein, a cationic protein that activates phospholipase and thus increases bacterial membrane permeability; major basic protein, a cationic eosinophil-derived peptide that injures parasites; and the defensin family of cationic peptides, which damage a number of microorganisms.

Oxygen-dependent mechanisms

The bulk of phagocyte-mediated microbial killing occurs by means of oxygen-dependent mechanisms.[33,34] Although small quantities of ROIs are produced as byproducts of a number of enzymatic reactions, the chief source of ROIs released into phagocytic vacuoles (and into the extracellular milieu) is the activation of reduced nicotinamide adenine dinucleotide phosphate (NADPH) oxidase.[35] The NADPH oxidase enzyme complex oxidizes NADPH and reduces molecular oxygen (O_2) to superoxide anion (O_2^-).[34,35] In turn, O_2^- is converted by dismutation (either spontaneously or through catalyzation by superoxide dismutase) into hydrogen peroxide (H_2O_2). NADPH oxidase is a complex assembly that consists of multiple subunits, which in quiescent cells are physically separated into the cytoplasmic and plasma membrane compartments.[34,36-39] On assembly and activation of the oxidase, the cytosolic components translocate to the plasma membrane (which may face the extracellular milieu or the inside of a phagocytic vacuole), where formation of a functional complex occurs.[34,35] A large array of ROIs derive from O_2^- and H_2O_2. Perhaps the most important microbicidal products are the hypohalites (eg, HOCl), which are formed by the action of myeloperoxidase (MPO), H_2O_2, and halide ions, such as Cl^-.[33] MPO is stored within azurophilic granules that fuse with phagocytic vacuoles, where the H_2O_2-MPO-halide system constitutes the most efficient bactericidal system in neutrophils. Catalase and glutathione peroxidase catalyze the degradation of H_2O_2 and thus limit its actions. Specific defects in oxygen-dependent mechanisms of microbial killing are addressed below.

Human Phagocyte Dysfunction Diseases

Chronic Granulomatous Disease (CGD): CGD is a rare, genetically heterogenous, congenital immunodeficiency marked by a complete or nearly complete absence of the respiratory burst that normally occurs on phagocyte activation.[34] As described above, the NADPH oxidase-dependent respiratory burst in phagocytes results in the generation of O_2^-, which in turn gives rise to a variety of ROIs and ROI derivatives. Because of the importance of ROIs in phagocyte-mediated microbial killing, patients who cannot generate NADPH

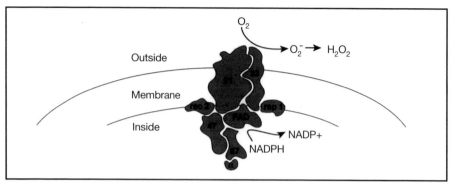

Figure 16-3

Leukocyte reduced nicotinamide adenine dinucleotide phosphate oxidase activation. Activation of quiescent neutrophils results in the activation of reduced nicotinamide adenine dinucleotide phosphate oxidase, a cytosolic and cell membrane-associated assembly of proteins that function in concert to catalyze the reduction of oxygen to superoxide anion. Mutations in genes that encode 4 major reduced nicotinamide adenine dinucleotide phosphate oxidase subunits (gp91^{phox}, p22^{phox}, p47^{phox}, and p67^{phox}) can result in a defective respiratory burst and the chronic granulomatous disease phenotype.

oxidase–derived O_2^- are susceptible to recurrent, serious bacterial and fungal infections.[34] From recognition in 1957 of the clinical entity referred to as "fatal granulomatous disease of childhood" (because of its high mortality rate and the striking granulomas that contained yellow-brown pigment-bearing macrophages)[40,41] to the current level of understanding of its molecular basis, the investigation of mechanisms responsible for CGD represents a true tour de force in biomedical research.[34]

The clinical, genetic, and molecular heterogeneity of CGD can be best understood in terms of NADPH oxidase (**Figure 16-3**). NADPH oxidase consists of 4 subunits, gp91^{phox}, p22^{phox}, p47^{phox}, and p67^{phox}, as well as a number of associated regulatory proteins (p40^{phox}, *rap*1A, *rac*1, and *rac*2).[34] Various types of mutations occur within each of the genes that encode the 4 major subunits.[34] Mutations within *CYBB* on chromosome Xp21.1 account for the X-linked form of CGD and approximately 65% of all cases. Mutations in the genes that encode p22^{phox} (*CYBA*), p47^{phox} (*NCF1*), and p67^{phox} (*NCF2*) are located on different autosomal chromosomes and account for the remaining 35% of CGD cases. Biochemical analyses carried out during the 1970s and 1980s revealed that gp91^{phox} and p22^{phox} are membrane-associated in resting phagocytes and contain a cytochrome (b-$_{245}$ or b$_{558}$), whereas p47^{phox} and p67^{phos} are located in the cytosol in inactive cells.[34,42-45] Phagocyte activation, either through phagocytosis or receptor-mediated pathways, results in the regulated translocation of the cytosolic component of NADPH oxidase to the membrane component. By the mid-1980s, most patients with CGD could be classified as having either X-linked/cytochrome-negative (X$^-$), autosomal recessive/cytochrome b-positive (A$^+$), or autosomal recessive/cytochrome b-negative (A$^-$) disease.[46] Patients are currently classified according to the component of the NADPH oxidase, which is affected as gp91^{phox}, p22^{phox}, p47^{phox}, p67^{phox}.[34] Other than a small number of patients in whom mutations in the promotor region of *CYBB* have been identified,[47,48] the defects in CGD all involve the genes that encode these 4 subunits.

Patients affected by CGD experience a wide variety of recurrent bacterial and fungal infections.[34] The most common include pneumonia, lymphadenitis, skin infections, hepatic and perihepatic abscesses, osteomyelitis, perirectal abscesses, otitis media, conjunctivitis, gastrointestinal infections, and septicemia. Patients with CGD also undergo a variety of infectious complications, including failure to thrive, anemia of chronic disease, short stature, chronic diarrhea, and hepatosplenomegaly. Although most patients present with clear-cut infectious diseases, patients may present with complications that are not immediately recognized as sequelae of chronic infections (eg, dermatitis, gastrointestinal or urinary tract stenosis caused by encroaching granulomatous tissue, iron-deficiency anemia, or bloody diarrhea associated with failure to thrive). The array of bacteria and fungi that infect patients with CGD have in common the ability to produce catalase. It is believed that microbial catalase degrades H_2O_2 produced by the infecting microorganisms, thereby essentially eliminating all or nearly all ROI accumulation within a phagolysosome. In contrast, microbes that produce H_2O_2, but not catalase, provide an alternative ROI source for hypohalite production. The most common microbial isolates include *Staphylococcus aureus*, gram-negative enterics, *Aspergillus* species, *Burkholderia cepacia* (formerly *Pseudomonas*), *Serratia marcescens*, *Candida albicans*, *Streptococcus* species, and *Nocardia* species.[34]

Diagnosis of CGD requires recognition of both typical and unusual clinical features, followed by demonstration of a defective phagocyte respiratory burst. A number of assays that measure the ability of neutrophils to produce O_2^- by means of NADPH oxidase have been developed.[34] The oxygen burst can be measured in leukocyte preparations by direct analysis of phagocytosis or soluble mediator-induced neutrophil activation (eg, formyl peptides, phorbol ester, and zymosan-activated serum) and oxygen consumption, by measurement of (superoxide dismutase-inhibitable) O_2^- generation and ferricytochrome c reduction, by measurement of H_2O_2 generation (oxidation of homovanillic acid), and by using a variety of chemiluminescence assays.[34] The classic nitroblue tetrazolium slide test is useful because it usually allows for identification of carriers, as well as most affected patients. Finally, flow cytometric assays (eg, dihydrorhodamine as a sensitive marker of H_2O_2 production) are particularly useful because they are sensitive, quantitative, allow analysis of individual cells (thus allowing carrier detection), and can be performed on whole blood up to 48 hours after collection (**Figure 16-4**).[49] CGD subgroup identification is usually achieved by analysis of immunoblot assays (all 4 NADPH oxidase subunits can be identified), cell-free NADPH oxidase functional assays, and molecular assays (polymerase chain reaction, restriction fragment length polymorphism, and DNA sequencing).[34]

The treatment and prognosis for patients with CGD have improved markedly. Effective treatment, addressed elsewhere, includes prevention of infection through immunizations and prophylaxis, use of recombinant interferon gamma, and aggressive medical and surgical management of infections. A few patients have successfully undergone bone marrow transplantation, and CGD is believed to be an excellent candidate disease for effective gene therapy.[23]

Myeloperoxidase Deficiency (MPO): MPO deficiency is a relatively common (1/2000-4000 persons) disorder in which granulocytes produce O_2^- and H_2O_2 but cannot generate normal levels of MPO-dependent hypohalite (HOCl) or HOCl-derived chloramines.[33] Patients with complete MPO deficiency, with partial MPO deficiency, and with acquired MPO deficiency have been described. Several different mutations that result in defective posttranslational processing of MPO have been described. Acquired partial MPO deficiency occurs in some patients with M2, M3, and M4 acute myelogenous leukemia, in patients with chronic myelogenous leukemia, and in patients with myelodysplastic syndromes.[33] In vitro leukocyte function assays reveal that affected cells exhibit delayed neutrophil-mediated microbial killing. Clinically affected patients, usually diabetics, primarily experience recurrent candidal infections. This disorder may involve other factors that are as yet not well-defined because most affected individuals are asymptomatic. Flow cytometric analysis may reveal an augmented respiratory burst, but diagnosis is usually made by using cytochemical staining procedures.[33]

Leukocyte Glucose-6-Phosphate Dehydrogenase Deficiency: More than 400 polymorphic variants of glucose-6-phosphate dehydrogenase (G6PD) are known.[33] Worldwide, G6PD deficiency is the most common cause of hemolytic anemia associated with a red cell enzyme deficiency. Episodes of hemolysis are most often triggered by infection, exposure to a drug that produces oxidative stress (eg, antimalarials, such as Primaquine [Sanofi-Winthrop, New York, NY], sulfa drugs, others), or ingestion of fava beans. Severe forms of G6PD deficiency in which patients present with a CGD-like syndrome have been described.[33] G6PD, which is part of the hexose monophosphate shunt, is an X-linked heterodimer that catalyzes the generation of NADPH from glucose-6-phosphate

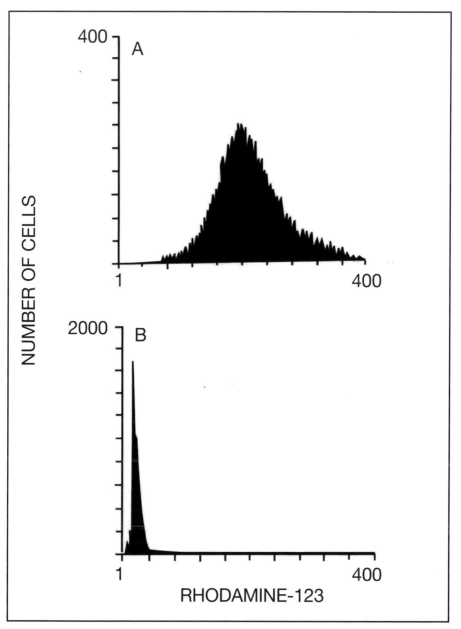

Figure 16-4

Fluorescence distribution of rhodamine 123, an oxidation product of dihydrorhodamine exposed to intracellular hydrogen peroxide. **A** depicts normal control neutrophils stimulated with phorbol ester. **B** depicts chronic granulomatous disease neutrophils stimulated with phorbol ester.

and the oxidized form of nicotinamide adenine dinucleotide phosphate. The G6PD expressed in leukocytes is encoded by the same gene as the G6PD expressed in red blood cells but is usually expressed at high enough levels that leukocyte dysfunction does not occur. Patients with recurrent infections possess very low concentrations of leukocyte NADPH and exhibit leukocyte enzyme activity levels that are usually less than 5% of normal. Mostly male patients have been reported.

As in patients with typical forms of CGD, patients with severe leukocyte G6PD deficiency experience recurrent coagulase-positive *Staphylococcus aureus* infections, infections with *Escherichia coli*, and infections with *Serratia marcescens*. Sites of infections typically include cervical lymph nodes, lungs, skin, and mucous membranes. Not surprisingly, these patients also have hemolytic anemia attributable to red blood cell G6PD deficiency. As in the case of CGD, leukocytes from profoundly G6PD-deficient patients fail to reduce nitroblue tetrazolium or produce H_2O_2.[33] As in patients with CGD, H_2O_2-mediated dye oxidation (dihydrorhodamine) is abnormal.[33]

Summary

The importance of host defense systems in the well-being of individuals has been recognized for many years. The clinical features of many immunodeficiency disorders have provided great insight into the biology of host defense and the inflammatory response. The widespread application of modern diagnostic techniques has allowed a more detailed understanding of the biologic bases of many immunodeficiency disorders.

Case Studies

Case 16-1

History

A 7-year-old boy presented with a poorly-healing soft tissue infection involving the left paratonsillar area. *Streptococcus pyogenes* had been isolated from the lesion 3 weeks earlier. A more detailed history revealed that the patient had been hospitalized 4 different times for cutaneous and perioral bacterial soft tissue infections. The patient also suffered from severe gingivitis. A diagnostic procedure was performed.

Frames A and B of **Figure 16-5** depict unstimulated neutrophils from a healthy control subject and the patient, respectively. Frames C and D depict phorbol ester-stimulated neutrophils from a healthy control subject and the patient, respectively. In this case, cells were analyzed with PE-labeled monoclonal antibodies directed against CD11b.

Interpretation

This patient suffers from leukocyte adhesion deficiency (LAD) I, an autosomal recessive disorder in which a mutation in *ITGB2* results in reduced expression of leukocyte integrins. The patient's clinical presentation and flow cytometric analysis results support the diagnosis of "moderate deficiency" phenotype. Patients with the "severe deficiency" often suffer from more severe and generalized infections and typically exhibit less than 1% of normal surface beta-2 integrin levels (**Figure 16-2**), while patients with the moderate deficiency phenotype exhibit 2.5% to 30% of normal expression.

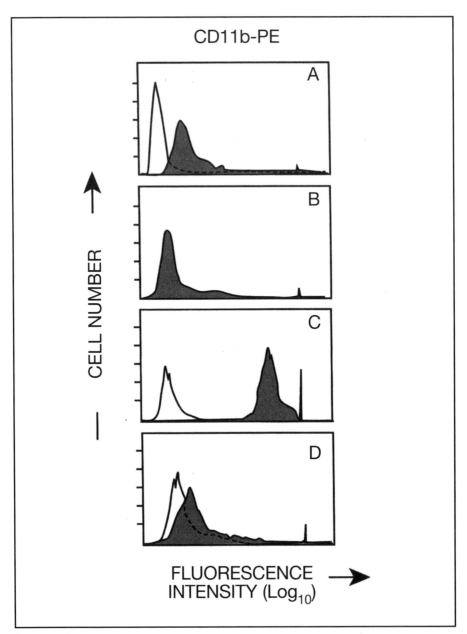

Figure 16-5

Case 16-2

History

A 23-year-old woman was referred for genetic counseling because her 3-month-old son had died from *Aspergillus* sepsis. The child had been born at term and had no grossly apparent malformations. A procedure was performed using the mother's peripheral blood.

Frames A and B of **Figure 16-6** depict control neutrophils and phorbol ester-stimulated neutrophils from the mother, respectively. The histograms depict the fluorescence distribution of rhodamine-123.

Interpretation

The 3-month-old boy who died from *Aspergillus* sepsis presumably suffered from X-linked chronic granulomatous disease. The approximately 50:50 distribution of maternal neutrophils which exhibit a defective oxidative burst versus those which exhibit a normal response suggests that the mother is a CGD carrier. As discussed in the text, the most common X-linked mutations that lead to CGD involve the *CYBB* gene located on the short arm of the X chromosome. *CYBB* encodes the gp91^{phox} subunit of NADPH oxidase. It should be emphasized that non-random X chromosome inactivation in maternal carriers of X-linked CGD may lead to abnormal-to-normal neutrophil rations of other than 50:50. Molecular diagnostic testing to prove that an X-linked mutation is carried by the mother has important genetic counseling implications.

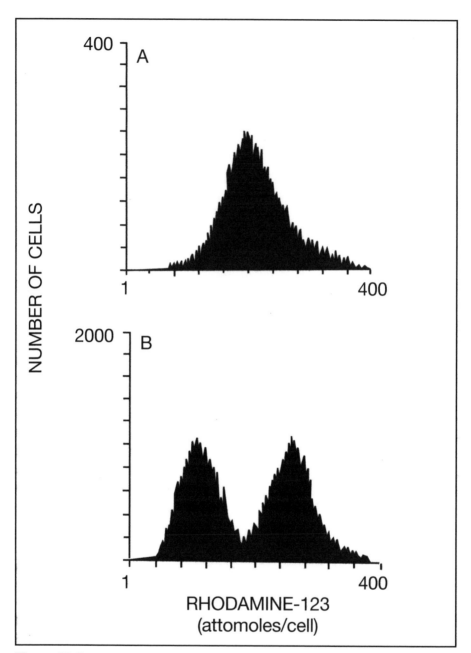

Figure 16-6

References

1. Weissman G. Inflammation: historical perspectives. In: Gallin JI, Henson PM, Wilson PD, eds. *Inflammation: Basic Principles and Clinical Correlates*. 2nd ed. New York: Raven Press, 1992:5-13.

2. Janeway CA, Cragi J, Davidson M, et al. Hypergammaglobulinemia associated with severe recurrent and chronic nonspecific infection. *Am J Dis Child.* 1954;88:388-397.

3. Butcher EC. Leukocyte-endothelial cell recognition: three (or more) steps to specificity and diversity. *Cell.* 1991;67:1033-1036.

4. Bevilacqua MP, Nelson RM. Selectins. *J Clin Invest.* 1993;91:379-387.

5. Tedder TF, Steeber DA, Chen A, et al. The selectins: vascular adhesion molecules. *FASEB J.* 1995;9:866-873.

6. Springer TA. Traffic signals for lymphocyte recruitment and leukocyte emigration: the multistep paradigm. *Cell.* 1994;76:301-314.

7. Hynes RO. Integrins: versatility, modulation, and signaling in cell adhesion. *Cell.* 1992;69:11-25.

8. Van der Vieren M, Le Trong HL, Wood CL, et al. A novel leukointegrin , adb2, binds preferentially to ICAM-3. *Immunity.* 1995;3:683-690.

9. Kishimoto TK, Rothlein R. Adhesion molecules which guide neutrophil endothelial cell interaction at site of inflammation. In: Gupta S, Griscelli C, eds. *New Concepts in Immunodeficiency Diseases*. New York: John Wiley; 1993:131-152.

10. Varki A. Selectin ligands. *Proc Natl Acad Sci USA.* 1994;91:7390-7397.

11. Muller WA, Weigle SA, Deng X, et al. PECAM-1 is required for transendothelial migration of leukocytes. *J Exp Med.* 1993;178:449-457.

12. Anderson DC, Springer TA. Leukocyte adhesion deficiency: an inherited defect in the Mac-1, LFA-1, and p150,95 glycoproteins. *Annu Rev Med.* 1987;38:175-194.

13. Etzioni A, Harlan JM. Cell adhesion and leukocyte adhesion defects. In: Ochs HD, Edvard Smith CI, Puck JM, eds. *Primary Immunodeficiency Diseases*. 1st ed. New York: Oxford University Press; 1999:375-388.

14. Springer TA. Mac-1 glycoprotein family and its deficiency in an inherited disease. *Fed Proc.* 1985;44:2660-2665.

15. Fischer A, Lisowska-Grospierre B, Anderson DC, et al. Leukocyte adhesion deficiency: molecular basis and functional consequences. *Immunodefic Rev.* 1988;1:39-54.

16. Solomon E, Palmer RW, Hing S, et al. Regional localization of CD18, the b-subunit of the cell surface adhesion molecule LFA-1, on human chromosome 21 by in situ hybridization. *Ann Hum Genet.* 1988;52:123-128.

17. Kuijpers TW, van Lier RAW, Hamann D, et al. Leukocyte adhesion deficiency type I (LAD-1)/variant. *J Clin Invest.* 1997;100:1725-1733.

18. Hayward AR, Leonard J, Wood CBS, et al. Delayed separation of the umbilical cord, wide spread infections, and defective neutrophil mobility. *Lancet.* 1979;1:1099-2002.

19. Crowley CA, Curnutte JT, Rosin RE, et al. An inherited abnormality of neutrophil adhesion: its genetic transmission and its association with a missing protein. *N Engl J Med.* 1980;302:1163-1167.

20. Bowen TJ, Ochs HD, Altman LC, et al. Severe recurrent bacterial infections associated with defective adherence and chemotaxis in two patients with neutrophils deficient in a cell associated glycoprotein. *J Pediatr.* 1982;101:932-939.

21. Schwartz BR, Harlan JM. Consequence of deficient granulocyte endothelium interaction. In: Gordon JL, ed. *Vascular Endothelium Interactions with Circulating Cells.* Amsterdam: Elsevier Biomedical; 1991:231-252.

22. Weening RS, Bredius RGM, Wolf H, et al. Prenatal diagnostic procedure for leukocyte adhesion deficiency. *Prenat Diagn.* 1991;11:193-197.

23. Fischer A, Landais P, Friedrich W. Bone marrow transplantation (BMT) in Europe for primary immunodeficiencies other than severe combined immunodeficiency. *Blood.* 1994;83:1149-1154.

24. Frydman M, Etzioni A, Eidilitz-Markus T, et al. Rambam-Hasharon syndrome of psychomotor retardation, short stature, defective neutrophil motility and Bombay phenotype. *Am J Med Genet.* 1992;44:297-302.

25. Etzioni A, Harlan JM, Pollack S, et al. Leukocyte adhesion deficiency (LAD) II: a new adhesion defect due to absence of sialyl Lewis x, the ligand for selectins. *Immunodeficiency.* 1993;4:307-308.

26. Shechter Y, Etzioni A, Levene C, et al. A Bombay individual lacking H and Le antigens but expressing normal levels of a-2-and a-fucosyltransferases. *Transfusion.* 1995;35:773-776.

27. Karsan A, Cornejo CJ, Winn RK, et al. Leukocyte adhesion deficiency type II is a generalized defect of de novo GDP-fucose biosynthesis. *J Clin Invest.* 1998;101:2438-2445.

28. Anderson DC. Neonatal neutrophil dysfunction. *Am J Pediatr Hematol Oncol.* 1989;11:224-237.

29. Anderson DC, Kishimoto TK, Smith CW. Leukocyte adhesion deficiency and other disorders of leukocyte adherence and motility. In: Scriver CR, Beaudet AL, Sly WS, et al, eds. *The Metabolic and Molecular Basis of Inherited Diseases.* 7th ed. New York: McGraw-Hill; 1995:3955-3995.

30. Spitznagel JK, Cooper MR, McCall AE, et al. Selective deficiency of granules associated with lysozyme and lactoferrin in human polymorphs (PMN) [abstract]. *J Clin Invest.* 1972;51:93A.

31. Boxer LA, Coates TD, Haak RA, et al. Lactoferrin deficiency associated with granulocyte function. *N Engl J Med.* 1982;307:404-411.

32. Gallin JI. Neutrophil specific granule deficiency. *Annu Rev Med.* 1985;36:263-275.

33. Yang KD, Quie PG, Hill HR. Phagocytic system. In: Ochs HD, Edvard Smith CI, Puck JM, eds. *Primary Immunodeficiency Diseases.* 1st ed. New York: Oxford University Press; 1999:82-96.

34. Ross D, Curnutte JT. Chronic granulomatous disease. In: Ochs HD, Edward Smith CI, Puck JM, eds. *Primary Immunodeficiency Diseases.* 1st ed. New York: Oxford University Press; 1999:353-374.

35. Curnutte JT, Kipnes RS, Babior BM. Detect in pyridine nucleotide dependent superoxide production by a particulate fraction from the granulocytes of patients with chronic granulomatous disease. *N Engl J Med.* 1975;293:628-632.

36. Bromberg Y, Pick E. Unsaturated fatty acids stimulate NADPH-dependent superoxide production by cell-free system derived from macrophages. *Cell Immunol.* 1984;88:213-221.

37. Heyneman RA, Vercauteren RE. Activation of a NADPH oxidase from horse polymorphonuclear leukocytes in a cell-free system. *J Leukoc Biol.* 1984;36:751-759.

38. Curnutte JT. Activation of human neutrophil nicotinamide adenine dinucleotide phosphate, reduced (triphosphopyridine nucleotide, reduced) oxidase by arachidonic acid in a cell-free system. *J Clin Invest.* 1985;75:1740-1743.

39. McPhail LC, Shirley PS, Clayton CC, et al. Activation of the respiratory burst enzyme from human neutrophils in a cell-free system. *J Clin Invest.* 1985;75:1735-1739.

40. Berendes H, Bridges RA, Good RA. Fatal granulomatous of childhood: clinical study of new syndrome. *Minn Med.* 1957;40:309-312.

41. Landing BH, Shirkey HS. A syndrome of recurrent infection and infiltration of viscera by pigmented lipid histiocytes. *Pediatrics.* 1957;20:431-438.

42. Segal AW, Jones OTG, Webster D, et al. Absence of a newly described cytochrome *b* from neutrophils of patients with chronic granulomatous disease. *Lancet.* 1978;2:446-449.

43. Segal AW, Cross AR, Garcia RC, et al. Absence of cytochrome *b*-245 in chronic granulomatous disease: a multicenter European evaluation of its incidence and relevance. *N Engl J Med.* 1983;308:245-251.

44. Segal AW. Absence of both cytochrome b-245 subunits from neutrophils in X-linked chronic granulomatous disease. *Nature.* 1987;326:88-92.

45. Curnutte JT, Scott PJ, Mayo LA. Cytosolic components of the respiratory burst oxidase: Resolution of four components, two of which are missing in complementing types of chronic granulomatous disease. *Proc Natl Acad Sci USA.* 1989;86:825-829.

46. Hamers MN, de Boer M, Meerhof LJ, et al. Complementation in monocyte hybrids revealing genetic heterogeneity in chronic granulomatous disease. *Nature.* 1984;307:553-555.

47. Newburger PE, Skalnik DG, Hopkins PJ, et al. Mutations in the promoter region of the gene for gp$^{91-phox}$ in X-linked chronic granulomatous disease with decreased expression of cytochrome *b*. *J Clin Invest.* 1994;94:1205-1211.

48. Woodman RC, Newburger PE, Anklesaria P, et al. A new X-linked variant of chronic granulomatous disease characterized by the existence of a normal clone of respiratory burst-component phagocytic cells. *Blood.* 1995;85:231-241.

49. Emmendörffer A, Nakamura M, Rothe G, et al. Evaluation of flow cytometric methods for diagnosis of chronic granulomatous disease variants under routine laboratory conditions. *Cytometry.* 1994;18:147-155.

17

Evaluation of Immunologic Dysfunction

David F. Keren
Irene J. Check

Introduction

The ability of flow cytometry to define the numbers of lymphocyte sub-populations in peripheral blood or other fluids has encouraged the use of this technique to help diagnose and improve our understanding of diseases that are thought to have an immunologic basis. Although research investigations into the mechanisms of immunologically mediated diseases are worthwhile when conducted under careful research protocols, they may or may not be useful for routine patient care. In this chapter we review proposed uses of flow cytometry to perform immunophenotyping on a variety of conditions associated with immune dysfunction.

Flow Cytometry as an Immunoserologic Technique

A wide variety of serologic assays are currently performed in clinical laboratories to aid in the detection of autoimmune phenomena that may correlate with clinical disease. For instance, the antinuclear antibody (ANA) test has been a standard for the past 40 years. It has been used to screen patients suspected of having systemic lupus erythematosus. The test is not specific enough to establish the diagnosis, but because 95% to 98% of patients with systemic lupus erythematosus possess ANAs in their sera, it is highly sensitive in identifying individuals who would benefit from more extensive laboratory and clinical evaluation. The test to detect ANAs may be performed by using indirect immunofluorescence (IIF) or by using enzyme immunoassay (EIA).[1]

The IIF test requires that the patient's serum, after dilution (anywhere from 1:20 to 1:160 depending on the kit used and laboratory studies) in buffer, be layered on a substrate-containing nuclei. The substrate may be a frozen section of rodent kidney or liver. Alternatively, tissue culture cell lines, especially HEp-2 cells, provide nuclei and nucleoli that are larger and easier to visualize than those with frozen section substrates. After incubation of the diluted serum on the substrate in a moisture chamber for about 30 minutes, the substrate is washed thoroughly with buffer. Then the substrate is incubated with fluorescein-conjugated anti-human immunoglobulin G (IgG), followed by another washing step. The substrate is examined under a fluorescence microscope, and the presence of fluorescence and the pattern (homogeneous-peripheral, speckled, nucleolar, or centromere) is recorded.

The EIA makes use of microtiter wells coated with nuclear antigens. The patients' sera are added to these wells and incubated for about 30 minutes. After a thorough wash with buffer, an enzyme-conjugated anti-human IgG is added, followed by another washing step. A chromogenic substrate is added and allowed to react with the enzyme. The amount of colored product resulting correlates with the presence of ANAs. Several investigators have found that both IIF and EIA work well as general screens for ANA reactivity.[1-3] Some recommend using EIA as a general screen and IIF to provide more specificity, along with titer and pattern.[4]

IIF and EIA formats are available as tests for detecting many different types of autoantibodies. Some authors have attempted to use flow cytometry to improve the automation, sensitivity, or objectivity of information resulting from autoantibody testing. The most prominent of these applications has been for the detection of antineutrophil cytoplasmic antibody (ANCA).

ANCA may occur as 2 major types of IIF patterns: cytoplasmic (C-ANCA) and perinuclear (P-ANCA). This reflects reactivity against 2 major antigens (serine protease 3 [PR3] and myeloperoxidase [MPO]) that are responsible for the C and P patterns, respectively. C-ANCA is found mainly in serum from patients with Wegener granulomatosis, whereas P-ANCA is found in a wide variety of conditions with small-vessel (microscopic) vasculitis.[5,6] As with the ANA assay,

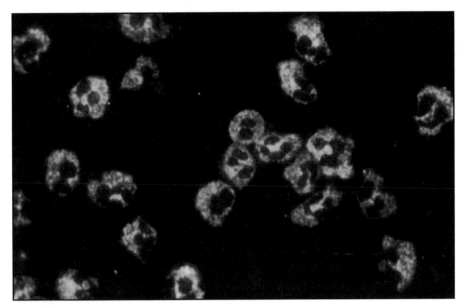

Figure 17-1
Dark-field photomicrograph of C-ANCA.

some investigators recommend use of both IIF and EIA assays to maximize specificity.[7]

In the authors' laboratories we offer ANCA testing on a rapid turn-around (STAT) basis because the presence of these antibodies in a patient with renal and respiratory tract involvement requires aggressive chemotherapy to prevent further tissue damage. Unfortunately, because the titers of the antibodies rise and fall with flare-ups of the disease, the absence of these antibodies cannot rule out these conditions. Also, whereas C-ANCA is highly specific for Wegener granulomatosis, P-ANCA has been described in several other conditions, including ulcerative colitis and primary sclerosing cholangitis, as well as among relatives of patients with ulcerative colitis and even in some patients with respiratory infections. Nonetheless, ANCA testing is one of the most vital autoimmune serology tests available today.

The IIF assay uses human neutrophils fixed in ethanol for the initial screening test. Because PR3 is fixed in the cytoplasmic granules with this fixative, a granular cytoplasmic pattern results when the IIF procedure (as above for the ANA test) is carried out (**Figure 17-1**). MPO escapes from the granules when ethanol is used as a fixative and binds to the electronegative nuclear membrane. This is why a perinuclear pattern results when the IIF procedure is carried out on a patient with positive test results for these antibodies (**Figure 17-2**). As with

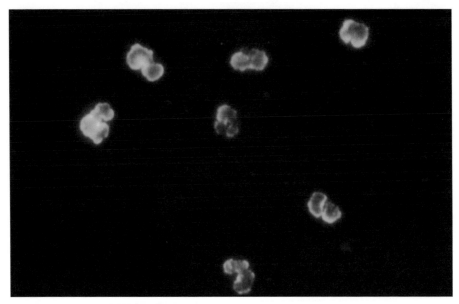

Figure 17-2
Dark-field photomicrograph of P-ANCA.

all IIF methods, the interpretation is subjective. However, with sufficient experience, the assay is highly reproducible.

To provide objective information about ANCA, Suzuki et al[8] proposed the use of flow cytometry for its detection in serum. Their method used heparinized blood from healthy volunteers. They took advantage of the fact that PR3 and MPO are expressed on the surface of neutrophils that have been primed.[9] The neutrophils were incubated with recombinant tumor necrosis factor a to prime the neutrophils. After this step, their staining procedure resembles that of IIF. Patient sera is incubated with the primed neutrophils, followed by a washing step in phosphate-buffered saline. This is followed by an immunofluorescence-labeled anti-human IgG and a second washing step. Using this technique, they detected all 30 sera positive for ANCA studied. However, 2 false-positive results were found in sera from patients with ANA. The latter could be distinguished by a second peak on the histogram (**Figure 17-3**).

Flow cytometric analysis has also been used to study the effect of ANCA on neutrophils. Kettritz et al[10] found that both C-ANCA and P-ANCA are able to bind to ANCA antigens on the cytoplasmic membranes of neutrophils. This results in a cross-linking of the antigens and stimulates oxygen burst from those cells. Interestingly, Fab fragments from C-ANCA and P-ANCA were not able to stimulate this response. These observations suggest a role for intact ANCA in

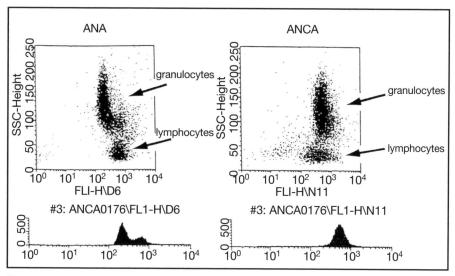

Figure 17-3

Histogram with ANA-positive serum *(left panel)* contrasted with ANCA-positive serum *(right panel)*.

Reprinted with permission from: Suzuki Y, Kaneko K, Saionji K. A novel method for detection of anti-neutrophil cytoplasmic antibody (ANCA) using flow cytometry. *Nippon Jinzo Gakkai Shi.* 1995;37:71-76.

the pathogenesis of the vasculitis that occurs in these patients, although the specific role is still unclear.[11] Because neutrophils are regularly stimulated in response to some host challenge (eg, infections, foreign bodies, and response to degenerating cells), ANCA antigens would be available on the cytoplasmic membrane of neutrophils to bind ANCA in the circulation. Alternatively, apoptotic neutrophils have been shown to express primary granule constituents on their surfaces and can bind to ANCA in the circulation.[12] Lastly, there is evidence that the expression of PR3 on the cytoplasmic membrane of neutrophils fluctuates with disease activity in patients with Wegener granulomatosis.[13]

Although the use of flow cytometry can provide more objective information for interpreting ANCA serology, the loss of the visualization of the different patterns seen is a significant price to pay. Our laboratories currently prefer to use IIF combined with EIA confirmation to provide pattern, titer interpretations, and immunologic confirmation of antigenic specificity. Recent guidelines on the performance and interpretation of ANCA testing recommend the combination of IIF and EIA confirmation.[7] Therefore, although it is of interest for research settings, the authors do not endorse the use of flow cytometry for detecting and quantifying ANCA in serum.

Immunophenotyping and Autoimmune Disease

The term *autoimmune disease* is a misnomer. A wide variety of conditions have been classified as autoimmune diseases, with an implication that the immune system is somehow responsible for the pathology seen. In fact, only occasionally has the immune system been proven to play a role in the pathogenesis of these conditions. However, typically there are autoreactive phenomena, usually autoantibodies but occasionally cell-mediated immune responses, which can be detected in these patients. Autoantibodies are useful in confirming the clinical diagnosis but may not relate to the pathogenesis of the disease.

For instance, in primary biliary cirrhosis, antimitochondrial antibodies (AMAs) are usually present in the serum. The presence of AMAs in the appropriate clinical setting is strong laboratory evidence supporting the diagnosis of primary biliary cirrhosis. However, it is extremely unlikely that the AMAs have anything to do with the pathogenesis of that disease.

Perhaps because the pathogenesis of autoimmune diseases is so poorly understood, some of the conditions included in this category have relatively vague definitions and may in fact represent a constellation of conditions. Others are quite specific.

In the past few years, some studies produced data suggesting that immunophenotyping may be useful in diagnosis or prognosis for some patients with these conditions. In this section, we review evidence for the use of immunophenotyping in such conditions and provide our perspective on the utility of this testing in a routine clinical setting.

Celiac Disease

Absorption of nutrients in the small intestine is dependent on a large functional surface area. This is provided by the extensive microvillus folds of the surface epithelial cells that line the finger-like villi that project into the lumen of the small intestine. Any loss of surface area decreases the absorption of nutrients by the body. In celiac disease, surface epithelial cells are damaged when gluten is ingested and is absorbed by the surface epithelial cells. Celiac disease occurs in about 1 in 500 individuals in most countries.[14] Patients with celiac disease have antibodies and cellular reactivity against gluten (actually against the alpha-gliaden component of gluten). This process may be responsible for the increased small intestinal apoptosis that results in the atrophy of villi and hyperplasia of crypts seen in biopsy specimens from patients with celiac disease.[15] Thus this is one of the autoimmune diseases in which the antibodies or cellular reactivity against gluten may logically be related to the resulting disease.

In the past, the mainstay of establishing the diagnosis of celiac disease required an intestinal biopsy before and after removing gluten from the diet to document an improvement in the histology. Before gluten is removed from the diet, the villi are markedly shortened, and the crypts are increased, with large numbers of mitotic cells.[16] After gluten is removed from the diet, the villi are restored to their normal height, and there is a decrease in crypt depth and number of mitoses. These features reflect the damage to the surface epithelium and the response of the crypt cells to divide in an attempt to repopulate the villi. After restoration of the villi, a brief challenge with gluten was necessary to document that this specific agent could reinduce damage. This latter step was needed to be certain that one was not dealing with another form of malabsorption that may have fortuitously regressed during the abstinence from gluten.[17]

Histologically, there are also noticeable derangements in the lymphocyte and plasma cell populations in the small bowel. Increased numbers of interepithelial lymphocytes and increased numbers of lamina propria plasma cells are characteristic of celiac disease.[18] These immunologic features of the small intestinal biopsy specimen help distinguish celiac disease from autoimmune enteropathy in children. Like celiac disease, autoimmune enteropathy is characterized by atrophy of villi and hyperplasia of crypts, but it lacks the increased numbers of plasma cells usually seen in celiac disease. In addition, children with autoimmune enteropathy usually have anti-goblet cell antibodies, and Paneth cells may be absent.[19] Because this condition is not related to gluten sensitivity, a gluten-free diet has no affect on the malabsorption.[20]

Although still somewhat controversial in clinical practice, IgA antiendomysium (tissue transglutaminase) against gliaden are useful screening tests in several studies for patients with malabsorption who display symptoms of celiac disease,[21-23] yet the cellular response is more likely to be related to the pathologic features of the disease. The fact that the interepithelial T lymphocytes increase locally in the small intestine after challenge with gluten provides a possible mediator of the cytologic damage observed.[24] The local T lymphocytes that increase in celiac disease are known to be gamma-delta T cell receptor (TCR)-bearing lympocytes.[25] These are thought to be regulatory cells that may be able to circumvent the normal suppressor cell activity that prevents the development of harmful immunologic reactions to innocuous food antigens in the intestine.[26] Indeed, the presence of increased numbers of TCR gamma-delta lymphocytes with decreased numbers of CD3$^-$, CD7$^+$ cells is typical of the small bowel lymphocyte phenotype from these patients (**Table 17-1**).[27]

Table 17-1

Increased Gamma-Delta-Positive TCR and Decreased CD3⁻, CD7⁺ Cells among Interepithelial Lymphocytes in Patients with Celiac Disease Compared with Control Subjects

Clinical Status (n) (SD)	gamma-delta⁺ TCR (SD)	CD3–, CD7⁺ (SD)	Age, y
Active celiac disease (15)	34.3 (15.5)	2.2 (2.9)	7.1 (4.3)
Treated celiac disease (5)	34.2 (10.9)	6.3 (4.6)	6.4 (2.9)
Control subjects (20)	6.7 (6.6)	41.4 (21.8)	5.3 (4.5)

Data adapted from Table 2 of Eiras P, Roldan E, Camarero C, et al. Flow cytometry description of a novel CD3-/CD7+ intraepithelial lymphocytes subset in human duodenal biopsies: potential diagnostic value in celiac disease. Cytometry. 1998;34:95-102.
Abbreviations: TCR = T cell receptor; SD = Standard deviation.

The functional significance of the decrease of the CD3⁻, CD7⁺ subset is not known. Therefore its use as a diagnostic test is not recommended at this time.

In the peripheral blood, however, Kerttula et al[28] found no significant differences in the number of TCR gamma-delta lymphocytes in patients with active untreated celiac disease compared with those found in healthy age- and sex-matched control subjects. Although Kerttula et al did note an increase in the CD45RO⁺ population of T cells, this finding is not a sufficiently specific feature to obviate the need for biopsy confirmation of the diagnosis. Therefore the only immunologic diagnostic tests we recommend are the use of IgA antiendomysium (tissue transglutaminase) and IgG antigliaden as an adjunct to selecting patients who may benefit from biopsy confirmation of the disease. However, biopsy confirmation is still optimal for this disease. Flow cytometric studies of the peripheral blood and/or intestinal biopsy specimens are intriguing research methods that are not yet part of routine care.

Patients with Silicone Implants

The study of a variety of immunologic and inflammatory disorders in patients with silicone implants has been a highly controversial subject that has been politicized and distorted in early lay news reports. Unfortunately, because of the hysteria created from these reports, some laboratories began offering a wide variety of useless tests for these women.

A brief background on the issue may be useful in understanding the nature of the controversy. Silicone (polydimethylsiloxane) is a relatively inert substance that was first used in 1962 for tubing to shunt fluid from the ventricles of patients with hydrocephalus. The key phrase here is "relatively inert." As with other foreign substances, silicone will evoke a usually mild foreign-body reaction. Because of its relatively inert nature, silicone has found widespread applications in medicine, including coating syringe needles, in ophthalmic and joint surgery, and as the key ingredient of a variety of prosthetic devices, including breast, penile, and testicular implants.[29] In addition to its medical uses, silicone is widely available for use by the general public as Silly Putty (Binney & Smith, Eaton, PA) and in antacids, processed foods, caulking materials, hand lotions, and hair sprays.[30]

In the early 1960s, primarily in Japan, liquid silicone was used to augment breast size by directly injecting it into the breast.[31] Because it is a foreign substance, the classic inflammatory response that can lead to fibrosis and scarring usually followed. This resulted in the development of dense fibrosis and scarring at the sites of injection. To control the distribution and foreign-body reaction, liquid silicone was later encased in an envelope of hardened silicone. Although this decreased the inflammation caused by direct injection, it did not eliminate the problem. All of the envelopes permitted liquid silicone to leak through.[32] This resulted in the formation of fibrous capsules around the implants. Furthermore, the liquid silicone could travel to regional lymph nodes and even spread widely throughout the body. Lastly, with time, the envelopes were subject to rupture, thereby releasing large quantities of silicone that could recapitulate the poor results obtained from the direct injections performed 2 decades earlier.

The potential inflammatory consequences of the implants were not thoroughly appreciated by early advocates, and many patients did not understand the potential for fibrosis, scarring, and leakage. As many as 25% of women receiving these silicone-filled implants reported having fibrous contractures.[33] Thus when scarring, fibrosis, and pain developed in women with these complications, litigation resulted.

Although these consequences were disturbing, a large public outcry developed after the appearance of anecdotal reports that speculated that there might be a connection between the presence of silicone and the development of an unusual autoimmune disease, progressive systemic sclerosis (scleroderma).[34] Unfortunately, the reports often emphasized the association of the silicone implants with the presence of the disease and did not place sufficient emphasis on the widespread use of implants and the number of cases of scleroderma that one would predict in such a large population.[35]

Careful epidemiologic studies from The Johns Hopkins Hospital, The Mayo Clinic, and Harvard University demonstrating the improbability of any

Table 17-2
Phenotype of Lymphocytes in Patients with Silicone Implants—
Peripheral Blood Studies

Phenotype	Patients with implants (± SD)	Control subjects (± SD)
CD3	71 ± 9 .1	75 ± 3.5
CD3 and DR	5.5 ± 2.5	3.9 ± 2.3
CD4 and CD29	41 ± 10	45 ± 9.2
CD8	30 ± 7.6	25 ± 7.1
CD19	12 ± 8.3	15 ± 4.1
CD3 and CD16/CD56	15 ± 7.2	11 ± 5.0

Data obtained from Katzin WE, Feng L, Abbuhl M, et al. Phenotype of lymphocytes associated with the inflammatory reaction to silicone gel breast implants. Clin Diagn Lab Immunol. *1996;3:156–161. Abbreviation: SD = Standard deviation.*

significant relationship took several years to be published.[36-39] Unfortunately, in the intervening years, there was a wide acceptance by the news media, the lay public, and many clinicians of the idea that the implants somehow were responsible for scleroderma or other autoimmune diseases. In more recent years, as a result of the lack of scientific evidence linking breast implants to the better-defined autoimmune diseases, plaintiffs' attorneys have concentrated on vaguer conditions, such as fibromyalgia (see below).

A handful of laboratories offered (and some chose to widely advertise) immunophenotyping of peripheral blood lymphocytes for studying these patients, despite the lack of a scientific basis for these clinical projects outside of formal research protocols. Most data in the literature found no significant differences in the immunophenotypes of control populations and those of women with silicone breast implants. When Granchi et al[40] looked at peripheral blood lymphocytes from patients with silicone implants with various levels of contracture, they found no difference in the number of CD19, CD3, CD4, CD8, CD25, CD16, $CD3^+DR^+$, $CD4^+DR^+$, or $CD8^+DR^+$ cells between patients with minimal contracture and non-implanted control subjects. Although a modest increase in CD57 lymphocytes was found in some of the patients, this trivial finding does not justify the use of flow cytometry to evaluate these patients. Furthermore, no differences in the number of $CD57^+$ natural killer cells were reported in an abstract published by Morse and Spiera.[41] This older abstract noted an increase in the CD4/CD8 ratio, an increase in the number of B lymphocytes, and decreased numbers of CD2 cells among the 30 patients with silicone implants on whom they reported. Unfortunately, a complete manuscript as a follow-up to this data was not found in our review of the literature. Katzin et al[42] (like Granchi

Table 17-3
Symptoms of Chronic Fatigue Syndrome

Memory lapses
Sore throat
Painful lymph nodes
Painful muscles
Painful joints
Headaches
No relief of fatigue by rest
Fatigue following exercise that persists for at least one day

---

Note: At Least 4 Symptoms Must Be Present for Inclusion
Data obtained from Fukuda K, Straus SE, Hickie I, et al. for the International Chronic Fatigue
Syndrome Study Group. The chronic fatigue syndrome: a comprehensive approach to its definition
and study. Ann Intern Med. 1994;121:953-959; and McKenzie R, O'Fallon A, Dale J, et al. Low-dose
hydrocortisone for treatment of chronic fatigue syndrome. JAMA. 1998;280:1061-1066.

et al[40]) found no compelling differences in the immunophenotypes of the peripheral blood lymphocytes from patients with implants compared with control subjects (**Table 17-2**).

The authors believe that the use of flow cytometry is a wasteful exercise in the routine clinical evaluation of these individuals.

Chronic Fatigue Syndrome

Patients with complaints of severe chronic fatigue probably represent a wide variety of conditions that result in those complaints.[43] Although the immune system may be involved, especially in viral infections, there is compelling evidence that endocrine dysfunction can lead to symptoms of chronic fatigue.

To be included in the category of chronic fatigue syndrome, an individual must be able to document severe chronic fatigue (unexplained) for at least 6 months in duration. In addition, the fatigue must not be related to obvious physical exertion and must not respond to rest.[44] The international study group provided 8 symptoms, requiring at least 4 to be present for inclusion of a patient as a patient with chronic fatigue syndrome (**Table 17-3**).[44,45]

Significantly, none of the current definitions of chronic fatigue syndrome puts weight in immunophenotyping of individuals for any single marker or any panel of markers. McKenzie et al[45] presented convincing evidence for the role of a deficiency in the endocrine system as a pathogenesis for at least some of these cases. Demitrack et al[46] noted problems in the hypothalamic-pituitary-adrenal axis resulting in reduced basal cortisol levels in serum, which is associated with depression in many patients. Indeed, use of low-dose hydrocortisone was found to be helpful for some of the patients with chronic fatigue syndrome (although the resulting suppression of adrenal responsiveness precluded their recommendation of this therapy for clinical purposes).[45]

This is not to say that there are not some articles reporting changes in immunologic indices in some patients with chronic fatigue syndrome. For instance, in 1991, Landay et al[47] reported a decrease in CD8 cells that reached significance among the patients they classified as having "major symptoms" of the disease compared with healthy control subjects. Furthermore, they noted increased expression of CD38 and HLA-DR (so-called activation markers) on these cells. Tirelli et al,[48] however, found no differences in the numbers of $CD3^+$, $CD4^+$, or $CD8^+$ T lymphocytes among those patients with chronic fatigue syndrome compared with healthy age- and sex-matched control subjects. They did note an increase in the numbers of CD19 lymphocytes and suspected the presence of increased expression of activation markers on $CD56^-$ natural killer cells. These findings are of interest and may deserve further investigation but are not of sufficient clarity to provide useful diagnostic or prognostic information in individual cases.

More recent information from Peakman et al[49] noted 43 individuals with chronic fatigue syndrome who were studied as part of a controlled, randomized clinical trial of therapy. They found that the percentages of CD3, CD4, and CD8 cells did not differ between the patients and the control subjects. They also found no difference between naive ($CD45RA^+RO^-$) and memory ($CD45RA^-RO^+$) T lymphocytes in the patients compared with the control subjects. An increase was recorded in the number of natural killer cells ($CD16^+/CD56^+/CD3^-$) in the patients versus the control subjects. Nonetheless, they concluded that there was no "important association" between the clinical status of patients with chronic fatigue or their response to treatment and the immunophenotype panels that they studied. Zhang et al[50] also found no significant differences in the immunophenotype parameters comparing nonmilitary patients with chronic fatigue syndrome with control subjects (**Table 17-4**). They did note a slight increase in the total T cells among Gulf War veterans who returned with severe fatigue. This finding, however, did not have general application to the civilian population with or without chronic fatigue syndrome.

Routine immunophenotyping of the peripheral blood lymphocytes from patients with complaints consistent with chronic fatigue syndrome does not add to the diagnostic evaluation of individual patients. If one wishes to perform immunophenotyping on these patients, it should only be performed in the context of a controlled, funded research trial.

Table 17-4

Immunophenotype from Patients with Chronic Fatigue Versus Control Subjects

Immunophenotype	Chronic fatigue* (n = 68)	Control subjects* (n = 53)
CD3+	75.53 ± 1.21	75.87 ± 0.97
CD3+ CD4+	48.60 ± 1.03	49.59 ± 1.18
CD3+ CD8+	24.81 ± 0.97	25.72 ± 1.20
CD19+	14.23 ± 0.80	13.38 ± 0.66
CD16+/CD56+	10.19 ± 0.73	10.62 ± 0.76

*Nonmilitary patients and control subjects. Data are expressed as the percentage of lymphocytes ± SE (standard error).
Data obtained from Zhang Q, Zhou X, Denny T, et al. Changes in immune parameters seen in Gulf War veterans but not in civilians with chronic fatigue syndrome. Clin Diagn Lab Immunol. 1999;6:6-13.

Fibromyalgia

This is a complex, poorly understood condition characterized by pain in joints and muscles, point tenderness, occasional depression, occasional chronic fatigue, and often poor sleep, and it is usually seen in middle-aged women. Laboratory findings among the patients with these complaints do not differ significantly from those of control subjects, and therefore this is a clinical diagnosis. The American College of Rheumatology published criteria in 1990 for the classification of fibromyalgia.[51] They require a history of diffuse musculoskeletal pain and pain in at least 11 of 18 specific points.

As is the case with other laboratory tests, flow cytometry is not recommended for evaluating these individuals for diagnosis. In one research study Hernanz et al[52] reported an increase in T lymphocytes that expressed activation CD69 and CD25 activation markers. Their CD3, CD4, CD8, CD19, CD16, and CD4/CD8 ratio findings did not differ between their patient and control populations. Consequently, the authors do not recommend that immunophenotyping be performed on this patient population.

Immunophenotyping of Bronchoalveolar Lavage Fluid

The respiratory tract is an important potential portal of entry for pathogenic microorganisms. A sophisticated mucosal defense system has evolved along this and other mucosal surfaces. Lymphocytes exist in several compartments within the respiratory tract: interepithelial lymphocytes, lamina propria lymphocytes, intra-alveolar lymphocytes, and aggregates of lymphoid follicles termed *bronchus-associated lymphoid tissue* (BALT).[53] The lymphocyte populations in these compartments parallel those found in similar compartments along the gastrointestinal tract.[54] In these mucosal surfaces the lymphocytes that exist between the epithelial cells are mainly CD8+ T lymphocytes, whereas those within the lamina propria have a CD4/CD8 ratio similar to that found in the peripheral blood. B lymphocytes are uncommon in the interepithelial compartment.

BALT follicles may be counterparts to the Peyer patches in the bowel. Although they are commonly present in the bronchi of younger individuals, their presence in the bronchi of older adults seems to correlate with the quantity of antigen to which the respiratory tract is exposed. For instance, Hiller et al[55] reported that BALT follicles were found in 40% of consecutive autopsies on individuals younger than 20 years but only rarely in older patients. These follicular structures persist in the larynx, however, in approximately 50% of adults over 20 years of age.

During bronchoalveolar lavage (BAL), sterile saline solution is instilled by means of a fiberoptic bronchoscope into a specific segment of the lung. Withdrawal of this fluid provides a sampling of both inflammatory and epithelial cells of that portion of the lung. To process cells for flow cytometry, samples with heavy mucus content must be filtered. The use of filters to remove the mucus varies considerably, but Hiller et al[55] use filtration sparingly, and only when heavy mucus content interferes with the analysis. Loss of cells by the filtration could distort the percentage of phenotypes present.

The largest single use for BAL fluid analysis by immunophenotyping is diagnosis of sarcoidosis. Alveolar macrophages form 80% to 90% of the total cells from most BAL fluid. In sarcoidosis the alveolar macrophages coexpress high levels of the T-cell activation-related markers CD86, CD40, and CD30L.[56] This has been associated with their functioning as effective antigen-presenting cells, whereas normal alveolar macrophages do not. Although macrophages predominate in most BAL fluid, the percentage of total lymphocytes is much greater in BAL fluid from patients with sarcoidosis (approximately 50% of the cells are lymphocytes) compared with control BAL fluid (less than 20% are lymphocytes).[53] Furthermore, among patients with sarcoidosis, the CD4/CD8 ratio is usually elevated as high as 20:1, which may help distinguish sarcoidosis from hypersensitivity pneumonitis or idiopathic pulmonary fibrosis, in which CD8 cells usually predominate.[53,57]

BAL fluid from patients with diffuse panbronchiolitis contains larger numbers of neutrophils than such samples from patients with sarcoidosis.[58] Indeed, 90% of BAL fluid from diffuse panbronchiolitis patients consisted of neutrophils in the study by Kikawada et al.[58] Furthermore, the CD4/CD8 ratio was useful in distinguishing their patients with diffuse panbronchiolitis who would respond to therapy (mean value, 1.35 ± 0.42) from those patients who were refractory to therapy (mean value, 0.45 ± 0.16). Their control subjects had a CD4/CD8 ratio of 2.54 ± 0.76.

Other workers have looked at a variety of activation, cytokine, and adhesion molecules as diagnostic or prognostic tools among patients with sarcoidosis.[59-61] Assays for none of these molecules have yet achieved general acceptance, although some show clinical promise. Suzuki et al[62] found that patients in whom at least 40% of $CD3^+$ cells were Ia^+ were more likely to have progressive disease than individuals whose $CD3^+$ cells were less than 40% Ia^+. Unfortunately, the group with more than 40% Ia^+ CD3 cells was relatively small. Furthermore, it is unlikely that this would alter how the patients are followed in the interim.

Summary

In summary, the use of flow cytometry as a tool to document several conditions classified as having to do with immunologic dysfunction is quite variable. Flow cytometry is most useful in defining cell populations in BAL fluid from patients with sarcoidosis or diffuse panbronchiolitis, where it helps in both diagnosis and in estimating response to therapy. The immunoserologic use of flow cytometry has not gained widespread acceptance. It can provide more objective information than IIF techniques but does not seem to offer significant advantage over EIA technology for most autoimmune diseases. The authors do not recommend the use of flow cytometry to evaluate patients with silicone breast implants, fibromyalgia, or chronic fatigue syndrome. Although it may be frustrating for clinicians to deal with poorly defined immunologic conditions, bad information is worse than no information. As we point out in this chapter, the immunophenotyping data for those conditions does not enable better diagnostic or prognostic conclusions. Although research investigations into the mechanisms of immunologically mediated diseases are worthwhile when conducted under careful research protocols, they may or may not be useful for routine patient care.

References

1. Keren DF, Hedstrom DL. Contemporary approaches to anti-nuclear antibody serology. *J Clin Ligand Assay.* 1999;22:50-55.

2. Gniewek RA, Sandbulte C, Fox PC. Comparison of antinuclear antibody testing methods by ROC analysis with reference to disease diagnosis. *Clin Chem.* 1997;43:1987-1989.

3. Homburder HA, Cahen YD, Griffiths J, et al. Detection of antinuclear antibodies. Comparative evaluation of enzyme immunoassay and indirect immunofluorescence methods. *Arch Pathol Lab Med.* 1998;122:993-999.

4. Reisner BA, DiBlasi J, Goel N. Comparison of enzyme immunoassay to an indirect fluorescent immunoassay for the detection of antinuclear antibodies. *Am J Clin Pathol.* 1999;111:503-506.

5. Jennette JC, Falk RJ. Small-vessel vasculitis. *N Engl J Med.* 1997;337:1512-1523.

6. Goeken JA. Antineutrophil cytoplasmic antibody—a useful serological marker for vasculitis. *J Clin Immunol.* 1991;11:161-174.

7. Lim LCL, Taylor JG III, Schmitz JL, et al. Diagnostic usefulness of antineutrophil cytoplasmic autoantibody serology. Comparative evaluation of commercial indirect fluorescent antibody kits and enzyme immunoassay kits. *Am J Clin Pathol.* 1999;111:363-369.

8. Suzuki Y, Kaneko K, Saionji K. A novel method for detection of anti-neutrophil cytoplasmic antibody (ANCA) using flow cytometry. *Nippon Jinzo Gakkai Shi.* 1995;37:71-76.

9. Mulder AH, Heeringa P, Brouwer E, et al. Activation of granulocytes by anti-neutrophil cytoplasmic antibodies (ANCA): a Fc gamma RII-dependent process. *Cell Exp Immunol.* 1994;98:270-278.

10. Kettritz R, Jennette JC, Falk RJ. Crosslinking of ANCA-antigens stimulates superoxide release by human neutrophils. *J Am Soc Nephrol.* 1997;8:386-394.

11. Salant DJ. ANCA: fuel for the fire or the spark that ignites the flame? *Kidney Int.* 1999;55:1125-1127.

12. Yang JJ, Tuttle RH, Hogan SL, et al: Target antigens for anti-neturophil cytoplasmic autoantibodies (ANCA) are on the surface of primed and apoptotic but not unstimulated neutrophils. *Clin Exp Immunol.* 2000;121:165-172.

13. Kobold ACM, Kallenberg CGM, Tervaert JWC. Leucocyte membrane expression of proteinase 3 correlates with disease activity in patients with Wegener's granulomatosis. *Br J Rheumatol.* 1998;37:901-907.

14. Murray JA. Serodiagnosis of celiac disease. In: Keren DF, Nakamura R, eds. Progress and Controversies in Autoimmune Disease Testing. *Clin Lab Med.* 1997;17:445-464.

15. Moss SF, Attia L, Scholes JV, et al. Increased small intestinal apoptosis in celiac disease. *Gut.* 1996;39:811-814.

16. Michalski JP, McCombs CC. Celiac disease: clinical features and pathogenesis. *Am J Med Sci.* 1994;307:204-211.

17. Trier JS. Celiac sprue. *N Engl J Med.* 1991;325:1709-1719.

18. Scott BB, Goodall A, Stephenson P, et al. Small intestinal plasma cells in celiac disease. *Gut.* 1984;25:41-46.

19. Moore L, Xu X, Davidson G, et al. Autoimmune enteropathy with anti-goblet cell antibodies. *Hum Pathol.* 1995;26:1162-1168.

20. Bousvaros A, Leichtner AM, Book L, et al. Treatment of pediatric autoimmune enteropathy with tacrolimus (FK506). *Gastroenterology.* 1996;111:237-243.

21. Nakachi K, Swift G, Wilmot D, et al: Antibodies to tissue transglutaminase: comparison of ELISA and immunoprecipitation assay in the presence and the absence of calcium ions. *Clin Chim Acta.* 2001;304:75-84.

22. Rostami K, Kerckhaert J, Tiemessen R, et al. Sensitivity of antiendomysium and antigliadin antibodies in untreated celiac disease: disappointing in clinical practice. *Am J Gastroenterol.* 1999;94:888-894.

23. Volta U, Molinaro N, De Franceschi L, et al. IgA anti-endomysial antibodies on human umbilical cord tissue for celiac disease screening. Save both money and monkeys. *Dig Dis Sci.* 1995;40:1902-1905.

24. Marsh MN. Studies of intestinal lymphoid tissue: IV. The predictive value of raised mitotic indices among jejunal epithelial lymphocytes in the diagnosis of gluten-sensitive enteropathy. *J Clin Pathol.* 1992;35:517-525.

25. Maki M, Holm K, Collin P, et al. Increase in gamma delta T cell receptor bearing lymphocytes in normal small bowel mucosa in latent celiac disease. *Gut.* 1991;32:1412-1414.

26. Fujihashi K, Taguchi T, McGhee JR, et al. Regulatory function for murine intraepithelial lymphocytes. Two subsets of CD3+ TCR-1 IEL T cells abrogate oral tolerance. *J Immunol.* 1990;145:2010-2019.

27. Eiras P, Roldan E, Camarero C, et al. Flow cytometry description of a novel CD3-/CD7+ intraepithelial lymphocytes subset in humanduodenal biopsies: potential diagnostic value in celiac disease. *Cytometry.* 1998;34:95-102.

28. Kerttula TO, Hallstrom O, Maki M. Phenotypical characterization of peripheral blood T cells in patients with celiac disease: elevation of antigen-primed CD45RO+ T lymphocytes. *Immunology.* 1995;86:104-109.

29. Cook RR, Harrison MC, LeVier RR. The breast implant controversy. *Arthritis Rheum.* 1994;37:153-157.

30. Sanchez-Guerrero J, Schur PH, Sergent JS, et al. Silicone breast implants and rheumatic disease. Clinical, immunologic, and epidemiologic studies. *Arthritis Rheum.* 1994;37:158-168.

31. Hirmand H, Latrenta GS, Hoffman LA. Autoimmune disease and silicone breast implants. *Oncology.* 1993;7:17-28.

32. Yu LT, Latorre G, Marotta J, et al. In vitro measurement of silicone bleed from breast implants. *Plast Reconstr Surg.* 1996;97:756-764.

33. Kossovsky N, Freiman CJ. Silicone breast implant pathology. Clinical data and immunologic consequences. *Arch Pathol Lab Med.* 1994;118:686-693.

34. Spiera H, Kerr LD. Scleroderma following silicone implantation: a cumulative experience of 11 cases. *J Rheumatol.* 1993;20:958-961.

35. Angell M. Shattuck Lecture—evaluating the health risks of breast implants: the interplay of medical science, the law and public opinion. *N Engl J Med.* 1996;334:1513-1516.

36. Hochberg MC, Miller R, Wigley FM. Frequency of augmentation mammoplasty in patients with systemic sclerosis: data from the Johns Hopkins-University of Maryland Scleroderma Center. *J Clin Epidemiol.* 1995;48:565-569.

37. Gabriel SE, O'Fallon WM, Kurland LT, et al. Risk of connective tissue diseases and other disorders after breast implantation. *N Engl J Med.* 1994;330:1697-1702.

38. Sanchez-Guerrero J, Colditz G, Karlson EW, et al. Silicone breast implants and the risk of connective-tissue diseases and symptoms. *N Engl J Med.* 1995;332:1666-1670.

39. Hennekens CH, Lee I, Cook NR, et al. Self-reported breast implants and connective-tissue diseases in female health professionals. A retrospective cohort study. *JAMA.* 1996;275:616-621.

40. Granchi D, Cavedagna D, Ciapetti G, et al. Silicone breast implants: the role of immune system on capsular contracture formation. *J Biomed Mater Res.* 1995;29:197-202.

41. Morse JH, Spiera H. Autoimmune diseases, immunoglobulin isotypes and lymphocyte subsets in 30 females with breast augmentation mammoplasty [abstract]. *Arthritis Rheum.* 1992;35(Suppl 9):S65.

42. Katzin WE, Feng L, Abbuhl M, et al. Phenotype of lymphocytes associated with the inflammatory reaction to silicone gel breast implants. *Clin Diagn Lab Immunol.* 1996;3:156-161.

43. Streeten DHP. The nature of chronic fatigue [editorial]. *JAMA.* 1998;280:1094-1095.

44. Fukuda K, Straus SE, Hickie I, et al. for the International Chronic Fatigue Syndrome Study Group. The chronic fatigue syndrome: a comprehensive approach to its definition and study. *Ann Intern Med.* 1994;121:953-959.

45. McKenzie R, O'Fallon A, Dale J, et al. Low-dose hydrocortisone for treatment of chronic fatigue syndrome. *JAMA.* 1998;280:1061-1066.

46. Demitrack MA, Dale JK, Strauss SE, et al. Evidence for impaired activation of the hypothalamic-pituitary-adrenal axis in patients with chronic fatigue syndrome. *J Clin Endocrinol Metab.* 1991;73:1224-1234.

47. Landay AL, Jessop C, Lennette ET, et al. Chronic fatigue syndrome: clinical condition associated with immune activation. *Lancet.* 1991;338:707-712.

48. Tirelli U, Marotta G, Improta S, et al. Immunological abnormalities in patients with chronic fatigue syndrome. *Scand J Immunol.* 1994;40:601-608.

49. Peakman M, Deale A, Field R, et al. Clinical improvement in chronic fatigue syndrome is not associated with lymphocyte subsets of function or activation. *Clin Immunol Immunopathol.* 1997;82:83-91.

50. Zhang Q, Zhou X, Denny T, et al. Changes in immune parameters seen in Gulf War veterans but not in civilians with chronic fatigue syndrome. *Clin Diagn Lab Immunol.* 1999;6:6-13.

51. Wolfe F, Smythe HA, Yunus MB, et al. The American College of Rheumatology criteria for the classification of fibromyalgia: report of the Multicenter Criteria Committee. *Arthritis Rheum.* 1990;33:160-172.

52. Hernanz W, Valenzuela A, Quijada J, et al. Lymphocyte subpopulations in patients with primary fibromyalgia. *J Rheumatol.* 1994;21:2122-2124.

53. Harbeck RJ. Immunophenotyping of bronchoalveolar lavage lymphocytes. *Clin Diagn Lab Immunol.* 1998;5:271-277.

54. Silbart LK, Keren DF. Structure and function of the immunologic system of the gastrointestinal tract. In: Ming S, Goldman H, eds. *The Pathology of the Gastrointestinal Tract.* 2nd ed. Baltimore: Williams & Wilkins; 1998:99-112.

55. Hiller AS, Tschernig T, Kleemann WJ, et al. Bronchus-associated lymphoid tissue (BALT) and larynx-associated lymphoid tissue (LALT) are found at different frequencies in children, adolescents and adults. *Scand J Immunol.* 1998;47:159-162.

56. Nicod LP, Isler P. Alveolar macrophages in sarcoidosis coexpress high levels of CD86 (B7.2), CD40, and CD30L. *Am J Respir Cell Mol Biol.* 1997;17:91-96.

57. Gruber R, Pforte A, Beer B, et al. Determination of gamma/delta and other T-lymphocyte subsets in bronchoalveolar lavage fluid and peripheral blood from patients with sarcoidosis and idiopathic fibrosis of the lung. *APMIS.* 1996;104:199-205.

58. Kikawada M, Ichinose Y, Minemura K, et al. A study of peripheral airway findings using an ultrathin bronchofiberscope and bronchoalveolar lavage fluid with diffuse panbronchiolitis. *Respiration.* 1998;65:433-440.

59. Iida K, Kadota J, Kawakami K, et al. Analysis of T cell subsets and beta chemokines in patients with pulmonary sarcoidosis. *Thorax.* 1997;52:431-437.

60. Nakamura H, Fujishima S, Soejima K, et al. Flow cytometric detection of cell-associated cytokines in alveolar macrophages. *Eur Respir J.* 1996;9:1181-1187.

61. Hol BE, Hintzen RQ, Van Lier RA, et al. Soluble and cellular markers of T cell activation in patients with pulmonary sarcoidosis. *Am Rev Respir Dis.* 1993;148:643-649.

62. Suzuki K, Tamura N, Iwase A, et al. Prognostic value of Ia+ T lymphocytes in bronchoalveolar lavage fluid in pulmonary sarcoidosis. *Am J Respir Crit Care Med.* 1997;154:707-712.

18

Clinical Applications of DNA Content Analysis

Irene Check

Introduction

Flow or image cytometry analysis of DNA content (DNA ploidy and S-phase) has shown that up to 70% of human cancers show aneuploidy and/or changes in the proportion of cells that are synthesizing DNA.[1] How to use such DNA content data to manage individual patients remains unresolved. Ultimately, the issue is not whether a tumor is aneuploid or highly proliferating but whether the test results can be used to define outcome or predict prognosis. The clinical value of DNA content analysis often disappears when considered after multivariate analysis that includes traditional prognostic factors, such as tumor grade or stage.[2]

Knowledge of the test result should contribute to a clinical decision that results in a more favorable clinical outcome for the patient, according to the proposed Tumor Marker Utility Grading System.[3] Outcomes may include increased overall survival, disease-free survival, improvement in quality of life, or reduction in cost of care. To place DNA flow cytometry of solid tumors into this context, clinicians must be convinced that the DNA result confers therapeutic alternatives.

A number of clinical groups have proposed general guidelines for use of clinical tumor markers.[3-6] If these guidelines were applied to DNA content analysis, the test would exhibit significant and independent predictive value that has been validated by clinical testing; that is, it would not be implemented solely on the basis of retrospective data analysis. The assays would be feasible, reproducible, widely available, and subject to quality control. The DNA analysis would provide data, with therapeutic implications, that are readily interpretable by the clinician, and the measurement would not consume tumor needed for other tests. Unfortunately, the existing DNA flow cytometry studies usually fall short on one or more of these counts. Despite hundreds of publications on DNA flow cytometry in cancer, few reach contemporary evidence-based clinical criteria for use as a diagnostic test.[7-10]

Obviously, sufficient tumor must be preserved for careful cytologic and/or histologic analysis. Furthermore, in the molecular era genes, or their encoded products, are more likely to provide therapeutically relevant information than DNA content analysis. The risk of consuming tumor material to measure DNA content, especially if the test result has marginal clinical utility, is the loss of future opportunity to measure a critical gene or its encoded product, which may be the target of a novel therapeutic drug. For example, in 1998, the FDA approved Herceptin (Trastuzumab; Genentech, Inc, South San Francisco, CA), a humanized monoclonal antibody that directly targets erbB-2-associated growth promotion for the treatment of metastatic breast cancer.[11-13] The approval occurred in 5 months. Although there is considerable discussion about how to select patients most likely to benefit from this treatment, most physicians believe that breast cancers without erbB-2 alterations will not respond to Herceptin. High expression of the *ERBB2* gene in breast cancer was associated with patient response to a dose-intensive doxorubicin-based (Ben Venue Laboratories, Beford, OH) chemotherapy treatment in an initial analysis of 397 patients,[14] although the results were more difficult to interpret in an additional cohort of 595 patients.[15] The measurement of erbB-2 in tumor samples, either by means of immunohistochemical staining or fluorescent in situ hybridization (FISH) has rapidly moved into widespread practice.[16,17]

This experience illustrates the value of preserving clinical material to the benefit of the individual patient. Archival tissue is now examined for erbB-2, a test that did not exist when many surviving patients with breast cancer had their initial surgery, to assist in deciding whether a patient whose disease has progressed now has a new therapeutic option. An argument could also be made that archival tissue should remain for testing markers that might increase our understanding of the underlying biology, whether it be to measure other existing growth factor receptor genes, oncogenes, or tumor suppressor genes or those yet to be discovered.[18]

No consideration of the clinical utility of a test can be made without taking financial reimbursement into account. In the United States state-to-state variability in Medicare reimbursement for clinical flow cytometry testing has been reported.[19] According to the Balanced Budget Act of 1997, Public Law 105-33 mandates adoption, beginning January 1, 1999, of national coverage and administrative policies for clinical diagnostic laboratory tests using negotiated rulemaking. A committee of parties who may be affected by the rule is convened, and the goal is to reach consensus on the content of the proposed rule that is then published for comment. The Recommended Medicare National Coverage Policy for Flow Cytometry is published on the HCFA web site.[20] It lists carcinomas as an indication for DNA analysis of tumor for ploidy and percentage of S-phase cells, specifically in patients with early-stage carcinomas (ovarian, breast, colon, endometrium, prostate, and carcinoma of unknown primary site) and advanced ovarian carcinoma. The disposition of the recommendations is yet to be determined.

Confounding the clinical acceptance of flow cytometry data for DNA content analysis is the fact that different investigators using similar types of clinical specimens have come to significantly different conclusions regarding the clinical utility of the measurements. The flow cytometry community has long recognized the need for a systematic review of the literature, with an eye toward both the quality of the study design and the technical aspects of tissue analysis. Whereas some divergent results were attributed to poorly designed studies lacking appropriate numbers of patients or follow-up, many were the result of technical factors. Earlier warnings about the potential effect of methodologic differences on the interpretation of clinical studies[21,22] were not heeded. Interlaboratory proficiency surveys conducted from 1990 to 1992 showed that from as few as 58% to 97% of laboratories reported the correct number of aneuploid peaks, depending on the specimen; S-phase results varied greatly.[23]

A consensus conference was convened in 1992 to begin to address these issues.[24] The organizers limited consideration to tumors of the breast, bladder, colon and rectum, prostate, and hematopoietic system. They produced consensus statements for each of these organ systems. In addition, they acknowledged that successful clinical implementation of cell DNA content measurement depends on the development of standards and standardization of the techniques. The published guideline recommended standardized terminology (*DNA diploid*, *DNA aneuploid*, and *DNA index*) and addressed a number of technical issues, ranging from tissue sampling and sample processing and staining to instrument standardization and data or histogram analysis.[25] A European consensus report[26] and guideline for image cytometry[27] have also been published. From the technical perspective, interlaboratory standardization can be improved,[28] but recent proficiency survey data still show considerable variability in important factors, such as specimen preparation, gating, and use of debris and aggregation modeling.[29]

The clinical utility of DNA flow cytometry studies has been stymied by the lack of progress in standardization, the lack of consistent methods to separate malignant from normal and inflammatory cells during analysis, and the lack of prospective longitudinal outcome studies. This chapter will review the current status of the clinical utility of these tests for patients with breast, bladder, prostate, and colorectal cancers, in which the outcomes have been best studied. For an analysis of the clinical implications of DNA ploidy and cell cycle analyses in the full spectrum of human malignancies, the reader is directed to the chapter by Witzig and Katzmann in this book[30] and to the review by Jeffrey Ross.[2]

Breast Cancer

In the first major retrospective study of the prognostic value of DNA flow cytometry in breast cancer, Auer et al[31] studied archival fine-needle aspiration biopsy material from 112 patients with breast cancer. The flow cytometric histograms were classified into 4 groups (sometimes still referred to as Auer groups) according to DNA content. Patients with diploid tumors were found to have had an excellent prognosis, whereas those with aneuploid tumors had increased relapse and mortality rates. The 1992 consensus review of the clinical utility of DNA cytometry in carcinoma of the breast concluded that operable breast cancers with a diploid DNA index have a favorable prognosis but that the magnitude of the advantage over aneuploid tumors is small.[32] This conclusion was based on a number of studies that included substantial numbers of patients.[33-49] However, more recent reviews question the independent prognostic value of DNA ploidy,[50,51] particularly in advanced breast cancer.[52]

The correlation of high S-phase fraction (SPF) with increased risk of recurrence and mortality for both node-negative and node-positive invasive cancer has been more consistent. The 1992 consensus conference concluded that the literature "clearly supports" such an association,[32] citing some studies that found favorable results with DNA ploidy[39,40,42] and others in which SPF emerged as the key variable.[53-58] Although the predictive power of SPF was retained after multivariate analysis with adjustment for a number of prognostic variables, it is strongly associated with tumor grade. The study by Witzig et al[59] of 502 patients with node-positive breast cancer showed no independent prognostic value for DNA content or SPF. Another study of 280 women with axillary lymph node-negative invasive cancer showed histologic grade to be the only independent predictor of relapse,[60] whereas tumor diameter and SPF did predict mortality. Nevertheless, flow cytometric data might provide an objective marker to assist in deciding whether to treat patients with pathologic stage I disease with systemic adjuvant therapy. Patients with node-negative cancer with small tumors (< 1 cm) have an excellent prognosis and do not require adjuvant therapy, whereas patients with larger (> 2 cm) tumors or involved nodes usually do. It is in the patients with node-negative cancer with tumors between 1.1 and 2 cm in diameter and who are not candidates for prospective trials that the test may be beneficial.[61]

Unfortunately, the measurement of SPF is highly subject to technical factors. In a substantial proportion of the published cases, the SPF was considered to be not evaluable because of technical reasons (eg, excess debris).[62] Results from a recent College of American Pathologists (CAP) flow cytometry proficiency survey illustrate the persistent magnitude of the problem. Although over 99% of the more than 200 participating laboratories correctly identified a single aneuploid peak with a median DNA index of 2.1 (range, 1.9-2.4; measured SPF ranged from 5.2% to 38.1%[63]), one may predict that the variability could be much higher in actual clinical specimens, in which factors such as the method of tissue disaggregation and the proportion of malignant cells play an important role. In addition, Baldetorp et al[64] recently demonstrated that different methods of calculating SPF produced different mean values of SPF (ranging from 4.3%-9.4% for 350 patients with breast cancer), although they did not affect the correlations with lymph node involvement, tumor size, or estrogen receptor content. A similar but larger multicenter study concluded that different calculation models yielded different prognostic results.[65]

The pros and cons of fresh versus frozen material are debatable. Fresh-frozen material provides better quality DNA histograms but cannot be used in studies of small mammogram-detected tumors. Paraffin sections make it possible for the pathologist to verify that the actual tissue submitted for analysis contains a substantial proportion (at least 20%) of malignant cells and consume a smaller amount of tumor. Whether the tissue source is fresh or frozen, artifacts arising from apoptotic or necrotic tumor cells, as well as dilution with benign stromal or inflammatory cells, limit the interpretation of DNA histograms. Multiparametric flow techniques with tumor cell suspensions stained for both cytokeratin and DNA have been reported to improve the accuracy of SPF calculations and to enhance the prognostic value of the test.[66,67] Recent improvements in techniques to extract nuclei with sufficient residual cytoplasm to detect cytokeratin, coupled with the use of a cocktail of 2 anticytokeratin clones, make it possible to analyze the DNA of deparaffinized breast cancers with cytokeratin gating of epithelial cells.[68] In their comparison of flow cytometric analyses of fresh-frozen versus archival tissue from 82 patients with breast cancer, McCormick et al[68] obtained better results than those obtained in earlier studies in terms of coefficient of variation (CV) and the amount of histogram background aggregates and debris found with the paraffin method.

The selection of clinically significant cutoff points for SPF is a point of serious concern. In addition to the fact that 2 different laboratories are highly likely to obtain 2 different SPF values for the same tumor, different published series have assigned different proportions of tumors to the high- and low-risk SPF groups. Thus when reporting the risk assessment of the percentage of SPF in a particular patient, the laboratory must avoid simply using published SPF cutoff points. The 1992 consensus conference recommended that each laboratory validate its own SPF values by correlating them to clinical outcome. At a minimum, each laboratory must establish its own distribution of SPF values for diploid and aneuploid tumors and interpret the breakpoint for low- versus high-risk SPF in the context of these distributions. One suggested solution is to simply report the SPF as a percentile result for breast tumors studied within the individual laboratory.[61] Another approach is to establish 3 prognostic groups: high, low, and intermediate risk. This classification scheme recognizes the fact that flow cytometric measurements of SPF contain a significant margin of error. It minimizes the chance that 2 patients may be placed in opposite prognostic categories on the basis of values that differ by insignificant amounts (eg, SPF estimates of 6.9% vs 7.1% when the cutoff point is 7%).[69]

The unresolved issues of standardization have strongly contributed to the reluctance of clinicians to adopt the use of SPF for making treatment decisions. The fact that a particular SPF value may be classified as high in one published series and low in another series has understandably confused clinicians. This lack of consistency prevented the National Institutes of Health Consensus Meeting on Early Breast Cancer, held in May 1990, from recommending the use of this marker in clinical practice, according to Merkel.[61,70] The American Society of Clinical Oncology excluded the routine use of DNA index and DNA flow cytometric proliferation analysis from their clinical practice guidelines in 1996 and recommended no change in the 1997 update.[71,72]

Wenger and Clark[73] recently reviewed 273 published articles and concluded that the measurement of SPF does have clinical utility for patients with breast cancer. Despite different techniques and cutoff points, correlations between SPF and other prognostic markers are relatively consistent across studies. Higher SPF is associated with worse tumor grade, larger tumors, positive axillary lymph nodes, and lack of estrogen receptors. It predicts worse disease-free and overall survival in multivariate analyses. Nevertheless, Wenger and Clark insisted that standardization and quality control must be improved before the test can be routinely used in community settings. In the meantime, alternative methods to measure cellular proliferation on tissue sections are emerging, although they are certainly not well validated. These range from simple mitotic counts[74] to immunohistochemical stains for cell cycle-related antigens, such as mitosin, a nuclear protein that is expressed in late G1, S, G2, and M phases of the cell cycle but not in the G0 phase.[75]

Bladder Cancer

The application of DNA flow cytometry to bladder washing and urine cytology in the early 1980s was the first attempt to apply this technique to improving the sensitivity of diagnostic cytology.[76] Early studies suggested that detection of aneuploidy using flow cytometry could identify nearly all cases of transitional cell carcinoma in situ and invasive carcinoma of the bladder.[77] A series of studies to examine whether flow cytometry improves the sensitivity of routine cytology studies ensued.[78-87] The DNA Cytometry Consensus Conference concluded that the specificity of flow cytometry was too low for use in screening low-risk patients, even though the data obtained with bladder irrigation specimens suggested that flow cytometry does improve the sensitivity of conventional cytology in detecting cancer. The need for invasive cystoscopy to obtain the specimens is also prohibitive. Hence, DNA cytometry should not be used for screening for bladder cancer nor for investigating microscopic hematuria.[88]

DNA ploidy status has been consistently linked to grade and stage in bladder cancer.[76] It has also been associated with biologic markers, such as loss of blood group antigen expression, and ras oncoprotein overexpression,[89] and p53 gene mutation.[90] The consensus panel recommended that DNA cytometry be used only to study patients with tumor or strong suspicion of tumor, with maximum utility in stratifying grade 2 superficial tumors. The interpretation of results differs depending on whether the analysis is performed at the time of a tumor event or at follow-up.

The clinical value of DNA analysis performed at the time of a tumor event is limited to grade 2 superficial (T_a, T_1, and tumor in situ) tumors.[82,91] Grade 1 tumors are usually DNA diploid, grade 3 tumors are usually aneuploid, and grade 2 tumors vary. Paired analysis of bladder irrigation specimens obtained before resection versus tumor tissue may provide prognostic information for progression to muscle invasion and metastases. The presence of multiple DNA aneuploid populations carries the worst prognosis, whereas the absence of aneuploidy is best. When the DNA indexes of the aneuploid populations of the paired specimens are different, the risk of progression to invasive or metastatic disease is high. When the irrigation sample is aneuploid, but the biopsy is diploid, the probability of tumor in situ is high.

The presence of a clear, nontetraploid, DNA aneuploid population in bladder irrigation samples after conservative treatment (transurethral resection) of early-stage disease is diagnostic for recurrent tumor.[83,92] Similarly, the presence of a DNA aneuploid population in bladder irrigation samples at 6 months after intravesical bacille Calmette-Guerin treatment predicts progression and treatment failure, whereas the presence of DNA diploid cells is a strong indicator of response.[91,93,94] However, a recent prospective study found no incremental value of DNA analysis over cytology.[95] Because none of the clinical studies directly assess the effect of treatment modality on the relative clinical value of DNA ploidy, it is not possible to evaluate whether the absence of predictive value in some studies[96] is due to differences in treatment (eg, preoperative radiation followed by cystectomy) or to other factors.

It is generally agreed that specificity and sensitivity of DNA flow cytometry in the context of bladder cancer might be improved by multiparameter analysis aimed at enriching for urothelial cells. In addition to light scatter-based approaches,[97] the combination of DNA cytometry with various monoclonal antibodies against urothelial cell or differentiation antigens continues to be tested with variable results.[98-101] Few clinical laboratories are currently performing these tests.

Prostate Cancer

The detection of prostate cancer has increased as a result of enhanced patient awareness and the use of prostate-specific antigen measurements in addition to digital rectal examination. Elevated serum prostate-specific antigen may be the only abnormality that ultimately results in transrectal, ultrasonography-guided, needle biopsy of the prostate. Important clinical questions include how to (1) identify those patients with prostatic intraepithelial neoplasia or stage T1 tumors who are at greatest risk of disease progression, (2) predict which patients with stage T2 cancers will respond to radiation monotherapy, (3) determine the optimal adjuvant therapy for patients with advanced stage disease that was not detected before radical prostatectomy, and (4) predict which patients with advanced disease are likely to respond poorly to androgen ablative therapy.[102]

As in the case of breast and bladder cancer, the 1992 consensus review of DNA cytometry in prostate cancer noted a number of limitations to existing studies, including the lack of sufficiently long follow-up periods, the small numbers of patients in many studies, and technical issues.[24] Nevertheless, most of the retrospective studies of DNA flow cytometry in prostate cancer have shown that DNA diploidy is associated with a favorable outcome, whereas aneuploidy is strongly associated with poor outcome regardless of stage or therapy.[24,76] A World Health Organization consensus panel on Early Diagnosis and Prognostic Parameters in Localized Prostate Cancer concluded that knowledge of DNA ploidy before treatment was valuable in making treatment decisions, especially when surveillance is a treatment option.[103] The World Health Organization panel concluded that aneuploid tumors can be expected to respond very poorly to either irradiation or endocrine therapy. The presence of aneuploid tumor, either on pretreatment biopsy specimens or in radical prostatectomy specimens, was considered an ominous sign. (However, it is important to recognize that aneuploidy may be present in the absence of malignancy if a seminal vesicle is present.[104,105]) The panel expressed a "strong opinion" that DNA ploidy should be uniformly studied in clinical trials, particularly in patients with localized prostate cancer. DNA content should be taken into account as a stratification variable in future randomized clinical trials.[24]

The 1992 consensus panel noted geographic differences in the extent of staging and the effect of this on the utility of DNA content analysis in prostate cancer. For example, in European studies where radical prostatectomy was uncommon, pathologic staging was not routinely determined. Thus in the absence of complete staging, DNA ploidy was a useful predictor of disease course, survival, and hormonal therapy.

Longitudinal studies of the ability of DNA ploidy to predict outcome in patients undergoing radical prostatectomy are still needed.[106] In a recent Danish study of 120 patients with clinically localized prostate cancer treated without intent to cure, DNA studies provided additional prognostic information only in patients with low-grade tumors.[107]

There are some data showing that DNA content analysis predicts outcome in advanced prostate cancer, but it is difficult to evaluate the effect of DNA results on therapeutic decisions. In patients with node-positive (stage D) prostate cancer treated with androgen ablation, disease progression rates were higher and survival rates lower in a small study of patients with aneuploid tumors.[108,109]

The significance of SPF analysis in prostate cancer has not been well established. SPF values were predictive for progression but not survival in one study[110] and were a strong independent predictor of long-term survival in another study.[111] More recently, SPF was found to be a prognostic factor for patients with localized cancer.[112]

One unresolved issue is the extent and clinical significance of tumor heterogeneity within a single prostate. It is recognized that solid tumors are phenotypically and genetically heterogeneous.[113,114] At the DNA content level, comparisons of primary tumors, transurethral prostate resection specimens, and needle biopsy samples have been recommended,[24] but few have been done. There is still little data on the utility of DNA content analysis in early-stage tumors, although the hope that this data might be useful for making therapeutic decisions persists.[115] A working group has been constituted to define the concept of intratumor heterogeneity and agree on how to measure it,[116] although the aim of the project is toward studying the biology of cancers rather than providing direct clinical application.

A notable feature of prostate tumors is the high frequency of DNA tetraploid cancers (4C, DNA index of 1.9-2.1). Some studies suggest that the prognosis of DNA tetraploid tumors in advanced disease is different from that of diploid tumors,[108,117] but not all studies have evaluated this group separately. The 1992 consensus conference recommended reporting tetraploid tumors as a separate category of DNA aneuploidy. They recommended defining as tetraploid those tumors in which the proportion of 4C events, when corrected for aggregated nuclei, is greater than 3 standard deviations above the mean for control prostate tissue. There has been no further clarification of the clinical significance of tetraploid tumors.

Image cytometry appears to be more successful at identifying rare DNA aneuploid populations than flow cytometry and may be the only means to measure DNA ploidy of small specimens, such as needle biopsy specimens.[118,119] Interestingly, one study of 124 patients with localized prostate cancer found that the postoperative pathologist-defined Gleason score was a strong univariate predictor of progression, but both DNA ploidy and HER-2/neu (erbB-2) antigen expression offered additional predictive value for progression in patients with low Gleason scores.[120] Image cytometry, however, like flow cytometry, has a number of unresolved standardization issues, including sample fixation, selection of cell populations, and histogram interpretation. A variety of techniques based on analysis of small numbers (50-100) of cells have been used to classify histograms.[121,122]

A novel approach to detecting aneuploidy in prostate tumors and one that would be amenable to small biopsy specimens is the use of FISH analysis with one or more DNA centromeric probes.[112,123] One study of 21 patients found that FISH analysis of alterations in the numbers of chromosomes 7 and 8 was more sensitive than flow cytometry in detecting aneuploid prostate tumors.[123] However, because tumors are heterogeneous, no matter what part of the tumor one obtains, FISH is unlikely to adequately sample the cells in which the genetic changes that may predict invasive potential or response to therapy have taken place.

DNA analysis of prostate tumors has played an important role in addressing the clinical problems encountered by urologists who treat patients with prostate cancer, but newer technologies are more appealing, if only because they are still in the promising stage of the test cycle. One low-technology approach is to measure the volume of lymph node metastases.[124] Researchers have also noted that in patients with low-stage disease, a decrease in alpha-catenin, one of the intracellular elements of the E-cadherin-catenin complex of adhesion molecules, as measured by using immunohistochemistry, was independently associated with poor survival.[125] Other investigators are using magnetic cell sorting with anticytokeratin monoclonal antibodies[126] or reverse transcriptase-polymerase chain reaction[127] to identify prostate cells in peripheral blood.

Colorectal Cancer

Colorectal cancer is the second most common cancer in the United States, with an annual incidence of 140,000 with 60,000 deaths. Because most patients with Duke stage A disease have an excellent prognosis, prognostic tests are likely to be of little benefit at this stage. Within the last decade, clinicians have desired more accurate prognostic information for patients with advanced but resectable cancer.[128] Clinicians would like to identify which tumors are likely to recur after surgical treatment of patients with stage B or C colon cancer, as well as to identify patients who would benefit from adjuvant chemotherapy and to spare those with an excellent prognosis.

DNA content studies in the 1980s generally concluded that DNA ploidy provides no additional significant prognostic information for colorectal cancers, particularly when subjected to multivariate analysis that includes traditional prognostic factors. [2,129-33]

Several studies found SPF to be a significant prognostic factor,[129,134-137] but others did not,[138] including a number making use of alternative measures of proliferation rate, such as Ki-67 and PCNA immunostaining.[139-141]

The 1992 consensus conference observed that contradictory study results of the utility of DNA content data in the prognosis of colorectal cancer reflected a broad range of technical and analytic methods, many of which were considered to compromise accurate flow cytometric results.[142] The study sizes ranged widely (from 33 to 694 patients in a review of 28 studies), and the panel recommended that subsequent studies include at least 300 patients because of the apparently modest effect of DNA content data and the large number of patient variables. Patient selection was also noted to be crucial, especially in light of the different biologic behavior of colon tumors versus rectal tumors. In 22 studies of survival in relation to DNA ploidy in colorectal carcinoma, the panel noted that the study populations were widely different, with the percentage of patients with cancer of the colon vs cancer of the rectum ranging from 0%[134] to 100%.[130] Other variables the panel observed among the studies included methods of tissue disaggregation, the use of archival versus fresh material, instrumentation, and data analysis, and further investigation of their effects was deemed necessary. Furthermore, the analysis of multiple samples from a tumor was supported to evaluate the significance of tumor heterogeneity.[143] Finally, the need for prospective analyses with fresh tissues using multiparameter flow cytometric techniques to focus the analyses on the malignant cells was emphasized.

In the meantime, other groups who were perhaps less tolerant of the idiosyncracies of the technical issues in flow cytometry developed their own consensus statements. In 1994, the Colorectal Cancer Working Group (consisting of pathologists, investigators, and surgeons) examined prognostic factors for adenocarcinoma of the large gut. The group concluded that the only items it could recommend for routine clinical use were pathologic TNM information and stage, tumor type, tumor grade, extramural venous invasion, and preoperative serum carcinoembryonic antigen level.[144] In 1996, a panel of the American Society of Clinical Oncology concluded that data were insufficient to recommend routine use of DNA index, DNA flow cytometric proliferation analysis, and several genetic measurements, including p53 tumor suppressor gene and ras oncogene in the treatment of colorectal cancer.[71] The recommendations were reviewed in 1997, and they were not changed.[72]

Recently, a prospective series of 309 cases of colorectal cancer was reported, with attention to the recommendations of the 1992 consensus conference.[145] It was found that neither DNA ploidy nor proliferation measurements predicted survival in any stage of colorectal carcinoma. Tumor heterogeneity probably contributes to the lack of predictive value, as suggested by the Flyger et al[146] multicenter study of 145 patients operated on for colorectal cancer. The authors analyzed a portion of the central core and 4 peripheral sections of each resected tumor and found that only 11% of tumors were solely diploid. The Kaplan-Meier survival curves varied, depending on whether the results of 1 to 5 biopsies were included. One big hypertetraploid or hypodiploid population in all biopsy specimens predicted a poor prognosis. Patients whose tumors showed the most divergent range of aneuploid DNA content had the poorest survival rate. Patients with diploid tumors, as defined by absence of near-diploid (DNA Index 0.97-1.15) tumor in any of the 5 samples, had the best outcome. Although these results provide interesting information about the complexity of the patterns of DNA aberrations in colorectal cancer, they cast further doubt on the value of conventional analyses. Concomitantly, the availability of long-term results of adjuvant chemotherapy trials, with a 33% reduction in death rate, compels the use of fluorouracil (Pharmacia-Upjohn, Peapack, NJ) plus levamisole (Zymed Laboratories, South San Francisco, CA) as standard treatment in high-risk colon cancer.[147]

References

1. Williams NN, Daly JM. Flow cytometry and prognostic implications in patients with solid tumors. *Surg Gynecol Obstet*. 1990;171:257-266.

2. Ross JS. DNA ploidy and cell cycle analysis: prediction of tumor aggressiveness and clinical outcome. In: Ross, JS, ed. *DNA Ploidy and Cell Cycle Analysis in Pathology*. New York: Igaku-Shoin; 1996:47-60.

3. Hayes DF, Bast RC, Desch CE, et al. Tumor marker utility grading system: a framework to evaluate clinical utility of tumor markers [see comments]. *J Natl Cancer Inst*. 1996;88:1456-1466.

4. Gasparini G, Pozza F, Harris AL. Evaluating the potential usefulness of new prognostic and predictive indicators in node-negative breast cancer patients [published correction appears in *J Natl Cancer Inst*. 1993;85:1605]. *J Natl Cancer Inst*. 1993;85:1206-1219.

5. NIH consensus conference. Treatment of early-stage breast cancer. *JAMA*. 1991;265:391-395.

6. Thor AD, II DM. Prognostic and predictive markers in breast cancer. In: Winchester DJ, Winchester DP, eds. *Breast Cancer: Atlas of Clinical Oncology*. Hamilton, Ontario, Canada: B.C. Decker; 2000:113-130.

7. Jaeschke R, Guyatt G, Sackett DL. Users' guides to the medical literature. III. How to use an article about a diagnostic test. A. Are the results of the study valid? Evidence-Based Medicine Working Group. *JAMA*. 1994;271:389-391.

8. Jaeschke R, Guyatt GH, Sackett DL. Users' guides to the medical literature. III. How to use an article about a diagnostic test. B. What are the results and will they help me in caring for my patients? The Evidence-Based Medicine Working Group. *JAMA*. 1994;271:703-707.

9. Sackett D, Straus S. On some clinically useful measures of the accuracy of diagnostic tests. *ACP J Club*. 1998;129:A17-A19.

10. van der Schouw YT, Verbeek AL, Ruijs SH. Guidelines for the assessment of new diagnostic tests. *Invest Radiol*. 1995;30:334-340.

11. Park JW, Hong K, Carter P, et al. Development of anti-p185HER2 immunoliposomes for cancer therapy. *Proc Natl Acad Sci U S A*. 1995;92:1327-1331.

12. McNeil C. Herceptin raises its sights beyond advanced breast cancer. *J Natl Cancer Inst*. 1998;90:882-883.

13. Pegram MD, Lipton A, Hayes DF, et al. Phase II study of receptor-enhanced chemosensitivity using recombinant humanized anti-p185HER2/neu monoclonal antibody plus cisplatin in patients with HER2/neu-overexpressing metastatic breast cancer refractory to chemotherapy treatment. *J Clin Oncol*. 1998;16:2659-2671.

14. Muss HB, Thor AD, Berry DA, et al. c-erbB-2 expression and response to adjuvant therapy in women with node- positive early breast cancer [published correction appears in *N Engl J Med*. 1994;331:211]. *N Engl J Med*. 1994;330:1260-1266.

15. Thor AD, Berry DA, Budman DR, et al. erbB-2, p53, and efficacy of adjuvant therapy in lymph node-positive breast cancer [see comments]. *J Natl Cancer Inst*. 1998;90:1346-1360.

16. Graziano C. HER-2 breast assay, linked to Herceptin, wins FDA's okay. *CAP Today*. 1998;12:14-16.

17. Check W. More than one way to look for HER2. *CAP Today*. 1999;13:40-42, 46.

18. Kononen J, Bubendorf L, Kallioniemi A, et al. Tissue microarrays for high-throughput molecular profiling of tumor specimens [see comments]. *Nat Med*. 1998;4:844-847.

19. Stelzer GT, Grimaud DL. Reimbursement for clinical flow cytometry testing. *Ann N Y Acad Sci*. 1993;677:21-27.

20. Quality of Care Information. Coverage Policies. Clinical Diagnostic Laboratory Tests. *Recommended Medicare National Coverage Policy for Flow Cytometry*. HCFA: Washington, DC; 1999.

21. Coon JS, Deitch AD, de Vere White RW, et al. Interinstitutional variability in DNA flow cytometric analysis of tumors. The National Cancer Institute's Flow Cytometry Network Experience. *Cancer*. 1988;61:126-130.

22. Wheeless LL, Coon JS, Cox C, et al. Measurement variability in DNA flow cytometry of replicate samples. *Cytometry*. 1989;10:731-738.

23. Coon JS, Paxton H, Lucy L, et al. Interlaboratory variation in DNA flow cytometry. Results of the College of American Pathologists' Survey. *Arch Pathol Lab Med*. 1994;118:681-685.

24. Shankey TV, Kallioniemi OP, Koslowski JM, et al. Consensus review of the clinical utility of DNA content cytometry in prostate cancer. *Cytometry*. 1993;14:497-500.

25. Shankey TV, Rabinovitch PS, Bagwell B, et al. Guidelines for implementation of clinical DNA cytometry. International Society for Analytical Cytology [published correction appears in *Cytometry.* 1993;14:842]. *Cytometry.* 1993;14:472-477.

26. Ormerod MG, Tribukait B, Giaretti W. Consensus report of the task force on standardisation of DNA flow cytometry in clinical pathology. *Anal Cell Pathol.* 1998;17:103-110.

27. Bocking A, Giroud F, Reith A. Consensus report of the European Society for Analytical Cellular Pathology task force on standardization of diagnostic DNA image cytometry. *Anal Quant Cytol Histol.* 1995;17:1-7.

28. D'Hautcourt JL, Spyratos F, Chassevent A. Quality control study by the French Cytometry Association on flow cytometric DNA content and S-phase fraction (S%). The Association Francaise de Cytometrie [published correction appears in *Cytometry.* 1996;26:183]. *Cytometry.* 1996;26:32-39.

29. Pathologists CoA. *Flow Cytometry Cytometry Survey Set FL-B.* Northfield, IL: College of American Pathologists; 1998.

30. Witzig T, Katzmann J. Clinical Utility of DNA Ploidy and %S-phase analysis of malignant cells by flow cytometry. In: Keren D, ed. *Flow Cytometry and Clinical Diagnosis.* 3rd ed. Chicago, IL: ASCP Press; 2001.

31. Auer GU, Caspersson TO, Wallgren AS. DNA content and survival in mammary carcinoma. *Anal Quant Cytol.* 1980;2:161-165.

32. Hedley DW, Clark GM, Cornelisse CJ, et al. Consensus review of the clinical utility of DNA cytometry in carcinoma of the breast. Report of the DNA Cytometry Consensus Conference. *Cytometry.* 1993;14:482-485.

33. Toikkanen S, Joensuu H, Klemi P. Nuclear DNA content as a prognostic factor in T1-2N0 breast cancer. *Am J Clin Pathol.* 1990;93:471-479.

34. Baak JP, Chin D, van Diest PJ, et al. Comparative long-term prognostic value of quantitative HER-2/neu protein expression, DNA ploidy, and morphometric and clinical features in paraffin-embedded invasive breast cancer. *Lab Invest.* 1991;64:215-223.

35. Beerman H, Kluin PM, Hermans J, et al. Prognostic significance of DNA-ploidy in a series of 690 primary breast cancer patients. *Int J Cancer.* 1990;45:34-39.

36. Cornelisse CJ, van de Velde CJ, Caspers RJ, et al. DNA ploidy and survival in breast cancer patients. *Cytometry.* 1987;8:225-234.

37. Dowle CS, Owainati A, Robins A, et al. Prognostic significance of the DNA content of human breast cancer. *Br J Surg.* 1987;74:133-136.

38. Eskelinen M, Lipponen P, Papinaho S, et al. DNA flow cytometry, nuclear morphometry, mitotic indices and steroid receptors as independent prognostic factors in female breast cancer. *Int J Cancer.* 1992;51:555-561.

39. Ferno M, Baldetorp B, Borg A, et al. Flow cytometric DNA index and S-phase fraction in breast cancer in relation to other prognostic variables and to clinical outcome. *Acta Oncol.* 1992;31:157-165.

40. Fisher B, Gunduz N, Costantino J, et al. DNA flow cytometric analysis of primary operable breast cancer. Relation of ploidy and S-phase fraction to outcome of patients in NSABP B-04. *Cancer.* 1991;68:1465-1475.

41. Gnant MF, Blijham G, Reiner A, et al. DNA ploidy and other results of DNA flow cytometry as prognostic factors in operable breast cancer: 10 year results of a randomised study. *Eur J Cancer*. 1992;28:711-716.

42. Hedley DW, Rugg CA, Gelber RD. Association of DNA index and S-phase fraction with prognosis of nodes positive early breast cancer. *Cancer Res*. 1987;47:4729-4735.

43. Kallioniemi OP, Blanco G, Alavaikko M, et al. Tumour DNA ploidy as an independent prognostic factor in breast cancer. *Br J Cancer*. 1987;56:637-642.

44. Muss HB, Kute TE, Case LD, et al. The relation of flow cytometry to clinical and biologic characteristics in women with node negative primary breast cancer. *Cancer*. 1989;64:1894-1900.

45. Noguchi M, Taniya T, Ohta N, et al. Lymph node metastases versus DNA ploidy as prognostic factors for invasive ductal carcinoma of the breast. *Breast Cancer Res Treat*. 1991;19:23-31.

46. O'Reilly SM, Camplejohn RS, Barnes DM, et al. DNA index, S-phase fraction, histological grade and prognosis in breast cancer. *Br J Cancer*. 1990;61:671-674.

47. Sharma S, Mishra MC, Kapur BM, et al. The prognostic significance of ploidy analysis in operable breast cancer. *Cancer*. 1991;68:2612-2616.

48. Clark GM, Dressler LG, Owens MA, et al. Prediction of relapse or survival in patients with node-negative breast cancer by DNA flow cytometry [see comments]. *N Engl J Med*. 1989;320:627-633.

49. Fallenius AG, Auer GU, Carstensen JM. Prognostic significance of DNA measurements in 409 consecutive breast cancer patients. *Cancer*. 1988;62:331-341.

50. Witzig TE, Ingle JN, Cha SS, et al. DNA ploidy and the percentage of cells in S-phase as prognostic factors for women with lymph node negative breast cancer. *Cancer*. 1994;74:1752-1761.

51. Bergers E, Baak JP, van Diest PJ, et al. Prognostic value of DNA ploidy using flow cytometry in 1301 breast cancer patients: results of the prospective Multicenter Morphometric Mammary Carcinoma Project. *Mod Pathol*. 1997;10:762-768.

52. Leivonen M, Krogerus L, Nordling S. DNA analysis in advanced breast cancer. *Cancer Detect Prev*. 1994;18:87-96.

53. Clark GM, Mathieu MC, Owens MA, et al. Prognostic significance of S-phase fraction in good-risk, node-negative breast cancer patients. *J Clin Oncol*. 1992;10:428-432.

54. Kallioniemi OP, Blanco G, Alavaikko M, et al. Improving the prognostic value of DNA flow cytometry in breast cancer by combining DNA index and S-phase fraction. A proposed classification of DNA histograms in breast cancer. *Cancer*. 1988;62:2183-2190.

55. O'Reilly SM, Camplejohn RS, Barnes DM, et al. Node-negative breast cancer: prognostic subgroups defined by tumor size and flow cytometry [see comments]. *J Clin Oncol*. 1990;8:2040-2046.

56. Sigurdsson H, Baldetorp B, Borg A, et al. Indicators of prognosis in node-negative breast cancer [see comments]. *N Engl J Med*. 1990;322:1045-1053.

57. Sigurdsson H, Baldetorp B, Borg A, et al. Flow cytometry in primary breast cancer: improving the prognostic value of the fraction of cells in the S-phase by optimal categorisation of cut-off levels [see comments]. *Br J Cancer*. 1990;62:786-790.

58. Toikkanen S, Joensuu H, Klemi P. The prognostic significance of nuclear DNA content in invasive breast cancer—a study with long-term follow-up. *Br J Cancer*. 1989;60:693-700.

59. Witzig TE, Ingle JN, Schaid DJ, et al. DNA ploidy and percent S-phase as prognostic factors in node-positive breast cancer: results from patients enrolled in two prospective randomized trials. *J Clin Oncol*. 1993;11:351-359.

60. Merkel DE, Winchester DJ, Goldschmidt RA, et al. DNA flow cytometry and pathologic grading as prognostic guides in axillary lymph node-negative breast cancer. *Cancer*. 1993;72:1926-1932.

61. Merkel DE. Breast Cancer. Clinical Commentary. In: Bauer KD, Duque RE, Shankey TV, eds. *Clinical Flow Cytometry. Principles and Application*. Baltimore: Williams & Wilkins; 1993:260-261.

62. Romero H, Schneider J, Burgos J, et al. S-phase fraction identifies high-risk subgroups among DNA-diploid breast cancers. *Breast Cancer Res Treat*. 1996;38:265-275.

63. *Flow Cytometry Survey Set FL-B. Participant Summary*. Northfield, IL: College of American Pathologists; 1999:25.

64. Baldetorp B, Stal O, Ahrens O, et al. Different calculation methods for flow cytometric S-phase fraction: prognostic implications in breast cancer? The Swedish Society of Cancer Study Group. *Cytometry*. 1998;33:385-393.

65. Bergers E, Baak JP, van Diest PJ, et al. Prognostic implications of different cell cycle analysis models of flow cytometric DNA histograms of 1,301 breast cancer patients: results from the Multicenter Morphometric Mammary Carcinoma Project (MMMCP). *Int J Cancer*. 1997;74:260-269.

66. Wingren S, Stal O, Nordenskjold B. Flow cytometric analysis of S-phase fraction in breast carcinomas using gating on cells containing cytokeratin. South East Sweden Breast Cancer Group. *Br J Cancer*. 1994;69:546-549.

67. Wingren S, Stal O, Sullivan S, et al. S-phase fraction after gating on epithelial cells predicts recurrence in node-negative breast cancer. *Int J Cancer*. 1994;59:7-10.

68. McCormick SR, Peters AA, Schrauth JB. Flow cytometric DNA analysis with cytokeratin gating of formalin-fixed deparaffinized breast cancer nuclei. *Am J Clin Pathol*. 1998;110:227-237.

69. Rabinovitch PS. Practical considerations for DNA content and cell cycle analysis. In: Bauer KD, Duque RE, Shankey TV, eds. *Clinical Flow Cytometry. Principles and Application*. Baltimore: Williams & Wilkins; 1993:117-142.

70. Veronesi U. NIH consensus meeting on early breast cancer. *Eur J Cancer*. 1990;26:843-844.

71. Clinical practice guidelines for the use of tumor markers in breast and colorectal cancer. Adopted on May 17, 1996 by the American Society of Clinical Oncology [see comments]. *J Clin Oncol*. 1996;14:2843-2877.

72. 1997 update of recommendations for the use of tumor markers in breast and colorectal cancer. Adopted on November 7, 1997 by the American Society of Clinical Oncology. *J Clin Oncol*. 1998;16:793-795.

73. Wenger CR, Clark GM. S-phase fraction and breast cancer—a decade of experience. *Breast Cancer Res Treat*. 1998;51:255-265.

74. Thor AD, Liu S, Moore DH 2nd, et al. Comparison of mitotic index, in vitro bromodeoxyuridine labeling, and MIB-1 assays to quantitate proliferation in breast cancer. *J Clin Oncol.* 1999;17:470-477.

75. Clark GM, Allred DC, Hilsenbeck SG, et al. Mitosin (a new proliferation marker) correlates with clinical outcome in node-negative breast cancer. *Cancer Res.* 1997;57:5505-5508.

76. Ross JS. Clinical applications of DNA ploidy and cell cycle analysis: role in cancer diagnosis and diagnostic cytopathology. In: Ross JS, ed. *DNA Ploidy and Cell Cycle Analysis in Pathology.* New York: Igaku-Shoin; 1996:47-60.

77. Klein FA, Herr HW, Sogani PC, et al. Detection and follow-up of carcinoma of the urinary bladder by flow cytometry. *Cancer.* 1982;50:389-395.

78. Murphy WM, Emerson LD, Chandler RW, et al. Flow cytometry versus urinary cytology in the evaluation of patients with bladder cancer. *J Urol.* 1986;136:815-819.

79. Badalament RA, Gay H, Whitmore WF Jr, et al. Monitoring intravesical bacillus Calmette-Guerin treatment of superficial bladder carcinoma by serial flow cytometry. *Cancer.* 1986;58:2751-2757.

80. Badalament RA, Kimmel M, Gay H, et al. The sensitivity of flow cytometry compared with conventional cytology in the detection of superficial bladder carcinoma. *Cancer.* 1987;59:2078-2085.

81. Badalament RA, Hermansen DK, Kimmel M, et al. The sensitivity of bladder wash flow cytometry, bladder wash cytology, and voided cytology in the detection of bladder carcinoma. *Cancer.* 1987;60:1423-1427.

82. Badalament RA, Fair WR, Whitmore WF Jr, et al. The relative value of cytometry and cytology in the management of bladder cancer: the Memorial Sloan-Kettering Cancer Center experience. *Semin Urol.* 1988;6:22-30.

83. de Vere White RW, Olsson CA, Deitch AD. Flow cytometry: role in monitoring transitional cell carcinoma of bladder. *Urology.* 1986;28:15-20.

84. Giella JG, Ring K, Olsson CA, et al. The predictive value of flow cytometry and urinary cytology in the followup of patients with transitional cell carcinoma of the bladder. *J Urol.* 1992;148:293-296.

85. Hermansen DK, Badalament RA, Fair WR, et al. Detection of bladder carcinoma in females by flow cytometry and cytology. *Cytometry.* 1989;10:739-742.

86. Klein FA, White FK. Flow cytometry deoxyribonucleic acid determinations and cytology of bladder washings: practical experience. *J Urol.* 1988;139:275-278.

87. Konchuba AM, Schellhammer PF, Alexander JP, et al. Flow cytometric study comparing paired bladder washing and voided urine for bladder cancer detection. *Urology.* 1989;33:89-96.

88. Wheeless LL, Badalament RA, de Vere White RW, et al. Consensus review of the clinical utility of DNA cytometry in bladder cancer. Report of the DNA Cytometry Consensus Conference. *Cytometry.* 1993;14:478-481.

89. Lopez-Beltran A, Croghan GA, Croghan I, et al. Prognostic factors in bladder cancer. A pathologic, immunohistochemical, and DNA flow-cytometric study. *Am J Clin Pathol.* 1994;102:109-114.

90. Kroft SH, Oyasu R. Urinary bladder cancer: mechanisms of development and progression. *Lab Invest.* 1994;71:158-174.

91. Norming U, Tribukait B, Nyman CR, et al. Prognostic significance of mucosal aneuploidy in stage Ta/T1 grade 3 carcinoma of the bladder. *J Urol.* 1992;148:1420-1427.

92. Gustafson H, Tribukait B, Esposti PL. DNA pattern, histological grade and multiplicity related to recurrence rate in superficial bladder tumours. *Scand J Urol Nephrol.* 1982;16:135-139.

93. Bretton PR, Herr HW, Kimmel M, et al. Flow cytometry as a predictor of response and progression in patients with superficial bladder cancer treated with bacillus Calmette-Guerin. *J Urol.* 1989;141:1332-1336.

94. Norming U. DNA flow cytometry: an update of its use in assessing prognosis for transitional cell cancer of the bladder. *Semin Urol.* 1993;11:154-163.

95. Gregoire M, Fradet Y, Meyer F, et al. Diagnostic accuracy of urinary cytology, and deoxyribonucleic acid flow cytometry and cytology on bladder washings during followup for bladder tumors. *J Urol.* 1997;157:1660-1664.

96. Granfors T, Duchek M, Tomic R, et al. Predictive value of DNA ploidy in bladder cancer treated with preoperative radiation therapy and cystectomy. *Scand J Urol Nephrol.* 1996;30:281-285.

97. Wheeless LL, Reeder JE, O'Connell MJ, et al. DNA slit-scan flow cytometry of bladder irrigation specimens and the importance of recognizing urothelial cells. *Cytometry.* 1991;12:140-146.

98. Planz B, Striepecke E, Jakse G, et al. Use of Lewis X antigen and deoxyribonucleic acid image cytometry to increase sensitivity of urinary cytology in transitional cell carcinoma of the bladder. *J Urol.* 1998;159:384-388.

99. Jankevicius F, Shibayama T, Decken K, et al. Dual-parameter immunoflow cytometry in diagnosis and follow-up of patients with bladder cancer. *Eur Urol.* 1998;34:492-499.

100. Konchuba AM, Clements MC, Schellhammer PF, et al. Failure of anticytokeratin 18 antibody to improve flow cytometric detection of bladder cancer. *Cancer.* 1992;70:2879-2884.

101. Fradet Y, Tardif M, Bourget L, et al. Clinical cancer progression in urinary bladder tumors evaluated by multiparameter flow cytometry with monoclonal antibodies. Laval University Urology Group. *Cancer Res.* 1990;50:432-437.

102. Kozlowski JM. Clinical Commentary. In: Bauer KD, Duque RE, Shankey TV, eds. *Clinical Flow Cytometry. Principles and Application.* Baltimore: Williams and Wilkins; 1993:301-305.

103. Schroder F, Tribukait B, Bocking A, et al. Clinical utility of cellular DNA measurements in prostate carcinoma. Consensus Conference on Diagnosis and Prognostic Parameters in Localized Prostate Cancer. Stockholm, Sweden, May 12-13, 1993. *Scand J Urol Nephrol Suppl.* 1994;162:51-63.

104. Arber DA, Speights VO. Aneuploidy in benign seminal vesicle epithelium: an example of the paradox of ploidy studies. *Mod Pathol.* 1991;4:687-689.

105. Wojcik EM, Bassler TJ Jr, Orozco R. DNA ploidy in seminal vesicle cells. A potential diagnostic pitfall in urine cytology. *Anal Quant Cytol Histol.* 1999;21:29-34.

106. Shockley KF, Maatman TJ, Carothers GC, et al. Comparative analysis of prognostic factors in men undergoing radical prostatectomy for adenocarcinoma of the prostate, including DNA ploidy, surgical tumor stage, prostatic specific antigen, Gleason grade, and age. *Prostate*. 1996;29:46-50.

107. Borre M, Hoyer M, Nerstrom B, et al. DNA ploidy and survival of patients with clinically localized prostate cancer treated without intent to cure. *Prostate*. 1998;36:244-249.

108. Zincke H, Bergstralh EJ, Larson-Keller JJ, et al. Stage D1 prostate cancer treated by radical prostatectomy and adjuvant hormonal treatment. Evidence for favorable survival in patients with DNA diploid tumors. *Cancer*. 1992;70:311-323.

109. Pollack A, Troncoso P, Zagars GK, et al. The significance of DNA-ploidy and S-phase fraction in node-positive (stage D1) prostate cancer treated with androgen ablation. *Prostate*. 1997;31:21-28.

110. Eskelinen M, Lipponen P, Majapuro R, et al. DNA ploidy, S phase fraction and G2 fraction as prognostic determinants in prostatic adenocarcinoma. *Eur Urol*. 1991;20:62-66.

111. Visakorpi T, Kallioniemi OP, Paronen IY, et al. Flow cytometric analysis of DNA ploidy and S-phase fraction from prostatic carcinomas: implications for prognosis and response to endocrine therapy. *Br J Cancer*. 1991;64:578-582.

112. Astrom L, Weimarck A, Aldenborg F, et al. S-phase fraction related to prognosis in localised prostate cancer. No specific significance of chromosome 7 gain or deletion of 7q31.1. *Int J Cancer*. 1998;79:553-559.

113. Beerman H, Smit VT, Kluin PM, et al. Flow cytometric analysis of DNA stemline heterogeneity in primary and metastatic breast cancer [see comments]. *Cytometry*. 1991;12:147-154.

114. Shankey TV, Jin JK, Dougherty S, et al. DNA ploidy and proliferation heterogeneity in human prostate cancers. *Cytometry*. 1995;21:30-39.

115. Leisinger HJ. Cancer of the prostate stage T1. Incidental carcinoma. Review of the literature and an appraisal of the classification. *Ann Urol*. 1994;28:229-234.

116. Chapman JA, Wolman E, Wolman SR, et al. Assessing genetic markers of tumour progression in the context of intratumour heterogeneity. *Cytometry*. 1998;31:67-73.

117. Montgomery BT, Nativ O, Blute ML, et al. Stage B prostate adenocarcinoma. Flow cytometric nuclear DNA ploidy analysis. *Arch Surg*. 1990;125:327-331.

118. Falkmer UG. Methodologic sources of errors in image and flow cytometric DNA assessments of the malignancy potential of prostatic carcinoma. *Hum Pathol*. 1992;23:360-367.

119. Ross JS, Figge H, Bui HX, et al. Prediction of pathologic stage and postprostatectomy disease recurrence by DNA ploidy analysis of initial needle biopsy specimens of prostate cancer. *Cancer*. 1994;74:2811-2818.

120. Veltri RW, Partin AW, Epstein JE, et al. Quantitative nuclear morphometry, Markovian texture descriptors, and DNA content captured on a CAS-200 Image analysis system, combined with PCNA and HER-2/neu immunohistochemistry for prediction of prostate cancer progression. *J Cell Biochem Suppl*. 1994;19:249-258.

121. Forsslund G, Zetterberg A. Ploidy level determinations in high-grade and low-grade malignant variants of prostatic carcinoma. *Cancer Res*. 1990;50:4281-4285.

122. Ahlgren G, Lindholm K, Falkmer U, et al. A DNA cytometric proliferation index improves the value of the DNA ploidy pattern as a prognosticating tool in patients with carcinoma of the prostate. *Urology*. 1997;50:379-384.

123. Barranco MA, Alcaraz A, Corral JM, et al. Numeric alterations in chromosomes 7 and 8 detected by fluorescent in situ hybridization correlate with high-grade localized prostate cancer. *Eur Urol*. 1998;34:419-425.

124. Cheng L, Bergstralh EJ, Cheville JC, et al. Cancer volume of lymph node metastasis predicts progression in prostate cancer. *Am J Surg Pathol*. 1998;22:1491-1500.

125. Aaltomaa S, Lipponen P, Ala-Opas M, et al. Alpha-catenin expression has prognostic value in local and locally advanced prostate cancer. *Br J Cancer*. 1999;80:477-482.

126. Martin VM, Siewert C, Scharl A, et al. Immunomagnetic enrichment of disseminated epithelial tumor cells from peripheral blood by MACS. *Exp Hematol*. 1998;26:252-264.

127. Ignatoff JM, Oefelein MG, Watkin W, et al. Prostate specific antigen reverse transcriptase-polymerase chain reaction assay in preoperative staging of prostate cancer. *J Urol*. 1997;158:1870-1875.

128. Merkel DE, Locker GY. Colorectal neoplasia. Clinical commentary. In: Bauer KD, Duque RE, Shankey TV, eds. *Clinical Flow Cytometry. Principles and Application*. Baltimore: Williams & Wilkins; 1993:316-317.

129. Bauer KD, Lincoln ST, Vera-Roman JM, et al. Prognostic implications of proliferative activity and DNA aneuploidy in colonic adenocarcinomas. *Lab Invest*. 1987;57:329-335.

130. Bauer DC, Bagwell CB, Giaretti W, et al. Consensus review of the clinical utility of DNA flow cytometry in colorectal cancer. *Cytometry*. 1993;14:486-491.

131. Visscher DW, Zarbo RJ, Ma CK, et al. Flow cytometric DNA and clinicopathologic analysis of Dukes' A&B colonic adenocarcinomas: a retrospective study. *Mod Pathol*. 1990;3:709-712.

132. Hood DL, Petras RE, Edinger M, et al. Deoxyribonucleic acid ploidy and cell cycle analysis of colorectal carcinoma by flow cytometry. A prospective study of 137 cases using fresh whole cell suspensions. *Am J Clin Pathol*. 1990;93:615-620.

133. Fisher ER, Siderits RH, Sass R, et al. Value of assessment of ploidy in rectal cancers. *Arch Pathol Lab Med*. 1989;113:525-528.

134. Quirke P, Dixon MF, Clayden AD, et al. Prognostic significance of DNA aneuploidy and cell proliferation in rectal adenocarcinomas. *J Pathol*. 1987;151:285-291.

135. Schutte B, Reynders MM, Wiggers T, et al. Retrospective analysis of the prognostic significance of DNA content and proliferative activity in large bowel carcinoma. *Cancer Res*. 1987;47:5494-5496.

136. Harlow SP, Eriksen BL, Poggensee L, et al. Prognostic implications of proliferative activity and DNA aneuploidy in Astler-Coller Dukes stage C colonic adenocarcinomas. *Cancer Res*. 1991;51:2403-2409.

137. Witzig TE, Loprinzi CL, Gonchoroff NJ, et al. DNA ploidy and cell kinetic measurements as predictors of recurrence and survival in stages B2 and C colorectal adenocarcinoma. *Cancer*. 1991;68:879-888.

138. Enker WE, Kimmel M, Cibas ES, et al. DNA/RNA content and proliferative fractions of colorectal carcinomas: a five-year prospective study relating flow cytometry to survival. *J Natl Cancer Inst*. 1991;83:701-707.

139. Kram N, Nessim S, Geller SA. A study of colonic adenocarcinoma, with comparison of histopathology, DNA flow cytometric data, and number of nucleolar organizer regions (NORs). *Mod Pathol*. 1989;2:468-472.

140. Porschen R, Lohe B, Hengels KJ, et al. Assessment of cell proliferation in colorectal carcinomas using the monoclonal antibody Ki-67. Correlation with pathohistologic criteria and influence of irradiation. *Cancer*. 1989;64:2501-2505.

141. Kubota Y, Petras RE, Easley KA, et al. Ki-67-determined growth fraction versus standard staging and grading parameters in colorectal carcinoma. A multivariate analysis. *Cancer*. 1992;70:2602-2609.

142. Bauer KD, Bagwell CB, Giaretti W, et al. Consensus review of the clinical utility of DNA flow cytometry in colorectal cancer. *Cytometry*. 1993;14:486-491.

143. Wersto RP, Liblit RL, Deitch D, et al. Variability in DNA measurements in multiple tumor samples of human colonic carcinoma. *Cancer*. 1991;67:106-115.

144. Fielding LP, Pettigrew N. College of American Pathologists Conference XXVI on clinical relevance of prognostic markers in solid tumors. Report of the Colorectal Cancer Working Group. *Arch Pathol Lab Med*. 1995;119:1115-1121.

145. Zarbo RJ, Nakhleh RE, Brown RD, et al. Prognostic significance of DNA ploidy and proliferation in 309 colorectal carcinomas as determined by two-color multiparametric DNA flow cytometry. *Cancer*. 1997;79:2073-2086.

146. Flyger HL, Larsen JK, Nielsen HJ, et al. DNA ploidy in colorectal cancer, heterogeneity within and between tumors and relation to survival. *Cytometry*. 1999;38:293-300.

147. Moertel CG, Fleming TR, Macdonald JS, et al. Fluorouracil plus levamisole as effective adjuvant therapy after resection of stage III colon carcinoma: a final report. *Ann Intern Med*. 1995;122:321-326.

19

Clinical Utility of DNA Ploidy and Cell Proliferation Measurements by Flow Cytometry

Thomas E. Witzig
Jerry A. Katzmann

Introduction

One of the earliest clinical applications of the flow cytometer was the analysis of DNA content of malignant tissues. Innovations in 3 key areas made these measurements practical: (1) hardware—the development of commercial flow cytometers, (2) laboratory techniques—staining with DNA binding dyes such as propidium iodide, and (3) computer software —designs that simplified and automated analysis of DNA content histograms. DNA content analysis was initially applied to "liquid cancers" such as leukemia, because cells from these cancers are easily obtained and processed. The ability to recover nuclei from paraffin-embedded tumors and determine the DNA content by flow cytometry was a major advance in clinical pathology because it allowed the rapid analysis of large numbers of tumors from patients in whom the long-term outcome was already known.[1]

The 2 main results of DNA content analysis are the DNA ploidy classification (DNA diploid, DNA tetraploid, or DNA aneuploid) and a measurement of cell proliferation (%S-phase). Determination of the chromosome content of a tumor has usually been performed by cytogenetic analysis of metaphases induced in fresh, viable tumor cells. Measuring DNA ploidy by flow cytometry after staining with a DNA binding dye such as propidium iodide can detect aneuploid clones with significant changes in DNA content, but it cannot detect small DNA gains or losses, or detect chromosomal translocations. Fluorescent in situ hybridization (FISH) is a new technique that can provide information on ploidy and specific chromosomal abnormalities in paraffin-embedded material. FISH is currently primarily a research tool but is likely to be increasingly used in clinical medicine. A drawback of cytogenetics and FISH is that they are labor-intensive tests that must be performed by highly trained personnel, which makes them costly clinical tests. Determining DNA content by flow cytometry, however, provides a rapid result at relatively low cost (approx. $225).

In the 1980s a flurry of publications applied DNA-content flow cytometry analysis to tissue from virtually every major tumor type. However, most of these studies reported DNA ploidy results alone; cell proliferation measurements were either not performed or not reported. With the availability of automated software that analyzes complex DNA-content histograms, studies began to appear that included cell proliferation measurements. The classical method of measuring cell proliferation is the labeling index, which detects cells synthesizing DNA (S-phase). This involves incubating fresh cells with tritiated thymidine or bromodeoxyuridine for a set period of time (usually 1 hour) and then determining the incorporation of DNA precursors by autoradiography or immunofluorescence microscopy in which 500 cells are enumerated and the percentage of labeled cells are determined. This test also requires trained lab personnel, and is currently performed as a clinical test in only a few clinical laboratories. The development of assays to detect proliferation markers on cells has led to the development of antibodies such as Ki-67, MIB-1, and proliferating cell nuclear antigen (PCNA). Ki-67 reacts with cells in late G1, S, G2, and M phases of the cell cycle; therefore, it will stain a higher percentage of cells than the labeling index technique will on the same sample. MIB-1 is similar to Ki-67, but can be used on paraffin-embedded tissue. PCNA is expressed primarily during S-phase; results from stains made with this marker correlate well with those obtained with the labeling index technique.[2]

The number of new studies published using DNA-content flow cytometry is now waning, as studies of the use of molecular markers as diagnostic and prognostic factors become more popular and interesting. Although these new markers are of great scientific interest, many have not undergone comparison with traditional prognostic factors nor been subjected to careful multivariate analysis.

Predicting Prognosis with DNA-Content Analysis

The main usefulness of DNA ploidy and %S measurements has been not in the diagnosis of tumors, but rather in predicting prognosis. Knowledge of the patient's prognosis can be helpful to the clinician in several ways. First, patients are usually interested in learning about the risk of recurrence and death from their cancer, and prognostic factor analysis can assist the physician in counseling the patient. In addition, patients may need this information to make important decisions regarding their family, work, and finances. Second, prognostic factors can help determine which patients may benefit from adjuvant therapy. Third, measurements such as DNA ploidy may be useful as predictive factors (ie, predicting response to certain types of treatment). Fourth, prognostic factors are important for proper patient stratification in randomized clinical trials to ensure proper balance in treatment arms. The decision to perform a laboratory test for prognostic or predictive (rather than diagnostic) purposes depends on several factors:

Who is Requesting the Test?

The patient may request the test after he or she has researched the disease. The physician may desire the information to help in patient treatment planning and in counseling the patient about his or her prognosis. A clinical trial may require the test for stratification purposes or to learn whether the presence of a factor predicts response to a certain therapy.

How Difficult is it to Perform the Test?

Ideal tests for prognosis are those that can be performed after the patient has a definitive tumor diagnosis and that can use paraffin-embedded tissue or a blood sample. The test should also be able to be performed locally or easily sent to a reference laboratory. Results should be available within 2 weeks so that the information can be used in treatment planning.

What Does the Test Cost?

The cost of the test and the frequency with which it must be performed also deserve consideration. Obviously, the cost must be viewed in light of the level of importance the information provides. For example, if the results of the test can spare the patient expensive adjuvant therapy, then its overall cost may be minor.

Will the Results Help Make a Treatment Decision?

Unfortunately, although knowledge of the prognosis may be of some usefulness, in the case of many solid tumors, there is limited ability to prevent tumor progression or relapse after surgery. Therefore, many physicians do not ask for additional prognostic testing because it will not help them make a treatment decision. This will change as more effective therapy for these malignancies is developed.

DNA-content analysis by flow cytometry fulfills many of the above criteria for a useful test. It can be readily performed on paraffin-embedded material, is easily sent to a reference laboratory, is inexpensive, and the results are available in 1 to 2 days.

DNA-Content Measurement of Specific Tumors

A DNA Cytometry Consensus Conference in 1992 identified a number of tumors in which DNA-content measurements were able to provide statistically significant independent prognostic information.[3-9] The focus of this review is to discuss key publications in the field since the Consensus Conference and summarize the current clinical indications for DNA ploidy and %S-phase analysis. Each of the main tumor areas will be discussed, and summary information regarding the prognostic utility of DNA ploidy and cell proliferation measurements will be presented. In general, the authors have restricted our review to DNA ploidy determined by flow cytometry rather than image analysis. Only articles that had information on patient survival were included.

Two key survival measurements are important to clinicians and patients: relapse-free survival (RFS) or disease-free survival (DFS) are terms used to measure the time from diagnosis (or end of therapy) until the cancer relapses, whereas overall survival (OS) refers to the elapsed time from diagnosis (or the initiation of a new therapy) until death from any cause. Because everybody eventually dies from some cause, some studies measure cancer-free survival (CFS), which refers to the time elapsed until death from cancer. For most malignancies, the pathologist will assign a *tumor grade*, which is based on the light-microscopic features of the tumor. *Tumor stage* is usually determined by a combination of pathologic examination of the tissue (eg, to discern the level of invasion and check for the presence of nodal metastases), physical exam by the physician, and radiographic tests or scans. Tumor grade and stage are often important prognostic factors, and, because they are part of the routine evaluation of the patient, do not require further testing. Therefore, grade and stage should be included in the statistical analyses to make certain that any new prognostic variable provides more information about prognosis than is already provided by grade or stage.

Bladder Cancer

The Consensus Conference concluded that DNA ploidy correlated with grade and stage and that the most useful groups of bladder cancers to study were grade 2 superficial (Ta, T1, TIS) tumors.[9] Patients in this group with tumors that are DNA aneuploid have a higher risk that their cancer will progress to muscle invasion and metastasis than patients with tumors that are DNA diploid. **Table 19-1** outlines the results of some recently published trials in this disease group. DNA ploidy analysis can provide prognostic information when performed on the initial resected bladder tumor sample. Bittard et al demonstrated that DNA ploidy was an independent prognostic factor for patients with transitional cell carcinoma; however, it was not particularly helpful in clinical decision-making at the time of diagnosis.[10] Alderisio et al recently demonstrated that cell proliferation was also an independent prognostic factor.[11] However, 2 recent studies on bladder washings did not show DNA ploidy analysis to be of benefit.[12,13] A number of these studies suggest that ploidy and proliferation analysis on the primary tumor may be useful as monitoring algorithms regarding the frequency of cystoscopy because of their correlations with recurrence. Further studies examining cell proliferation measurements are needed.

Table 19-1
Summary of Selected Recent Publications in Bladder Cancer

Author	Year	N	Method	Prognostic Significance		Comment
				Ploidy	Proliferation	
Alderisio[11]	1998	94	FC	Yes, DFS and OS (m)	Yes, DFS and OS (m)	Transitional cell carcinoma stages Ta – T3
Bittard[10]	1996	275	FC	Yes, OS (m)	ND	Transitional cell carcinoma stages Ta – T4; ploidy most useful in T1 grade 3 disease
Song[14]	1990	38	FC	Yes, DFS	ND	Adenocarcinoma
Corrado[15]	1991	92	FC	Yes, OS (m)	ND	Transitional cell carcinoma of the upper urinary tract
Blute[16]	1988	109	FC	Yes, OS (u); No, OS (m)	ND	Transitional cell carcinoma of the upper urinary tract. Ploidy correlated with grade and stage; helpful in low-grade, low-stage patients.
Winkler[17]	1989	73	FC	Yes, DFS	ND	Primary squamous cell carcinoma of the bladder
Gregoire[12]	1997	66	FC	No, DFS	ND	Bladder washings from patients with previous bladder tumors in whom cystoscopy was normal. Found no additional benefit to cytology.
Tetu[18]	1996	199	FC	No, DFS	No, DFS	PTa/pT1 transitional cell carcinoma tumors of the bladder
Granfors[13]	1996	43	FC	No, OS	ND	Bladder washings from patients who then underwent radiotherapy followed by cystectomy

Abbreviations: FC = flow cytometry; ND = not done; RFS = relapse-free survival;
DFS = disease-free survival; OS = overall survival; u = univariate analysis; m = multivariate analysis.

Prostate Cancer

The conclusions of the Consensus Conference[6] regarding prostate cancer were that patients with DNA-diploid prostate tumors had an improved overall survival rate and response to anti-androgen therapy compared with patients with DNA-aneuploid tumors. The Conference recommended that S-phase be further studied to learn whether that parameter was also prognostic. Since 1993, several important studies have further validated the clinical utility of DNA ploidy analysis (**Table 19-2**) in prostate cancer. Ross et al[19] demonstrated

Table 19-2
Summary of Selected Recent Publications in Prostate Cancer

Author	Year	N	Method	Prognostic Significance Ploidy	Proliferation	Comment
Hawkins[22]	1995	894	FC	Yes	ND	Stage pT3; ploidy was not significant for predicting local recurrence, but was for systemic progression
Ross[19]	1999	111	IA	Yes, DFS	ND	Needle biopsy DNA ploidy status independently predicted disease recurrence
Amling[21]	1999	108	FC	Yes, PCS and DFS (m)	ND	Patients who had RRP after failing RT; DNA ploidy strongest predictor of cancer-specific and progression-free survival
Åström[23]	1998	153	FC	Yes, PCS (m)	Yes, DFS and OS (m)	Mean SPF higher in DNA aneuploid tumors; SPF cut-off was 5%.
Cheng[24]	1998	86	FC	Yes, PCS (m)	ND	Patients with recurrent prostate cancer after RT who then underwent an RRP
Di Silverio[25]	1996	85	FC	Yes, PCS (m)	ND	Stages C-D1 only
Borre[26]	1998	96	FC	Yes, PCS (m); No, OS	ND	Low grade tumors. Ploidy not siginficant for OS.
Ahlgren[20]	1997	96	IA	Yes, OS (m)	Yes, OS (m)	Combining proliferative index with DNA ploidy added prognostic information
Azua[27]	1996	54	IA	Yes, OS	ND	
Pollack[28]	1997	33	FC	Yes, RFS	No	Stage D2
Mora[29]	1999	55	FC	Yes, RFS (u)	Yes, RFS (m)	Stage B only
Zincke[30]	1992	370	FC	Yes, PCS, DFS, and OS (m)	ND	Stage D1 patients only adjuvant hormonal therapy benefitted only patients with DNA diploid tumors
Montgomery[31]	1990	261	FC	Yes, DFS	ND	Stage B only
Nativ[32]	1989	146	FC	Yes, DFS	ND	Stage C only

Abbreviation: PCS = prostate cancer survival

that DNA ploidy analysis of needle biopsy samples could independently predict disease recurrence. This is an important finding because most prostate cancers are first diagnosed by needle biopsy and the patient is then treated with either radical retropubic prostatectomy (RRP) or radiation therapy (RT). Two studies, both using image analysis, have demonstrated that cell proliferation is also an important prognostic variable in prostate cancer.[19,20] There continues to be a lack of data regarding cell proliferation and prognosis determined by the flow cytometry technique.

DNA ploidy was also shown to have prognostic importance in a specific group of patients who underwent RRP after relapsing following RT.[21] DNA ploidy analysis remains an important tool for predicting response to hormonal therapy and survival in prostate cancer. DNA content and cell proliferation determination by flow cytometry or image analysis is part of the routine work-up of newly diagnosed prostate cancer patients. It should also be part of the stratification process for patients entering clinical trials.

Renal Cell Carcinoma

Studies of DNA ploidy analysis as a predictive factor for prognosis in renal cell carcinoma (RCC) patients have traditionally shown variable results. Recently, several additional reports have again shown variable results. Some studies indicate that ploidy is an independent factor for survival, whereas others have not demonstrated that determining ploidy provides any benefit (**Table 19-3**). Two of 3 recent studies suggest that measuring cell proliferation may also be of value.[33-35] In summary, these variable results justify the inclusion of DNA ploidy and S-phase analysis in the assessment of a newly-diagnosed patient with RCC to assist in determining prognosis and interpreting the results of new treatment modalities.

Ovarian Cancer

DNA ploidy as a prognostic factor has been the subject of several recently reported trials in stage III and stage IV ovarian cancer (**Table 19-4**). Most studies demonstrated that DNA ploidy is a prognostic factor for relapse, but not for OS. Cell proliferation in ovarian cancer has not been extensively studied as a prognostic factor by flow cytometry; the limited results that do exist are variable. A recent editorial by Braly[40] concludes that "additional prospective, well-controlled studies are needed to conclusively determine the impact of DNA content and S-phase fraction as prognostic factors for ovarian cancer."

Table 19-3
Summary of Selected Recent Publications in Renal Cell Cancer

Author	Year	N	Method	Prognostic Significance Ploidy	Proliferation	Comment
Del Vecchio[36]	1998	37	FC	Yes, OS (m)	ND	Papillary renal cell carcinoma (a variant of RCC)
Ruiz-Cerda[37]	1996	108	FC	Yes, DFS (m)	ND	Surgically resected with no adjuvant therapy
Gelb[33]	1997	52	FC	No, OS (m)	No, DFS (m)	Mib1, intratumoral microvessel density, and p53 also were not significant predictors of OS
Jochum[38]	1996	58	IA	Yes, OS (u)	ND	Proliferation measured by Mib1 was also significant. Good review of studies prior to 1996.
Larsson[35]	1993	69	FC	Yes, OS (u); No, OS (m)	Yes, OS (u, m)	
Nakano[39]	1993	72	FC	No, OS	ND	
Grignon[34]	1995	44	FC	No, OS	Yes, OS	

Table 19-4
Summary of Selected Recent Publications in Ovarian Cancer

Author	Year	N	Method	Prognostic Significance Ploidy	Proliferation	Comment
Zanetta[41]	1996	282	FC	Yes, DFS (m); No, OS (m)	No, DFS and OS (u)	Stages 3, 4
Reles[42]	1998	103	IA	No, DFS and OS (m)	Yes, DFS and OS (u); No, DFS, OS (m)	
Zanetta[43]	1996	27	FC	Yes, OS (u)	ND	Limited to Stage III patients who had no macroscopic residual disease at surgery
Pfisterer[44]	1994	184	FC	Yes, OS (u); No, OS (m)	ND	

Endometrial Carcinoma

A number of large studies have confirmed the prognostic significance of DNA ploidy in endometrial carcinoma. Britton et al[45] demonstrated that histo-

Table 19-5
Summary of Selected Recent Publications in Endometrial Cancer

Author	Year	N	Method	Prognostic Significance		Comment
				Ploidy	Proliferation	
Britton[45]	1990	256	FC	Yes, DFS (m)	ND	All stages
Hamel[47]	1996	221	FC	Yes, DFS (m)	ND	All stages
Nordstrom[48]	1996	266	FC	Yes, OS (m)	ND	
Nordstrom[49]	1996	297	FC	ND	Yes, OS (m)	
Britton[46]	1989	203	FC	Yes, DFS	ND	
Podratz[50]	1993	140	FC	Yes, DFS (m)	Yes, DFS (m)	Pretreatment uterine curettage samples

logic subtype and DNA ploidy were significant predictors in a multivariate analysis of disease-free survival, whereas tumor grade, depth of invasion, and surgical stage were not. DNA ploidy also constituted a significant factor for survival in patients with stage I disease.[46] Hamel et al[47] extended these studies to include evaluation of tumors by p53 and HER2/neu expression and cell proliferation by PCNA staining, and found in a multivariate analysis that strong p53 expression, HER2/neu expression, histologic subtype, and DNA ploidy were independent prognostic factors for disease-free survival. Nordstrom et al have also demonstrated DNA ploidy to be an independent factor for survival.[48] These authors also evaluated %S-phase by flow cytometry and cell proliferation by Ki-67 and PCNA staining, and demonstrated by multivariate analysis that %S-phase was the strongest predictor of survival.[49] An important study by Podratz et al[50] has demonstrated that DNA ploidy and proliferative fraction in pretreatment endometrial curettage samples identified patients at high risk for extrauterine metastasis and relapse. Patients at risk for aggressive disease can therefore be referred to physicians with expertise in managing patients with high-risk endometrial cancer. The evidence supports the routine use of DNA ploidy and cell proliferation analysis in endometrial carcinoma.

Breast Cancer

The wide variation in the clinical course of patients with breast cancer makes this tumor type ideal for an analysis of prognostic factors. Indeed, the technique of DNA-content analysis on paraffin-embedded samples by flow cytometry was first applied to breast cancer samples.[51] The DNA Consensus Conference[5] suggested that the studies reported up to that time indicated that patients with DNA-diploid tumors had a small survival advantage over those with DNA-aneuploid tumors. Tumors with a high S-phase fraction were associated with a significantly increased risk of recurrence and shorter overall survival times.

Recent studies continue to demonstrate that cell proliferation, but not DNA ploidy, is a significant independent prognostic factor for breast cancer survival. Bergers et al[52] reported a very large study of DNA ploidy analysis by flow cytometry. They found a definite decrease in relapse-free survival and overall survival in patients with nondiploid tumors compared with patients with diploid tumors. Tetraploid tumors behaved as aneuploid tumors and therefore were grouped as such. In a multivariate analysis, however, DNA ploidy did not retain significance after tumor size and lymph node status were known. This report contains an excellent reference list of prior publications in this area. Pinto et al[53] examined a group of 51 women whose tumors were hypertetraploid. These tumors represented 5.9% of a series of 860 breast cancers subjected to DNA-content flow cytometry. When compared with 138 women who had tumors that were nonhypertetraploid, the group of women with hypertetraploid tumors had larger tumors and tumors of higher histologic grade, were more likely to be hormonal receptor-negative, and had a poorer overall survival rate. DNA-content flow cytometry has also been studied with primary breast tumors to learn whether DNA ploidy or %S-phase could predict the likelihood of axillary node metastases.[54] Of tumors measuring 2 cm, 22% were node-positive. If the tumor was DNA-diploid and 2 cm, only 4% of patients were node-positive. If the %S-phase was <7% and the tumor size was 2 cm, only 16% of patients were node-positive. All patients in whom the primary breast tumor was 2 cm, %S-phase <7%, and DNA-diploid were found to have axillary nodes free of tumor metastases.

Bryant et al[55] evaluated paraffin blocks from women who had axillary node-negative and estrogen receptor-positive breast cancer and who were treated with placebo vs tamoxifen on NSABP trial B-14. S-phase calculated by DNA flow cytometry was found to be an independent prognostic factor for disease-free and overall survival; ploidy was not significant. Further evidence of the usefulness of S-phase was provided in a recent study by Thor et al[56], in which the bromodeoxyuridine labeling index was compared with mitotic index and MIB 1 staining. The proliferation rate was found to be an independent prognostic factor for overall survival, and MIB 1 staining was a stronger prognostic factor than the labeling index. Wenger and Clark conducted a review of the literature regarding the use of S-phase as a prognostic factor in breast cancer.[57] They concluded that S-phase is a useful prognostic factor and has clinical utility; however, they felt that further standardization of S-phase analysis is needed.

Table 19-6
Summary of Selected Recent Publications in Breast Cancer

Author	Year	N	Method	Prognostic Significance		Comment
				Ploidy	Proliferation	
Eissa[58]	1997	100	FC	No	ND	Fresh tissue
Railo[59]	1997	212	FC	No, DFS	No, OS	All were pT1N0 diagnosed between 1975 and 89. No adjuvant chemotherapy. Ki-67 10% was significant for relapse.
Bergers[52]	1997	1301	FC	Yes (u), DFS and OS; No (m)	ND	Fresh-frozen samples; patients diagnosed between 1987 and 1990
Frost[60]	1996	51	FC	No	Yes, DFS	Infiltrating lobular
Brown[61]	1996	674	FC	No, DFS and OS	Yes (m), 5-year DFS	Node-negative only; Ki-67 also significant
Cufer[62]	1997	169	FC	No, DFS	ND	Stages 1 and 2
Bryant[55]	1998	1249	FC	No, DFS and OS	Yes (m), DFS and OS	Node-negative, ER+ pts treated on NSABP B-14

It is apparent from the recent literature that DNA content flow cytometry is a reasonable test to perform in the evaluation of a newly diagnosed case of breast cancer. Because DNA ploidy has not been shown to be prognostic, the goal of flow cytometry in breast cancer should be to obtain an accurate %S-phase.

Cancers of the Central Nervous System

Recent studies of DNA content and cell proliferation measurements by flow cytometry have shown that cell proliferation is the more important measurement for central nervous system (CNS) malignancies. Coons et al,[63] in a study of 230 astrocytomas, found cell proliferation determined by flow cytometry to be an independent prognostic factor for survival. Similar results were found for oligodendrogliomas,[64] but not for astrocytomas.[65]

In studies of benign meningiomas, the focus has been on how to predict recurrence rather than overall survival. Maíllo et al[66] found %S-phase to be an independent factor for relapse. A study by Meixensberger did find DNA ploidy to be useful in a series of 134 patients.[67] A large study by Perry et al[68] examined MIB-1 (Ki-67) staining on sections of menigiomas and quantified the area of staining using image analysis. This parameter was compared with DNA ploidy

Table 19-7
Summary of Selected Recent Publications in CNS Tumors

Author	Year	N	Method	Prognostic Significance		Comment
				Ploidy	Proliferation	
Coons[63]	1994	230	FC	Yes, OS (m)	Yes, OS (m)	Astrocytomas; S-phase a stronger prognostic factor
Coons[64]	1994	60	FC	No	Yes, OS (m)	Oligodendrogliomas
Perry[68]	1998	425	FC	No	No	Meningiomas; cell proliferation by MIB-1 staining was a predictor of relapse-free survival
Meixens-berger[67]	1996	134	FC	Yes, RFS	ND	Meningiomas
Mathew[69]	1996	57	FC	No	ND	Pediatric gliomas
Perry[65]	1999	85	FC	Yes, OS (u); No, OS (m)	ND	66 astrocytomas and 19 oligoastrocytomas; age the best prognostic factor
Maíllo[66]	1999	105	FC	No	Yes, RFS (m)	Meningiomas

and cell proliferation determined by flow cytometry. The researchers found MIB-1 to be a better predictor of relapse-free survival than S-phase; DNA ploidy was not a significant predictor of relapse-free survival.

In CNS tumors it appears that cell proliferative rate is more important as a diagnostic or predictive factor than is DNA ploidy. Most biopsies of CNS tumors (other than meningiomas, which are usually simply resected) are small; therefore, it may be simpler and more practical to determine proliferative activity using MIB-1 staining.

Lung Cancer

The clinical utility of DNA content and cell proliferation measurements in lung cancer was not reviewed at the Consensus Conference; however, there have been a number of reports in the 1990s concerning lung cancer that are summarized in **Table 19-8.** Tumor stage is a powerful predictor of relapse and survival in lung cancer, and it has been difficult to demonstrate consistent clinical utility for DNA ploidy and cell proliferation measurements. Current clinical practice does not include DNA content measurements by flow cytometry in either small cell or non-small cell lung cancer. Most reported studies have included small numbers of patients; therefore, it would be useful to perform DNA content measurements on a large cohort of patients who were being uniformly treated as part of a clinical trial to definitively answer the question of the clinical utility of these factors for predicting prognosis. Performing such a study

Table 19-8
Summary of Selected Recent Publications in Lung Tumors

| Author | Year | N | Method | Prognostic Significance | | Comment |
				Ploidy	Proliferation	
Roberts[71]	1998	45	FC	Yes, RFS, OS, and predicted brain metastases	No, RFS or OS, but did predict local recurrence	All were stage I adenocarcinomas. Good review of literature.
Pujol[72]	1996	137	Static	No, OS	ND	Majority were non-small cell lung cancer. Ki67 immuno-histochemical not prognostic.
Costa[73]	1996	102	FC	No, RFS	ND	Non-small cell lung cancer. %S-phase measured by tritiated thymidine labeling index and found to be significant.
Desinan[74]	1996	72	FC	No, RFS	No, RFS	Non-small cell lung cancer. No overall survival data provided. Good review of literature.
Mugüerza[70]	1997	132	FC	Yes, RFS, OS (m)	No, OS	Non-small cell lung cancer. %S-phase calculations performed only on diploid samples.
Virén[75]	1997	36	FC	No, OS	No, OS	All cases were small cell carcinoma
Huang[76]	1996	97	FC	No, OS	ND	All cases were broncho-alveolar carcinoma
Kim[77]	1996	52	FC	No, OS	No, OS	Non-small cell lung cancer
Schmidt[78]	1992	102	FC	No, DFS	No, DFS	T1N0 non-small cell lung cancers
Filderman[79]	1992	44	FC	Yes, OS	Yes, OS (m)	T1 and T2N0 non-small cell lung cancers
Rice[80]	1993	272	FC	No, OS	No, OS	Stages I-IV non-small cell lung cancers
Tanaka[81]	1995	160	FC	Yes, OS	ND	Stages I-III adenocarcinoma

would require significant resources, however, and these efforts are probably better focused on newer techniques of genetic analysis. A commentary by Rice and Farver in 1997 summarized the current situation well: "…the key to predicting patient outcome and developing future therapies is not measuring aneuploidy but understanding the genes that control cell proliferation."

Melanoma

DNA aneuploidy in melanomas has been shown to be associated with the development of metastases and a lower overall survival rate.[82] DNA-content results have typically correlated with tumor thickness and Clark level of invasion, but ploidy has been shown to be an independent prognostic factor for recurrence in stage I cutaneous melanoma.[82] As detailed in **Table 19-9**, studies continue to demonstrate that DNA ploidy determined by flow cytometry is a prognostic factor in melanoma; however, because of its correlation with Clark level and tumor thickness, which are easily measured in routine pathologic examination, DNA-content flow cytometry is not routinely performed in non-study situations.

Table 19-9
Summary of Selected Recent Publications in Melanoma

Author	N	Method	Prognostic Significance Ploidy	Proliferation	Comment
Kheir[82], 1988	162	FC	Yes, RFS (m)	ND	Stage I cutaneous melanomas
Tralongo[83], 1998	78	FC	Yes, OS (u); multivariate analysis not done	ND	Ploidy correlated with tumor thickness and level of invasion (Clark level)
Toti[84], 1998	61	FC	Yes, OS (u); multivariate analysis not done	ND	Choroidal melanomas; no correlation between ploidy and cell type
Karlsson[85], 1996	79	FC	Yes, OS (m)	Yes, OS (m) when performed with Ki-67	Uveal melanoma
Scheistrøen[86], 1996	43	FC	Yes, OS (m)	ND	Melanoma of the vulva
Richardson[87], 1997	51	FC	No	No	Uveal melanomas

Colon and Rectal Cancer

In the 1990s, there was a concerted effort to understand the molecular pathogenesis of colon cancer.[88] It has become apparent that at least 2 genetic pathways can lead to colon cancer:microsatellite instability (MIN) and chromosomal instability (CIN). Tumors with CIN tend to have allelic imbalance and are DNA aneuploid when examined through flow cytometry,[89] whereas tumors with MIN are more likely to be DNA diploid.[90,91] Tumors arising in the proximal colon are more likely to be DNA diploid, whereas distal tumors are more likely to be DNA nondiploid.[92] In future large studies of molecular markers it will be important to relate the findings to DNA ploidy and cell proliferation, because these measurements may be surrogate markers for the molecular genetic abnormalities. In daily practice the performance of DNA content and cell proliferation analysis by flow cytometry may be more cost effective and more widely available than molecular markers.

The wide variation in the clinical course of patients with adenocarcinoma of the colon or rectum and the variable efficacy of adjuvant therapy increases the value of prognostic factors. The Consensus Conference document on colorectal cancer summarizes the important publications in the field up to the early 1990s. The committee agreed that the evidence supported DNA ploidy as a prognostic factor in Dukes stage B (Astler-Coller B2) and stage C colorectal cancers and encouraged additional studies.[8] **Table 19-10** summarizes the key findings of 5 studies of DNA ploidy and cell proliferation in colon cancer. In 4 out of the 5 studies DNA ploidy was a significant prognostic factor for survival. In the other study, by Sinicrope et al,[93] DNA ploidy was of borderline significance (p=0.06) for all other cases, but was a significant prognostic factor for adenocarcinomas of the proximal colon. DNA ploidy was not significant in cases in which the cancer was located in the distal colon.

The importance of cell proliferation in colon and rectal cancer is still not completely known. Sinicrope et al[93] studied cell proliferation by DNA-content flow cytometry (via the proliferative index) and by measuring the mitotic index. They found that the proliferative index and mitotic index correlate with each other (p=0.02), and the mitotic index proved significant in multivariate analysis. This study therefore substantiates the usefulness of some measure of cell proliferation in colorectal carcinomas for predicting relapse and survival. The actual method used (flow cytometry, mitotic index, Ki-67, or MIB-1 staining) is one of choice for the investigator. Currently, in the authors' institution, DNA ploidy and cell proliferation measurements are performed routinely by flow cytometry on all Dukes B2 colorectal carcinomas. If the tumor is DNA-nondiploid or is diploid with a high proliferative rate (20% S + G2M calculated without debris

Table 19-10
Summary of Selected Recent Publications in Adenocarcinomas of the Colon or Rectum

Author	Year	N	Method	Prognostic Significance		Comment
				Ploidy	Proliferation	
Sinicrope[93]	1999	150	FC	All cases: No, RFS (u,m) (p=0.06); No, OS (u, m) (p=0.06)	No, RFS (p=0.06); No, OS (p=0.07)	Stages I or II (majority were stage II). No adjuvant therapy. Used 15% as cutoff for proliferative index.
Sinicrope[93]				Yes, RFS (p=0.03); Yes, OS (p=0.05)	No, RFS p=0.17; No, OS p=0.33	Cases of proximal colon cancer
Sinicrope[93]				No, RFS (p=0.88); No, OS (p=0.73)	No, RFS (p=0.39); Yes, OS (p=0.03)	Cases of distal colon cancer
Takanishi[94]	1996	210	FC	Yes, OS (u,m)	Yes, OS (u) No, OS (m)	Astler-Coller modified Dukes B
Lanza[95]	1996	204	FC	Yes, OS (u,m)	ND	All stages and locations
Lanza[96]	1998	191	FC	Yes, DFS (u,m); Yes, OS (u,m)	ND	Stages II and III. Used frozen tumor samples.
Baretton[97]	1996	86	FC	No, DFS; No, OS	ND	P53 overexpression and chromosome 17 aneusomy correlated with DNA nondiploid

subtraction), the patient is considered a candidate for adjuvant therapy. If the tumor is Dukes C, the patient is offered adjuvant therapy irrespective of DNA ploidy or cell proliferation, which makes the routine performance of flow cytometry unnecessary. Studies are needed to learn whether DNA ploidy and cell proliferation can be used to predict not only prognosis but also response to therapy.

Gastric Cancer

Recent studies in gastric cancer indicate that both DNA ploidy and %S-phase are useful prognostic factors for survival (**Table 19-11**); however, these measurements have not been routinely used in clinical practice.

Table 19-11
Summary of Selected Recent Publications in Gastric Cancer

Author	Year	N	Method	Prognostic Significance		Comment
				Ploidy	Proliferation	
Omejc[98]	1997	79	FC	No, OS	ND	Specimens from patients with potentially curative resections
Abad[99]	1998	76	FC	Yes, OS (m)	No, OS	
Setala[100]	1997	289	FC	Yes, OS (m)	Yes, OS (u); No, OS (m) (p=0.58)	

Table 19-12
Summary of Selected Recent Publications in Adenocarcinoma of the Pancreas

Author	Year	N	Method	Prognostic Significance		Comment
				Ploidy	Proliferation	
Park[103]	1996	32	FC	No	No	
Rugge[102]	1996	60	FC	Yes, OS (m)	ND	
Allison[101]	1998	96	FC	Yes, OS (m)	ND	

Pancreatic Cancer

Adenocarcinoma of the pancreas continues to be a tumor with a poor prognosis. The results of DNA ploidy and cell proliferation analysis of these tumors have been derived from small studies that often provide discordant results (**Table 19-12**). However, 2 recent large studies have shown DNA ploidy to be an independent factor for OS.[101,102] It is therefore appropriate to perform this analysis on patients with newly diagnosed pancreatic cancers. Future studies should also analyze %S-phase as a prognostic factor.

Cancers of the Head and Neck

The clinical utility of DNA ploidy and cell proliferation markers in head and neck cancer was most recently reviewed in 1996.[104] Since then, a number of additional studies have been published (**Table 19-13**). The results demonstrate

Table 19-13
Summary of Selected Recent Publications in Tumors of the Head and Neck

Author	Year	N	Method	Prognostic Significance Ploidy	Proliferation	Comment
Melchiorri[105]	1996	24	FC	Yes, DFS and OS (m)	ND	Squamous cell carcinoma of oral and maxillofacial region
Gemryd[106]	1997	28	FC	Yes, RFS and OS (u)	No, RFS	Mucoepidermoid carcinomas
Rubio Bueno[107]	1998	109	FC	Yes, DFS and OS (m)	ND	Squamous cell carcinomas of oral cavity and base of tongue
Yip[108]	1998	51	FC	Yes, OS (m)	Yes, OS (m)	Nasopharyngeal carcinoma
Takashima[109]	1996	46	FC	Yes, DFS (m)	No, RFS	Major salivary gland tumors
Staibano[110]	1998	25	FC	Yes, OS	ND	Oral squamous cell carcinoma
Schimming[111]	1997	52	IA	Yes, (u)	ND	Oral squamous cell carcinoma
Del Valle-Zapico[112]	1998	51	FC	No, OS	No, OS	Squamous cell carcinoma of the pyriform sinus

that DNA ploidy is useful as a prognostic factor; however, most of the evidence derives from small studies. Until more data is collected, it is appropriate to perform DNA ploidy and cell proliferation measurements on the primary tumor sample from patients entering large clinical trials for this tumor site.

Thyroid Cancer

DNA-content flow cytometry has been applied to different types of thyroid cancer. There have been several recent studies (**Table 19-14**), and the consensus is that these measurements can add important information regarding risk of tumor relapse or OS in these cancers.[113,114]

Table 19-14
Summary of Selected Recent Publications in Thyroid Cancer

Author	Year	N	Method	Prognostic Significance		Comment
				Ploidy	Proliferation	
Pasieka[114]	1992	73	IA	Yes, RFS and OS (m)	ND	Primary or relapsed papillary thyroid cancer. Fine-needle aspirations.
Kurozumi[115]	1998	131	FC	Yes, CFS (m)	Yes, CFS (m)	Papillary thyroid cancer
Dineen[116]	1995	100	FC	Yes, OS (u); No, OS (m)	ND	All patients had papillary thyroid cancer and distant metastases
Nishida[117]	1996	100	FC	Yes, RFS and OS (m)	Yes, (u); No (m)	Follicular and papillary thyroid cancer
Hay[118]	1990	119	FC	Yes, OS (m)	Yes, OS (m)	Medullary thyroid carcinoma
Grant[119]	1990	64	FC	Yes ,OS (m)	No	Follicular carcinomas

Sarcoma

Sarcomas are unusual tumors with a varied clinical course. Early studies of leiomyosarcomas in the 1980s had indicated that DNA ploidy was an important prognostic factor.[120] More recent studies, as summarized in **Table 19-15** below, tend to show prognostic value for DNA ploidy and cell proliferation analysis in this tumor type.

Multiple Myeloma

There has been significant interest in the cytogenetics and cell proliferation of the malignant plasma cells in the bone marrow of patients with multiple myeloma (MM). In contrast to solid tumors, MM lends itself to relatively easy and repeated access to the tumor cells. Aneuploidy is the hallmark of MM cells, whether it is detected by flow cytometry, fluorescence in-situ hybridization (FISH), or classical cytogenetics. Drach et al demonstrated aneuploidy in 90% of cases of MM by use of interphase FISH.[129] High rates of aneuploidy have been demonstrated by FISH in bone marrow plasma cells from patients with AL-primary systemic amyloidosis and monoclonal gammopathy of undetermined significance (MGUS).[130]

Table 19-15

Summary of Selected Recent Publications in Sarcomas.

Author	Year	N	Method	Prognostic Significance		Comment
				Ploidy	Proliferation	
Golouh[121]	1996	60	FC	Yes, OS (m)	ND by FC	Spindle-cell sarcomas of soft tissue
Gustafson[122]	1997	160	FC	Yes, RFS (u);	Yes, RFS (m) No, RFS (m)	Extremity soft-tissue sarcomas
Blom[123]	1998	49	FC	Yes, OS (m)	Yes, OS (m)	Uterine leiomyo–sarcomas
De Zen[124]	1997	59	FC	Yes, OS (m); unusual finding that patients with diploid tumors did worse	Yes, OS (m)	Childhood rhabdomyosarcoma
Lopes[125]	1998	49	FC	Yes, RFS (u) and OS (u); No, RFS (m) and OS (m)	Not significant by FC	Synovial sarcoma. High proliferative rate by PCNA staining was an independent factor for OS.
Nordal[126]	1996	48	FC	No	ND	Endometrial stromal cell sarcoma
Oliveira[127]	1997	17	FC	No	ND	Osteosarcoma of the jaw
Plaat[128]	1997	44	FC	No	ND	Soft-tissue sarcoma

Using classical cytogenetic techniques, Rajkumar et al[131] detected a chromosomally abnormal clone in 43% of patients with relapsed MM who were being treated with autologous transplant. Interestingly, these researchers found a positive correlation between aneuploidy and a high plasma cell proliferative rate. Calasanz et al[132] studied 111 cases of new MM and found aneuploidy (specifically hypodiploidy) to be an adverse factor for RFS and OS. A recent study by Greipp et al[133] detected hypodiploidy by flow cytometry in only 1.4% of 349 cases of new MM; the cases with hypodiploid clones had a prognosis similar to the other cases.

In plasma cell malignancies, the rate of marrow plasma cell proliferation can be determined by either the plasma cell labeling index (PCLI) or flow cytometry. The PCLI is typically measured with the bromodeoxyuridine labeling

Table 19-16
Summary of Selected Recent Publications in Multiple Myeloma.

| Author | Year | N | Method | Prognostic Significance | | Comment |
				Ploidy	Proliferation	
San Miguel[140]	1995	120	FC	ND	Yes, OS (m)	
Garcia-Sanz[143]	1999	26	FC	ND	Yes, OS (m)	Plasma cell leukemia
Trendle[138]	1999	210	FC	ND	Yes, OS (m)	%S-phase by FC not independent if PCLI known

index. This is a 2-color, slide-based assay that stains the cytoplasmic light chain with FITC-conjugated anti-kappa or anti-lambda; the S-phase cells are detected by an antibody to bromodeoxyuridine and a secondary goat anti-mouse rhodamine antibody. The PCLI has been shown to be an independent prognostic factor for MM survival in multiple clinical trials.[134-139] CD38 and CD138 have been used along with propidium iodide in a flow cytometric procedure to determine DNA content and S-phase of malignant marrow plasma cells (**Table 19-16**).[140-142] Using this method, 60% of patients with MM and 73% of those with MGUS have aneuploid plasma cells. The %S-phase from DNA content histogram was an independent prognostic factor.[140,141] In summary, both cytogenetics and %S-phase are important prognostic markers in MM. At this time, FISH is the preferred strategy over flow cytometry DNA-content measurements to detect precise genetic abnormalities. In addition, the PCLI is preferred over flow cytometry because it can be performed on marrow samples with <5% plasma cells. However, if the expertise is available, %S-phase can be calculated by flow cytometry as discussed above.[138-140]

Leukemia

Cytogenetic analysis of acute leukemia cells has been of demonstrated clinical and research utility for many years. Aneuploidy is typically determined by FISH and classical cytogenetic techniques;[144-146] DNA-content analysis by flow cytometry is not typically performed in the initial evaluation of acute leukemia.

Lymphoma

The non-Hodgkin's lymphomas (NHL) are a group of diseases with very diverse prognosis. In the 1980s, it was anticipated that ploidy or cell proliferation might serve as useful markers of prognosis in this disease. The International Prognostic Index (IPI), which uses age, stage, performance status, serum LDH, and the number of extranodal sites involved with NHL to predict prognosis, was developed in 1993 and has been in widespread use ever since. To be useful, any new prognostic factor for lymphoma must be proven to be independent of the IPI. In 1996 Winter et al[147] published their results on 242 patients with aggressive NHL who were treated with chemotherapy as part of a cooperative group trial. The researchers were unable to demonstrate independent significance for DNA ploidy or cell proliferation over the IPI. Other studies have also not found independent significance for DNA ploidy or S-phase as prognostic factors.[148] Witzig et al[149] have demonstrated that the bromodeoxyuridine labeling index is a prognostic factor for survival in low-grade NHL but not diffuse large cell (intermediate-grade) NHL.[150] Other studies using flow cytometry also found cell proliferation to be predictive in low-grade NHL[151,152] and in peripheral T-cell NHL.[153] It appears that cell proliferation measurements may be useful in NHL (especially in low-grade NHL) and can be determined by immunohistochemistry (MIB-1), flow cytometry, or the bromodeoxyuridine labeling index. Because the labeling index requires immediate cell processing, the most practical methods for measuring cell proliferation are flow cytometry on paraffin-embedded material or MIB-1 staining. At this time, neither DNA ploidy nor cell proliferation measurements are indicated for routine clinical evaluation and treatment of typical large cell NHL. The cell proliferative rate is useful for predicting prognosis in patients with low-grade NHL, and will be useful in a research setting for evaluating the cell cycle consequences of molecular genetic abnormalities.

Conclusions

Over the last 15 years the evidence from multiple studies has demonstrated the clinical utility of DNA ploidy and cell proliferation measurements by flow cytometry. As demonstrated in the summary tables above, these tests have clinical utility for many different tumors. The use of flow cytometry to perform these tests is advantageous in that flow cytometry can be performed electively on paraffin-embedded tissue, it is widely available in most large medical centers or can be performed in reference laboratories, results are available within days, and the cost is low. It is likely that in the next decade this test will be replaced with more precise measurements of chromosome number and specific chromosomal abnormalities which should enhance our ability to predict tumor behavior, improve our understanding of the pathogenesis of malignant tumors, and, hopefully, lead to improved treatment and prognosis of patients with malignant disease.

References

1. Hedley DW, Friedlander ML, Taylor IW, et al. Method for analysis of cellular DNA content of paraffin-embedded pathological material using flow cytometry. *J Histochem Cytochem*. 1983;31:1333-1335.

2. Sebo TJ, Roche PC, Witzig TE, et al. Proliferative activity in non-Hodgkin's lymphomas. A comparison of the bromodeoxyuridine labeling index with PCNA immunostaining and quantitative image analysis. *Am J Clin Path*. 1993;99:668-672.

3. Duque RE, Andreeff M, Braylan RC, et al. Consensus review of the clinical utility of DNA flow cytometry in neoplastic hematopathology. *Cytometry*. 1993;14:492-496.

4. Hedley D, Shankey T, Wheeless L. DNA cytometry consensus conference. *Cytometry*. 1993;14:471.

5. Hedley DW, Clark GM, Cornelisse CJ, et al. Consensus review of the clinical utility of DNA cytometry in carcinoma of the breast. Report of the DNA Cytometry Consensus Conference. *Cytometry*. 1993;14:482-485.

6. Shankey TV, Kallioniemi OP, Koslowski JM, et al. Consensus review of the clinical utility of DNA content cytometry in prostate cancer. *Cytometry*. 1993;14:497-500.

7. Shankey TV, Rabinovitch PS, Bagwell B, et al. Guidelines for implementation of clinical DNA cytometry. International Society for Analytical Cytology [published correction appears in *Cytometry*. 1993;14:842]. *Cytometry*. 1993;14:472-477.

8. Bauer KD, Bagwell CB, Giaretti W, et al. Consensus review of the clinical utility of DNA flow cytometry in colorectal cancer. *Cytometry*. 1993;14:486-491.

9. Wheeless LL, Badalament RA, de Vere White RW, et al. Consensus review of the clinical utility of DNA cytometry in bladder cancer. Report of the DNA Cytometry Consensus Conference. *Cytometry*. 1993;14:478-481.

10. Bittard H, Lamy B, Billery C. Clinical evaluation of cell deoxyribonucleic acid content measured by flow cytometry in bladder cancer. *J Urol*. 1996;155:1887-1891.

11. Alderisio M, Cenci M, Valli C, et al. Nm23-H1 protein, DNA-ploidy and S-phase fraction in relation to overall survival and disease free survival in transitional cell carcinoma of the bladder. *Anticancer Res*. 1998;18:4225-4230.

12. Gregoire M, Fradet Y, Meyer F, et al. Diagnostic accuracy of urinary cytology, and deoxyribonucleic acid flow cytometry and cytology on bladder washings during followup for bladder tumors. *J Urol*. 1997;157:1660-1664.

13. Granfors T, Duchek M, Tomic R, et al. Predictive value of DNA ploidy in bladder cancer treated with preoperative radiation therapy and cystectomy. *Scand J Urol Nephrol*. 1996;30:281-285.

14. Song J, Farrow GM, Lieber MM. Primary adenocarcinoma of the bladder: favorable prognostic significance of deoxyribonucleic acid diploidy measured by flow cytometry. *J Urol*. 1990;144:1115-1118.

15. Corrado F, Ferri C, Mannini D, et al. Transitional cell carcinoma of the upper urinary tract: evaluation of prognostic factors by histopathology and flow cytometric analysis. *J Urol*. 1991;145:1159-1163.

16. Blute ML, Tsushima K, Farrow GM, et al. Transitional cell carcinoma of the renal pelvis: nuclear deoxyribonucleic acid ploidy studied by flow cytometry. *J Urol*. 1988;140:944-949.

17. Winkler HZ, Nativ O, Hosaka Y, et al. Nuclear deoxyribonucleic acid ploidy in squamous cell bladder cancer. *J Urol*. 1989;141:297-302.

18. Tetu B, Allard P, Fradet Y, et al. Prognostic significance of nuclear DNA content and S-phase fraction by flow cytometry in primary papillary superficial bladder cancer. *Hum Pathol*. 1996;27:922-926.

19. Ross JS, Sheehan CE, Ambros RA, et al. Needle biopsy DNA ploidy status predicts grade shifting in prostate cancer. *Am J Surg Pathol*. 1999;23:296-301.

20. Ahlgren G, Lindholm K, Falkmer U, et al. A DNA cytometric proliferation index improves the value of the DNA ploidy pattern as a prognosticating tool in patients with carcinoma of the prostate. *Urol*. 1997;50:379-384.

21. Amling CL, Lerner SE, Martin SK, et al. Deoxyribonucleic acid ploidy and serum prostate specific antigen predict outcome following salvage prostatectomy for radiation refractory prostate cancer. *J Urol*. 1999;161:857-862, discussion 862-863.

22. Hawkins CA, Bergstralh EJ, Lieber MM, et al. Influence of DNA ploidy and adjuvant treatment on progression and survival in patients with pathologic stage T3 (PT3) prostate cancer after radical retropubic prostatectomy. *Urol*. 1995;46:356-364.

23. Astrom L, Weimarck A, Aldenborg F, et al. S-phase fraction related to prognosis in localised prostate cancer. No specific significance of chromosome 7 gain or deletion of 7q31.1. *Int J Cancer*. 1998;79:553-559.

24. Cheng L, Sebo TJ, Slezak J, et al. Predictors of survival for prostate carcinoma patients treated with salvage radical prostatectomy after radiation therapy. *Cancer*. 1998;83:2164-2171.

25. Di Silverio F, D'Eramo G, Buscarini M, et al. DNA ploidy, Gleason score, pathological stage and serum PSA levels as predictors of disease-free survival in C-D1 prostatic cancer patients submitted to radical retropubic prostatectomy. *Eur Urol.* 1996;30:316-321.

26. Borre M, Hoyer M, Nerstrom B, et al. DNA ploidy and survival of patients with clinically localized prostate cancer treated without intent to cure. *Prostate.* 1998;36:244-249.

27. Azua J, Romeo P, Valle J, et al. DNA quantification as a prognostic factor in prostatic adenocarcinoma. *Anal Quant Cytol Histol.* 1996;18:330-336.

28. Pollack A, Troncoso P, Zagars GK, et al. The significance of DNA-ploidy and S-phase fraction in node-positive (stage D1) prostate cancer treated with androgen ablation. *Prostate.* 1997;31:21-28.

29. Mora L, Moscinski L, Diaz J, et al. Stage B prostate cancer: correlation of DNA ploidy analysis with histological and clinical parameters. *Cancer Control.* 1999;6:587-591.

30. Zincke H, Bergstralh EJ, Larson-Keller JJ, et al. Stage D1 prostate cancer treated by radical prostatectomy and adjuvant hormonal treatment. Evidence for favorable survival in patients with DNA diploid tumors. *Cancer.* 1992;70:311-323.

31. Montgomery BT, Nativ O, Blute ML, et al. Stage B prostate adenocarcinoma. Flow cytometric nuclear DNA ploidy analysis. *Arch Surg.* 1990;125:327-331.

32. Nativ O, Winkler HZ, Raz Y, et al. Stage C prostatic adenocarcinoma: flow cytometric nuclear DNA ploidy analysis. *Mayo Clin Proc.* 1989;64:911-919.

33. Gelb AB, Sudilovsky D, Wu CD, et al. Appraisal of intratumoral microvessel density, MIB-1 score, DNA content, and p53 protein expression as prognostic indicators in patients with locally confined renal cell carcinoma. *Cancer.* 1997;80:1768-1775.

34. Grignon DJ, Abdel-Malak M, Mertens W, et al. Prognostic significance of cellular proliferation in renal cell carcinoma: a comparison of synthesis-phase fraction and proliferating cell nuclear antigen index. *Mod Pathol.* 1995;8:18-24.

35. Larsson P, Roos G, Stenling R, et al. Tumor-cell proliferation and prognosis in renal-cell carcinoma. *Int J Cancer.* 1993;55:566-570.

36. del Vecchio MT, Lazzi S, Bruni A, et al. DNA ploidy pattern in papillary renal cell carcinoma. Correlation with clinicopathological parameters and survival. *Pathol Res Pract.* 1998;194:325-333.

37. Ruiz-Cerda JL, Hernandez M, Gomis F, et al. Value of deoxyribonucleic acid ploidy and nuclear morphometry for prediction of disease progression in renal cell carcinoma. *J Urol.* 1996;155:459-465.

38. Jochum W, Schroder S, al-Taha R, et al. Prognostic significance of nuclear DNA content and proliferative activity in renal cell carcinomas. A clinicopathologic study of 58 patients using mitotic count, MIB-1 staining, and DNA cytophotometry. *Cancer.* 1996;77:514-521.

39. Nakano E, Kondoh M, Okatani K, et al. Flow cytometric analysis of nuclear DNA content of renal cell carcinoma correlated with histologic and clinical features. *Cancer.* 1993;72:1319-1323.

40. Braly P. DNA content and S-phase fraction in epithelial ovarian cancer: what information do they really add [editorial]? *Gynecol Oncol.* 1998;71:1-2.

41. Zanetta G, Keeney GL, Cha SS, et al. Flow-cytometric analysis of deoxyribonucleic acid content in advanced ovarian carcinoma: its importance in long-term survival. *Am J Obstet Gynecol.* 1996;175:1217-1225.

42. Reles AE, Gee C, Schellschmidt I, et al. Prognostic significance of DNA content and S-phase fraction in epithelial ovarian carcinomas analyzed by image cytometry [see also comments]. *Gynecol Oncol.* 1998;71:3-13.

43. Zanetta G, Keeney GL, Cha SS, et al. DNA index by flow cytometric analysis: an additional prognostic factor in advanced ovarian carcinoma without residual disease after primary operation. *Gynecol Oncol.* 1996;62:208-212.

44. Pfisterer J, Kommoss F, Sauerbrei W, et al. Cellular DNA content and survival in advanced ovarian carcinoma. *Cancer.* 1994;74:2509-2515.

45. Britton LC, Wilson TO, Gaffey TA, et al. DNA ploidy in endometrial carcinoma: major objective prognostic factor. *Mayo Clin Proc.* 1990;65:643-650.

46. Britton LC, Wilson TO, Gaffey TA, et al. Flow cytometric DNA analysis of stage I endometrial carcinoma. *Gynecol Oncol.* 1989;34:317-322.

47. Hamel NW, Sebo TJ, Wilson TO, et al. Prognostic value of p53 and proliferating cell nuclear antigen expression in endometrial carcinoma. *Gynecol Oncol.* 1996;62:192-198.

48. Nordstrom B, Strang P, Lindgren A, et al. Carcinoma of the endometrium: do the nuclear grade and DNA ploidy provide more prognostic information than do the FIGO and WHO classifications? *Int J Gynecol Pathol.* 1996;15:191-201.

49. Nordstrom B, Strang P, Bergstrom R, et al. A comparison of proliferation markers and their prognostic value for women with endometrial carcinoma. Ki-67, proliferating cell nuclear antigen, and flow cytometric S-phase fraction. *Cancer.* 1996;78:1942-1951.

50. Podratz KC, Wilson TO, Gaffey TA, et al. Deoxyribonucleic acid analysis facilitates the pretreatment identification of high-risk endometrial cancer patients. *Am J Obstet Gynecol.* 1993;168:1206-1213, discussion 1213-1215.

51. Hedley DW, Rugg CA, Ng AB, et al. Influence of cellular DNA content on disease-free survival of Stage II breast cancer patients. *Cancer Res.* 1984;44:5395-5398.

52. Bergers E, Baak JP, van Diest PJ, et al. Prognostic value of DNA ploidy using flow cytometry in 1301 breast cancer patients: results of the prospective Multicenter Morphometric Mammary Carcinoma Project. *Mod Pathol.* 1997;10:762-768.

53. Pinto AE, Andre S, Nogueira M, et al. Flow cytometric DNA hypertetraploidy is associated with unfavourable prognostic features in breast cancer. *J Clin Pathol.* 1997;50:591-595.

54. Zanon C, Durando A, Geuna M, et al. Flow cytometry in breast cancer: prognostic and surgical indications of the sparing of axillary lymph node dissection. *Am J Clin Oncol.* 1998;21:392-397.

55. Bryant J, Fisher B, Gunduz N, et al. S-phase fraction combined with other patient and tumor characteristics for the prognosis of node-negative, estrogen-receptor-positive breast cancer. *Breast Cancer Res Treatment.* 1998;51:239-253.

56. Thor AD, Liu S, Moore DH 2nd, et al. Comparison of mitotic index, in vitro bromodeoxyuridine labeling, and MIB-1 assays to quantitate proliferation in breast cancer. *J Clin Oncol.* 1999;17:470-477.

57. Wenger CR, Clark GM. S-phase fraction and breast cancer—a decade of experience. *Breast Cancer Res Treatment.* 1998;51:255-265.

58. Eissa S, Khalifa A, el-Gharib A, et al. Multivariate analysis of DNA ploidy, p53, c-erbB-2 proteins, EGFR, and steroid hormone receptors for short-term prognosis in breast cancer. *Anticancer Res.* 1997;17:3091-3097.

59. Railo M, Lundin J, Haglund C, et al. Ki-67, p53, Er-receptors, ploidy and S-phase as prognostic factors in T1 node negative breast cancer. *Acta Oncologica.* 1997;36:369-374.

60. Frost AR, Karcher DS, Terahata S, et al. DNA analysis and S-phase fraction determination by flow cytometric analysis of infiltrating lobular carcinoma of the breast. *Mod Pathol.* 1996;9:930-937.

61. Brown RW, Allred CD, Clark GM, et al. Prognostic value of Ki-67 compared to S-phase fraction in axillary node-negative breast cancer. *Clin Cancer Res.* 1996;2:585-592.

62. Cufer T, Lamovec J, Bracko M, et al. Prognostic value of DNA ploidy in breast cancer stage I-II. *Neoplasma.* 1997;44:127-132.

63. Coons SW, Johnson PC, Pearl DK. Prognostic significance of flow cytometry deoxyribonucleic acid analysis of human astrocytomas. *Neurosurg.* 1994;35:119-125, discussion 125-126.

64. Coons SW, Johnson PC, Pearl DK, et al. Prognostic significance of flow cytometry deoxyribonucleic acid analysis of human oligodendrogliomas. *Neurosurg.* 1994;34:680-687, discussion 687.

65. Perry A, Jenkins RB, O'Fallon JR, et al. Clinicopathologic study of 85 similarly treated patients with anaplastic astrocytic tumors. An analysis of DNA content (ploidy), cellular proliferation, and p53 expression. *Cancer.* 1999;86:672-683.

66. Maíllo A, Díaz P, Blanco A, et al. Proportion of S-phase tumor cells measured by flow cytometry is an independent prognostic factor in meningioma tumors. *Cytometry (Comm Clin Cytometry).* 1999;38:118-123.

67. Meixensberger J, Janka M, Zellner A, et al. Prognostic significance of nuclear DNA content in human meningiomas: a prospective study. *Acta Neurochirurgica.* 1996;65(suppl):70-72.

68. Perry A, Stafford SL, Scheithauer BW, et al. The prognostic significance of MIB-1, p53, and DNA flow cytometry in completely resected primary meningiomas. *Cancer.* 1998;82:2262-2269.

69. Mathew P, Look T, Luo X, et al. DNA index of glial tumors in children. Correlation with tumor grade and prognosis. *Cancer.* 1996;78:881-886.

70. Muguerza JM, Diez M, Torres AJ, et al. Prognostic value of flow cytometric DNA analysis in non-small-cell lung cancer: rationale of sequential processing of frozen and paraffin-embedded tissue. *World J Surg.* 1997;21:323-329.

71. Roberts HL, Komaki R, Allen P, et al. Prognostic significance of DNA content in stage I adenocarcinoma of the lung. *Int J Rad Oncol Biol Phys.* 1998;41:573-578.

72. Pujol JL, Simony J, Jolimoy G, et al. Hypodiploidy, Ki-67 growth fraction and prognosis of surgically resected lung cancers. *Br J Cancer*. 1996;74:964-970.

73. Costa A, Silvestrini R, Mochen C, et al. P53 expression, DNA ploidy and S-phase cell fraction in operable locally advanced non-small-cell lung cancer. *Br J Cancer*. 1996;73:914-919.

74. Desinan L, Scott CA, Pizzolitto S, et al. Non-small cell lung cancer. Morphology and DNA flow cytometry. *Anal Quant Cytol Histol*. 1996;18:438-452.

75. Viren MM, Ojala AT, Kataja VV, et al. Flow cytometric analysis of tumor DNA profile related to response to treatment and survival in small-cell lung cancer. *Med Oncol*. 1997;14:35-38.

76. Huang MS, Colby TV, Therneau TM, et al. DNA ploidy and protein content in bronchioloalveolar carcinoma multi-variable flow cytometry. *Cytometry*. 1996;26:253-259.

77. Kim YC, Park KO, Kim HJ, et al. DNA ploidy and proliferative activity in bcl-2 expressed non-small cell lung cancer. *Kor J Intern Med*. 1996;11:101-107.

78. Schmidt RA, Rusch VW, Piantadosi S. A flow cytometric study of non-small cell lung cancer classified as T1N0. *Cancer*. 1992;69:78-85.

79. Filderman AE, Silvestri GA, Gatsonis C, et al. Prognostic significance of tumor proliferative fraction and DNA content in stage I non-small cell lung cancer. Am *Rev Respir Dis*. 1992;146:707-710.

80. Rice TW, Bauer TW, Gephardt GN, et al. Prognostic significance of flow cytometry in non-small-cell lung cancer. *J Thorac Cardiovasc Surg*. 1993;106:210-217.

81. Tanaka I, Masuda R, Furuhata Y, et al. Flow cytometric analysis of the DNA content of adenocarcinoma of the lung, especially for patients with stage 1 disease with long term follow-up. *Cancer*. 1995;75:2461-2465.

82. Kheir SM, Bines SD, Vonroenn JH, et al. Prognostic significance of DNA aneuploidy in stage I cutaneous melanoma. *Ann Surg*. 1988;207:455-461.

83. Tralongo V, Daniele E, Leonardi V, et al. Prognostic value of clinicopathologic variables and DNA ploidy in stage I cutaneous malignant melanoma. *Oncol Rep*. 1998;5:1095-1098.

84. Toti P, Greco G, Mangiavacchi P, et al. DNA ploidy pattern in choroidal melanoma: correlation with survival. A flow cytometry study on archival material [also see comments]. *Br J Ophthalmol*. 1998;82:1433-1437.

85. Karlsson M, Boeryd B, Carstensen J, et al. Correlations of Ki-67 and PCNA to DNA ploidy, S-phase fraction and survival in uveal melanoma. *Eur J Cancer*. 1996;32A:357-362.

86. Scheistroen M, Trope C, Kaern J, et al. Malignant melanoma of the vulva FIGO stage I: evaluation of prognostic factors in 43 patients with emphasis on DNA ploidy and surgical treatment. Gynecol Oncol. 1996;61:253-258.

87. Richardson RP, Lawry L, Rees RC, et al. DNA index and %S phase fraction in posterior uveal melanoma: a 5 year prospective study of fresh tissue using flow cytometry. *Eye*. 1997;11:629-634.

88. Nicholl I, Dunlop M. Molecular markers of prognosis in colorectal cancer. *J Natl Cancer Inst*. 1999;91:1267-1269.

89. Miyazaki M, Furuya T, Shiraki A, et al. The relationship of DNA ploidy to chromosomal instability in primary human colorectal cancers. *Cancer Res.* 1999;59:5283-5285.

90. Halling K, French A, McDonnell S, et al. Microsatellite instability and 8p allelic imbalance in stage B2 and C colorectal cancers. *J Natl Cancer Inst.* 1999;91:1295-1303.

91. Thibodeau SN, French AJ, Roche PC, et al. Altered expression of hMSH2 and hMLH1 in tumors with microsatellite instability and genetic alterations in mismatch repair genes. *Cancer Res.* 1996;56:4836-4840.

92. Changchien CR, Wang JY, Tang R, et al. Pathogenetic implications of DNA nondiploidy in colorectal cancers. *Dis Colon Rectum.* 1997;40:1244-1247.

93. Sinicrope FA, Hart J, Hsu HA, et al. Apoptotic and mitotic indices predict survival rates in lymph node-negative colon carcinomas. *Clin Cancer Res.* 1999;5:1793-1804.

94. Takanishi DM Jr, Hart J, Covarelli P, et al. Ploidy as a prognostic feature in colonic adenocarcinoma. *Arch Surg.* 1996;131:587-592.

95. Lanza G Jr, Maestri I, Dubini A, et al. p53 expression in colorectal cancer: relation to tumor type, DNA ploidy pattern and short-term survival. *Am J Clin Pathol.* 1996;105:604-612.

96. Lanza G, Gafa R, Santini A, et al. Prognostic significance of DNA ploidy in patients with stage II and stage III colon carcinoma: a prospective flow cytometric study. *Cancer.* 1998;82:49-59.

97. Baretton GB, Vogt M, Muller C, et al. Prognostic significance of p53 expression, chromosome 17 copy number, and DNA ploidy in non-metastasized colorectal carcinomas (stages IB and II). *Scand J Gastroenterol.* 1996;31:481-489.

98. Omejc M, Repse S, Bracko M. DNA flow cytometry in gastric carcinoma: implication in patients with potentially curative resection. *J Surg Oncol.* 1997;65:237-241.

99. Abad M, Ciudad J, Rincon MR, et al. DNA aneuploidy by flow cytometry is an independent prognostic factor in gastric cancer. *Analytical Cell Pathol.* 1998;16:223-231.

100. Setala LP, Nordling S, Kosma VM, et al. Comparison of DNA ploidy and S-phase fraction with prognostic factors in gastric cancer. *Anal Quant Cytol Histol.* 1997;19:524-532.

101. Allison DC, Piantadosi S, Hruban RH, et al. DNA content and other factors associated with ten-year survival after resection of pancreatic carcinoma. *J Surg Oncol.* 1998;67:151-159.

102. Rugge M, Sonego F, Sessa F, et al. Nuclear DNA content and pathology in radically treated pancreatic carcinoma. The prognostic significance of DNA ploidy, histology and nuclear grade. *Cancer.* 1996;77:459-466.

103. Park CS, Wiebke EA, Sidner RA, et al. The role of flow cytometric DNA analysis in determining prognosis of resectable ductal adenocarcinoma of the pancreas. *Am Surg.* 1996;62:609-615, discussion 615-616.

104. Ensley JF. The clinical application of DNA content and kinetic parameters in the treatment of patients with squamous cell carcinomas of the head and neck. *Cancer Metastasis Rev.* 1996;15:133-141.

105. Melchiorri C, Cattini L, Lalli E, et al. DNA ploidy analysis of squamous cell carcinomas of the oral and maxillofacial region: clinical and pathologic correlations. *Oral Surg Oral Med Oral Pathol Oral Radiol Endodontics*. 1996;82:308-314.

106. Gemryd P, Lundquist PG, Tytor M, et al. Prognostic significance of DNA ploidy in mucoepidermoid carcinoma. *Eur Arch Otorhinolaryngol*. 1997;254:180-185.

107. Rubio Bueno P, Naval Gias L, Garcia Delgado R, et al. Tumor DNA content as a prognostic indicator in squamous cell carcinoma of the oral cavity and tongue base. *Head Neck*. 1998;20:232-239.

108. Yip TT, Lau WH, Chan JK, et al. Prognostic significance of DNA flow cytometric analysis in patients with nasopharyngeal carcinoma. *Cancer*. 1998;83:2284-2292.

109. Takashima S, Sone S, Horii A, et al. Major salivary gland lesions: correlation of MR findings with flow cytometric DNA analysis and prognosis. *Am J Roentgenol*. 1996;167:1297-1304.

110. Staibano S, Mignogna MD, Lo Muzio L, et al. Overexpression of cyclin-D1, bcl-2, and bax proteins, proliferating cell nuclear antigen (PCNA), and DNA-ploidy in squamous cell carcinoma of the oral cavity. *Hum Pathol*. 1998;29:1189-1194.

111. Schimming R, Hlawitschka M, Haroske G. DNA analysis of squamous cell carcinoma in the oral cavity by image cytometry and its rating in the assessment of tumor prognosis. *Mund-, Kiefer- und Gesichtschirurgie*. 1997;1:108-110.

112. Del Valle-Zapico A, Fernandez FF, Suarez AR, et al. Prognostic value of histopathologic parameters and DNA flow cytometry in squamous cell carcinoma of the pyriform sinus. *Laryngoscope*. 1998;108:269-272.

113. Hay ID. Papillary thyroid carcinoma. *Endocrinol Metab Clin North Am*. 1990;19:545-576.

114. Pasieka JL, Zedenius J, Auer G, et al. Addition of nuclear DNA content to the AMES risk-group classification for papillary thyroid cancer. *Surg*. 1992;112:1154-1159, discussion 1159-1160.

115. Kurozumi K, Nakao K, Nishida T, et al. Significance of biologic aggressiveness and proliferating activity in papillary thyroid carcinoma. *World J Surg*. 1998;22:1237-1242.

116. Dinneen SF, Valimaki MJ, Bergstralh EJ, et al. Distant metastases in papillary thyroid carcinoma: 100 cases observed at one institution during 5 decades. *J Clin Endocrinol Metab*. 1995;80:2041-2045.

117. Nishida T, Nakao K, Hamaji M, et al. Overexpression of p53 protein and DNA content are important biologic prognostic factors for thyroid cancer. *Surg*. 1996;119:568-575.

118. Hay ID, Ryan JJ, Grant CS, et al. Prognostic significance of nondiploid DNA determined by flow cytometry in sporadic and familial medullary thyroid carcinoma. *Surg*. 1990;108:972-979, discussion 979-980.

119. Grant CS, Hay ID, Ryan JJ, et al. Diagnostic and prognostic utility of flow cytometric DNA measurements in follicular thyroid tumors. *World J Surg*. 1990;14:283-289, discussion 289-290.

120. Tsushima K, Rainwater LM, Goellner R, et al. Leiomyosarcomas and benign smooth muscle tumors of the stomach: nuclear DNA patterns studied by flow cytometry. *Mayo Clin Proc*. 1987;62:275-280.

121. Golouh R, Bracko M, Novak J. Predictive value of proliferation-related markers, p53, and DNA ploidy for survival in patients with soft tissue spindle-cell sarcomas. *Mod Pathol.* 1996;9:919-924.

122. Gustafson P, Ferno M, Akerman M, et al. Flow cytometric S-phase fraction in soft-tissue sarcoma: prognostic importance analysed in 160 patients. *Br J Cancer.* 1997;75:94-100.

123. Blom R, Guerrieri C, Stal O, et al. Leiomyosarcoma of the uterus: A clinicopathologic, DNA flow cytometric, p53, and mdm-2 analysis of 49 cases. *Gynecol Oncol.* 1998;68:54-61.

124. De Zen L, Sommaggio A, d'Amore ES, et al. Clinical relevance of DNA ploidy and proliferative activity in childhood rhabdomyosarcoma: a retrospective analysis of patients enrolled onto the Italian Cooperative Rhabdomyosarcoma Study RMS88. *J Clin Oncol.* 1997;15:1198-1205.

125. Lopes JM, Hannisdal E, Bjerkehagen B, et al. Synovial sarcoma. Evaluation of prognosis with emphasis on the study of DNA ploidy and proliferation (PCNA and Ki-67) markers. *Analytical Cell Pathol.* 1998;16:45-62.

126. Nordal RR, Kristensen GB, Kaern J, et al. The prognostic significance of surgery, tumor size, malignancy grade, menopausal status, and DNA ploidy in endometrial stromal sarcoma. *Gynecol Oncol.* 1996;62:254-259.

127. Oliveira P, Nogueira M, Pinto A, et al. Analysis of p53 expression in osteosarcoma of the jaw: correlation with clinicopathologic and DNA ploidy findings. *Hum Pathol.* 1997;28:1361-1365.

128. Plaat BE, Muntinghe FL, Molenaar WM, et al. Clinical outcome of patients with previously untreated soft tissue sarcomas in relation to tumor grade, DNA ploidy and karyotype. *Int Cancer.* 1997;74:396-402.

129. Drach J, Schuster J, Nowotny H, et al. Multiple myeloma: high incidence of chromosomal aneuploidy as detected by interphase fluorescence in situ hybridization. *Cancer Res.* 1995;55:3854-3859.

130. Fonseca R, Ahmann GJ, Jalal SM, et al. Chromosomal abnormalities in systemic amyloidosis. *Br J Haematol.* 1998;103:704-710.

131. Rajkumar SV, Fonseca R, Dewald GW, et al. Cytogenetic abnormalities correlate with the plasma cell labeling index and extent of bone marrow involvement in myeloma. *Cancer Genet Cytogenet.* 1999;113:73-77.

132. Calasanz MJ, Cigudosa JC, Odero MD, et al. Hypodiploidy and 22q11 rearrangements at diagnosis are associated with poor prognosis in patients with multiple myeloma. *Br J Haematol.* 1997;98:418-425.

133. Greipp PR, Trendle MC, Leong T, et al. Is flow cytometric DNA content hypodiploidy prognostic in multiple myeloma? *Leukemia Lymphoma.* 1999;35:83-89.

134. Gertz MA, Lacy MQ, Inwards DJ, et al. Early harvest and late transplantation as an effective therapeutic strategy in multiple myeloma. *Bone Marrow Transplantation.* 1999;23:221-226.

135. Gertz MA, Witzig TE, Pineda AA, et al. Monoclonal plasma cells in the blood stem cell harvest from patients with multiple myeloma are associated with shortened relapse-free survival after transplantation. *Bone Marrow Transplantation.* 1997;19:337-342.

136. Greipp P, Lust J, O'Fallon M, et al. Plasma cell labeling index and b2-microglobulin predict survival independent of thymidine kinase and C-reactive protein in multiple myeloma. *Blood*. 1993;81:3382-3387.

137. Joshua D, Ioannidis R, Brown R, et al. Multiple myeloma: relationship between light chain isotype suppression, labeling index of plasma cells and CD38 expression on peripheral blood lymphocytes. *Am J Hematol*. 1988;29:5-11.

138. Trendle MC, Leong T, Kyle RA, et al. Prognostic significance of the S-phase fraction of light-chain-restricted cytoplasmic immunoglobulin (cIg) positive plasma cells in patients with newly diagnosed multiple myeloma enrolled on Eastern Cooperative Oncology Group treatment trial E9486. *American J Hematol*. 1999;61:232-237.

139. Boccadoro M, Gallamini A, Fruttero A, et al. Plasma cell acid phosphatase activity as prognostic factor in multiple myeloma: relationship to the thymidine-labeling index. *J Clin Oncol*. 1985;3:1503-1507.

140. San Miguel J, García-Sanz R, González M, et al. A new staging system for multiple myeloma based on the number of S-phase plasma cells. *Blood*. 1995;85:448-455.

141. Almeida J, Orfao A, Mateo G, et al. Immunophenotypic and DNA content characteristics of plasma cells in multiple myeloma and monoclonal gammopathy of undetermined significance. *Pathologie Biologie*. 1999;47:119-127.

142. San Miguel JF, Garcia-Sanz R, Gonzalez M, et al. DNA cell content studies in multiple myeloma. Leukemia Lymphoma. 1996;23:33-41.

143. Garcia-Sanz R, Orfao A, Gonzalez M, et al. Primary plasma cell leukemia: clinical, immunophenotypic, DNA ploidy, and cytogenetic characteristics. *Blood*. 1999;93:1032-1037.

144. Pajor L, Szuhai K, Mehes G, et al. Combined metaphase, interphase cytogenetic, and flow cytometric analysis of DNA content of pediatric acute lymphoblastic leukemia. *Cytometry*. 1998;34:87-94.

145. Martin PL, Look AT, Schnell S, et al. Comparison of fluorescence in situ hybridization, cytogenetic analysis, and DNA index analysis to detect chromosomes 4 and 10 aneuploidy in pediatric acute lymphoblastic leukemia: a Pediatric Oncology Group study. *J Pediatr Hematol Oncol*. 1996;18:113-121.

146. Mertens F, Johansson B, Mitelman F. Dichotomy of hyperdiploid acute lymphoblastic leukemia on the basis of the distribution of gained chromosomes. *Cancer Genet Cytogenet*. 1996;92:8-10.

147. Winter JN, Andersen J, Variakojis D, et al. Prognostic implications of ploidy and proliferative activity in the diffuse, aggressive non-Hodgkin's lymphomas. *Blood*. 1996;88:3919-3925.

148. Czader M, Mazur J, Pettersson M, et al. Prognostic significance of proliferative and apoptotic fractions in low grade follicle center cell-derived non-Hodgkin's lymphomas. *Cancer*. 1996;77:1180-1188.

149. Witzig T, Habermann T, Kurtin P, et al. S-phase fraction by the labeling index as a predictive factor for progression and survival in low grade non-Hodgkin's lymphoma. *Cancer*. 1995;76:1059-1064.

150. Ansell S, PJ K, Stenson M, et al. Evaluation of the proliferative index as a prognostic factor in diffuse large cell lymphoma: correlation with the International Index. *Leukemia Lymphoma*. 1999;34:529-537.

151. Macartney JC, Camplejohn RS, Morris R, et al. DNA flow cytometry of follicular non-Hodgkin's lymphoma. *J Clin Pathol.* 1991;44:215-218.

152. Lackowska B, Gruchala A, Niezabitowski A, et al. Prognostic and predictive evaluation of DNA content, S-phase fraction and immunophenotyping in non-Hodgkin's lymphomas in adults. A prospective study. *Polish J Pathol.* 1999;50:23-29.

153. Grierson HL, Wooldridge TN, Purtilo DT, et al. Low proliferative activity is associated with a favorable prognosis in peripheral T-cell lymphoma. *Cancer Res.* 1990;50:4845-4848.

Reference Range Appendix

J. Philip McCoy, Jr.

Cord Blood — Percentages
95% Confidence Interval

CD	Mean	Minimum	Maximum
CD3	64	48	81
CD3$^+$CD4$^+$	46	30	62
CD3$^+$CD8$^+$	18	8	28
CD19$^+$CD3-	17	5	29
CD56$^+$CD3-	8	0	15
CD56$^+$CD3$^+$	0	0	1
CD8$^+$CD3-	5	0	11
CD29$^+$CD4^{+*}	55	21	89
CD45RA$^+$CD4^{+*}	87	75	98
CD19$^+$CD10^{+**}	5	1	12

All values expressed as a percentage of lymphocytes except where noted otherwise.
* expressed as a percentage of CD4$^+$ lymphocytes
** expressed as a percentage of CD19$^+$ lymphocytes
From Motley D, Meyer MP, King RA, et al. Determination of lymphocyte immunophenotype values for normal full-term cord blood. Am J Clin Pathol. *1996;105:38-43.*

Additional cord blood reference ranges have been published in D'Arena G, Musto P, Cascavilla N, et al. Flow cytometric characterization of human umbilical cord blood lymphocytes: immunophenotypic features. Haematologica. *1998;83(3):197-203.*

Neonatal Peripheral Blood—Percentages (and Absolute Counts)
10th and 90th Percentiles

CD	Median	10th Percentile	90th Percentile
CD3	82.7 (3697)	72.2 (2537)	90.3 (5785)
CD3+CD4+	63 (2710)	52.4 (1971)	72 (4355)
CD3+CD8+	23 (1054)	15.8 (539)	29.2 (1752)
CD19+CD3-	14 (579)	6 (233)	21.6 (1188)
CD56+CD16+CD3-	4 (200)	2 (64)	8.3 (376)
CD10+CD19+	1.5 (not calc.)	1 (not calc.)	4 (not calc.)
CD5+CD20+	13 (not calc.)	5 (not calc.)	18 (not calc.)
CD3+HLADr+	2 (not calc.)	1 (not calc.)	3 (not calc.)
CD3+CD25+	7 (not calc.)	5 (not calc.)	9.8 (not calc.)
CD8+HLADr+	2 (not calc.)	0 (not calc.)	3 (not calc.)
CD8+CD57+	0 (not calc.)	0 (not calc.)	1 (not calc.)
CD8+CD28+	19 (not calc.)	13.5 (not calc.)	27 (not calc.)
CD8+CD38+	21 (not calc.)	16.7 (not calc.)	29 (not calc.)

All values expressed as a percentage of lymphocytes except where noted otherwise, with absolute counts given in parentheses.
Abbreviations: not calc. = not calculated

From O'Gorman MRG, Millard DD, Lowder JN, et al. Lymphocyte subpopulations in healthy 1-3 day old infants. Cytometry. *1998;34:235-241.*

Pediatric Peripheral Blood—Percentages (and Absolute Counts)
95% Confidence Interval

CD	Age	Minimum	Maximum
CD2	0–6 months	55 (3900)	88 (5300)
	6–12 months	55 (3800)	88 (4900)
	12–18 months	55 (3500)	88 (4200)
	18–24 months	55 (3100)	88 (3900)
	24–30 months	55 (2600)	88 (3600)
	30–36 months	55 (2200)	88 (3500)
	3–17 years	65 (1200)	84 (4100)
CD3	0–6 months	55 (3500)	82 (5000)
	6–12 months	55 (3400)	82 (4600)
	12–18 months	55 (3200)	82 (3900)
	18–24 months	55 (2800)	82 (3500)
	24–30 months	55 (2300)	82 (3300)
	30–36 months	55 (1900)	82 (3100)
	3–17 years	55 (1000)	82 (3900)
CD4+	0–6 months	50 (2800)	57 (3900)
	6–12 months	49 (2600)	55 (3500)
	12–18 months	46 (2300)	51 (2900)
	18–24 months	42 (1900)	48 (2500)
	24–30 months	38 (1500)	46 (2200)
	30–36 months	33 (1200)	44 (2000)
	3-17 years	27 (560)	57 (2700)
CD8+	0–6 months	8 (350)	31 (2500)
	6–12 months	8 (350)	31 (2500)
	12–18 months	8 (350)	31 (2500)
	18–24 months	8 (350)	31 (2500)
	24–30 months	8 (350)	31 (2500)
	30–36 months	8 (350)	31 (2500)
	3–17 years	14 (330)	34 (1400)
CD19+	0–6 months	11 (430)	45 (3300)
	6–12 months	11 (430)	45 (3300)
	12–18 months	11 (430)	45 (3300)
	18–24 months	11 (430)	45 (3300)
	24–30 months	11 (430)	45 (3300)
	30–36 months	11 (430)	45 (3300)
	3–17 years	9 (200)	29 (1300)

Data derived from Kotylo PK, Fineberg NS, Freeman KS, et al. Reference ranges for lymphocyte subsets in pediatric patients. Am J Clin Pathol. *1993;100:111-115.*

Pediatric Peripheral Blood—Percentages (and Absolute Counts)
95% Confidence Interval

CD	Age	Minimum	Maximum
CD3	2–3 months	60 (2070)	87 (6540)
	4–6 months	57 (2280)	84 (6450)
	12–23 months	53 (1460)	81 (5440)
	24–59 months	62 (1610)	80 (4230)
CD4	2–3 months	41 (1460)	64 (5110)
	4–6 months	36 (1690)	61 (4600)
	12–23 months	31 (1020)	54 (3600)
	24–59 months	35 (900)	51 (2860)
CD8	2–3 months	16 (650)	35 (6540)
	4–6 months	16 (720)	34 (6450)
	12–23 months	16 (570)	38 (5440)
	24–59 months	22 (630)	38 (4230)

Data derived from Denny T, Yogev R, Gelman R, et al. Lymphocyte subsets in healthy children during the first 5 years of life. JAMA. 1992;267:1484-1488.

Pediatric Peripheral Blood—Percentages (and Absolute Counts)
5% and 95% Percentiles

CD	Age	Minimum	Maximum
CD19	neonatal (cord blood)	5 (400)	22 (1100)
	1 week—2 months	4 (600)	26 (1900)
	2–5 months	14 (600)	39 (3000)
	5–9 months	13 (700)	35 (2500)
	9–15 months	15 (600)	39 (2700)
	15–24 months	17 (600)	41 (3100)
	2–5 years	14 (200)	44 (2100)
	5–10 years	10 (200)	31 (1600)
	10–16 years	8 (200)	24 (600)
	>16 years	6 (100)	19 (500)
CD3	neonatal (cord blood)	28 (600)	76 (5000)
	1 week—2 months	60 (2300)	85 (7000)
	2–5 months	48 (2300)	75 (6500)
	5–9 months	50 (2400)	77 (6900)
	9–15 months	54 (1600)	76 (6700)
	15–24 months	39 (1400)	73 (8000)
	2–5 years	43 (900)	76 (4500)
	5–10 years	55 (700)	78 (4200)
	10–16 years	52 (800)	78 (3500)
	>16 years	55 (700)	83 (2100)
CD3+CD4+	neonatal (cord blood)	17 (400)	52 (3500)
	1 week—2 months	41 (1700)	68 (5300)
	2–5 months	33 (1500)	58 (5000)
	5–9 months	33 (1400)	58 (5100)
	9–15 months	31 (1000	54 (4600)
	15–24 months	25 (900)	50 (5500)
	2–5 years	23 (500)	48 (2400)
	5–10 years	27 (300)	53 (2000)
	10–16 years	25 (400)	48 (2100)
	>16 years	28 (300)	57 (1400)
CD3+CD8+	neonatal (cord blood)	10 (200)	41 (1900)
	1 week—2 months	9 (400)	23 (1700)
	2–5 months	11 (500)	25 (1600)
	5–9 months	13 (600)	26 (2200)
	9–15 months	12 (400)	28 (2100)
	15–24 months	11 (400)	32 (2300)
	2–5 years	14 (300)	33 (1600)
	5–10 years	19 (300)	34 (1800)
	10–16 years	9 (200)	35 (1200)
	>16 years	10 (200)	39 (900)

(continued on next page)

Pediatric Peripheral Blood—Percentages (and Absolute Counts) *(continued)*
5% and 95% Percentiles

CD	Age	Minimum	Maximum
CD3+HLA-Dr+	neonatal (cord blood)	1 (30)	6 (400)
	1 week—2 months	1 (30)	38 (3400)
	2–5 months	1 (70)	9 (500)
	5–9 months	1 (70)	7 (500)
	9–15 months	2 (100)	8 (600)
	15–24 months	3 (100)	12 (700)
	2–5 years	3 (80)	13 (400)
	5–10 years	3 (50)	14 (700)
	10–16 years	1 (20)	8 (200)
	>16 years	2 (30)	12 (200)
CD3-CD16+CD56+	neonatal (cord blood)	6 (100)	58 (1900)
	1 week—2 months	3 (200)	23 (1400)
	2–5 months	2 (100)	14 (1300)
	5–9 months	2 (100)	13 (1000)
	9–15 months	3 (200)	17 (1200)
	15–24 months	3 (100)	16 (1400)
	2–5 years	4 (100)	23 (1000)
	5–10 years	4 (90)	26 (900)
	10–16 years	6 (70)	27 (1200)
	>16 years	7 (90)	31 (600)

Data from Comans-Bitter WM, de Groot R, van den Beemd, et al. Immunophenotyping of blood lymphocytes in childhood. J Pediatr. *1997;130:388-393.*

Adult Peripheral Blood—Percentages (and Absolute Counts)
Mean ± (1.96 × SD)

Immunophenotype	Minimum	Maximum
CD3+	49 (411)	85 (2061)
CD3+CD4+CD8-	26 (212)	61 (1391)
CD3+CD4+CD8+	0 (0)	3 (67)
CD3+CD4-CD8+	10 (59)	31 (699)
CD3+CD4-CD8-	0 (0)	6 (122)
CD56+	5 (71)	28 (499)
CD3-CD8+CD56+	0 (0)	4 (72)
CD3+CD8-CD56+	0 (0)	3 (34)
CD3-CD8+CD56+	0 (0)	4 (63)
CD5+	47 (394)	95 (2235)
CD5+CD10+	0 (0)	2 (431)
CD19+	4 (32)	17 (341)
CD19+CD5+	0 (0)	6 (132)
CD19+CD10+	0 (0)	1 (17)
CD20+	3 (0)	27 (559)
CD20+lambda+	0 (0)	12 (243)
CD20+kappa+	1 (3)	9 (161)

Data derived from Stewart CC, Stewart SJ. Immunological monitoring utilizing novel probes. Ann NY Acad Sci. *1993;677:94-112.*

Adult Peripheral Blood and Bone Marrow—Percentages
95% Confidence Interval

CD	Specimen	Minimum	Maximum
CD1	peripheral blood	0	6
	bone marrow aspirate	0	4
	bone marrow biopsy	0	10
CD3	peripheral blood	57	94
	bone marrow aspirate	21	72
	bone marrow biopsy	9	32
CD4	peripheral blood	27	60
	bone marrow aspirate	16	40
	bone marrow biopsy	0	12
CD5	peripheral blood	57	90
	bone marrow aspirate	3	80
	bone marrow biopsy	10	33
CD8	peripheral blood	12	38
	bone marrow aspirate	13	37
	bone marrow biopsy	9	22
CD10	peripheral blood	0	10
	bone marrow aspirate	2	15
	bone marrow biopsy	0	24
CD14	peripheral blood	0	8
	bone marrow aspirate	0	6
	bone marrow biopsy	0	7
CD15	peripheral blood	0	10
	bone marrow aspirate	0	11
	bone marrow biopsy	0	11
CD16	peripheral blood	0	6
	bone marrow aspirate	0	4
	bone marrow biopsy	0	10
CD19	peripheral blood	1	16
	bone marrow aspirate	4	28
	bone marrow biopsy	0	27
HLA-Dr	peripheral blood	1	24
	bone marrow aspirate	8	46
	bone marrow biopsy	7	32

Data derived from Clark P, Normansell DE, Innes DJ, et al. Lymphocyte subsets in normal marrow. Blood. 1986;67:1600-1606.

Pediatric Bone Marrow Aspirates—Percentages
Mean ± (1.96 × SD)

Cluster Designation	Age	Minimum	Maximum
CD2	1–5 years	16	51
	6–10 years	37	72
	11–15 years	43	76
CD4	1–5 years	6	33
	6–10 years	15	39
	11–15 years	25	48
CD8	1–5 years	4	22
	6–10 years	14	33
	11–15 years	11	30
CD10	1–5 years	13	41
	6–10 years	7	28
	11–15 years	7	23
CD19	1–5 years	20	68
	6–10 years	22	44
	11–15 years	13	32
CD20	1–5 years	19	40
	6–10 years	11	31
	11–15 years	4	17
CD21	1–5 years	0	14
	6–10 years	1	14
	11–15 years	2	14

Derived from Caldwell CW, Poje E, Helikson MA. B-cell precursors in normal pediatric bone marrow. Am J Clin Pathol. 1991;95:816-823.

Pediatric Bone Marrow Biopsies—Percentages
25th and 75th Percentiles

Cluster Designation	Age	25th Percentile	75th Percentile
CD2+	Less than 1 year	4.6	23.7
	1 to 4 years	8.5	16.9
	4 to 15 years	15.3	23.6
	Over 15 years	26.1	51.5
CD3+	Less than 1 year	5.3	24.8
	1 to 4 years	6.8	17.5
	4 to 15 years	16.6	25.2
	Over 15 years	22.6	50.6
CD4+	Less than 1 year	2.0	9.3
	1 to 4 years	2.1	5.2
	4 to 15 years	4.2	7.3
	Over 15 years	8	13.9
CD7+	Less than 1 year	5	24.4
	1 to 4 years	6.2	16.7
	4 to 15 years	13.4	20.8
	Over 15 years	20.6	39.9
CD8+	Less than 1 year	2.3	11.4
	1 to 4 years	4.1	10.1
	4 to 15 years	10.0	18.5
	Over 15 years	20.3	37.2
CD14+	Less than 1 year	0.0	4.7
	1 to 4 years	0.7	5.0
	4 to 15 years	0.4	4.5
	Over 15 years	1.0	7.0
CD19+	Less than 1 year	44.1	70.4
	1 to 4 years	53.5	78.1
	4 to 15 years	41.6	58.4
	Over 15 years	16.5	40.3
CD19+CD10+	Less than 1 year	23.1	64.7
	1 to 4 years	39.8	67.2
	4 to 15 years	32.7	53.1
	Over 15 years	6.0	19.1
CD19+CD20+	Less than 1 year	6.0	30.2
	1 to 4 years	25.8	38.6
	4 to 15 years	24.2	32.0
	Over 15 years	12.3	22.7
CD3-CD16,56+	Less than 1 year	2.3	7.5
	1 to 4 years	1.6	5.3
	4 to 15 years	1.1	4.6
	Over 15 years	3.2	7.1
CD33+CD34-	Less than 1 year	2.0	9.7
	1 to 4 years	2.2	9.0
	4 to 15 years	3.0	9.5
	Over 15 years	5.4	6.8
CD33-CD34+	Less than 1 year	2.3	9.8
	1 to 4 years	2.8	8.7
	4 to 15 years	2.0	9.5
	Over 15 years	5.3	9.5

From Rego EM, Garcia AB, Viana SR, et al. Age-related changes of lymphocyte subsets in normal bone marrow biopsies. Cytometry. 1998;34:22-29.

Lymph Node—Percentages
95% Confidence Interval

CD	Minimum normal/hyperplastic	Maximum normal/hyperplastic
CD1	0/0	11/5
CD2	41/33	89/83
CD3	41/31	89/81
CD4	29/21	68/68
CD5	44/np	84/np
CD8	6/7	26/41
CD9	0/np	16/np
CD10	0/np	0/np
CD19	8/16	48/73
CD20	9/np	49/np
CD21	0/np	46/np
CD22	0/np	35/np
CD24	5/np	47/np
CD38	2/np	30/np
CD56	0/np	4/np
CD71	0/1	18/51
kappa	6/9	26/39
lambda	0/4	24/26

Abbreviations: np = test not performed on hyperplastic nodes
Derived from Bryan CF, Eastman PJ, Conner JB, et al. Clinical utility of a lymph node normal range obtained by flow cytometry. Ann NY Acad Sci. 1993;677:404-406 and Self SE, Burdash NM, Ponzio AD, et al. Lymphocyte subsets in lymph node hyperplasias and B cell neoplasms as determined by fluoresceinated antibodies and flow cytometry. Ann NY Acad Sci. 1986;486:195-210.

Additional Reference Ranges of Interest:

Sugiyama M, Yamane H, Konishi K, et al: Subsets of tonsillar lymphocytes and activated cells in each subset analyzed by two color flow cytometry. *Acta Otolaryngol (Stockholm)*. 1987;104:342-350.

Plum P, van Cauwenberge P, De Smedt M, et al. Phenotyping of mononuclear cells from tonsils and corresponding biopsies using a cytofluorimeter. *Acta Otolaryngol (Stockholm)*. 1986;101:129-134.

McCoy JP, Overton WR, Schroeder K, et al. Immunophenotypic analysis of the T cell receptor Vβ repertoire in normal peripheral blood: survey of expression in CD4+ and CD8+ lymphocytes. *Cytometry*. 1996;26(2):148-153.

Howard RR, Fasano CS, Frey L, et al. Reference intervals of CD3, CD4, CD8, CD4/CD8, and absolute CD4 values in Asian and Non-Asian populations. *Cytometry*. 1996;26:231-232.

Shahabuddin S, al Ayed IH, el-Rad MO, et al. Lymphocyte subset reference ranges in healthy Saudi Arabian children. *Pediatr Allergy Immunol*. 1998;9:44-48.

Vithayasai V, Sirisanthana T, Sakonwasun C, et al. Flow cytometric analysis of T-lymphocyte subsets in adult Thais. *Asian-Pacific J Allergy Immunol*. 1997;15:141-146.

Choong ML, Ton SH, Cheong SK. Influence of race, age, and sex on the lymphocyte subsets in peripheral blood of healthy Malaysian adults. *Ann Clin Biochem*. 1995;32:532-539.

Index

A

7-AAD. *See* 7-Aminoactinomycin D
ABC. *See* Antibody-bind capacity
ABN. *See* Advance beneficiary notice
Absolute cell count, 53, 109
Accuracy, 131-134, 493
ACD. *See* Acid citrate dextrose
Acetylcholinesterase, *553-554*
Acid citrate dextrose (ACD), 228, *228*
Acquired immune deficiency syndrome.
    See Human immunodeficiency virus
    infection
Acridine orange, 52, *560*
Acrodermatitis enteropathica, *384*, 418-419
Actin, 422
Acute leukemia. *See also* specific types
  antigen phenotyping for diagnosis,
    348-362
  differential diagnosis of, 265
  drug resistant, 362-364
  flow cytometric analysis of, *339-369*
  gating for acute leukemia blasts, 341-343
  immunophenotyping in
    cytoplasmic flow analysis, 346-347, *347*
    membrane (cell surface) analysis, 344-346,
     345
    method selection, 341
    panels and analysis, 343-347
  triage, 340

Acute lymphoblastic leukemia (ALL), 339
  B-lineage. *See* B-lineage acute lymphoblastic
    leukemia
  changes in phenotype at relapse, 354-355
  cytogenetic analysis in, 368
  DNA content analysis in, 368-369
  DNA ploidy in, 369
  gating for acute leukemia blasts, 341-343
  immunophenotyping in
    cytoplasmic flow analysis, 346-347, *347*
    membrane (cell surface) analysis, 344-346,
     345
    method selection, 341
    panels and analysis, 343-344
  karyotypic analysis in, 368-369
  L3, 350
  medical triage, 340
  minimal residual disease in, 343-344, 364-
    368
  myeloid antigen-positive, 361
  proliferative fraction in, 369
  S-phase fraction in, 368
  T-lineage. *See* T-lineage acute lymphoblastic
    leukemia
  typing of, 348-355
Acute megakaryocytic leukemia. *See* Acute
    myelogenous leukemia, M7
Acute mixed lineage leukemia, 361-362
Acute myelogenous leukemia (AML), 208, 339

in sarcoidosis, 634
in Sézary syndrome/mycosis fungoides, 286
in silicone implant recipient, 630, *630*
in T-large granular lymphocytic leukemia, 285
in T-lineage acute lymphoblastic leukemia, 352, *353*, 354
in T/NK-cell lymphoma, 322-324, *323-324*
in T-prolymphocytic leukemia, 287
in ZAP-70 deficiency, 400
CD9, 79, 91
in B-lineage acute lymphoblastic leukemia, 351
in B-lineage prolymphocytic leukemia, 269
reference ranges for, 707
CD10 (CALLA), 55, 69-70, 72, *73-74*, 74-77, 77, 91, 246, *247-248*
in acute lymphoblastic leukemia, 344, *345*
in acute myelogenous leukemia, 344, *345*, 357
in B-chronic lymphocytic leukemia/small lymphocytic lymphoma, 258, 260, *262*
in B-lineage acute lymphoblastic leukemia, *349*, 350-351
in Burkitt's lymphoma/leukemia, 282
in follicular center lymphoma, *254*, 266, 304, *305*, 306, *307*
in hematogones, 366, 368
in mantle-cell lymphoma, *254*, 264
in myeloma, 278-279
ontogeny of B cells, 429-430
reference ranges for, 697-698, 703-707
in small-cleaved-cell lymphoma, *254*
in splenic lymphoma with veiled lymphocytes, 276
in variant hairy-cell leukemia, *271*, 274
CD11
correlation with older surface marker assays, *21*
defect in leukocyte adhesion deficiency I, 602, *603*
CD11a (LFA-1, integrin alpha), 72, 77-78, 91, 420-421, 600-602
in neonate, 424, 434, 436
CD11b (mac-1), 72, 76-78, 77-78, 80, 91, 421, 600-602
in acute myelogenous leukemia, 358
deficiency of, 606
in leukocyte adhesion deficiency I, 613, *614*
in neonate, 424, 436, 439, 605
in T-prolymphocytic leukemia, 287
CD11c, 72, 77-78, 78, 91, 246, *247-248*
in acute myelogenous leukemia, 361
in B-chronic lymphocytic leukemia/small lymphocytic lymphoma, *254*, 257, *270*, 295-296, *297*, 298, 299i
in hairy-cell leukemia, *270*, 271, 273-274

in marginal zone lymphoma, 310-312, *311*
in monocytoid B-cell lymphoma, 268
in neonate, 424
in splenic lymphoma with veiled lymphocytes, *270*, 276
in splenic marginal zone lymphoma, *270*
in variant hairy-cell leukemia, 271, 274
CD11d, 72
CDw12, 91
CD13 (aminopeptidase N), 76, 77-78, 91, 130
in acute lymphoblastic leukemia, 344, *345*
in acute myelogenous leukemia, 344, *345*, 355-360, *356*
in B-lineage acute lymphoblastic leukemia, 350-351
in T-lineage acute lymphoblastic leukemia, 352, 355
CD14, 78, 78, 91, 130, *553*
in acute lymphoblastic leukemia, 343-344, *345*
in acute myelogenous leukemia, 343-344, *345*, 357-360
CD45/glycophorin A/CD14 surveillance tube, 234, *235*
correction of results for CD45/CD14 staining, 129-130
in HIV infection, 485-486, *486*
in neonate, 423-424
in paroxysmal nocturnal hemoglobinuria, 555, *556-557*
reference ranges for, 704, 706
CD15, 76, 77, 78, 78, 91
in acute myelogenous leukemia, 357, 359-360
in B-lineage acute lymphoblastic leukemia, 351
reference ranges for, 704
CD16 (FcāRIII), 19-20, 71, 76, 77-78, 78, 91, 130, 246, *248-249*, *553*
in acute myelogenous leukemia, 357
in chronic fatigue syndrome, 632, 633
correlation with older surface marker assays, 21
in HIV infection, *486*, 489, *489-490*, 491, 492
in neonate, 436, 439-440
in paroxysmal nocturnal hemoglobinuria, 555, *556-557*
in plasma-cell leukemia, *313*, 315
reference ranges for, 698, 702, 704
in T-prolymphocytic leukemia, 287
CDw17 (lactoceramide), 92
CD18 (LFA-1; integrin beta-chain), 72, 77, 92, 421, 600
in leukocyte adhesion deficiency, 417, 602
CD19, 19, 72-74, *73-74*, 92, 130, *233*, 234, 241-242, *247-249*

CDw128 (IL-8R type I), 96
CD130 (cytokine R), 96
CDw131 (cytokine R), 96
CD132 (cytokine R gamma chain), 96
CD134 (OX40), 96
CD135 (FLT3), 96
CDw136 (MSP-R), 96
CDw137, 96
CD138 (syndecan-1), *73*, 76, 96, 238-239
  in monoclonal gammopathies of
    undetermined significance, 278
  in myeloma, 278-279
  in plasma-cell leukemia, 278
  in plasmacytoma, 278
CD139, 96
CD140 (PDGF-R), 96
CD141 (thrombomodulin), 96
CD142 (tissue factor), 96
CD143, 97
CD144 (cadherin-5), 97
CDw145, 97
CD146 (MCAM), 97
CD147 (EMMPRIN), 97
CD148, 97
CDw149, 97
CDw150 (SLAM), 97
CD151 (PETA-3), 79-80, 97
CD152 (CTLA-4), 97
CD153 (CD30 ligand), 97
CD154 (CD40 ligand), 97
CD155 (PVR), 97
CD156, 97
CD157, 97
CD158, 97
CD158a, *72*, 97
CD158b, *72*, 97
CD161 (NKR-P1A), 97
CD162, 97
CD163, 97
CD164, 97
CD165, 97
CD166 (CD6 ligand), 97
CD-Chex Plus, *128*
CD monoclonal antibodies, 137
Celiac disease, 626-628
Cell count, absolute, 53, 109
Cell cycle analysis, 109-110
  laboratories performing tests by flow
    cytometry, 23, *23*
  Cell granularity, 38
  Cell proliferation measurement. *See also*
    S-phase fraction
  in acute leukemia, 369
  in bladder cancer, 667, *668*
  in breast cancer, 672-674, *674*
  in central nervous system cancer, 674-675,
    675

clinical utility of, 663-686
  in colorectal cancer, 678-679, *679*
  in endometrial cancer, 671-672, *672*
  in gastric cancer, 679, *680*
  in head and neck cancer, 680-681, *681*
  in lung cancer, 675-677, *677*
  in lymphoma, 685
  in melanoma, 677, *677*
  in myeloma, 682-684, *684*
  in ovarian cancer, 670, *671*
  in pancreatic cancer, 680, *680*
  in prostate cancer, 668-670, *669*
  in renal cell carcinoma, 670, *671*
  in sarcoma, 682, *683*
  in thyroid cancer, 681, *682*
CELLQuest software, 100, *101*, *105*,
    107-108, 108-111
Cell size, light scatter and, 38
Cell sorting
  high-speed sorters, 50
  low-speed sorters, 50
  preparative, 49-50
Cellular analysis
  basic concepts of, *33*-34
  population, *33*
  single-cell, *33*
Cellular cytotoxicity, evaluation of, 445
Cellular immunity
  defects in, 396-415
  development of, 432-440
  evaluation of patient with suspected
    immune deficiency, *442*
  laboratory evaluation of, 444-445
  in neonate, 432-440
Cellular immunodeficiency with
    immunoglobulins. *See* Nezelof syndrome
Cellular viability, monitoring of, 52, 123-124
Centers for Disease Control and Prevention
    (CDC), guidelines for flow cytometry, 146
Central nervous system cancer, DNA content
    analysis in, 674-675, *675*
Centroblasts, 75
Centrocytes, 75
Cervical cancer, 201
CFS. *See* Cancer-free survival
CGD. *See* Chronic granulomatous disease
Channel number, 102
Channel shift, 514
Channel value, 514-515
CHARGE anomalad. *See* DiGeorge anomaly
Chemically preserved cells, as target cells in
    quality control, 126-128, *128-129*
Chemokines, 527
CHH. *See* Cartilage-hair hypoplasia
Child
  normal values for T lymphocytes, 435-436,
    436

in breast cancer, 22, 642, 644-647,
672-674, *674*
in central nervous system cancer, 674-675,
675
clinical applications of, 641-653
clinical utility of, 642-644, 663-686
in colorectal cancer, 22, 651-653, 678-679,
679
consensus conference on, 643
cost of, 664, 666
difficulty of performing test, 665
dyes for, 52
economics of, *190*
in endometrial cancer, 671-672, *672*
in gastric cancer, 679, *680*
in head and neck cancer, 680-681, *681*
in leukemia, 684
in lung cancer, 675-677, *677*
in lymphoma, 685
in melanoma, 677, *677*
in myeloma, 682-684, *684*
in ovarian cancer, 670, *671*
in pancreatic cancer, 680, *680*
person requesting test, 665
prognostic value of, 665-666
in prostate cancer, 648-651, 668-670, *669*
quality control in, 55-56, *56*
in renal cell carcinoma, 670, *671*
in sarcoma, 682, *683*
software for, 109
in thyroid cancer, 681, *682*
treatment decisions and, 666
DNA ploidy, 21-22, 56-57, 641
in acute lymphoblastic leukemia, 369
in acute myelogenous leukemia, 369
in bladder cancer, 647-648, 667, *668*
in breast cancer, 644-645, 672-674, *674*
in central nervous system cancer, 674-675,
675
clinical utility of, 663-686
in colorectal cancer, 651-653, 678-679, *679*
in endometrial cancer, 671-672, *672*
FISH analysis, 651
in gastric cancer, 679, *680*
in head and neck cancer, 680-681, *681*
laboratories performing tests by flow
cytometry, 23, *23*
in lung cancer, 675-677, *677*
in lymphoma, 685
in melanoma, 677, *677*
in myeloma, 682-684, *684*
in ovarian cancer, 670, *671*
in pancreatic cancer, 680, *680*
in prostate cancer, 649-650, 668-670, *669*
in renal cell carcinoma, 670, *671*
in sarcoma, 682, *683*
in thyroid cancer, 681, *682*

Domain, in relational database, 160-161
Donor-specific hyporesponsiveness, 531
Dot-plot, 39, 102, *103, 105, 107*, 110
Down syndrome, *384*, 418
DRG. *See* Diagnosis-related groups
Drop-down list box, 172
Drug resistance
in acute leukemia, 362-364
in HIV infection, 479
Dyes, *46*, 51-52
detection of immature red blood cells,
559-560, *560*
Dyserythropoeisis, 549

E

EBV. *See* Epstein-Barr virus
Economics
of DNA content analysis, 664, 666
of flow cytometry, 60-61, 187-195
cost analysis, 187-188, *189-191*
diagnosis codes and, 194-195, *194*
reimbursement and CPT coding,
192-194, *194*
of HIV care, 476
of lymphocyte immunophenotyping in HIV
infection, 493-494
Ecto-apyrase. *See* CD39
Ecto-5¢-nucleotidase, 429
EDTA. *See* Ethylenediaminetetraacetic acid
Electronic compensation. *See* Compensation
Electronic gating. *See* Gating
Electronics, of flow cytometer, 34, 41-42
Emerging technologies, 22-26
EMMPRIN. *See* CD147
Endometrial cancer, 201
DNA content analysis in, 671-672, 672
Endometrial stromal cell sarcoma, *683*
Endothelium
CD markers for, 93, 95-97
leukocyte-endothelial adhesion, 598-601,
599
Enteropathy, autoimmune, 627
Entity integrity rule, 170
Entity-relationship diagram, 159, 174, *175*
Enzyme histochemistry, 11
Enzyme immunoassay
for antineutrophil cytoplasmic antibodies,
625
for antinuclear antibodies, 622
Epitope, 12, 14, 18
Epstein-Barr virus (EBV), 209, 212, 272,
408-409
ERBB2 gene, 642
Erythroblast(s), 76, 81
Erythroblastic leukemia. *See* Acute
myelogenous leukemia, M6

Fluorescein di-B-D-galactoside, 206
Fluorescein isothiocyanate (FITC), *39*, 46-47, *46*, *48*, 52, 82, 121, 584
Fluorescence, 38-39, 41, 45-46
  intensity of, 50-51
  sensitivity of, 120
  standardization of, 120-122, *121*, *123*
Fluorescence compensation, 121-122. *See also* Compensation
Fluorescence in situ hybridization (FISH), 216, 664
  cellular-based, 211
  detection of aneuploidy, 651
  detection of specific DNA sequences, 211-212
  detection of specific RNA sequences, 212-213, *213*
  with in situ PCR, 214
  testing for minimal residual disease, 365
Fluorescence intensity, 149-150
"Fluorescence triggering," 59
Fluorescence units, calibrated, 109
Fluorescent techniques
  direct, 82
  indirect, 82
Fluorochromes, 38-40, 45-46, *46*, 51-52
  "bleeding over," 47-48
  for CD34 stem cell enumeration, 584
  ratios of, 108
  spectral overlap of, 106
  stability/variability of, 138, *139*
  tandem, 46
Fluorouracil, 653
FluoTrol, *128*
FMC7, 246, *247-248*
  in B-chronic lymphocytic leukemia/small lymphocytic lymphoma, 254, 257, 260, *261*, *270*
  in B-lineage prolymphocytic leukemia, 269-271, *270*
  in follicular center lymphoma, *254*, 266, 304, *305*, *306*, *307*
  in hairy-cell leukemia, *270*, 273
  in mantle-cell lymphoma, *254*, 263-264, 271, 302, *303*
  in marginal zone lymphoma, 254, 310-312, *311*
  in small-cleaved-cell lymphoma, *254*
  in splenic lymphoma with veiled lymphocytes, *270*, 276
  in splenic marginal zone lymphoma, *270*, 308, 309
  in variant hairy-cell leukemia, *271*, 274
  in Waldenström's macroglobulinemia, 280
FMH. *See* Fetal-maternal hemorrhage
f-MLP. *See* Formyl-methionyl-leucyl-phenylalanine

Folate deficiency, *559*, 562
Follicular center lymphoma (FCL), *233*, *247*, 252, 259, 264
  case study of, 304, *305*, *306*, *307*
  clinical and morphologic features of, 265-266
  differential diagnosis of, 264-266, 268, 271, 273, 282
  immunophenotyping in, *254*, 266
  leukemic phase of, 266
Follicular dendritic cells, 75
Follicular thyroid cancer, *682*
Foreign key, 160-161, *161*, 170, 175
Form(s) (database), 173, *174*, 176
Formaldehyde fixation, to prevent red blood cell agglutination, 545, *545*
Formyl-methionyl-leucyl-phenylalanine (f-MLP), 422-423
Forward-angle light scatter, 38, 122
Fucosylation defect, 604-605

G

Gas ion laser, 37
Gastric cancer, DNA content analysis in, 679, *680*
Gate, definition of, 44
Gating, 34, *39*, 44, *45*, 58-59, 232, 488
  for flow cytometric crossmatch, 510, *512*
  of mature lymphocytes, 232-234, *233-237*
  of plasma cells, 234-239, *238-239*
GC/AT ratio, of individual chromosomes, 210
G-CSF. *See* Granulocyte colony stimulating factor
Gelsolin, 422
Gene expression, *33*
Gene product analysis, 198-207
General integrity rules, 170-171, *171*
Gene rearrangements, T-cell receptor, 199-201, *200*
Gene therapy, 205-207, 380
Glioma, *675*
Globotriasylceramide. *See* CD77
Glucose-6-phosphate dehydrogenase (G6PD) deficiency, leukocyte, 610-612
Glutaraldehyde fixation, to prevent red blood cell agglutination, 545, *545*
GlyCAM-1, 600-601
Glycogen storage disease, type 2, *384*
Glycophorin A (GPA), *80*, *81*, 562-563
  in acute lymphoblastic leukemia, 343-344, *345*
  in acute myelogenous leukemia, 343-344, *345*, *346*, 359
CD45/glycophorin A/CD14 surveillance tube, 234, *235*
Glycosylphosphatidylinositol-associated proteins, 553, *553*

GM-CSF. *See* Granulocyte-monocyte colony stimulating factor
Goat antimouse-phycoerythrin, 82
Gold therapy, 392
Good syndrome, 396
gp120, 472
GPA. *See* Glycophorin A
G6PD deficiency. *See* Glucose-6-phosphate dehydrogenase deficiency
Graft-versus-host disease (GvHD), 398-399, 407, 441-443
Granulocyte(s)
  CD markers for, 91-92, 94, 96-97
  differentiation of, 76-77, *77*
  light scattering characteristics of, *38*, *39*
Granulocyte colony stimulating factor (G-CSF), *423*
Granulocyte-monocyte colony stimulating factor (GM-CSF), 422
Green fluorescent protein, 206-207
Growth factors, 527
GvHD. *See* Graft-versus-host disease

H

Hairy-cell leukemia (HCL), 234, *247*, 259, 268
  clinical and morphologic features of, *270*, 271-272
  differential diagnosis of, 268, 271, 273-276
  immunophenotyping in, *270*, 272-273
  variant (vHCL), *247*, *256*, 268, 273
    case study of, 310-312, *311*
    clinical and morphologic features of, 274
    differential diagnosis of, 275
    immunophenotyping in, *270*, 274
HAM test, in paroxysmal nocturnal hemoglobinuria, 554-555, *554-555*
Hardware compensation, 106
HCFA. *See* Health Care Financing Administration
HCL. *See* Hairy-cell leukemia
Head and neck cancer, DNA content analysis in, 680-681, *681*
Health Care Financing Administration (HCFA), billing for flow cytometry, 193-194
Health maintenance organization (HMO), payment for flow cytometry, 193
Heavy-chain isotype switching, 75
Heavy chain rearrangements, 428
Helium-neon laser, 37, *46*
Hematogones, 366-368, *367*
Hematology analyzer, 43
  CD4 enumeration with, 495-498
Hematopoietic cells, differentiation of, 65-84
Hematopoietic stem cells. *See also* CD34 stem cells

CD markers for, 92
  definition of, 582
  sources of, 582-583
Hemoglobin
  detection of hemoglobin variants, 25
  fetal. *See* Fetal hemoglobin
Hemolytic anemia, 549, 562
  autoimmune, *545*, 547-548, *559*
Hemosiderin, urine, *554*
Heparin, 228, *228*
HER2/neu, in endometrial cancer, 672
Herceptin, 642
Hereditary persistence of hemoglobin F, *552*
HGPRT. *See* Hypoxanthine/guanine phosphoribosyl transferase
Histogram, 34, *35*, *39*, 42, *107*, 110
  overlaid, *103*
  single-parameter, 102, *102*
Histogram subtraction, 109
Histology, correlation with flow cytometry, 143, 152
Historical database, for flow cytometer, 54
HIV infection. *See* Human immunodeficiency virus infection
HLA antibody, posttransplant development of, 531
HLA-B7, 567-568, *568*, 570
HLA-B13, 567, *568*
HLA-B22, 567, *568*
HLA-B27
  assays for
    external proficiency testing, 571
    quality assurance, 571
  cross-reactive epitopes and allele associations of MoAbs to, 567-568, *568-570*, 571
  detection in disease states, 563-571, *564*
  flow cytometric assay for, 564-571, *566*, 568-570
  laboratories performing tests by flow cytometry, 23, *23*
  lymphocytotoxicity assay for, 564
  PCR-SSP genotyping for, 564, 567
HLA-B37, *568*
HLA-B39, *568*
HLA-B40, 567
HLA-B41, 567, *568*
HLA-B42, 567, *568*
HLA-B44, *537*, *538*, 567-568, *568*
HLA-B47, 567
HLA-B48, 567
HLA-B55, *568*
HLA-B57, 567, *568*
HLA-B60, *568*
HLA-B62, *568*
HLA-B73, *568*
HLA-CW1, 564

in Burkitt's lymphoma/leukemia, 282
chain rearrangements, 428
Light scatter, 58
forward-angle, 38, 122
side scatter, 38, 44, 122
standardization of, 122, *123*
Light scatter gating, for mature lymphocytes,
232-234, *233*
Linking table, 163-164, *163*
List box, 172
Listmode analysis, 41-42
Liver transplantation, 24
Long-pass filter, 40, *40*
Lookup table, 162
data entry into, 174-179, *176-178*
LRP. *See* Lung resistance-related protein
L-selectin, *93*, 599-601
abnormalities in neonate, 605
Lung cancer, DNA content analysis in,
675-677, *676*
Lung resistance-related protein (LRP),
202-203
Lymph nodes, reference ranges for, 135, 707
Lymphoblast(s), *45, 73, 366*
Lymphoblastic lymphoma, 265
Lymphocyte(s). *See also* specific types
alternative methods of immunophenotyping,
493-499
advantages of, 493
limitations of, 494
microtiter plate technologies, 498-499
single-platform cytometry methods,
494-498, *496-498*
in bone marrow, *45*
flow cytometric identification of, 232-234,
233-236
light scattering characteristics of, 38, *39*
Lymphocyte-inhibiting factor (LIF), 439
Lymphocytic leukemia/lymphoma, 252
Lymphocytosis, reactive, 291, *292*
Lymphocytotoxicity assay, for HLA-B27,
564
Lymphoid lineage, differentiation of, 67-68
Lymphokine-activated killer (LAK) cells, 440
Lymphoma. *See also* specific types of
lymphoma
DNA content analysis in, 685
immunophenotyping in, 23, *23, 248-249*
quality control, 147-148
mature, 227-327
Lymphoplasmacytic lymphoma/small
lymphocytic lymphoma with
plasmacytoid features, 276
Lymphoproliferations, benign NK, 283-286
Lymphoproliferative disease, X-linked, *381*,
408-409
Lymphosum, 130, 149-150

Lyophilized cells, as target cells in quality
control, 126
Lysing process, quality control/quality
assurance, 139-140
Lysozyme, 606-607

M

Mac-1. *See* CD11b
MacCycle software, 110
MacLAS software, 100, *101, 107-108*, 110-111
Macrophage(s), *78*
CD markers for, 91-97
development of, 420-426
functions of
antigen presentation, 425
chemotaxis, phagocytosis, and killing,
424-425
monokine production, 425-426
in neonate, 420-426
Macrophage-inhibiting factor (MIF), 439
MadCAM. *See* Mucosal addressin cell
adhesion molecule
Major basic protein, 607
Major histocompatibility complex (MHC)
antigen
class I, 70, 72, 403
class II, 70, 72, 403-404
defective expression of, 402-404
MALT lymphoma, 252, 258, 264, 267-268
Managed care organization (MCO), payment
for flow cytometry, 192-193
Mannan, 412
Mantle-cell lymphoma (MCL), *236*, 241, *247*,
252, 350
blastoid, 258, 263, 265, 345
case study of, 300, *301, 302, 303*
clinical and morphologic features of, 260-263
differential diagnosis of, 259, 264-266, 273
immunophenotyping in, *254*, 263
leukemic phase of, 258, 269, 271
Many-to-many relationships, in relational
database, 163-164, *163*
Marginal zone lymphoma (MZL), *247*, 252,
259, 264
case study of, 310-312, *311*
clinical and morphologic features of, 267
differential diagnosis of, 264-268, 273
immunophenotyping in, *254*, 267
leukemic phase of, 258
Mature leukemia
B lineage, 251-268
case studies of, 291-327
T lineage, 283-290, *284*
Mature lymphoid leukemia, 227-327. *See also*
specific types of leukemia
B-cell, *248*

diagnostic interpretation, 247-250
immunophenotyping panels for, 240-246
laboratory report, 250-251
medical triage, 231-232
natural killer cell, *248*
specimen collection, 227-230
T-cell, *248*
Mature lymphoid neoplasms, laboratory,
    morphologic, and clinical features, *240*
Mature lymphoma, 227-327. *See also* specific
    types of lymphoma
  B lineage, 251-268
  case studies of, 291-327
  diagnostic interpretation, 247-250
  immunophenotyping panels for, 240-246
  laboratory report, 250-251
  medical triage, 231-232
  specimen collection, 227-230
  T lineage, 283-290, *284*
MBCH. *See* Monocytoid B-cell hyperplasia
MBCL. *See* Monocytoid B-cell lymphoma
MCAM. *See* CD146
MCL. *See* Mantle-cell lymphoma
MCO. *See* Managed care organization
MDR1 gene, 202, 216, 364
Mean channel number, 120
Mean channel of fluorescence, 83
Mean equivalent of soluble fluorescein
    (MESF), 51
Medically useful tests, 231
Medical triage, 231-232, 340
Medicare, payment for flow cytometry, 188, 195
Medullary thyroid cancer, *682*
Megakaryoblasts, 79-80
Megakaryocytes, 76, 79-80, *79*, *93*
Megaloblastic anemia, *559*
Melanoma, DNA content analysis in, 677, *677*
Membrane inhibitor of reactive lysis. *See* CD59
Meningioma, 674-675, *675*
2-Mercaptoethanol, to prevent red blood cell
    agglutination, 545
MESF. *See* Mean equivalent of soluble
    fluorescein; Molecules of equivalent
    soluble fluorochrome
Messenger RNA, FISH detection of specific
    sequences, 212, 216
Metabolic disease, immunodeficiency
    associated with, 419
Metamyelocytes, *45*, *77*
MGUS. *See* Monoclonal gammopathies of
    undetermined significance
MHC antigens. *See* Major histocompatibility
    complex antigens
MIB-1, 664, 672
  in breast cancer, 673
  in lymphoma, 685
  in meningioma, 674

Microparticle flow cytometric PRA analysis,
    521-525, *523-528*, 537
Microsoft Access, 157
Microspheres, fluorescence-standard,
    120-122, *121*, 123
Microtiter plate immunoassay analysis, CD4,
    498-499
MIF. *See* Macrophage-inhibiting factor
Milan-Mulhouse protocol. *See* Milan
    protocol
Milan-Nordic protocol, for CD34 stem cell
    enumeration, 587
Milan protocol, for CD34 stem cell
    enumeration, *586*, 587-588, *588*
Minimal residual disease (MRD), 208-209
  in acute lymphoblastic leukemia, 343-344,
    364-368
  in acute myelogenous leukemia, 343-344,
    364-368
  oncogene products and, 203
  testing for
    FISH techniques, 365
    immunophenotyping, 365
    PCR-based methods, 365
MIRL. *See* CD59
Mitogen stimulation study, 23-24
  laboratories performing tests by flow
    cytometry, *23*, *23*
Mitotic count, 21
MLL gene, 351, 360
MoAb. *See* Monoclonal antibodies
ModFit software, *108*, 110
Molecular cytometry, clinical, 197-216
Molecular pathology, 197
Molecules of equivalent soluble fluorochrome
    (MESF), 120, 513-515, 567
Monoblast(s), 78, *78*
Monoblastic leukemia, 78
Monoclonal antibodies (MoAb), 65-66
  advantages of, 16, 65-66
  aliquoting/dilution of, 138-139
  analyte-specific reagents. *See* Analyte-
    specific reagents
  bacterial contamination of, 140
  CD, 137
  CD34, 582-584, *584*
  disadvantages of, 18-19
  isotype negative control, 136-138
  nomenclature of, 19
  production of, 16, *17*, 65
  quality control/quality assurance, 136-139
  reactivity of, 137-138
  reagents for flow cytometry, 65-66
    practical considerations, 81-84
  specificity of, 18
Monoclonal Antibody Information form
    (database), 176-177, *176-177*

730   Index

Surface immunoglobulin (sIg), 241-242
in acute lymphoblastic leukemia, 345
in B-chronic lymphocytic leukemia/small
lymphocytic lymphoma, 253, *254, 261,
270*, 293, *294*, 295, *297*, 298, *299*
in B-lineage prolymphocytic leukemia,
269-270
B lymphocyte differentiation, 72
in follicular center lymphoma, 266, 304,
305, 306, *307*
in hairy-cell leukemia, 273
in mantle-cell lymphoma, 265, 300, *301,
302, 303*
in marginal zone lymphoma, 267, 310-312,
311
in myeloma, 277
in plasma-cell leukemia, 277, *314*, 315
in splenic lymphoma with veiled
lymphocytes, 276
in splenic marginal zone lymphoma, 308, *309*
in Waldenström's macroglobulinemia, 280
Surface immunoglobulin assay
for B lymphocytes, 3-8, *4-5*, 19
problems with, 6-8
Surface marker assays
for B lymphocytes, 2-9
history and evolution of, 1-12, 32
problems with, *5*
techniques to improve, 6-7, *7*
for T lymphocytes, 2-9
Switchboard, 174
Syndecan-1. *See* CD138
Synovial sarcoma, 683
Systemic lupus erythematosus (SLE),
415-416, 622

T

Tables, in relational database, 159-160, *159*
Tamoxifen, 201, 673
Tandem conjugates, 46, *46*, 52
TAP2 gene, 403
TAPA-1. *See* CD81
Tartrate-resistant acid phosphatase (TRAP)
in B-chronic lymphocytic leukemia/small
lymphocytic lymphoma, 272
in B-lineage prolymphocytic leukemia, 272
in hairy-cell leukemia, *270*, 272
in variant hairy-cell leukemia, *270*
T-cell lineage, immunophenotyping panels
for, 240-241
T-cell lymphoma, *248*
T-cell receptor (TCR), 69-70, 216
alpha-beta, *248-249*, 407, 414, *433, 436*
in adult T-cell lymphoma, 290
in peripheral T-cell lymphoma, 290
in T-prolymphocytic leukemia, 287

alpha chain, 199, *200*
beta chain, 199, *200*, 201
in celiac disease, 627-628, *628*
in cutaneous T-cell lymphoma, 199
defects in recombination of, 407
deficiency of, *382*, 399, 404-405
detection of gene rearrangements, 199-201,
200
gamma-delta, *248-249*, 407, 414, *433-434*,
627-628, *628*
in HIV disease, 201
in neonate, *433, 436*
in Omenn syndrome, 407
in Sézary syndrome/mycosis fungoides,
286
T-cell-rich B-cell lymphoma (TCRBCL), 281
T-chronic lymphocytic leukemia (T-CLL)
case study of, 316-318, *317*
clinical and morphologic features of, 288
differential diagnosis of, 289
immunophenotyping in, *248*, 288
T-CLL. *See* T-chronic lymphocytic leukemia
TCR. *See* T-cell receptor
TCRBCL. *See* T-cell-rich B-cell lymphoma
TdT. *See* Terminal deoxynucleotidyl
transferase
TEL-AML1 fusion, 351
Terminal deoxynucleotidyl transferase (TdT),
68, *69*, 72, 73, 429
in acute lymphoblastic leukemia, 346-347
in acute myelogenous leukemia, 347
in B-lineage acute lymphoblastic leukemia,
271
in Burkitt's lymphoma/leukemia, 282
in hematogones, 366, 368
in T-lineage acute lymphoblastic leukemia,
354
Testicular implant, 628-631
Thalassemia, 549, 551, *562*
THI. *See* Transient hypogammaglobulinemia
of infancy
Thiazole orange, 560, 560
Third Normal Form, 168-170, *168-169*
Thrombocytopenia, X-linked, 409
Thrombomodulin. *See* CD141
Thymic epithelium, 97
Thymic hypoplasia, *381*, 396-398
Thymic selection, 70
Thymic stem cells, 68
Thymidine-labeling studies, for lymphocyte
function, 20-21
Thymocytes, *69*, 433
CD markers for, 91-93, 95, 97
Thymoma, immunodeficiency with, 396
Thymus, fetal, *433*
Thyroid cancer, DNA content analysis in,
681, *682*

U

Ulcerative colitis, 622
Umbilical cord blood, source of
    hematopoietic stem cells, 582-583
Undercompensation, *47*, 48-49
Update anomaly, 169
Uterine leiomyosarcoma, *683*
Uveal melanoma, *677*

V

Vaccine, AIDS, 479
Vascular cell adhesion molecule 1 (VCAM-1),
    95, 600
VCAM. *See* Vascular cell adhesion molecule
Velo-cardio-facial syndrome. *See* DiGeorge
    anomaly
Very late antigen 4 (VLA-4), 600-601
vHCL. *See* Hairy-cell leukemia, variant
Viability assessment, 52, 123-124
Viral load determination, 212-213
Viremia, in HIV infection, 473
Vital dye, 230
Vitamin B12 deficiency, *559, 562*
VLA. *See* Very late antigen
Volumetric capillary cytometry, 43
Volumetric cytometry, 31
Vulvar cancer, 201
Vulvar melanoma, *677*

W

Waldenström's macroglobulinemia (WM),
    266, 268, 277
    clinical and morphologic features of, 279
    differential diagnosis of, 280
    immunophenotyping in, 280
WAS. *See* Wiskott-Aldrich syndrome
Wegener granulomatosis, 622-623, 625
Weibel-Palade body, 601
Whole blood controls, 125

Whole blood lysis technique, 55, 82, 230, 484
WinFCM software, 100-101, *101, 107-108,*
    110-111
WinLAS software, 101, *101, 107-108,* 110-111
WinList software, 101, *101, 105-108,* 106,
    108-111
WinMDI software, 101, *101-102, 104-105,*
    107-108
WinReport software, *108,* 110
Wiskott-Aldrich syndrome (WAS), 383, *383,*
    409-411, 441, 444
"Wizards," 178
WM. *See* Waldenström's macroglobulinemia
Wright's stain, 2, *2*

X

XAG. *See* X-linked agammaglobulinemia
X box, 404
Xeroderma pigmentosum, 418
X-linked agammaglobulinemia (XAG), *381,*
    385-389, 429
X-linked agammaglobulinemia with
    hyper-IgM, *381*
X-linked chronic granulomatous disease, 608,
    615, *616*
X-linked immunodeficiency with hyper-IgM,
    388-389
X-linked lymphoproliferative disease (XLP),
    381, 408-409
X-linked severe combined immunodeficiency
    disease, *382,* 399-400
X-linked thrombocytopenia, 409
XLP. *See* X-linked lymphoproliferative disease

Z

ZAP-70 deficiency, *382,* 399-401
Zinc, inability to absorb, 418-419
Zygosity analysis, *547*
Zymune, 498